Neurorehabilitation for the
PHYSICAL THERAPIST ASSISTANT

Second Edition

Neurorehabilitation for the
PHYSICAL THERAPIST ASSISTANT
Second Edition

Edited by

Darcy A. Umphred, PT, PhD, FAPTA
Emeritus Professor
Retired Chair and Professor
Department of Physical Therapy
University of the Pacific
Stockton, California

Rolando T. Lazaro, PT, PhD, DPT, MS, GCS
Associate Professor and Co-Chair
Department of Physical Therapy
Samuel Merritt University
Oakland, California

Previously co-edited by Constance Carlson, PT, MS Ed

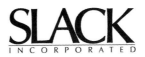

www.Healio.com/books

ISBN: 978-1-61711-073-3

Neurorehabilitation for the Physical Therapist Assistant, Second Edition includes ancillary materials specifically available for faculty use. Please visit www.efacultylounge.com to obtain access.

Published by: SLACK Incorporated
                   6900 Grove Road
                   Thorofare, NJ 08086 USA
                   Telephone: 856-848-1000
                   Fax: 856-848-6091
                   www.Healio.com/books

Contact SLACK Incorporated for more information about other books in this field or about the availability of our books from distributors outside the United States.

          Library of Congress Cataloging-in-Publication Data
Neurorehabilitation for the physical therapist assistant / edited by Darcy A. Umphred, Rolando T. Lazaro. -- Second edition.
     p. ; cm.
  Includes bibliographical references and index.
  ISBN 978-1-61711-073-3 (alk. paper)
  I. Umphred, Darcy Ann, editor of compilation. II. Lazaro, Rolando T., 1965- editor of compilation.
  [DNLM: 1. Nervous System Diseases--rehabilitation. 2. Physical Therapy Modalities. 3. Rehabilitation--methods. WL 140]
  RC350.P48
  616.8'046--dc23
                    2013037900

Printed in the United States of America.

Last digit is print number: 10   9   8   7   6   5   4   3   2

DEDICATION

This Second Edition of *Neurorehabilitation for the Physical Therapist Assistant* is dedicated to all those therapists, authors, and individuals who have identified and tried to clarify the role of the physical therapist assistant in the larger profession of physical therapy.

—Darcy and Rolando

As in the First Edition, I would also like to dedicate this edition to my immediate and extended family, whose support and encouragement has always given me energy to keep trying to provide to younger colleagues those materials that will help translate academic work into clinical competency. To my friends and colleagues who have deepened my belief in the empowerment of individuals to regain movement function in spite of body system problems, I truly thank all of you for your guidance in my evolution.

—Darcy

I dedicate this book to my mentors. Thank you for the support and encouragement, and for always believing in me. Most importantly, thank you for the friendship and love through the years. I honor your legacy by being the best mentor I could be to the next generation of physical therapy clinicians and educators.

—Rolando

Contents

Dedication .... *v*
Acknowledgments .... *ix*
About the Editors .... *xi*
Contributing Authors .... *xiii*
Preface... *xvii*
Introduction... *xix*

Chapter 1   Introduction to Neurorehabilitation for the Physical Therapist Assistant 1
             Rolando T. Lazaro, PT, PhD, DPT, MS, GCS; Nelson Marquez, PT, EdD;
             Darcy A. Umphred, PT, PhD, FAPTA; and Dennis Klima, PT, MS, PhD, GCS, NCS

Chapter 2   Normal Movement Development Across the Lifespan.. 15
             Dale Scalise-Smith, PT, PhD

Chapter 3   Motor Control, Motor Learning, and Neuroplasticity.. 45
             Darcy A. Umphred, PT, PhD, FAPTA and Fritzie Arce, PT, PhD

Chapter 4   Intervention Procedures.. 69
             Sharon L. Gorman, PT, DPTSc, GCS and Darcy A. Umphred, PT, PhD, FAPTA

Chapter 5   Examination Procedures 117
             Patricia Harris, PT, MS and Lisa Ferrin, PTA, AS

Chapter 6   Psychosocial and Cognitive Issues Affecting Therapy.. 151
             Gordon U. Burton, OT/L, PhD

Chapter 7   Documentation in Neurorehabilitation 165
             Shannon Ryals, PTA

Chapter 8   Children With Central Nervous System Insult.. 177
             Kristine N. Corn, PT, MS, DPT and Cynthia J. Hogan, PTA

Chapter 9   Clients With Genetic and Developmental Problems 211
             Esmerita Roceles Rotor, PT, MAEd, PTRP; Darcy A. Umphred, PT, PhD, FAPTA;
             Eunice Shen, PT, PhD, DPT, PCS; and Barbara H. Connolly, PT, DPT, EdD, C/NDT, FAPTA

Chapter 10   Clients With Spinal Cord Injury... 251
             Bret Kennedy, PT, DPT; Kelly Ryujin, PT, DPT; and Claire E. Beekman, PT, MS, NCS

Chapter 11   Clients With Traumatic Brain Injury 297
             Dennis Klima, PT, MS, PhD, GCS, NCS

Chapter 12   Clients With Stroke.. 325
             Becky S. McKnight, PT, MS and James M. Smith, PT, DPT, MA

Chapter 13   Clients With Degenerative Diseases: Parkinson's Disease,
             Multiple Sclerosis, and Amyotrophic Lateral Sclerosis.. 375
             Rolando T. Lazaro, PT, PhD, DPT, MS, GCS and Amanda A. Forster, PT, DPT, NCS

Chapter 14   Cardiopulmonary Issues Associated With Patients
                    Undergoing Neurorehabilitation 393
                    Ronald De Vera Barredo, PT, DPT, EdD, GCS

Chapter 15   Complementary Therapies or Integrative Health Care 411
                    Carol Davis, PT, DPT, EdD, MS, FAPTA and Megan E. Petrosky, PT, DPT

Financial Disclosures 425
Index 427

Neurorehabilitation for the Physical Therapist Assistant, Second Edition includes ancillary materials specifically available for faculty use. Please visit www.efacultylounge.com to obtain access.

ACKNOWLEDGMENTS

Dr. Lazaro and Dr. Umphred would like to thank all the authors in the Second Edition of *Neurorehabilitation for the Physical Therapist Assistant* who have shown such a commitment to the profession of physical therapy and to the evolution of practice for the physical therapist assistant (PTA). As this Second Edition has a new online video portion with actual video clips of both normal and problems in movement patterns, we would like to thank everyone who participated in this aspect of this edition. Also, thanks is expressed to everyone at SLACK Incorporated who has helped with this Second Edition in order to make it a visionary textbook for the PTA. We would especially like to thank Brien Cummings, Jennifer Cahill, April Billick, Michelle Gatt, and John Bond for their devoted time and energy at SLACK Incorporated and for making our jobs easier and without extreme stress.

ABOUT THE EDITORS

Darcy A. Umphred, PT, PhD, FAPTA graduated from the University of Washington with a BS in Physical Therapy, from Boston University with a MS in Allied Health Education, and from Syracuse University with a PhD in Theories of Learning and Teacher Education. She has taught in both physical and occupational therapy programs throughout the United States. At the time of her retirement she was professor and chair of the Department of Physical Therapy at the University of the Pacific and played a major role in its evolution to granting a Doctorate of Physical Therapy to its graduates. After retirement she was made an emeritus professor with all the honors that brings. Throughout her professional career and throughout the world, she taught courses, which combined theories of central nervous system function, movement science, and evidence-based practice into an integrated approach to analyzing individuals with central nervous system dysfunction creating functional movement problems. Her love of clinical practice and analyzing movement problems has driven her to question the "why's" behind patients' functional restrictions. Similarly, she has studied how our limbic, cognitive, and belief systems affect the interactions between the client and the therapist. She has been the primary editor of the textbook *Neurological Rehabilitation*, currently in its Sixth Edition and translated into many different languages throughout the world. She has received numerous awards at the local, state, and national levels within the American Physical Therapy Association and was made a Catherine Worthingham Fellow in 2003. Her respect for the profession of physical therapy and the 2 educated clinicians—the physical therapist and the physical therapist assistant—has been demonstrated by her commitment to the responsibilities and services both professionals play in the delivery of physical therapy services throughout the world. It is her belief that physical therapy can and should play a unique role in the delivery of services for individuals with functional movement problems whether those problems arise from disease or pathology or from everyday life experiences. Optimal quality of life is defined by each individual, and it is the therapist's role to help that person regain as much of that quality available.

Rolando T. Lazaro, PT, PhD, DPT, MS, GCS graduated from the College of Allied Medical Professions, University of the Philippines Manila with a BS in Physical Therapy, from the University of the Pacific with a MS in Physical Therapy, from Creighton University with a Postprofessional Doctor of Physical Therapy, and from the Touro University with a PhD in Health Science. Dr. Lazaro has coauthored many research articles and chapters for a variety of textbooks. He is coeditor of both this book and the Sixth Edition of *Neurological Rehabilitation*. His publications demonstrate his commitment to not only teaching but also contributing to the body of knowledge known as evidence-based practice within and outside the profession of physical therapy. Dr. Lazaro was awarded a Fulbright Senior Scholarship to the Philippines from June to November 2013. Dr. Lazaro is currently an associate professor and co-chair of the Department of Physical Therapy at Samuel Merritt University in Oakland, California. Previously, he was an assistant professor at the University of the Pacific in Stockton, California. He was also a part-time physical therapist assistant faculty at the Professional Skills Institute in Concord, California. Dr. Lazaro is committed to helping others provide evidence-based practice while remaining open to visionary ideas.

Contributing Authors

Fritzie Arce, PT, PhD (Chapter 3)
Post-Doctoral Scholar
Department of Organismal Biology and Anatomy
University of Chicago
Chicago, Illinois

Ronald De Vera Barredo, PT, DPT, EdD, GCS (Chapter 14)
Professor and Head
Department of Physical Therapy
Tennessee State University
Nashville, Tennessee

Claire E. Beekman, PT, MS, NCS (Chapter 10)
Retired Physical Therapy Manager
Spinal Injury Service
Rancho Los Amigos National Rehabilitation Center
Downey, California

Gordon U. Burton, OT/L, PhD (Chapter 6)
Professor Emeritus
Past Chair and Professor
Department of Occupational Therapy
San Jose State University
San Jose, California

Barbara H. Connolly, PT, DPT, EdD, C/NDT, FAPTA (Chapter 9)
Professor Emeritus
Department of Physical Therapy
University of Tennessee Health Science Center
Memphis, Tennessee

Kristine N. Corn, PT, MS, DPT (Chapter 8)
Owner and Clinician
Sierra Pediatrics
Roseville, California
Founder and Clinician
Ride To Walk: Therapeutic Horseback Riding
Granite Bay, California

Carol Davis, PT, DPT, EdD, MS, FAPTA (Chapter 15)
Professor Emerita
Department of Physical Therapy
University of Miami Miller School of Medicine
Coral Gables, Florida

Lisa Ferrin, PTA, AS (Chapter 5)
Physical Therapist Assistant
Outpatient Rehabilitation
Methodist Hospital
Sacramento, California

Amanda A. Forster, PT, DPT, NCS (Chapter 13)
Senior Physical Therapist
Kaiser Permanente
San Jose, California

Sharon L. Gorman, PT, DPTSc, GCS (Chapter 4)
Associate Professor
Department of Physical Therapy
Samuel Merritt University
Oakland, California

Patricia Harris, PT, MS (Chapter 5)
Professor
Physical Therapist Assistant Program
Sacramento City College
Sacramento, California

Cynthia J. Hogan, PTA (Chapter 8)
Sierra Pediatrics
Roseville, California

Bret Kennedy, PT, DPT (Chapter 10)
Adjunct Assistant Professor
Department of Physical Therapy
Samuel Merritt University
Oakland, California

Dennis Klima, PT, MS, PhD, GCS, NCS (Chapters 1 and 11)
Assistant Professor
Department of Physical Therapy
University of Maryland Eastern Shore
Princess Anne, Maryland

Nelson Marquez, PT, EdD (Chapter 1)
Chair
Physical Therapist Assistant Program
Polk State College
Winter Haven, Florida

Becky S. McKnight, PT, MS (Chapter 12)
Program Coordinator
Physical Therapist Assistant Program
Ozarks Technical Community College
Springfield, Missouri

Megan E. Petrosky, PT, DPT (Chapter 15)
Jupiter Medical Center
Jupiter, Florida

Esmerita Roceles Rotor, PT, MAEd, PTRP (Chapter 9)
Associate Professor
Department of Physical Therapy
College of Allied Medical Professions
University of the Philippines
Manila, Philippines

Shannon Ryals, PTA (Chapter 7)
Academic Coordinator of Clinical Education
Polk State College
Winter Haven, Florida

Kelly Ryujin, PT, DPT (Chapter 10)
Adjunct Assistant Professor
Department of Physical Therapy
Samuel Merritt University
Oakland, California

Dale Scalise-Smith, PT, PhD (Chapter 2)
Vice President for External Programs and Partnerships
Professor of Physical Therapy
Utica College
Utica, New York

Eunice Shen, PT, PhD, DPT, PCS (Chapter 9)
California Children's Services
County of Los Angeles
Department of Public Health
El Monte, California

James M. Smith, PT, DPT, MA (Chapter 12)
Associate Professor
Physical Therapy
Utica College
Utica, New York

PREFACE

This Second Edition of *Neurorehabilitation for the Physical Therapist Assistant* was written for the student physical therapist assistant (PTA), PTAs in practice, and for faculty who teach neurorehabilitation in PTA programs. The area of neurorehabilitation has evolved from specific approaches designed by master clinicians from around the world to an environment where treatment interventions are supported by evidence. Evidence-based practice is a process that considers 3 aspects: the available documented evidence, the patient's values, and the clinical judgment of the practitioner. Evidence-based practice leads to optimal outcomes. The physical therapist (PT) should not ask a PTA to perform an intervention that has no evidence to support that it will lead to the desired outcomes of the plan of care. In the future, evidence that is true today may become simplistic or proven to be ineffective. New evidence can only evolve into new practice when both the PT and PTA recognize that intervention approaches that they were taught are not working effectively or not working at all, and new ideas whether discovered by the PT or PTA seem to positively change the outcomes of the plan of care.

This Second Edition widens the role of the PTA and also the responsibility of that therapist in the evolution of intervention approaches that will best benefit the individual coming to physical therapy. Both editors have spent many years working in the area of neurorehabilitation as well as in the direct education of PTs who will be evaluating and setting up plans of care for individuals with movement dysfunctions arising from central nervous system (CNS) problems. The majority of the chapter authors of this book have been involved in the education of PTAs as well. Therefore, this book is specifically and purposely designed to be used by PTAs.

As physical therapy educators and clinicians, both editors understand the differences between disease/pathology and movement dysfunction. Thus, the medical model is only briefly introduced within this book. The major focus of this book is on approaches to gain or regain function. As therapists dealing with movement problems, both editors have clearly seen the potential of the human body to gain or regain function following a disease or pathology. Therapists do not correct the disease or damage to the CNS, but they do help in learning or relearning movement function lost to the individual coming to physical therapy. The plasticity of the CNS has now been shown in the literature as well as ways to learn or regain movement function and why those activities become best practice. Similarly, literature supports the concept that individual potential is dramatically improved when the person values the activities practiced and is actively engaged in the plan of care. For that reason, the PTA's role is not only to provide intervention or follow-up examinations, but also to be actively engaged in the interactions during those treatment sessions. As roles change so must the responsibility of the clinicians who either delegate or actively assume treatment of individuals under their care. The one specific concept that should be the foundation for neurorehabilitation is that there is potential in all of us to change and learn as long as we believe that change is possible.

INTRODUCTION

The conceptualization of this book began a decade ago and has evolved into the text seen in the Second Edition. This role of the physical therapist assistant (PTA) is enlarging and has become a critical link in successful outcomes of many interventions provided to individuals with movement dysfunctions. This Second Edition has been written to help students and colleagues who are working with individuals with movement dysfunction arising from central nervous system (CNS) problems. As the depth and breadth of the role of the PTA expands, so must textbooks that introduce, discuss, and explain both the interventions as well as examination tools that a PTA might be asked to implement within the plan of care for individuals with CNS movement deficits. Those problems can arise at birth, in early childhood, adolescence, adulthood, or as one ages toward and into geriatrics. The initial chapters lay the foundation for discussion of interventions and follow-up examinations that a PTA might be asked to perform throughout the plan of care. The model for PTA practice as identified by the American Physical Therapy Association has been used as a guide to direct the PTA toward appropriate interventions and examination tools that might be delegated to the assistant. For that reason, intervention precedes examination because the PTA will be asked to begin components of the plan of care designed by the physical therapist (PT) before being asked to perform selected examination procedures to generate information regarding the progress of a patient or client. As this model is different from the model used by PTs, the differentiation of those roles are identified throughout the book. The World Health Organization's International Classification of Functioning, Disability and Health has been adopted as the foundation for both the PT and PTA focus of care and now places the patient/client as the one who identifies value or quality to the various movement goals used in the plan of care.

The intervention chapters introduce and discuss common movement dysfunctions caused by CNS injury across the lifespan and the intervention approaches a PTA might be asked to perform as well as examination tools used to measure outcomes of those interventions. A discussion of the cardiopulmonary issues that might affect neurorehabilitation should help the PTA understand how other body systems can affect movement dysfunctions and complicate the plan of care. Similarly, a chapter on complementary approaches to intervention should help the reader understand when these techniques can be used under supervision of the PT, when a PTA who has obtained expertise in one of these approaches can use those clinical skills independently, and how these services can be part of the plan of care.

A thorough study guide has been developed to help the learner identify critical issues within each chapter. Study guide questions posed for specific case studies are found both within the text as well as online. Also, the reader will find online specific video clips of individuals with movement problems discussed in the various chapters along with treatment approaches. Video clips of specific handling or movement techniques have been developed by the editors to help the learner see how normal movements can be facilitated by a therapist. These video clips of handling techniques should assist the PTA in ways that he or she can empower his or her patients and clients to learn or regain motor control leading to greater function and, hopefully, a higher quality of life.

The evolution of this edition hopefully parallels the evolution of PTA practice. As more and more delegation is given to the PTA, continued education and potentially higher degrees will become a reality. This edition is not only a thoroughly written textbook regarding interventions and examination tools used by the PTA when working with patients with CNS problems; it also has a visionary component introducing the importance of visual analysis of movement problems and highlights the need for the PTA to develop visual recognition of specific problems found in the population of individuals with CNS deficits. This visual aspect of this textbook should help faculty introduce with consistency specific movement problems seen in this population.

In the end, physical therapy is all about providing excellent care to the patients and clients we serve. As editors, we are confident that this text will provide readers with excellent information that elevates their clinical practice.

1

Introduction to Neurorehabilitation for the Physical Therapist Assistant

Rolando T. Lazaro, PT, PhD, DPT, MS, GCS
Nelson Marquez, PT, EdD
Darcy A. Umphred, PT, PhD, FAPTA
Dennis Klima, PT, MS, PhD, GCS, NCS

KEY WORDS

- Activity
- Body structure and function
- Evaluation and examination
- Health condition
- International Classification of Functioning, Disability and Health (ICF) intervention and outcomes
- Neurorehabilitation
- Participation and quality of life
- Personal and environmental factors
- Physical therapist assistant (PTA)
- Physical therapy diagnosis
- Prognosis

CHAPTER OBJECTIVES

- Discuss the ICF model and its implications on physical therapy management.
- Discuss the difference between the western medical model and the ICF model used by physical therapists (PTs) and PTAs today.
- Discuss the factors involved when a PT determines which tests, measures, and interventions are appropriate to be delegated to a PTA.

Umphred DA, Lazaro RT, eds.
Neurorehabilitation for the Physical Therapist Assistant,
Second Edition (pp 1-14).
© 2014 SLACK Incorporated.

INTRODUCTION

The topic of neurological rehabilitation encompasses knowledge of the neurosciences, behavioral sciences, and social sciences. It requires an understanding of development across the lifespan and the pathologies or diseases relating to the nervous system. The causes and medical treatments for all known neurological pathologies or diseases fall within the domain of medical practice. Physical therapists (PTs) and physical therapist assistants (PTAs) do not treat those diseases, although understanding the pathologies is important in selecting the appropriate tests and measures, establishing goal expectations and parameters for interventions, and considering limitations on motor control, motor learning, and neuroplasticity.

A patient may present to physical therapy with impairments or abnormalities in body structures and functions, and/or activity limitations, or problems with performance of functional activities. These impairments and activity limitations may have developed from a combination of the pathology or disease of the nervous system and the preexisting health status of the individual. Traditionally, neurological rehabilitation (or neurorehabilitation) is the process of regaining optimal function following the pathology or disease of the peripheral nervous system (PNS) and central nervous system (CNS). Generally, patients with these problems are sent to physical therapy through a referral process from medical doctors and other health care professionals. The focus of this text will be on this scope of practice and the role of the PT and PTA when a referral has been made. Although the focus of this text is on neurorehabilitation following CNS insult, PTAs must also be aware of the role of physical therapy in wellness or pre-disease, as well as maintenance of motor function or quality of life of individuals following physical rehabilitation.

As many physical therapy clinics offer health promotion and wellness and risk reduction activities, individuals who at a prior date had a CNS problem may come into those clinics without a referral source but with a prior medical diagnosis. Again, PTs and PTAs may be involved in examining and establishing treatment protocols to enhance the wellness, promote the health, and reduce the risk of developing other impairments and activity limitations of this individual. Similarly, individuals may be placed in care facilities where a PT and PTA provide service to maintain mobility and optimize function. In those situations, the individual may first be evaluated by the PT, who establishes a plan of care. Then, the PTA may perform subsequent interventions and appropriate portions of reexaminations. The PT and PTA must closely collaborate to ensure that optimal care is provided to the patient or client. Similarly, the PT and PTA must understand and appreciate the models both professionals learn and use when interacting with the patient. The model used by a PT begins with examination, followed by drawing conclusions that lead to a physical therapy diagnosis, prognosis, and the plan of care. The model used by a PTA begins with discussion by both the PT and PTA of the plan of care, followed by the PTA interventions when appropriate and follow-up examinations at established intervals or when changes in the patient's motor skills would indicate it is appropriate. These practice models are different, and for that reason the intervention chapter precedes the chapter on examination when considering the PTA's responsibilities within neurological rehabilitation.

In the clinical setting, differentiation of the roles of the PT and PTA may not be as clear, especially when PTs or PTAs start at the particular practice setting as novice practitioners. Following graduation from an educational program, these practitioners must commit to becoming lifelong learners. Most PTAs continue their learning through continuing education courses, in-service education, mentorship opportunities, formal academic degree programs, and certification or licensure in other areas of health care delivery. For this reason, a PT may delegate certain interventions and reassessments of specific basic impairments to a novice PTA while delegating more complex interventions, reassessment of functional skills and more complex impairments, and a role in discharge planning to a more experienced PTA. Similarly, novice PTs may not realize that an experienced PTA could have advanced knowledge and skills and be able to competently provide high-quality care to individuals with even the most complex movement problems secondary to neurological pathologies. In both scenarios, it is critical that the PT and PTA closely communicate and collaborate to develop a plan of care that returns the patient to the highest level of physical functioning.

This chapter aims to present a conceptual understanding of the model of neurorehabilitation that is pertinent in current physical therapy practice. This provides the foundation for learning the specific neurological clinical problems presented in subsequent chapters of this text. These specific clinical problems, crossing a lifespan of development, will also play a role in determining what should and should not be delegated. The PTA must always remember that although a specific age population may be the focus of a pathology topic, many clinical problems can occur at any age. Obviously, those problems that occur in utero, at birth, or with a genetic link will set the stage for alternative paths to development. But these individuals who have neurological issues early in their lives can develop any of the other clinical problems discussed in this text. For example, someone with an early medical diagnosis of cerebral palsy (CP) can later have a stroke, a spinal injury, or a head injury or can develop some demyelinating disease as an adult. Thus, those interventions presented within each of the clinical problem chapters are within the scope of a PTA and might be delegated as part of the treatment plan for an individual on a PTA's caseload.

MODEL OF NEUROREHABILITATION: INTRODUCTION TO THE INTERNATIONAL CLASSIFICATION OF FUNCTIONING, DISABILITY AND HEALTH

Disablement Models of the Past (International Classification of Impairments, Disabilities, and Handicaps and Nagi Models)

Physical therapy, like many health professions throughout the world, analyzes and implements theoretical models to link the relationship between the acute disease and pathology to resulting movement dysfunctions and to explain how these problems can affect an individual's life. Therapists who work with movement problems can directly relate specific activity limitations to a pathology within the brain, but, just as frequently, many pathologies within the brain can lead to the same movement problem. As the profession of physical therapy moved from technique-based interventions to an evidence-based approach, it was natural to link our examinations and interventions to the pathology or disease that seemed to have caused those movement problems. For that reason, models that identified the medical condition with the specific movement problems began to be developed and accepted by PTs. Two specific models were embraced in the 1980s and 1990s that clearly differentiated the disease or pathologies treated by medical doctors from the functional problems treated by PTs. These two models, Nagi[1] and International Classification of Impairments, Disabilities, and Handicaps (ICIDH),[2] basically followed a linear, sequential model in which a medical condition/disease or pathology leads to impairments, which denote body system or subsystem abnormalities. These impairments lead to functional limitations (Nagi) or disability (ICIDH), which describe what the person **cannot** do functionally. These then lead to disability (Nagi) or handicaps (ICIDH), which are the person's perceived limitations in his or her ability to perform societal roles. Both models are based on a model of disablement and do not take into account the strengths of the patient that may assist in recovery and rehabilitation. The *Guide to Physical Therapist Practice* (the *Guide*) adopted the Nagi model in its First and Second Editions.[3]

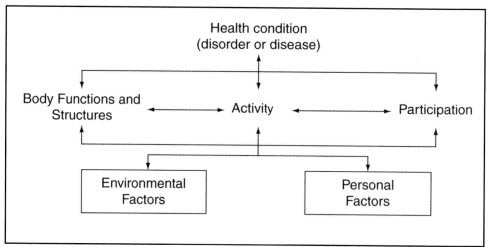

Figure 1-1. The International Classification of Functioning, Disability and Health model. (Reprinted with permission from World Health Organization. *Towards a Common Language for Functioning, Disability and Health.* Geneva, Switzerland: Author; 2002.)

Today's Enablement Model: The International Classification of Functioning, Disability and Health

In 2002, the World Health Organization (WHO) introduced the International Classification of Functioning, Disability and Health (ICF) model.[4] This is a model of enablement, which takes into consideration the strengths of the patient/client, in addition to the patient's problems or limitations. This model identifies the complex, multidirectional, and integrated relationship between medical pathology, body systems and functions, functional activity, and participation in life. It also takes into account contextual factors, which could be personal, societal, and/or environmental considerations that may influence the person's path of rehabilitation and return to optimal health and well-being. As such, the ICF subscribes to the biopsychosocial model of human functioning following a disease or illness.[4]

The ICF model is presented in Figure 1-1. In this model, the interaction between *health condition* and *contextual factors* forms the basis for disability and functioning. Also in the model, human functioning is classified according to 3 levels: (1) body or body part, (2) the person as a whole, and (3) the person in relation to the larger society. Starting from the left of the diagram, *body functions and structures* refers to the anatomical and physiological functioning of the human systems. *Impairments* denotes problems in body structures and functions. *Activities* refers to the ability of a person to perform functional tasks. *Activity limitations* indicates problems with performance of functional activities. *Participation* involves the ability of a person to be engaged in life situations. Problems with participation are termed *participation restrictions*.

A therapist could therefore assess each level of functioning of an individual in relation to the presenting strengths and weaknesses at each level. Body functions and structures, activities, and participation highlight dimensions of functioning that are normal for the individual, while impairments, activity limitations, and participation restrictions are problems that may be addressed by therapeutic intervention.

Moreover, contextual factors could also affect functioning. Environmental factors include the physical, social, and attitudinal attributes that may facilitate or hinder the return to optimal function. This return to function may also be facilitated or inhibited by personal factors or specific attributes of the individual.[4]

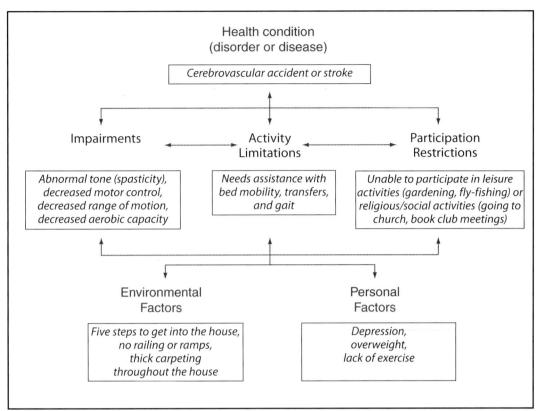

Figure 1-2. Application of the International Classification of Functioning, Disability and Health model to PT/PTA practice. The headings show the original model, and the italicized words and phrases in the boxes show how the model is applied to physical therapy practice.

Figure 1-2 provides an example of how the ICF model can be applied to physical therapy practice. Assume that the patient has a medical diagnosis of cerebrovascular accident or stroke (health condition/disorder or disease). This person may demonstrate activity limitations such as the need for assistance to perform bed mobility, transfers, and gait performance. The therapist must then hypothesize the possible impairments that may explain the noted activity limitations. The activity limitations may be due to impairments such as tone abnormalities, motor control problems, lack of range, decreased aerobic capacity, and possible cognitive deficits.[4] The patient or patient's family may also provide information about how the activity limitations and impairments limit the patient's ability to perform societal roles or participate in life (participation restrictions). The incorporation of personal and environmental factors will determine if such factors facilitate or hinder the rehabilitation process.

In 2008, the American Physical Therapy Association (APTA) joined various international health care entities and the WHO in endorsing the ICF model.[5] This model is now widely used in the national and international physical therapy communities; therefore, this model will be consistently used throughout this text. Also, the reader can always find new and expanded information regarding the clinical applications of the ICF model through various Web sites.[6,7]

GUIDE TO PHYSICAL THERAPIST PRACTICE

This book will also consistently incorporate the terminology and definitions of terms used in the *Guide*,[3] published by the APTA. The intent of the *Guide* is to discuss the common features

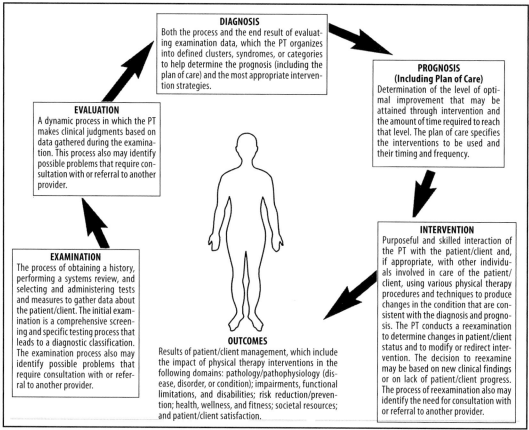

Figure 1-3. Elements of the Patient/Client Management Model. (Reprinted from *Guide to Physical Therapist Practice*. 2nd ed, 2003 with permission of the American Physical Therapy Association. This material is copyrighted, and any further reproduction or distribution requires written permission from APTA.)

that describe the physical therapy management of selected patient/client conditions and diagnostic groups. As of the writing of this text, the *Guide* is being revised to more consistently follow the ICF model.[8]

Central to the understanding of the *Guide* is the understanding of the elements of patient/client management, which are as follows: examination, evaluation, diagnosis, prognosis, intervention, and outcomes (Figure 1-3). The following describes each element and the role of the PTA.

Examination

A physical therapy examination includes obtaining a patient history, performing a systems review, and administering tests and measures to gather relevant data about the patient. The initial examination is comprehensive and leads to a diagnostic classification or identification of specific body systems, activity limitations, and participation restrictions that may benefit from physical therapy intervention. This process may also result in identification of problems that may require consultation with or referral to other health care providers.[3] The PT conducts the initial examination. The PTA may assist in collecting data as determined by the PT. If the PTA is asked to participate in this initial examination, then those data or results must be reported to the supervising PT in an effort to generate an appropriate plan of care.

Evaluation

This is a process in which the PT makes clinical judgments based on data gathered during the examination. The evaluation facilitates the determination of the systems or subsystems that may explain the corresponding functional loss. Through examination, the PT also identifies possible problems that may require consultation with or referral to other providers. This element is beyond the scope of practice for the PTA and is conducted by the supervising PT. However, the PTA may be present for the evaluation process.[3]

Diagnosis

The physical therapy diagnosis identifies the activity limitations and the impairments that may contribute to the functional problem. The physical therapy diagnosis also articulates the possible participation restriction resulting from the impairments and activity limitations. The physical therapy diagnosis may also contain a brief discussion of the contextual factors that affect function. It is a "process and the outcome of examination and evaluation"[3] and provides the basis for determining the patient/client prognosis and planning intervention strategies.

The referring physician is responsible for the medical diagnosis that should identify the disease and/or pathology, and the supervising PT determines the diagnosis of impairment, activity, and participation loss. The determination of both types of diagnoses are beyond the scope of PTA practice. However, it is the responsibility of the PTA to comprehend the meaning of the diagnosis and how it relates to intervention. It is the PTA's responsibility to communicate to the supervising PT the changes in the patient/client's functional performance to allow the PT to make the necessary changes in the treatment plan.[3] Although the roles and responsibilities of the PT and PTA will change in the future, the relationship and responsibilities to communicate with each other will always remain a key to best practice.

Prognosis

The prognosis identifies the predicted optimal improvement in function and the time parameters needed to change the existing limitations into functional activities the patient will be able to perform.[3] Part of the prognosis will deal with specific body systems that need changing before function can be expected. Examples of those body system problems may be as simple as strengthening a specific muscle group or increasing general range of motion in joints, or as complex as improving balance and postural control. Another part of the prognosis will deal with specific activities that the therapist, patient, and family have identified as needing improvement to regain optimal function. These activities may include moving in bed, walking, climbing stairs, getting in and out of the shower, dressing, and feeding. In some rehabilitation environments, specific activities of daily living (ADL) tasks may be the responsibility of other professionals, such as occupational therapists. Also, it is important to link therapy goals to those of the patient/family and what that individual wants and needs to do once leaving the rehabilitation environment. These future activities may include golfing, fly fishing, going to religious services, shopping, or other activities that allow the individual to participate in life. As such, those activities should be identified by the patient and the family and not determined by the therapist.

The prognosis also includes the plan of care established by the PT, which specifies the anticipated goals and expected outcomes, and the specific interventions to be used, including the timing and frequency. While the establishment of these goals is the responsibility of the PT, the PTA could provide input on the development of these goals and how they should be changed based on the patient's response to the interventions.

Regardless of the delegated responsibilities, the PTA is always responsible for communicating any changes in the patient's response to the plan of care. The PTA provides this input to allow the supervising PT to modify the prognosis and the treatment plan as appropriate. The observed changes may be due to development of new problems that may require reexamination or referral to other professionals.

Intervention

This element of the Patient/Client Management Model involves the use of various physical therapy procedures to achieve the patient goals. A reexamination may be conducted to determine any changes in the patient/client status, progress toward established goals, or the modification of the current plan of care.[3]

In the area of neurorehabilitation, common interventions delegated to PTAs include impairment training, such as strength training or range of motion (ROM) exercises, and functional training, such as task-specific exercises to improve bed mobility, sit to stand, walking, or sitting (see Chapter 4). The PTA may assist in data collection to determine if the current plan of care is on track in meeting the established goals or to determine if the plan of care needs to be modified.

The depth and breadth of the PTA scope of practice may change if the educational preparation for the PTA moves from an associate to a baccalaureate degree. The roles of the PTA may also be influenced by the acquisition of additional treatment skills through continuing education. The specific delegation to the PTA has to be based on the abilities of the PTA and the scope of practice identified within the respective state law. It is not clear in the future how the roles of the PT and PTA will change, but both professionals must work closely together to provide the best care for the patient.

Outcomes

Physical therapy outcomes refers to the product of the patient/client management process and the impact of physical therapy care on the impairments, activities, and participation, as well as patient/client satisfaction following the physical therapy intervention.[3] The PTA could participate in tracking outcomes by assisting in collecting objective and measurable data.

Physical Therapy Practice Areas

The *Guide* includes various practice patterns that provide details on the possible examination, intervention, and prognostic indications given specific practice patterns. The following lists 4 content (practice) areas under which these practice patterns are classified:

1. Musculoskeletal (muscles, joints, and bony structures)
2. Neuromuscular (sensory and motor peripheral nerves and CNS processing, including somatic and autonomic)
3. Cardiovascular and pulmonary (heart and lungs)
4. Integumentary (skin)

This text will focus on the clinical problems that develop out of the neuromuscular practice area. The reader must be aware that patients may have difficulty in more than one practice area, and the interactions may be significant. For example, a person with movement dysfunction following a neurological condition may also develop cardiopulmonary problems, or the person may already have a cardiopulmonary issue prior to the neurological insult (see Chapter 14 for more details). Both body systems must be considered when implementing appropriate physical therapy plans of care.

Although the *Guide*[3] clearly identifies the 4 practice patterns used by PTs, there are additional systems that can affect the habilitation or rehabilitation of those individuals. Organ systems can play a critical role in the effectiveness of the PT interventions. The gastrointestinal system plays a primary role in nutrition intake and elimination of waste. The hepatic and urinary systems play a vital role in filtering out chemical waste and excess fluid. The lymphatic system helps the vascular system with fluid elimination. Any one of these other systems can dramatically affect the cardiac, smooth, and striated muscles' metabolism and function.

Similarly, a dysfunction of the neuromuscular system can affect the function of other organ systems as well. For example, an individual may be referred to physical therapy with the medical diagnosis of early-stage Parkinson's disease. A patient may complain of constipation, which may be a result of decreased level of mobility, medication side effects, and rigidity of the trunk and the abdominal muscles. In this case, the patient may benefit from an increase in mobility and ambulation and interventions to decrease torso rigidity. The interventions may lead to an increased level of activity performance and participation and may also provide the added benefit of improvement of gastrointestinal function, leading to decreased complaints of constipation.

ROLE OF THE PHYSICAL THERAPIST AND PHYSICAL THERAPIST ASSISTANT

Although the role of the PTA within a clinical setting is dictated by the licensing board of the state, the specific types of delegation fall under the responsibilities of the PT and should directly relate to the needs of the patient. The PTA is the PT's assistant and should function within that scope of practice. The PT will have ultimate responsibility for the physical therapy provided to the patient.

Theoretical Framework

The authors have developed a theoretical framework to assist the reader in understanding the role of the PTA in working with patients/clients with neurological conditions. The theoretical framework is aligned with key components of the ICF model, the Patient/Client Management Model, and effective delegation principles (Figure 1-4).

Designated interventions for a patient recovering from neurological pathologies are directed at improving the patient's functional status through comprehensive interventions at both the activity and body systems and functions level. These interventions may simultaneously improve activity and participation (such as returning to leisure activities like golfing or fly-fishing) or may be directed at resolving impairments that could ultimately improve activity and participation.

For example, if the patient's ultimate goal is to be able to return to fly-fishing, the PTA can work with the client in sitting or standing and having the client hold or hold with assistance a fishing rod placed in a large can stabilized with sand. As the activity is performed, the client will, by virtue of the task, be working on range of motion, strength, balance, and postural control of the trunk, limbs, and shoulder girdle, all of which may need retraining after the neurological insult. In addition, the PTA must employ effective strategies to address the cognitive, musculoskeletal, and neuromuscular needs of the patient while working on specific activities selected by the patient or family.

Delegation Strategies: Decision Making Versus Doing

In the Patient/Client Management Model continuum, the PTA will ultimately be delegated selecting reexamination procedures and interventions.[3] As discussed previously, the determination of these interventions follows a thorough initial examination by the PT. The PT will summarize findings of the examination in the evaluation and will formulate a diagnosis and prognosis based on these findings. Designated interventions will then be indicated in the plan of care, and the PTA will perform select intervention activities in conjunction with ongoing communication with the supervising PT.

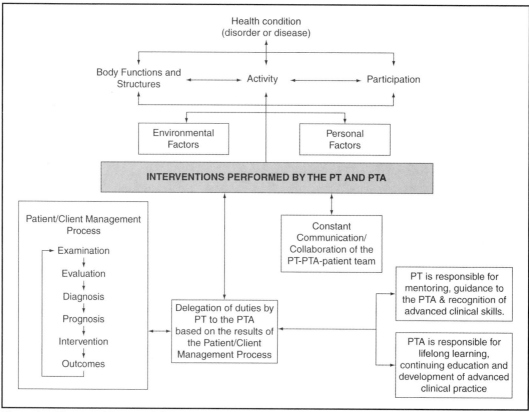

Figure 1-4. Theoretical framework for interventions provided by the PTA.

Effective delegation strategies were presented to our profession within a few years of the development of the PTA in an article by Nancy Watts, PT, PhD, FAPTA, in 1971.[9] The PT's responsibility for determination of the tasks that can be delegated to a PTA, including interventions and reexaminations, is a complex issue. Watts proposed a method for making such decisions that includes analyzing the physical therapy tasks involved in the interventions under consideration to determine the degree to which it represents decision making versus doing and the degree to which the elements are separable. She suggests that both components interact and both are necessary to quality care and best practice (Box 1-1).

The decision-making aspect of care requires evaluation and treatment planning skills. These skills require complex problem solving, up-to-date knowledge of the science of physical therapy, and a sophisticated ability to analyze and synthesize information from various sources in order to rationally choose the best alternative. To a large extent, these responsibilities fall into the PT's scope of practice.

The doing aspect of care requires excellence in skill, the knowledge of various therapeutic interventions, the capacity to recall correct treatment sequences, the artful manipulation of one's hands and body, and the ability to be sensitive to patient response moment to moment. Watts maintains that, in general, "decision-making skills involve dealing with data, while doing skills require dealing with people and things."[9] She also added that "the distinction drawn in this model between these 2 categories of skill should not be misconstrued as implying any hierarchy of importance nor any lack of interdependence between activities in the 2 realms."[9]

Watts also identifies 5 factors that are present in treatment that more adequately characterize the continuum that flows between deciding and doing:

Box 1-1

Delegation Strategies: Decision Making Versus Doing

1. Predictability of consequences: How uncertain is the situation? How confident can the decision maker be in the predictions about the consequences of action?
2. Stability of the situation: How much and how quickly is change likely to occur in the factors on which decisions are made?
3. Observability of basic indicators: How difficult is it to elicit the phenomena on which decisions are based? How easy are these phenomena to perceive or observe?
4. Ambiguity of basic indicators: How difficult are the key phenomena to interpret? How easily might they be confused with other phenomena?
5. Criticality of results: How serious are the consequences of a poor choice of method?

---

1. Predictability of consequences: How uncertain is the situation? How confident can the decision maker be in the predictions about the consequences of action?

   For example, a gait-training program for an individual with a sprained ankle with no other medical conditions is very different from a gait-training program for a person with a stroke, cardiac and pulmonary complications, uncontrolled diabetes, and a new orthotic device because of ankle weakness and instability.[9] The predictability of the probable consequences of gait-training decisions made for a patient with a sprained ankle seems more certain than those made for a person following a stroke with added complicating medical variables.

2. Stability of the situation: How much and how quickly is change likely to occur in the factors upon which decisions are made?

   For example, a mat exercise program for someone with a complete spinal cord injury (SCI) will remain relatively unchanged for a period of time compared with a mat program for an individual with an incomplete SCI. The person with the incomplete SCI may demonstrate significant functional improvement within a short period of time. However, considering the medical condition, a PTA with accurate visual recognition skills and experience and additional education in SCI management may be delegated intervention strategies but will be expected to report to the PT any changes that might indicate an alteration in the plan of care.

3. Observability of basic indicators: How difficult is it to elicit the phenomena on which decisions are based? How easy are these phenomena to perceive or observe?

   For example, an obligatory reflex may be easy to elicit and observe, whereas a maximal voluntary contraction requires full patient participation and may be more difficult to elicit.[9] The PT has been educated to recognize specific movement components and how they interact in functional activities, while the PTA is educated in providing interventions for specific body system problems and training of functional activities. When minor and major adjustments in treatment are needed on a moment-to-moment basis, the intervention should remain with the PT. As soon as those movements begin to stabilize and changes are easily recognized, then delegating to the PTA is appropriate.

4. Ambiguity of basic indicators: How difficult are the key phenomena to interpret? How easily might they be confused with other phenomena?

   For example, possible signs indicating the possibility of a cerebrovascular accident would be more difficult to identify and interpret than determining whether a muscle substitution was used in a manual muscle test.[9] A PTA can easily recognize muscle substitution and certainly an obvious stroke in transition, but subtle changes that reflect worsening of a medical problem is the responsibility of the PT, and a patient who may be that unstable should not be delegated.

5. Criticality of results: How serious are the consequences of a poor choice of method?

> For example, a wrong choice in a facilitation method that resulted in no response of the muscle would be of less consequence than the wrong choice in the amount of exercise without rest to be given to a patient with cardiac compromise.[9] If the intervention needs constant reexamination throughout the treatment, the PT should not be asking the PTA to make those decisions. On the other hand, a very skilled and experienced PTA might be able to monitor a patient and recognize when the PT is needed. Thus, the decision to delegate or retain control over the intervention should be made with serious consideration of the patient's needs and the stability of the vital organ systems of the patient.

These 5 factors are present to varying degrees in all treatment situations. In deciding which interventions and reexaminations to delegate to the PTA, the PT must clearly differentiate between the deciding and doing aspects of the intervention and then, using the factors listed previously, determine the extent to which these 2 aspects of care can be separated. These components will guide a PT regarding when to delegate select interventions for a client with CNS damage to a PTA. Obviously, the experiences and continuing education of the PTA may change how a PT decides to delegate. The patient must always be the one constant factor, and the belief that "we do no harm and provide best practice" should be the guiding factor in that decision making.

If the patient needs constant guarding and guidance in order to carry out a specific functional task, and the amount of guarding and guidance varies from moment to moment, delegation of that activity to a PTA may be inappropriate. On the other hand, if the patient is able to run a motor program, such as moving from sit to stand, but needs guidance to stay within a parameter of range of limits of stability or balance, delegation of the intervention to a PTA is appropriate. If the patient does not need guidance and only needs practice in order to overcome functional limitations, usually a family member or an aide can assist, and this may not be an appropriate use of the PTA. Although there are many overlapping variables that might determine when a PT versus a PTA should be responsible for the intervention, having time to provide a service should not be a reason. If the PTA is being asked to treat someone because he or she has time and not because the PTA is the best provider given the needs of the patient, then that delegation is inappropriate and is a misuse of the PTA within a clinical setting.

Effective delegation strategies are enhanced by ongoing communication with the supervising PT to optimize interventions performed by the PTA to enhance the plan of care. If an intervention is delegated to a PTA and the skill is outside of what the PTA has learned, it is always appropriate for the PTA to ask the PT for help or guidance. If what was delegated seems to contradict what the PTA has learned as contraindications, the PTA should always ask the PT for clarification before beginning treatment.

CAREER DEVELOPMENT AND CLINICAL INTERACTION ISSUES

Career development is important to every individual. Every person strives to perform work that provides a sense of satisfaction and purpose. In the case of a PTA, different career pathways have emerged with the advancement of the practice of physical therapy. It is, however, important to have a clear picture of the implications of these various career pathways in relation to the ethical and legal aspects of practice.

Within the profession itself, the APTA initiated the PTA Recognition of Advanced Proficiency. This is the equivalent of the clinical specialist certifications for PTs. This advanced proficiency designation recognizes PTAs who have furthered their careers beyond their entry-level preparation by achieving advanced skills through experience, leadership, and education.[10] This also recognizes the exceptional PT/PTA team collaboration that facilitates the provision of the best possible care to the patient or client. Currently, PTAs can obtain advanced proficiencies in the following: acute care, aquatic, cardiovascular/pulmonary, geriatric, integumentary, musculoskeletal, neuromuscular, oncology, and/or pediatric physical therapy. More information regarding Advanced Proficiency for the PTA can be found on the APTA Web site.

The following clinical scenarios describe potential areas of conflict in the PT/PTA dynamic. The first pertains to the clinical interactions between a PT and PTA from a business model. One scenario that has developed is the PTA owning a physical therapy practice that employs PTs and PTAs. Most state physical therapy licensing boards have identified the practice relationship of this business model. If the PTA owns the practice, then *that individual cannot function as a PTA within that setting.* The conflict of interest between the role of a boss to the PT and being the assistant to the same individual is self-explanatory and legally controlled by most state regulations governing the practice of physical therapy.

Another role the PTA may assume in a clinical setting is that of receiving certification or licensure in a complementary approach to patient management. Examples of these certifications or licensure include being a Feldenkrais practitioner, a Rolfer, or training in craniosacral techniques (refer to Chapter 15 for additional information). In these cases, the PTA may develop intervention skills outside the skills of the PT but complementary to providing intervention. Hopefully, open communication exists between the PT and PTA that encourages implementation of all interventions that can benefit the patient, but again, the PTA must remember that the PT is responsible for deciding which interventions are to be used and which interventions will be delegated to the PTA. The PTA should always make the PT aware of intervention strategies that may be helpful but are not already provided within the plan of care and never begin interventions without clarifying the intent with the PT. If the PTA is practicing as a complementary therapist independently of a physical therapy practice setting and outside the supervision of a PT, then she or he must remember that she or he is not practicing as a PTA and that what is offered is not physical therapy and cannot be billed as such. PTAs who have additional certification should also be aware of the legal and liability issues that may apply to them as licensed PTAs practicing in the complementary therapy arena. Discussion of these issues is beyond the scope of this text, but each PTA with complementary training must become familiar with the laws within the state in which he or she practices.

FUTURE ROLES

Physical therapy is a profession that has been evolving since its conception. The roles of the PT and PTA will change in the future, as they have changed over previous decades. Yet, the interactions should remain as 2 clinicians whose responsibility is to help guide patients toward functional recovery and higher quality of life. As PTs develop more wellness clinics and disease-prevention and risk-reduction programs, the roles of PTAs will enlarge in these practice areas as well. As the aging population copes with chronic diseases and the life-altering loss of functional skills, optimizing quality of life versus regaining function will become part of an ever-expanding scope of practice. As the population ages, maintaining as much independence as possible will decrease individuals' care costs. The PTA will continue to play an important role in that maintenance of functional skills in a cost-effective manner.

The role of the PTA has the potential of enlarging with increased responsibility in the areas of examination and intervention strategies and responsibilities for patient care. As these roles change, so will the educational requirements for entry-level practitioners, as seen in the move to an entry-level clinical doctorate as the terminal degree for PTs. PTA educational requirements may change to require a baccalaureate degree. PTAs of today may well be facing the same dilemma as PTs who graduated with bachelor's and master's degrees in the past. Younger graduates today may have a degree higher than the one a current practitioner has. This means only that the younger therapist, whether a PT or a PTA, may have new knowledge to teach the seasoned clinician, just as the clinician has skills to teach the novice. The key to not being caught with limitations in practice parameters is to continue with one's learning no matter the degree received that opened the door to entry into this profession. It is hoped that this text will provide a background to the PTA that will not only help during study as a student but also provide insight and guidance once the student moves into an exciting practice arena as a PTA.

REFERENCES

1. Nagi S. *Disability Concepts Revisited: Implication for Prevention.* Washington, DC: National Academy Press; 1991.
2. World Health Organization. *International Classification of Impairments, Disabilities and Handicaps* (ICIDH). Geneva, Switzerland: Author; 2001.
3. *Guide to Physical Therapist Practice.* 2nd ed. Alexandria, VA: American Physical Therapy Association; 2001.
4. The WHO International Classification of Functioning, Disability and Health. http://www3.who.int/icf/icftemplate.cfm?myurl=homepage.html &mytitle=Home%20Page. Accessed November 2, 2012.
5. American Physical Therapy Association. APTA Endorses World Health Organization ICF Model. http://www.apta.org/Media/Releases/APTA/2008/7/8/. Accessed November 2, 2012.
6. Sykes C. Health classifications 2: using the ICF in clinical practice. *WCPT Keynotes.* http://www.wcpt.org/sites/wcpt.org/files/files/KN-ICF-Clinical_practice.pdf. Accessed August 29, 2013.
7. Rauch A, Cieza A, Stucki G. How to apply the International Classification of Functioning, Disability and Health (ICF) for rehabilitation management in clinical practice. *Eur J Phys Rehabil Med.* 2008;44:329-342.
8. *Guide to Physical Therapist Practice.* Welcome to the Guide. http://guidetoptpractice.apta.org/site/misc/welcome.xhtml. Accessed November 16, 2012.
9. Watts NT. Task analysis and division of responsibility in physical therapy. *Phys Ther.* 1971;51(1):23-35.
10. American Physical Therapy Association. PTA recognition of advanced proficiency. http://www.apta.org/ptarecognition/. Accessed November 16, 2012.

Please see accompanying Web site at
www.healio.com/books/neuroptavideos

2

Normal Movement Development Across the Lifespan

Dale Scalise-Smith, PT, PhD

KEY WORDS

- Cognition
- Development
- Dynamic systems theory
- Innate motor behaviors
- Locomotion
- Motor development
- Osteoporosis

CHAPTER OBJECTIVES

- Recognize the interaction among multiple systems in performance of motor behaviors.
- Explain motor behaviors and changes that occur across the lifespan and variability of motor performance among individuals.
- Examine the impact of health and fitness (physical activity) sustained over the lifespan on motor skill performance.
- Discuss the impact of age and age-related changes in exercise and training programs.

INTRODUCTION

Effective practitioners recognize the interactional processes that lead to changes in motor development across the lifespan. The human motor system comprises more than 700 muscles and the nerves that supply them. Motor behaviors require coordinated efforts among these and other bodily systems to produce movements. Motor behavior, the study of how movement is learned and controlled and changes with increasing age, is divided into subdisciplines: motor control, motor development, and motor learning[1] (refer to Chapter 3 for additional information).

Umphred DA, Lazaro RT, eds.
Neurorehabilitation for the Physical Therapist Assistant,
Second Edition (pp 15-43).
© 2014 SLACK Incorporated.

This chapter provides an overview of motor development to help the reader (1) recognize typical and atypical changes in motor behaviors across the lifespan, (2) appreciate factors that influence motor development, and (3) apply knowledge of motor development, and associated mechanisms of change, to intervention strategies.

Until the late 1960s, research in motor development focused on infants and children. In the 1970s, developmentalists came to realize that changes in motor behaviors did not end in adolescence, but rather were dynamic processes with changes occurring through older adulthood. Thus, models of motor development have expanded to include changes that occur throughout the lifespan. Consequently, lifespan motor development now examines movement from early infancy through older adulthood. Motor development, a subdiscipline of motor behavior, is characterized by acquisition of motor skills during infancy (birth to 1 year) and childhood (1 to 10 years), followed by a period of stability from adolescence (10 to 19 years) through early and middle adulthood (20 to 59 years), and finally, a decline in execution of movements during late adulthood (60 years to death).

Lifespan motor development reflects motor behaviors observed from the prenatal period through older adulthood. The acquisition, control, and retention of motor skills is not confined to any one part of the lifespan. During early infancy, acquisition of postural control and grasping are primary foci. Later in infancy, mobility and object manipulation become primary objectives. During childhood, the skills acquired earlier are refined and coalesce to produce complex motor behaviors. Throughout adolescence and adulthood, opportunities to practice motor behaviors in different environmental contexts expand and motor skills mature. As individuals grow old, successful aging is the ability to control motor skills without decline. Whether this decline is due to aging, disuse, or a combination of both along with disease is open to debate. Within this context of motor development, the impact of internal and external factors on motor skill acquisition will be considered both individually and collectively.

THEORIES OF DEVELOPMENT

Development is defined as "the changes that occur in one's life from conception to death."[2] Development is described as a dynamic process focused on the individual adapting movements to physical changes in the system throughout the lifespan.[3] Changes in human behavior, including cognitive, motor, language, social-emotional, and physical characteristics, result from aging, life experiences, genetics, and their interactive effects.

Early studies of motor development were based on maturational models of central nervous system (CNS) organization.[4,5] These studies provided elegant descriptions of posture acquisition and a timeline for skill development. Most research development has focused on the emergence of cognitive and affective behaviors and neglected the processes and mechanisms involved in learning motor tasks.[6] Development was thought to occur in a fixed sequence, and behaviors observed were a direct reflection of the maturation of intrinsic mechanisms.[7]

This traditional model of development relied on motor milestones to evaluate ability levels in infants and children. While motor milestones provided an assessment of actual motor skills a child performed, they failed to provide information about the process of attaining motor skills.

Researchers have proposed theories on motor development that emphasize the forces behind behavioral changes. Some scientists[4,5] theorized that developmental changes arise from internal factors (genetics and/or maturation), while others associated changes with external variables (environmental, experience, and/or learning).[8,9] While sufficient evidence exists to support the idea that some predetermined processes occur at relatively similar points in development, not all motor behaviors emerge at the same biological, chronological, or psychological age in every individual. The traditional theories on development and maturation fail to adequately address the variation

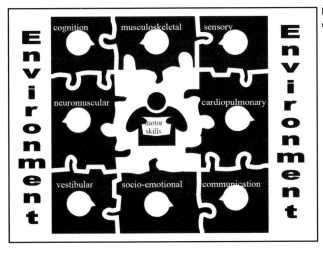

Figure 2-1. Interaction between intrinsic and extrinsic factors.

inherent in human motor development. Successful acquisition of motor skills may be directly related to the individual's need to solve a problem within the context of the environment.

Researchers who have focused on developing new models for motor skill acquisition in infants and young children include Heriza, Thelan, and Zelazo et al.[10-12] Rather than using traditional methods to measure changes in motor development and assess the outcomes, these researchers examined the process of motor skill acquisition.[13,14] These contemporary developmentalists support an interactive model of motor development in which both intrinsic and extrinsic variables impact the development and acquisition of motor skills (Figure 2-1). The primary foundation for this model is dynamic systems theory.

Dynamic systems theory states that an individual uses all possible strategies to accomplish a task, and as physiological systems are modified, the motor behavior changes.[15] Systems theorists purport that modifications in motor behaviors are the result of dynamic interactions between and among the musculoskeletal, neuromuscular, cardiovascular and pulmonary, and cognitive systems. Communicative and social-emotional aspects are equally considered. Interactive, multidimensional systems are susceptible to changes in organizational and behavioral capabilities as one ages.[16] As an individual acquires a skill, the organization of the behavior may change, thereby allowing the person to identify the most efficient strategy for effective functioning.

It is clear that a small change in any subsystem may result in a change in a motor behavior. For example, Thelan examined stepping in infants 8 weeks of age.[15] During the baseline phase of this study, the infants' feet were placed on a treadmill with trunk support in an upright position. When the treadmill was turned on, the infants stepped. Immediately afterward, weights were applied to each leg, and the infants were again placed on the treadmill. The treadmill was turned on, but no infant stepped. The author concluded that small changes in one subsystem—in this case, the musculoskeletal system—resulted in a change in the whole behavior: stepping. This evidence supported the premise that modifying one aspect of a multicomponent system, especially during a critical period, results in a change in behavior.

As one ages, organizational changes of bodily systems increase the complexity of the collective system, allowing for greater adaptability and more efficient functioning. Scott defined periods of rapid differentiation or change during development when an organism is most easily altered or modified as *critical periods*.[16] These periods are when physiological systems are most vulnerable and may be positively or negatively affected by intrinsic as well as extrinsic factors acting on the system.[17] Thelan and Smith[17] acknowledge that while behaviors appear in a fairly typical temporal sequence, individuals exhibit delayed or accelerated timing with different environmental contexts. These periods occur at different times for different systems throughout the body.

Understanding systems theory and the concept of critical periods is crucial to all aspects of motor development. These theories illustrate the complexity of development and the difficulty in identifying the variables that influence performance of motor behaviors across the lifespan and in identifying the most effective treatments to use when a motor skill is compromised.

AGE AND AGING

Just as changes in different intrinsic and extrinsic systems affect movement early in development, aging also affects motor performance. Age is defined in terms of chronological age and biological age.[18] Chronological age is the period of time that a person has been alive expressed in years and months. In infants, it is measured in days, weeks, or months, while in adults, it is expressed in terms of years.

Unlike chronological age, biological age is not measured according to the calendar. Instead, biological age measures functional age in different body systems in relation to chronological age.[19] For example, an individual who competes in marathons may have biologically younger cardiovascular and pulmonary systems than same-age peers who are not runners. As another example, a female may go through menopause prematurely. A postmenopausal woman experiences a decrease in estrogen levels that, in turn, negatively affects bone strength as measured by bone density. This woman has less dense bones than her same-age peers who will experience menopause later. No consistent method has been established for measuring biological age, but there is general agreement that a wide variability of biological aging exists among individuals.

"Aging refers to the time-sequential deterioration that occurs in most animals including weakness, increased susceptibility to disease and adverse environmental conditions, loss of mobility and agility, and age-related physiological changes."[20] Factors associated with aging are characterized as age dependent or age related. Age-dependent behaviors are physiological changes that affect different tissues, organ systems, and functions that, cumulatively, can affect activity and participation levels of older adults.

Age-related behaviors are observed in many people but may be accelerated or decelerated in individuals of the same chronological age. One reason why behaviors may be designated as age related rather than age dependent is that individuals of the same chronological age are not necessarily the same biological age. From a genetic perspective, structural and functional changes in general are thought to be a consequence of aging and are, therefore, predictable and consistent across physiological systems. Affecting the genetic potential for longevity are the strong effects of environmental factors, such as toxins, radiation, and oxygen-free radicals—highly reactive molecules produced as cells turn food and oxygen into energy.[21] Consequently, using biological age rather than chronological age may be a more accurate reflection of changes in a biological system.

Researchers are unsure how much of the decline in motor behaviors in older adults is due to a decline in physiological systems or to decreased practice and/or conditioning.[22] Rowe and Kahn found that "with advancing age, the relative contribution of genetic factors decreases and the nongenetic factors increases."[22] Nongenetic risk factors can be identified through screening and addressed through clinical intervention and patient education. Lifestyle choices, including diet, physical activity, and other health habits, as well as behavioral and social factors, have a potent effect on aging processes. Kaplan and colleagues reported that well-being later in life is affected by lifestyle established earlier in life.[23] This suggests that interventions focused on positively influencing aging are important to preventive care and reducing sequelae associated with disease or injury.

PHYSIOLOGICAL CHANGES IN BODY SYSTEMS ACROSS THE LIFESPAN

Following dynamic systems theory, researchers and clinicians who examine motor behaviors across the lifespan acknowledge that many biological systems involved in the execution of motor skills and their associated behaviors undergo physiological changes as a consequence of aging. Using a dynamic systems theory approach to lifespan development may explain how seemingly small changes in one system can affect an individual's functional abilities.

Musculoskeletal System

The musculoskeletal system is composed of muscles, bones, cartilage, tendons, and ligaments. The roles of the musculoskeletal system are to provide a structural framework for the body to move and to protect internal organs.

Development of the muscular system initiates in utero and continues into young adulthood as a direct result of growth in the number and size of the fibers. Differentiation and development of the fibers is first observed during the fifth and eighth weeks of fetal life.[24] Evidence of rapid differentiation in the musculoskeletal system translates to discernible, complex movements early in prenatal life.

Muscle tissue reportedly grows at a rate 2 times faster than bones between the ages of 5 months to 3 years.[25] Throughout development of the musculoskeletal system, changes occur in muscle length, width, and girth, but the overall outward appearance remains unchanged. There is considerable variation in this growth. The structural and functional capabilities of an infant's muscular system differ from those of an adult. One example of a structural difference between the infant and adult is in muscle fiber type. Compared with adults, a high prevalence of Type I muscle fibers are present in infant muscles that contain both Type I and Type II fibers. Functionally, the infants' predominance of Type I fibers results in a predominance of postural motor behaviors that rely on slow-twitch fibers, whereas adults are able use both muscle fiber types to produce ballistic movements and postural activities.

Differences exist in the temporal differentiation of muscular changes of same-age males and females. Males exhibit rapid increase in the number of muscle fibers during 2 periods: from birth to 2 years of age and again between 10 and 16 years.[26] Females experience a longer and more gradual increase in fiber size between the ages of 3.5 to 10 years. In addition, during adolescence males experience an overall fiber size increase of 14-fold compared with a 10-fold increase in females. While muscle fiber development continues into middle adulthood, the pace is slower in males and females.

Age-related changes in the musculoskeletal system include decreased fiber size, muscle fiber recruitment, and quantity of fast-twitch fibers.[27] By age 50, the muscle mass begins to decrease so that by age 80 muscle mass has deteriorated by as much as 40%.[28] Similarly, muscle force production decreases by up to 30% between the ages of 60 and 90 years.

Strength and flexibility are 2 areas of the muscular system central to an individual's level of activity and participation. Strength is defined as the ability of a muscle to generate force against a specific resistance or produce torque at a joint.[29] Flexibility is the ability to bend.

Strength increases because of higher levels of resistance applied gradually during a muscular contraction. Changes in the cross-sectional area of muscles directly influence the force production of a given muscle. As the cross-sectional area of the muscle fibers hypertrophy, the ability to produce force increases. Conversely, as the cross-section of muscles diminishes, the ability to produce force decreases.

Sarcopenia, the age-related loss of muscle mass, results in a loss of strength and power with decreased functional independence.[30] As an individual ages, the number and size of the muscle fibers decrease, resulting in a reduction in strength.[31] Although all muscles experience a reduction in strength as a consequence of age, the impact is greater on the lower rather than upper extremities.

While strength is critical to musculoskeletal function, flexibility is equally as important. Flexibility incorporates joint motion and the extensibility of the tissues that cross the joint.[29] Flexibility changes across the lifespan and is directly related to the amount, frequency, and variability of motor activity in which the individual participates.[9] Early in postnatal life, infants exhibit limited flexibility due to the environmental constraints of the uterine environment. As the infant ages, flexibility increases in direct relation to increased joint play and extensibility of surrounding tissues. Flexibility increases in males and females through early childhood. By 10 years of age for boys and 12 years for girls, flexibility begins to decrease. However, this may not be true of athletes, dancers, and other individuals involved in activities that incorporate flexibility training. The result is that as individuals age, strength and flexibility decrease. While this appears to be age dependent, it may be more likely that it is age related.[27] Regularly performing motor activities (exercise) directed toward improving strength and/or flexibility can reverse the effects of inactivity for most individuals, even those older than 90 years of age.[27] While it may take longer for older individuals to regain strength and/or flexibility than young adults or children, musculoskeletal tissue is modifiable. Modifying strength and flexibility in an older adult requires that other systems are capable of modifying performance levels to meet the increased needs of the musculoskeletal system.

Current research supports the premise that changes in the muscular system are more likely age related and attributable to decreased motor activity levels and not purely age dependent.[27,32] Thus, keeping physically active while progressing into older adulthood may be key to maintaining functional independence and may positively affect (decelerate) age-related changes.

The skeletal system, similarly to the muscular system, experiences phases of growth, stability, and degeneration. The skeletal system of infants and children is immature; bones are flexible and porous, with a strong periosteum.[33] Movement plays a key role as a "modeling force" in joint formation beginning in the prenatal period and continuing into postnatal development.[34] Early in prenatal development, the acetabulum is deep and surrounding the femoral head, whereas during prenatal development, the rate of growth in the femoral head is greater than the socket, and thus, by birth, the hip is the most unstable joint. Developmental changes of the acetabular socket may be attributed to the fetus' growth within a restricted uterine environment. These changes may in turn facilitate the infant's ability to successfully pass through the vaginal canal during birth.[34]

A primary difference between the child and adult skeletal system is the presence of the growth plate complex in children. Ossification centers appear from birth through skeletal maturity.[35] While primary ossification occurs in utero, secondary ossification is not complete until the individual reaches skeletal maturity, usually by 14 years in females and 16 years in males.

Even after bone length is complete, bones continue to grow on the surface. This is termed *appositional growth* and continues throughout most of life. During childhood and adolescence, new bone growth exceeds bone reabsorption and bone density increases. Until age 30, bone density increases in most individuals, and bone growth and reabsorption remain stable through middle adulthood. Later in adulthood, reabsorption exceeds new bone growth and bone density declines.[29]

Women exhibit more loss of bone mass than men. Decreased bone density in women is generally attributed to differences in the type and level of hormones present. While the difference is most significant during menopause, premenopausal women still lose bone density at a higher rate than their male peers do.

Osteopenia is the presence of a less-than-normal amount of bone and, if left untreated, can lead to osteoporosis. Progressive loss of bone density, observed into older adulthood, is commonly identified as osteoporosis. Osteoporosis is more common in women than in men and is a major cause of fractures and postural changes in both sexes.[31]

Overall, many of the changes in the musculoskeletal system relate to demands placed on the system. The extrinsic and intrinsic forces imposed on musculoskeletal systems of typically and atypically developing children may contribute to functional and structural differences in their musculoskeletal systems. Similarly, accelerated or decelerated age-related changes in the older adult may be the direct result of the individual's activity level.[36]

As an integral part of intervention, education is central to the client/patient recognizing the significance and long-term benefits of an active lifestyle. While all systems contribute to and are affected by one's lifestyle, the cardiovascular and pulmonary systems play an important role.

Cardiovascular and Pulmonary Systems

The cardiovascular and pulmonary systems comprise the heart, lungs, and associated vascular complex. The cardiovascular system is responsible for pumping blood through the pulmonary, coronary, cerebral, and systemic circulation for the purposes of perfusing tissues with oxygen and nutrients and removing waste products. The pulmonary system is responsible for oxygen transport and gas exchange.

The symbiotic relationship between the cardiovascular and pulmonary systems means that small changes in one system can significantly affect both systems and, by extension, all other systems. In addition, other internal and external factors are important to maintaining physiological stability.

Changes within the cardiovascular and pulmonary systems directly affect an organism's growth and development. With aging comes a change in the cardiovascular and pulmonary systems' ability to adapt the intrinsic and extrinsic factors that contribute to the functioning of the system.

Regardless of the age of the individual, therapeutic intervention directed toward prevention and wellness are critical to continuing to function, performing activities, and participating as an active member of a community.

From 3 to 8 weeks of prenatal life, all of the cardiac structures are formed.[37] All other structures of the cardiovascular system are fully developed and functional shortly after birth. At birth, the left and right ventricles are of similar size, but by 2 months of age, the muscle wall of the left ventricle is thicker than the right ventricle. The significance of the difference in thickness between the muscular wall of the left and right ventricles is related to function. The left ventricle is responsible for pumping blood to the whole body, while the right ventricle is responsible for pumping blood only to the lungs.

Structurally, the heart doubles by an infant's first birthday and increases its size 4-fold by age 5. Much of the changes associated with cardiac growth occur during childhood. As the size of the heart increases, the heartbeat decreases, and blood pressure (BP) increases.[38] Heart rate in a newborn is generally 120 to 140 beats per minute (bpm), 80 bpm by age 6, and 70 bpm by age 10. Systolic BP (defined as maximal pressure on the artery during left ventricular contraction or systole) increases from 40 to 75 mm Hg in the newborn to 95 mm Hg by age 5.[39] BP continues to rise into adolescence. The capacity to maintain exercise for longer periods and at greater intensities increases throughout early childhood. Children as young as 5 years of age who have not had opportunities for adequate aerobic exercise and nutritional intake may show signs of or be at risk for cardiovascular disease.[40]

Development of the pulmonary system occurs during later prenatal and postnatal life.[41] The weight of the lungs triples by 1 year of age. As the size of the lungs continues to grow, the capacity and efficiency of the lungs increase and respiratory rate decreases. The vital capacity of a 5-year-old is one-fifth that of an adult, but this is not usually a limiting factor during exercise. Overall, aerobic capacity increases during childhood and is slightly higher in males than females. The overall work capacity of children increases most dramatically from 6 to 12 years of age.[38] Peak oxygen consumption is achieved early in adulthood and changes in direct relation to activity levels.

As activity decreases in older adulthood, so do the structural and functional capacities of the cardiovascular and pulmonary systems. Many of these changes are the direct result of decreased elasticity of the tissues, decreased efficiency of the structures, and decreased ability to increase workload. Functional changes include a decrease in the overall maximum heart rate from 200+ bpm through young adulthood to 170 bpm by age 65. Older adults have less elastic vessels, and resistance to blood volume increases. Consequently, older adults reach peak cardiac output at lower levels than younger individuals do. These cardiovascular changes may be compounded by high levels of inactivity, and the result may be decreased capacity to perform activities that raise metabolic demands and increase the requirement for oxygen transport.[42] However, these normal aging responses can be reduced through aerobic activities.

Throughout life, performance of motor activities and activities of daily living (ADL) depends highly on the integrity of an individual's cardiopulmonary and cardiovascular systems. Introduction of aerobic activities during early childhood has implications for improved health and wellness across the lifespan. While aging affects the performance and efficiency of the cardiopulmonary and cardiovascular systems, aerobic exercise can improve the capacity and efficiency of the cardiovascular and cardiopulmonary systems. All of these changes in the cardiovascular and pulmonary systems have a significant impact on other systems and consequently on overall body function. Information from the cardiovascular and pulmonary systems (eg, BP and oxygen saturation rates) is communicated through the nervous system. The nervous system, in turn, regulates responses of the cardiovascular and pulmonary systems through the autonomic nervous system.

Neurological System

The nervous system is composed of the CNS and peripheral nervous system. The CNS includes the brain and spinal cord and directs all bodily functions. The peripheral nervous system includes both the autonomic and somatic nerves and is responsible for transporting impulses to and from the CNS.[43]

Development of the CNS occurs as an integration of intrinsic and extrinsic variables and environmental and genetic influences. The most critical and vulnerable period in CNS development is the first year of postnatal life, when the infant's brain develops from one-fourth to one-half the size of the adult brain. Much of the growth during this period is related to increases (1) in the number of glial cells, (2) in myelin in the brain, and (3) in the size of neurons. During this period, the cerebral cortex undergoes rapid growth. These structural changes observed in the brain are directly related to motor behaviors and cognitive development observed during the first few years of life. Growth in the CNS slows after 2 years of age, but it continues into adulthood. As the nervous system matures, the complexity of the gross and fine motor skills and cognitive processes increases. By adolescence, the brain has reached adult size, but myelination and differentiation continue into adulthood.

While the CNS, much like other bodily systems, has the capacity to compensate for some age-related changes, the extent of the compensation depends on the task and "practice" over time. Repetition of motor activities may stimulate activation of new growth in dendrites located proximal to neurons previously lost. Activation of new pathways may or may not result in improved functional ability (see Chapter 3, specifically Motor Learning and Neuroplasticity).

Neuromuscular systems of the older adult may be limited in the capacity to reorganize muscle synergies and produce variability in functional responses. Decline of the nervous system generally begins after age 30 and is characterized by the death of thousands of neurons and decreased brain weight. Loss of neurons in the centers controlling sensory information, long-term memory, abstract reasoning, and coordination of sensorimotor information negatively affect function. For some individuals, this may not have significant implications. For others, CNS changes have serious implications. Alterations in the CNS may play a role in postural instability and impaired sensation, and these changes can result in falls.[44]

Implicit in performance of many functional activities is cognition. If changes in cognition coexist with changes in other systems, it may be difficult to accurately interpret the underlying causes.

Cognitive System

Cognition may be defined as awareness, perception, reasoning, and judgment.[45] The cognitive system uses the 5 senses (sight, smell, sound, touch, and taste) to process, interpret, store, and retrieve information. Existing theories support the premise that sensory information is integrated and stored to allow for interpretation, storage, and retrieval.[45] Cognition is directly related to problem solving and information processing. Often, cognition is not measured directly but rather is inferred.

One of the most important skills that infants learn early in life is to differentiate familiar and unfamiliar people. The infant's ability to act on the environment improves as comprehension of cause-effect improves. Early in development, infants and young children are unable to recognize relevant cues when processing information and cannot chunk information for storage. Consequently, infants and young children may not use or interpret the information as efficiently as older children. An example may be a parent giving instructions to a young child. If the young child is given more than one instruction, he or she may be delayed in processing or may not accurately process the information. Consequently, the child produces an inaccurate response.

During childhood, higher-level cognitive processing skills emerge as the ability to accurately identify relevant cues, filter irrelevant information, and process information faster. Optimal higher-level processing begins in adolescence and continues into adulthood.

As an individual grows older, information is processed more slowly, and the time necessary to perform motor skills increases. Additionally, while learning may occur more slowly with age, once a behavior is learned, retention is no different from that of a younger individual. While the time necessary to perform the task may increase, older adults are able to execute many tasks without incident. Other motor tasks may be altered because of processing. One example is driving a motor vehicle. Delayed processing in individuals older than 70 years of age may significantly delay execution of the task and pose a danger to the driver, passengers, pedestrians, and individuals driving in other vehicles. While driving may be a longstanding activity of an older adult, impaired cognitive and/or motor abilities may make driving a vehicle unsafe. The associated risks of injury to self and others may outweigh the individual's desire to maintain community independence.[46]

While cognitive processing has shown to deteriorate in older adults, the degree or rate of deterioration is highly variable. Cognitive changes most frequently encountered in older adults include dual-task performance, word retrieval, recall, and rapid processing tasks. As a physical therapist assistant (PTA), you can reinforce the concept of "use it or lose it" as it relates to all CNS function, including, but not limited to, cognition and motor skills. The literature reinforces this simple phrase, and your patients can understand these simple words. There are many computer programs available to the general public that are not only fun activities but can challenge the individual's cognitive skills. Playing games like Sudoku, solitaire of various complexities, or any activity that challenges the "thinking ability" of your client will help to maintain the cognitive skills that once seemed easy.

Throughout life, growth and development of many body systems play an important role in the acquisition and performance of motor skills. The interactive and interdependent nature of systems supports the idea that changes in one system can affect, positively or negatively, performance of motor behaviors.

MOTOR DEVELOPMENT

"Motor development is the study of changes in human motor behavior over the lifespan, the processes that underlie these changes, and the factors that affect them."[47] Haywood referred to motor development as the gradual process of refining skills and integrating biomechanical principles of movement so that the result is a motor behavior that is consistent and efficient.[9] Efficiency is attained through practice of a behavior to reduce intra-individual variability and improve stability of performance.

Traditional developmental researchers regarded infants as passive beings that were acted on (stimulated) by external forces in the environment, more often reactive to external stimuli than actively producing purposeful movements. Infants were thought to produce responses that were stereotypic in nature and referred to as primitive and postural reflexes.

Contemporary research refutes the premise that infants are passive beings. Rather, infants are seen as competent beings capable of complex interactive behaviors beginning at birth.[48,49] One example of the infant's ability to produce purposeful interactions at birth is observed when the infant turns his or her head to his or her mother's voice.

Primitive reflexes represent an example of infant behaviors that classify infants as passive beings. These reflexes, now referred to as *innate motor behaviors*, are based on traditional models of CNS organization and motor development theories. More recently, researchers have produced evidence that these behaviors are not solely dependent on the CNS but are the result of interactions and interdependence of intrinsic and extrinsic factors.[50] One example of an innate motor behavior is sucking. Infants will generally suck if a stimulus is placed strategically in the infant's mouth. However, the stimulus may not produce a similar response if an infant has recently been fed and is sated. Innate motor behaviors, present at birth, are modifiable and represent functional behaviors observed in very young infants.

The extensive literature on motor development indicates that not all individuals acquire the same motor skills at the same chronological age, nor will every individual exhibit motor behaviors in a fixed sequence of activities.[7,49] Additionally, while most children acquire skills in a somewhat fixed order, the sequence in which motor behaviors emerge may also vary and does not affect functional independence later in life.

Changes in motor performance, measured both qualitatively and quantitatively, are evident throughout life. These changes are not thought to be purely age dependent, but rather age related. Practice of skills through repetition improves motor performance. Similarly, decreased frequency in performing activities as an individual ages may be the factor that most contributes to a decline in motor skills. Acquisition of motor skills is multifactorial, interweaving maturation and experience. Declines in motor skills may be attributable to changes that occur as part of the aging process. Equally as important is the frequency and level of activity and participation of the individual.[51] Changes in these behaviors do not occur at exactly the same time for any 2 individuals.

Aging is a process seen in all species on earth, and it varies within and among individuals. This variability depends on intrinsic factors, such as maturation of physiological systems, and extrinsic factors, such as environment. Motor development, seen as changes in motor behaviors, can be recognized across the lifespan (Table 2-1).

Prenatal (0 to 40 Weeks' Gestation)

Motor behaviors appear early in prenatal life. Technological advances enable health providers and family members to observe fetal movements such as reaching, grasping, thumb sucking, and kicking. These complex behaviors lend evidence to the theory that at birth, infants are competent beings. Postnatally, the extrauterine environment is quite different for the newborn infant. Behaviors observed in utero, through ultrasound, may not be observed immediately after birth,

Table 2-1

Motor Development

Age	Prone	Supine	Sitting	Locomotion	Hand
0 to 1 months	Lifts head. Turns to side.	Head turns side-to-side. Tracks objects. Prefers head to one side.	Head upright 1 to 2 seconds. Slumped in supported sitting.	Makes crawling movements.	Arm movements jerky.
2 to 3 months	Lifts head to 90 degrees. Chest elevated. Weight-bearing on arms. May begin rolling.	Hand to foot play.	Head upright bobs. Head lags in pull to sit. Requires support to sit. Rounded back.	Pivots 30 degrees prone.	Briefly holds toy placed in hand. Hand to mouth. Bats at bright objects. Hands to midline.
4 to 6 months	Reaches in prone. Pushes up onto extended arms.	Begins rolling supine to side-lying.	Propped to independent sitting (Figure 2-2).	Pivots in prone.	Retrieves object within reach. Holds 2 objects. Holds object with 2 hands. Brings toy to mouth.
7 to 10 months	Rocks on hands and knees. Moves into sitting.	Lifts head as in sit-up.	Moves from sitting to prone or quadruped. Rotates in sitting to retrieve object.	Moves forward on belly. Pushes up to hands and knees. Pulls to standing. Briefly stands independently.	Grasp progresses from radial to inferior to lateral pattern. Spontaneously releases objects.
11 to 12 months	Prone to standing (Figure 2-3).		Side-sits.	Walks, one hand held. Stands alone. Moves stand to sit.	Begins to use objects as tools.

(continued)

Table 2-1 (continued)

Motor Development

Age	Prone	Supine	Sitting	Locomotion	Hand
13 to 14 months	Moves to standing using half-kneel.			Walks without support. Stoops to retrieve objects, regains standing. Walks backward. Assists with feeding.	Holds 2 cubes in same hand. Grasps with thumb and first 2 fingers. Pats pictures in book.
15 to 18 months	Creeps up stairs. Walks up stairs with support.			Carries objects while walking. Walks sideways. Running immature.	Builds 3-cube tower. Propels ball. Pokes with finger.
19 to 22 months				Stoops and retrieves objects (Figure 2-4). Ascends stairs with step-to pattern.	Builds 5- to 6-cube tower.
24 months				Kicks ball. Throws ball forward. Jumps off low step.	
30 months				One foot leads jumping off step. Climbs on tricycle.	Builds 8-cube tower. Imitates circular and horizontal strokes with crayon.

(continued)

Table 2-1 (continued)
Motor Development

Age	Prone	Supine	Sitting	Locomotion	Hand
3 to 3.5 years				Propels self on tricycle. Balances one foot momentarily. Arms reciprocate in running. Independent on tricycle activities. Balances one foot > 3 seconds.	Builds 9-cube tower. Unbuttons and buttons. Attempts cutting. Dominant hand emerging. Builds bridge with blocks. Strings large beads.
4 to 4.5 years				Hops 2 to 3 times. Walks on tiptoes. Runs with arm swing. Catches large ball. Throws ball 8 to 12 inches. Jumps both feet 2 to 3 inches.	Tripod pencil grasp. Attempts to trace line. Hand preference established. Places raisins in jar. Cuts shapes from paper.
5 to 8 years				Jumps forward and sideways. Jumps over 6- to 8-inch object. Skips, gallops, bounces large ball, and jumps.	Draws letters, shapes, and numbers. Places small pegs in pegboard. Prints well. Buttons small buttons.
9 to 12 years				Mature patterns in running, jumping, and throwing.	Handwriting develops. Learns to draw.

Figure 2-2. Newborn with head turned to mother's voice.

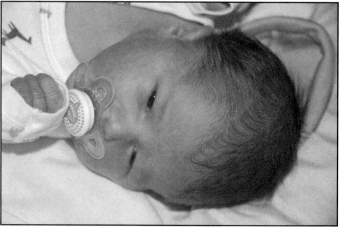

as the newborn must adapt to this new environment and modify movements given the new forces imposed by gravity. Consequently, the newborn must learn to perform these tasks under new environmental constraints.

Infancy (Birth to 12 Months)

Emergence of motor behaviors is more rapid during the first year of life than at any other time. At birth, the infant is an interactive, competent organism capable of purposeful movements. Brazelton reported that, even at birth, infants turn toward the sound of their mother's voice (see Figure 2-2) and visually focus on and track objects 8 to 12 inches from their faces.[48]

Taking into consideration the abilities and interactions of which a newborn is capable, behaviors previously referred to as reflexive movements are more likely functional motor behaviors that infants are capable of modifying. Motor skills emerge out of the infant's need to interact and solve problems within the new environment. As the repertoire of behaviors increases, the infant integrates feedback to refine behaviors and adapt to intrinsic (growth) or environmental parameters.[52]

During the first 3 months of life, infant motor behaviors focus on acquisition of head control (see Figures 2-3A and B) in all planes of movement. Gaining head control enables the infant to visually track people and objects and coordinate eye-hand activities during reaching activities. Manipulative skills acquired during this period include reaching for objects held 6 to 8 inches away and grasping an object placed in the infant's hand. Initially, both grasping and reaching are inefficient, but with practice, efficiency and accuracy improve.

By age 3 to 4 months, the infant achieves head control in the upright position and eye-hand coordination is first observed (see Figure 2-4). Reaching requires integration of information from the sensory, motor, and cognitive systems. Early reaching activities allow the infant to gather information about depth perception and use this in improving the accuracy of future reaching activities. As infants learn to vary the force and distance, their success in attaining the object improves.

When in the prone position, infants prop on their elbows and are able to roll. These motor behaviors represent the emergence of postural programming integrated with the power and range to maintain gravitational demand during upright holding and movement patterns.

At 4 to 6 months of age, infants begin to maintain an upright posture during supported sitting and, soon after, begin to prop sit and then sit independently (see Figure 2-5). Sitting is a functional behavior and serves as a prerequisite for performance of ADL as well as higher-level activities related to work, school, and play. As infants' independent sitting improves, so does their perspective of the world. These motor behaviors not only require postural programming but now integrate balance strategies as well. Manipulative skills that emerge from 4 to 6 months include retrieving objects if placed within reach, holding 2 objects (one in each hand), using

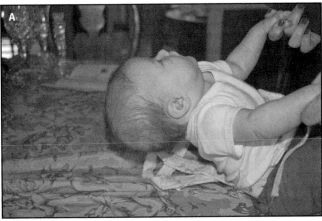

Figure 2-3A. Pulling to sit with head lag.

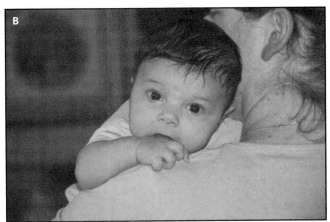

Figure 2-3B. Head control in upright.

Figure 2-4. Hands in midline with binocular control of the eyes.

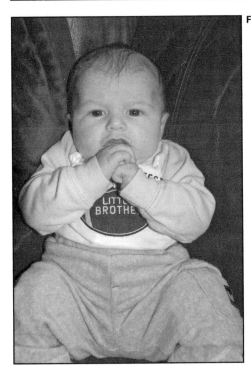

Figure 2-5. Prop sitting.

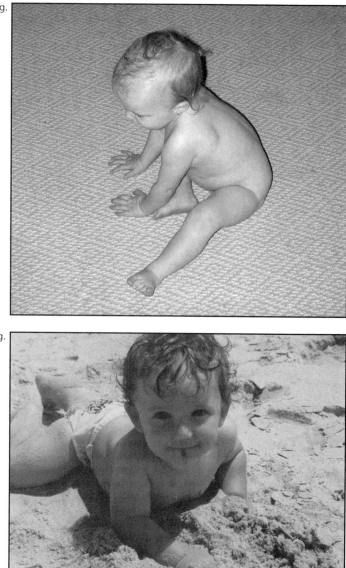

Figure 2-6. Belly crawling.

2 hands to hold an object (bottle), and holding a toy in one hand while retrieving another toy with the free hand.

During the second half of year 1, the primary focus is on mobility, as seen in rolling, belly crawling (Figure 2-6), creeping on all fours, cruising, and independent ambulation. Balance and posture (Figures 2-7A and B), as part of mobility tasks, incorporate sensory input and motor actions, including visual, vestibular, and somatosensory systems.

Infants use visual input to modulate reaching and grasping to accurately retrieve objects as manipulative skills by 8 months of age (Figure 2-8). By 9 months of age, an infant can grasp a spoon and bang it on the high chair tray but is not yet able to feed himself with the spoon (Figure 2-9). These patterns illustrate the development of trunk and axial posture and mobility control, but the child still needs to link the fine motor and corticospinal systems to accomplish intentional fine motor activities.

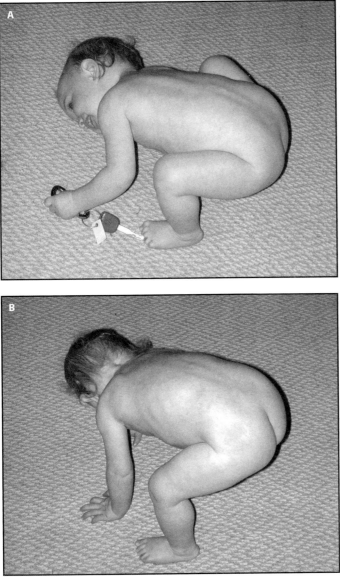

Figure 2-7. (A) and (B) Transition from sitting into standing.

Early Childhood (1 to 5 Years)

While the first year of life is described as a period of motor skills development, the second year of life is a time when skills are refined and higher-level motor function emerges. As infants develop independence in ambulation, they exhibit wide-based gait patterns with little rotation of the pelvis and little reciprocal movement of the upper extremities. While upright, infants begin to independently move sideways and backward in addition to moving forward. This allows them to maintain their center of gravity within a given base of support as well as gaining lateral hip control. Manipulative skills observed during this period include banging 2 blocks together; retrieving small objects using a rake, finger-thumb, or pincer grasp; and placing objects into a container.

As independent ambulation matures, dynamic balance in an upright bipedal posture evolves, allowing for new adventures and environmental exploration (Figures 2-10 and 2-11). With new

Figure 2-8. Developing prehension.

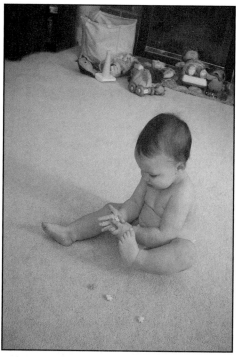

Figure 2-9. Finger feeding.

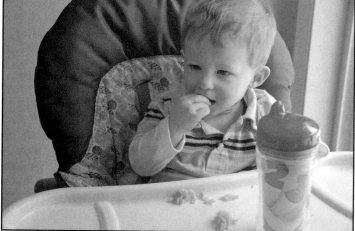

opportunities come motor challenges and the emergence of new motor behaviors, including running, climbing, and jumping. Toddlers find particular pleasure in throwing (Figure 2-12), kicking, and catching balls. Additionally, toddlers begin to propel themselves on ride-on toys (Figure 2-13). The focus on this period for toddlers is independence.

Fine motor skills emerging during this period include eating with a utensil (spoon usually) with fewer spills than before. Additionally, infants build small block towers, color with crayons, button large buttons, turn doorknobs, and open and close small jars. Integration of fine motor skills with cognitive spatial abilities and the desire to move are predicated on the emergence of postural control.[53]

Preschool-age children exhibit a mature gait pattern and ambulate using a narrow base of support, reciprocal arm swing, and a heel-to-toe gait pattern. Children mimic a true run but continue to have difficulty starting and stopping efficiently. In addition, receipt and propulsion of balls of all

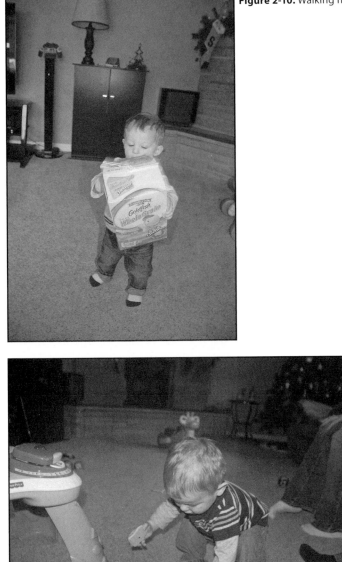

Figure 2-10. Walking holding an object.

Figure 2-11. Squatting in play to retrieve an object.

shapes and sizes improve qualitatively. By 3 years of age, children pedal a tricycle and ascends stairs, most using alternating feet, and by 4 years most children descend stairs alternately.

Fine motor behaviors emerge from environmental demands the child encounters in preschool and day care centers. Examples of the many fine motor skills observed during this period include cutting with scissors, copying circles or crosses, and matching colors, and some children demonstrate hand preference. These specific skills reflect innate ability, environmental demands, repetition, and motivation to succeed by the child.

Figure 2-12. Throwing a ball.

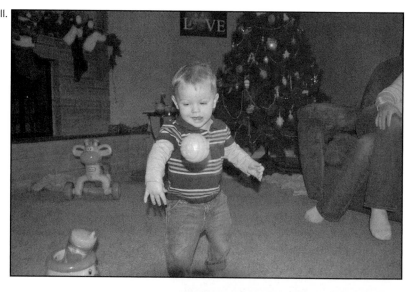

Figure 2-13. Mounting a riding toy.

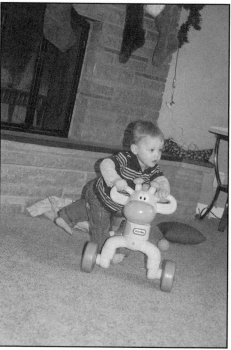

Childhood (5 to 10 Years)

School-age children, 5 to 8 years of age, experience rapid increases in muscle growth that account for much of the weight gained during this period. Girls continue to be physically more mature than boys. Children at this age are extremely flexible predominantly because muscle and ligamentous structures are not firmly attached to bones. Throughout development, acquisition of motor skills is directly related to practice and demand. A child who skis 6 months out of the year is developing different programs from a child who surfs daily.

Skills that emerge during this period include galloping, hopping on one foot for up to 10 hops (hopscotch), jumping rope, kicking a ball with improved control (soccer), and bouncing a large ball

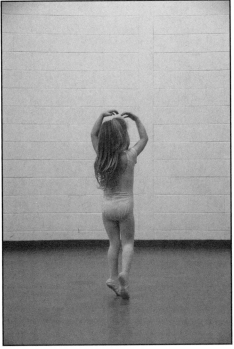

Figure 2-14. Early ballet training: tiptoes.

(basketball). Mobility, balance, and fine motor skills improve dramatically. Girls and boys exhibit similar abilities in speed up to age 7, but by age 8, boys begin to outperform girls.

Qualitative changes are observed in coordination, balance, speed, and strength while performing previously acquired skills. These qualitative improvements of motor skills may be due to children's limbs growing faster than the trunk. Consequently, they exhibit better leverage. Existing motor skills become more refined, more controlled, more efficient, and more complex.[54] Motor skills have a strong influence in social domains, as boys and girls begin to perform in organized sports teams in school and the community (Figure 2-14). Competition within sports becomes a powerful force in motivating children to practice motor skills or directing children away from organized sports. Children with poorly developed motor skills, due either to genetics or opportunity, may be excluded from team activities and experience social isolation.[54]

Between 5 and 8 years of age, manipulative skills increase exponentially. Hand preference is confirmed by this age. Children acquire and practice many manipulative and fine motor skills as part of their academic experience. Manipulative skills that improve dramatically include dressing self, particularly buttoning and unbuttoning clothing items; building with blocks; coloring with crayons; and handwriting and printing. As children move toward preadolescence (9 to 12 years of age), manipulative skills improve qualitatively. Children now progress to cursive handwriting and more complex drawings.

Adolescence (11 to 19 Years)

In early adolescence, motor skills are refined and, for most individuals, considered mature. Balance skills, coordination, eye-hand coordination, and endurance may plateau. Exceptions may be elite athletes who continue to improve motor skills into adulthood (Figure 2-15).

Motor skills continue to develop until 12 years of age. By then, individuals have achieved 90% of mobility and the reaction times of adults. While most motor skills are acquired throughout childhood, proficiency continues into adolescence consistent with musculoskeletal growth, leading to

Figure 2-15. Running with a mature gait pattern.

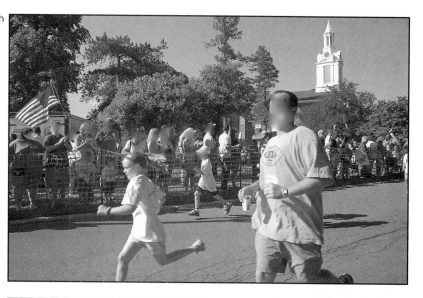

Figure 2-16. Advanced skill, ballet: young adult.

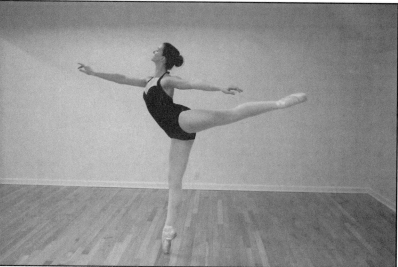

increased strength, endurance, and coordination. Previously acquired skills, like running, jumping, and throwing, progress quantitatively with respect to speed, distance, accuracy, and power (Figure 2-16). In adolescence, motor performance during competitive sports requires that basic skills are integrated and performed in more dynamic environments. During this period, children who may be genetically predisposed to performing high-level motor activities stand apart from their peers, as do children who are less competent in motor abilities. Always remember that practice and motivation to succeed also play a significant role in performance outcome. Similarly, environmental restraints also influence motor behavior. For example, a child who has the genetic predisposition for downhill skiing but lives in a warm climate may never ski and, thus, never actualize that ability.

By adolescence, manipulative skills are complex and resemble skills observed in adults. Greater dexterity of the fingers for more complex tasks, including art, sewing, crafts, knitting, and musical performance, enables adolescents to perform these motor tasks with greater precision and proficiency.

Adulthood (20 to 39 Years)

Motor performance is relatively stable in adulthood and directed at either leisure activities or high-level athletic competition. Exercise is probably one of the most easily modifiable behaviors affecting an individual's health and wellness. Adults perform various types of exercise to remain physically fit and to decrease the risk of degenerative diseases. For those who do not routinely exercise, obesity and associated syndromes emerge as primary health problems. For the many young adults who integrate fitness training as part of their leisure activities, fitness continues as a way of life. Maintaining a healthy lifestyle can have positive benefits into older adulthood, reducing or slowing degenerative disease processes.

The peak of muscular strength occurs between 25 and 30 years of age in males and females. After that period, muscle strength decreases as a result of reduction in the number and size of the muscle fibers.[53] Loss is related to genetic factors, nutritional intake, exercise regimen, and daily activities.

Middle Adulthood (40 to 59 Years)

Aging is associated with changes in the neuromuscular, musculoskeletal, and cardiovascular and pulmonary systems. Changes in these systems can greatly affect motor performance, although the degree of the impact is individually specific. Between 30 and 70 years of age, strength loss is thought to be moderate, with about 10% to 20% of total strength lost, which is, for most activities, insignificant and undetectable by the individual.[44,53] Mechanisms to counter muscle atrophy and assist in muscle strengthening include exercise regimens that emphasize aerobic and strengthening activities.

Older Adulthood (60+ Years)

Most older adults function reasonably well until an acute illness, a traumatic event such as a fall, or a compounding of small incidents results in an alteration of a motor skill or associated skills[30] (Figures 2-17 through 2-19).

While some effects are age associated and may be reduced with regular exercise and increased motor activity, not all are modifiable. Timing appears to affect performance of motor skills. As individuals age, they appear less able to modulate timing of muscles during contraction and relaxation phases. The outcome is that motor skills are performed more slowly, and agonist-antagonist movement is more poorly coordinated than earlier in adulthood. A consequence of these changes may be that while older adults are able to produce adequate force to counteract a perturbation, delay in response time may alter the outcome and result in a step strategy.[30] Mackey and Robinovitch reported that deficits in strength and speed are directly related to poorer outcomes when balance is perturbed in older adults.[55] Besides being less efficient in movement production, variability in performance of motor skills increases. These age-related changes have serious implications for older adults because these changes put them at increased risk for falls.

Thirty percent of individuals over the age of 65 experience at least one fall each year.[56] Factors thought to be associated with falls include slower muscle activation, sensory deficits associated with impaired balance, muscle weakness, and medication.[30,57] The risks associated with falls increase with age and the number of associated risk factors. The most significant intrinsic alterations in the older adult with implications for performance of motor skills occur when functions of the neuromuscular, musculoskeletal, cardiovascular, pulmonary, and sensory systems deteriorate.

Jette and colleagues examined manipulative skills in older adults.[58] They found that changes in hand function associated with muscle weakness and decreased range of motion negatively affected ADL performance.

Figure 2-17. Older adult ascending stairs holding the rail.

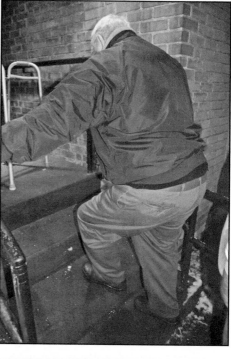

Figure 2-18. Older adult transitioning to sitting in a car.

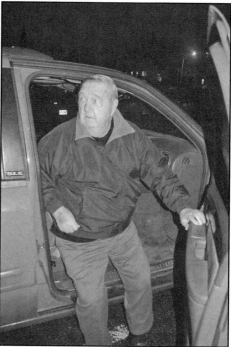

Age-related changes may be attributed to compensations in the neural mechanisms in response to changes between and within the different systems involved in motor skill performance.[59] The integrated effects may include slowing in movement production and increased activation of agonist-antagonist muscle groups. An example of agonist-antagonist activation is during dynamic balance activities.[60] After age 70, most individuals are said to incur losses in muscle strength of

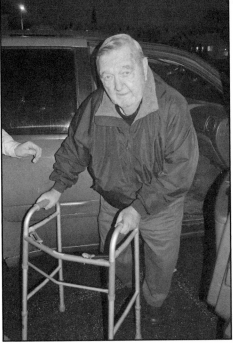

Figure 2-19. Older adult walking with a walker.

up to 30% over the next 10 years. Overall, the loss of muscle strength through adulthood may be as much as 40% to 50% by the time an individual reaches 80 years of age.[44] Again, the percentage will correlate with the demand by the individual for repetition of the movements. Additionally, performance of dual-task activities or conducting higher-level cognitive activities concurrent with a motor task has been shown to lead to delayed and altered balance responses in older adults. One thought is that executive functioning also declines with age.[61] While evidence supports the premise that decline in some systems leads to deterioration in motor behaviors, individual lifestyle choices, including playing tennis or golf, running, and downhill skiing, may result in slowing the percentage of loss and decline in successful performance of motor behaviors. The PTA should identify activities the older adult client enjoyed prior to a change or decline in motor abilities and use technology such as the Nintendo Wii system to allow the individual to successfully engage in motor activities, including bowling, skiing, and golfing, in a safe and supportive environment. As the older individual is able to execute the task in a supportive environment, the opportunity to participate in these real-life leisure activities may occur and provide additional social interactions.

PROMOTING MOTOR SKILL DEVELOPMENT IN A THERAPEUTIC ENVIRONMENT

Motor skill acquisition, refinement, and retention evolve from the individual's need and desire to interact in his or her environment. Through skill acquisition, the individual learns to meet the environmental demands contributing to the individual's function, activity, and participation in work, play, and leisure-time activities. Before intervening with clients or patients, clinicians must recognize motor behaviors that typically occur from infancy to older adulthood and factors that affect the performance of these behaviors. A comprehensive approach that considers the individual is the optimal strategy for intervention. Best practice integrates the combined perspectives and unique contributions of each professional involved with the patient. Interventions are directed toward motor learning and organized around activities that challenge individuals and motivate them to practice tasks. Activities must be functional and appropriate to age and participation level. Movement and activity should be the emphasis of the program. Practice is critical to acquisition and refinement of motor skills (see Chapter 3). The dilemma associated with this fact is that with practice comes repetition and boredom, and this may lead to decreased motivation. It is critical to vary tasks by frequently altering the environmental context to keep a child's or an adult's interest while practicing and refining a task. Initially, the professional provides feedback to the individual about results and performance. The goal is for the individual to develop the ability to detect and correct errors in movement without the clinician present. Visual feedback in the form of mirrors and recordings provide information about motor performance. Auditory feedback may be provided through verbal feedback or auditory switches.

The individual's desire to successfully perform a task and participate in activities may be the motivation needed for achieving the desired goal or outcome. Strategies that incorporate the target motor skills into the patient's daily life and encourage physical fitness as a lifelong activity to promote health and wellness of the body and spirit are important to prevention and wellness across the lifespan. During each therapeutic session, seeking client feedback on activity performance and participation emphasizes the valuable role and contribution the client contributes to achieving his or her desired outcomes. The PTA can engage the child in movements using music. Devise simple movement sequences, choreographed to music, with opportunities for expressive free movements. As the child begins to attempt motor skills and participation increases, add additional choreographed activities. Music facilitates the sequenced activities to integrate motor sequencing and cognitive skills.

PLAY AS THERAPY

Children perceive play time as an opportunity to engage in an enjoyable activity of their own choosing without any specific goal. Adults perceive play as a child-directed activity used to achieve a desired outcome. Children and adults use play as a social context to promote acquisition of motor skills. As infants and children grow older, techniques for utilizing play must be modified consistently with the children's cognitive and motor skill performance and social skills. While some genetic differences exist in play preferences between males and females, gender-neutral activities should be encouraged during play sessions. Given that children see practice, the primary strategy for acquisition and retention of motor skills, as the opportunity to achieve the desired goal, they are excited to repeatedly practice activities. Directing the activities to the developmental ability and interest of the child motivates the child to practice motor skills by varying the task and the environment. Play positively reinforces development of motor skills in a noncompetitive environment.

Older children and adults may require different strategies that challenge affective, sensory, and cognitive systems to practice motor skills. Engaging the client in selecting age-consistent activities validates his or her role and responsibility and promotes investment in achieving the desired goals. In reality, adults usually enjoy playing as well. It is important that the tasks not be considered child-like or beyond a person's potential for success, but games can increase in difficulty if the adult shows improvement in the specific task. Games in the newspaper, such as Sudoku and word puzzles, can be challenging, and success is a good motivator to keep practicing. Computer games that challenge motor skill can also be fun for adults no matter the age and can be incorporated into daily activities that are enjoyable as well as repetitive to encourage positive change in all areas of body function.

CONCLUSION

Development of motor skills occurs out of a need to solve specific motor problems in the environment. Effective practitioners work cooperatively with patients or clients to identify motor problems and develop strategies that solve the problems and promote functional interaction in the environment. While genetic and environmental factors play a role in acquiring motor skills, the relative importance of these factors changes across the lifespan. During early acquisition of motor behaviors, genetics plays a greater role. Later in life, environmental factors are stronger.

Systems theory provides a model for why individuals exhibit motor skills at different biological ages and why the quality of motor behavior varies.[62] It is the physical therapist's responsibility to examine the influence of sensory, musculoskeletal, neuromuscular, vestibular, and cognitive systems on motor development to provide an understanding of how different systems exert influence at different points in development. The delegation of specific interventions is within the role of the PTA. The human organism is complex and is composed of interactive and interdependent systems. The underlying theoretical constructs of systems theory may more fully explain development than traditional theories. Human systems do not function in a unidirectional fashion but collaboratively across the lifespan. Just as not all individuals exhibit motor behaviors such as sitting, creeping, or walking at the same time, not all individuals lose their ability to perform certain tasks (eg, driving a car or independently performing personal care) at the same biological, chronological, or even psychological age.

No one theory explains the development of complex motor behaviors completely, and none encompass the essence of inter- and intra-individual variability in aging. Aspects of theories provide evidence that an integrative perspective may be a more accurate reflection of aging. Lifestyle choices, including diet, physical activity, and other health habits, and behavioral and social factors have potent effects on aging processes.

An integrated approach to intervention addresses the complex nature of motor behaviors observed throughout life. All systems discussed here play significant roles in the acquisition, refinement, and retention of motor behaviors. Careful consideration of each system individually and the interactive effects among systems is important to understanding motor behaviors. Remember, if a child, adult, or elderly individual repetitively practices a stereotypic movement limited in function, that will become the program used by the individual. Thus, intervention can limit as well as expand the functional skill of the patient or client.

REFERENCES

1. Fairbrother JT. *Fundamentals of Motor Behavior.* Champaign, IL: Human Kinetics; 2010.
2. Short-DeGraf M. *Human Development.* New York, NY: John Wiley; 1988.
3. Jenkins SPR. *Sports Science Handbook: Volume 2: The Essential Guide to Kinesiology, Sport and Exercise Science.* Essex, UK: Multi-Science Publishing Co, Ltd; 2005.
4. Gesell A. *The First Five Years of Life.* New York, NY: Harper and Brothers Publishers; 1940.
5. McGraw MB. *Neuromuscular Maturation of the Human Infant.* 2nd ed. New York, NY: Hafner; 1943.
6. Singer RN. The readiness to learn skills necessary for participation in sport. In: Magill RA, Ash MJ, Smoll FL, eds. *Children in Sport: A Contemporary Anthology.* Champaign, IL: Human Kinetics; 1978.
7. Smith LB, Thelan E. *A Dynamic Systems Approach to Development.* Cambridge, MA: MIT Press; 1993.
8. Gibson JJ. *The Ecological Approach to Visual Perception.* Boston, MA: Houghton Mifflin; 1979.
9. Haywood KM. *Lifespan Motor Development.* Champaign, IL: Human Kinetics; 1986.
10. Heriza CB. Motor development: traditional and contemporary theories. In: MJ Lister, ed. *Contemporary Management of Motor Control Problems.* Alexandria, VA: Foundation for Physical Therapy; 1991.
11. Thelan E. Developmental origins of motor coordination: leg movements in human infants. *Dev Psychobiol.* 1985;18(1):1-22.

12. Zelazo PR, Weiss MJ, Leonard EL. The development of unaided walking: the acquisition of higher order control. In: Zelazo PR, Barr R, eds. *Challenges to Developmental Paradigms: Implications for Theory Assessment.* Hillsdale, NJ: Erlbaum Associates Inc; 1976.

13. Bradley NS. Animal models offer the opportunity to acquire a new perspective on motor development. *Phys Ther.* 1990;70(12):776-787.

14. Thelan E. The role of motor development in developmental psychology: a view of the past and an agenda for the future. In: Lockman J, Hazen N, eds. *Action in Social Context: Perspectives in Early Development.* New York, NY: Plenum; 1990.

15. Thelan E. The (re)discovery of motor development: learning new things from an old field. *Dev Psych.* 1989;25(6):946-949.

16. Scott JP. Critical periods in organizational processes. In: Faulkner F, Tanner JM, eds. *Human Growth.* New York, NY: Plenum Press; 1986:181-196.

17. Thelan E, Smith LB. *A Dynamic Systems Approach to the Development of Cognition and Action.* Cambridge, MA: MIT Press; 1994.

18. Chodzko-Zajko WJ. Biological theories of aging: implications for functional performance. In: Bonder BR, Wagner MB, eds. *Functional Performance in Older Adults.* 2nd ed. Philadelphia, PA: FA Davis; 2001:28-41.

19. Karasik D, Hannan MT, Cupples AL, Feslon DT, Kiel DP. Genetic contributions to biological aging: the Framingham study. *J Gerontol A Biol Sci Med Sci.* 2004;59(3):218-226.

20. Bengtson VL, Putney NM, Johnson ML. The problem of theory in gerontology today. In: Johnson ML, ed. *Cambridge Handbook of Age and Aging.* Cambridge, MA: Cambridge University Press; 2005:9.

21. Goldstein S, Gallo JJ, Reichel W. Biologic theories of aging. *Am Fam Physician.* 1989;40(30):195-200.

22. Rowe JW, Kahn RL. Successful aging. *J Gerontol.* 1997;37:433-450.

23. Kaplan MS, Huguet N, Orpana H, Feeny D, McFarland BH, Ross N. Prevalence and factors associated with thriving in older adulthood: a 10-year population-based study. *J Gerontol.* 2008;63(10):1097-1104.

24. Sadler TW. *Langeman's Medical Embryology.* Baltimore, MD: Williams & Wilkins; 1984.

25. Ashburn SS. Biophysical development during infancy. In: Schuster CS, Ashburn SS, eds. *The Process of Human Development: A Holistic Life-Span Approach.* Philadelphia, PA: Lippincott; 1992:118-140.

26. Wilder PA. Muscle development and function. In: Cech D, Martin S, eds. *Functional Movement Development Across the Lifespan.* Philadelphia, PA: Saunders; 1995:137-157.

27. Lieber RL. *Skeletal Muscle Structure, Function, and Plasticity: The Physiological Basis of Rehabilitation.* Philadelphia, PA: Lippincott Williams & Wilkins; 2002.

28. Thompson LV. Physiological changes associated with aging. In: Guccione AA, ed. *Geriatric Physical Therapy.* 2nd ed. St Louis, MO: Mosby; 2000:28-55.

29. Dutton M. *Orthopedic Examination, Evaluation, and Intervention.* 3rd ed. New York, NY: McGraw-Hill; 2012.

30. Sturnieks DL, Menant J, Vanrenterghem J, Delbaere K, Fitzpatrick RC, Lord SR. Sensorimotor and neuropsychological correlates of force perturbations that induce stepping in older adults. *Gait Posture.* 2012;36(3):356-360.

31. Lewis CB, Kellems S. Musculoskeletal changes with age: clinical implications. In: Lewis CB, ed. *Aging: The Health-Care Challenge.* 4th ed. Philadelphia, PA: FA Davis; 2002:104-126.

32. Candow DG, Chilibeck PD. Differences in size, strength, and power of upper and lower body muscle groups in young and older men. *J Gerontol A Biol Sci Med Sci.* 2005;60(2):148-156.

33. Carroll KL. Alterations of musculoskeletal function in children. In: McCance KL, Huether SE, eds. *Pathophysiology: The Biologic Basis for Disease in Adults and Children.* 6th ed. Maryland Heights, MO: Mosby; 2010:1618-1643.

34. Walker JM. Musculoskeletal development: a review. *Phys Ther.* 1991;71(12):878-889.

35. Sullivan JA. Introduction to the musculoskeletal system. In: Sullivan JA, Anderson SJ, eds. *Care of the Young Athlete.* Rosemont, IL: American Academy of Orthopedic Surgeons and American Academy of Pediatrics; 2000:242-258.

36. Willardson JM, Tudor-Locke C. Survival of the strongest: a brief review examining the association between muscular fitness and mortality. *Strength Cond J.* 2005;27(3):80-85.

37. Larsen WJ. *Human Embryology.* Singapore: Churchill Livingstone; 1993.

38. Stout J. Physical fitness during childhood and adolescence. In: Campbell S, ed. *Physical Therapy for Children.* 2nd ed. Philadelphia, PA: Saunders; 2000:141-169.

39. Jarvis C. *Physical Examination and Health Assessment.* St Louis, MO: WB Saunders; 2004.

40. Overbay JD, Purath J. Self-concept and health status in elementary-school-aged children. *Issues Compr Pediatr Nurs.* 1997;20:(2)89-101.

41. Kelly MK. Physical therapy associated with respiratory failure in the neonate. In: DeTurk WE, Cahalin LP, eds. *Cardiovascular and Pulmonary Physical Therapy: An Evidence-Based Approach.* New York, NY: McGraw-Hill; 2004.

42. Dean E. Cardiopulmonary development. In: Bonder BR, Wagner MB, eds. *Functional Performance in Older Adults.* 2nd ed. Philadelphia, PA: FA Davis; 2001:86-120.

43. Kandel ER, Schwartz JH, Jessel TM. *Principles of Neural Science.* 4th ed. New York, NY: McGraw-Hill; 2000.

44. Wagner MB, Kaufman TL. Mobility. In: Bonder BR, Wagner MB, eds. *Functional Performance in Older Adults.* 2nd ed. Philadelphia, PA: FA Davis; 2001:61-85.

45. Papalia DE, Olds SW, Feldman R. *Human Development.* 11th ed. New York, NY: McGraw-Hill; 2008.

46. Ekelman BA, Mitchell S, O'Dell-Rossi P. Driving and older adults. In: Bonder BR, Wagner MB, eds. *Functional Performance in Older Adults.* 2nd ed. Philadelphia, PA: FA Davis; 2001:448-477.

47. Payne VG, Isaacs LD. *Human Motor Development: A Lifespan Approach.* 7th ed. New York, NY: McGraw-Hill; 2008.

48. Brazelton TB. *Neonatal Behavioral Assessment Scale.* London, England: Blackwell Scientific Publications Ltd; 1984:3.

49. VanSant AF. Motor control, motor learning and motor development. In: Montgomery PC, Connolly BH, eds. *Clinical Applications for Motor Control.* Thorofare, NJ: SLACK Incorporated; 2003:26-50.

50. Shumway-Cook A, Woollacott MH. *Motor Control: Theory and Practical Applications.* Philadelphia, PA: Lippincott Williams & Wilkins; 2001.

51. Fischer KW. Relationship between brain and cognitive development. *Child Dev.* 1997;68:623-632.

52. Bertenthal B. Origins and early development of perception, action and representation. *Annu Rev Psychol.* 1996;47:431-459.

53. Ashburn SS. Biophysical development during early adulthood. In: Schuster CS, Ashburn SS, eds. *The Process of Human Development: A Holistic Life-Span Approach.* Philadelphia, PA: Lippincott; 1992:556-577.

54. Owens KB. *Child and Adolescent Development: An Integrated Approach.* Belmont, CA: Wadsworth; 2002.

55. Mackey D, Robinovitch SN. Mechanisms underlying age-related differences in ability to recover balance with the ankle strategy. *Gait Posture.* 2006;23(1):59-68.

56. Tinnetti ME, Baker DI, McAvay G, et al. A multifactorial intervention to reduce the risk of falling among elderly people living in the community. *N Engl J Med.* 1994;331(13):821-827.

57. Woollacott MH, Shumway-Cook A, Nashner LM. Aging and postural control: changes in sensory organization and muscular coordination. *Int J Aging Hum Dev.* 1986;23(2):97-114.

58. Jette AM, Branch LG, Berlin J. Musculoskeletal impairments and physical disablement among the aged. *J Gerontol.* 1990;45(6):M203.

59. Patten C, Craik RL. Sensorimotor changes and adaptation in the older adult. In: Guiccone AA, ed. *Geriatric Physical Therapy.* 2nd ed. St Louis, MO: Mosby; 2000:78-109.

60. Benjuva N, Melzer I, Kaplanski J. Aging-induced shifts from a reliance on sensory input to muscle cocontraction during balanced standing. *J Gerontol A Biol Sci Med Sci.* 2004;59(2):166-171.

61. Inzitari M, Baldereschi M, Di Carlo A, et al. Impaired attention predicts motor performance decline in older community-dwellers with normal baseline mobility: results from the Italian Longitudinal Study on Aging (ILSA). *J Gerontol A Biol Sci Med Sci.* 2007;62(2):837-843.

62. Adolph KE. Babies' steps make giant strides toward a science of development. *Infant Behavior and Development.* 2002;25(1):86-90.

Please see accompanying Web site at
www.healio.com/books/neuroptavideos

3

Motor Control, Motor Learning, and Neuroplasticity

Darcy A. Umphred, PT, PhD, FAPTA
Fritzie Arce, PT, PhD

KEY WORDS

- Extrinsic feedback
- Intrinsic feedback
- Motor control
- Motor learning
- Neuromechanisms
- Neuroplasticity
- Practice context
- Practice schedule
- Stages of motor learning

CHAPTER OBJECTIVES

- Identify the differences among motor learning, motor control, and neuroplasticity.

- Differentiate between practice context and practice schedule.

- Discuss the stages of motor learning and their implications on the intensity of practice and the degree of external feedback.

- Discuss the differences between external and internal feedback and identify which feedback schedule is appropriate for a patient's stage of motor learning.

- Conceptually differentiate between a cognitively run movement and an automatic/feedforward motor program controlled by the central nervous system (CNS).

- Discuss the difference between new motor learning, as seen in a child, and relearning of movement patterns, as seen in a patient with CNS dysfunction.

- Explain current theories of neuroplasticity and the critical elements that are needed to encourage motor control and motor learning.

- Identify the interactions among sensory processing, motor learning, and sensory input that can be used to retrain the motor system.

Umphred DA, Lazaro RT, eds.
Neurorehabilitation for the Physical Therapist Assistant,
Second Edition (pp 45-68).
© 2014 SLACK Incorporated.

INTRODUCTION

Motor control, motor learning, and neuroplasticity are 3 areas of interest to the physical therapist (PT) and physical therapist assistant (PTA) when working with patients of various ages diagnosed with disease or trauma to the central nervous system (CNS). New advances in research in the areas of neurophysiology, theories of motor control and learning, and adaptation of the nervous system following injury (termed *neuroplasticity*) are significantly affecting physical therapy management.[1-3] Although the specific rationale for each component of an intervention design is the responsibility of the PT, a general understanding of the theory within these 3 areas and their relationship to evaluation and treatment should enhance the PTA's knowledge and understanding for why specific interventions for a particular patient may or may not be delegated. In addition, similarly, explanations can be provided to justify why certain practice environments need to be the responsibility of a caregiver or family member. Lastly, knowledge of neuroplasticity principles can assist the PTA in selecting the appropriate intensity of treatment, saliency of the activity itself, need for a home program, and importance of patient adherence. Table 3-1 identifies the differences among these 3 conceptual areas of CNS function as well as the time parameters needed for the CNS to control, learn, and adapt to the motor requirements of the environment.

Theories within the areas of motor control, motor learning, and neuroplasticity will be introduced in this chapter. For theories of development and how they affect stages of learning, see Chapter 2. Before discussing how theories might guide examination and intervention decisions, a clear definition of each topic and the specific role it plays in activity and functional movement will be introduced. Once each topic has been discussed, the interaction of these theories will be presented through case examples as possible explanations for selected examination and treatment sequences and required intervention changes. For specific intervention techniques appropriate to the PTA, refer to Chapter 4. As the responsibility of the PTA enlarges and both the reexaminations and treatment protocols are falling under the PTA scope of practice, clinicians need to be able to identify signs of new motor control problems as well as progressions in motor learning when working with individuals with CNS problems. The goal of this chapter is the discussion of theory and its application to the practice of physical therapy and specifically to those concepts within the practice of the PTA.

The roles of the PT and PTA are directly linked to interventions that improve performance of functional activities, thus improving a person's quality of life. These activity limitations can often be linked to disease, pathology, trauma, or preexisting life experiences that affect a specific system and its interactions with the functions of the cardiopulmonary, integumentary, musculoskeletal, and neuromuscular systems. Regardless of the specific system involvement, the individual's ability to manage movement in functional activities (motor control), capacity to learn new movement options (motor learning), and capability to regain motor function following direct or indirect CNS insult (neuroplasticity) is regulated by the existing potential of an individual and by the environment created for learning. Although this chapter will focus on individuals who have identified CNS problems, PTs and PTAs need to remember that the theories presented within this chapter relate to motor output controlled by the nervous system and those functional movement problems seen in any one individual despite what the identified medical problems or diseases may be.

This chapter's organizational structure begins with a historical perspective and then proceeds to current theories of motor control, motor learning, and neuroplasticity. This order was selected to help the reader understand how treatment philosophies have evolved and to emphasize theory in the order consistent with CNS processing. An individual will need to learn a behavioral sequence or motor program before he or she will have the ability to control that motor pattern or behavior. Most motor learning uses sensory input initially to give the nervous system needed information that will be used to facilitate motor learning and to gain control over that movement. Sensory input is also needed when changes in programming are necessary. Thus, it is very important not

Table 3-1

Summary of Motor Control, Motor Learning, and Neuroplasticity Concepts and Implications for the PTA

	Control Function	*Neuromechanism and Implications for the PTA*
Motor control	Using existing synaptic connections and existing programming.	Neurotransmitters: 10th to 100th of milliseconds to respond. Neuropeptides: Hour or days for transmission to synapse; response can be hours, days, months, or lifetimes (in the case of certain drugs). Thus, PTA needs to give time to the patient once asked to perform before another instruction is given. PTA uses prior learning to regain motor control.
Motor learning	Modification of existing motor programs and synaptic firing patterns.	Repetition of practice of new motor program takes days, weeks, or months and needs continual practice to ensure permanent learning. Practice must continue from site to site as patient's skills improve. Variation of practice within the program is critical for adaptability. PT/PTA must first establish motor control before new learning can occur.
Neuroplasticity	Modification of surviving cellular structure to reform primary function, assume a different function, and enhance neuroplasticity.	Based on environmental demands placed on the organism and potential for the organism to regain control of sensory processing and motor programming. Repetition of practice takes weeks, months, or years and continual environmental demands. Internal motivation to regain function is paramount to this type of neurofunction. Thus, never say "never" because the "never" is up to the patient's internal motivation and potential.

to totally separate the concepts of sensory input from motor learning and motor control. Once motor control is programmed and accessible to the nervous system, however, unless changes in that programming are required, sensory input is no longer necessary to run those movements. Some motor learning occurs in utero and is often called *reflexive* or *preexisting* motor programs. In a 6-month gestational-aged infant born premature, the heart muscle and most autonomic smooth muscle control have already been established; however, the skeletal muscle tone characteristics observed will be hypotonic with no muscle control evident. These types of observations help therapists understand that motor learning begins very early in the development of a fetus. Motor learning will continue throughout life as long as the environment asks for change and the CNS has the pliability and desire to retain control over functional movements. As individuals grow during childhood; move into adolescence and adulthood selecting specific activities they enjoy or are required to perform, such as activities of daily living (ADL) or recreational sports; and progress into aging with structural changes within their frames or system deficits, such as heart conditions, circulatory problems, or respiratory function, motor control will need to adapt in order for each specific individual to maintain control over his or her life's environment. The role of therapists, whether that person is a PT or a PTA, is to help individuals learn initially to maintain or regain control over those functional movements. The ultimate goal of therapy is to provide and enhance an individual's opportunity to control those movement patterns that he or she values, which in turn enhances his or her respective quality of life.

HISTORICAL PERSPECTIVES

The science and practice of rehabilitation medicine has been shaped by the existing theories on motor control and learning. Since regaining movement function through therapeutic exercise has been a central theme for the field of physical therapy, the decision of how best to regain or learn motor skill in various functional activities has always been based on the best science theory of the time or the available evidence. Motor control models and their corresponding neurological rehabilitation models have evolved through the years. The motor control models attempt to answer 2 basic questions: "What are the control parameters?" and "What are the underlying processes involved in the generation of movement?" The neurorehabilitation models, on the other hand, incorporate the evaluation and treatment intervention that respond to the principles of the motor control model they adhere to.

In the first half of the 20th century, exercises were based on theories of reinforcement, existing muscle physiology, and practice schedules related to maximal and submaximal strength of existing muscles. In the mid-20th century, treatment techniques in the area of neurorehabilitation began to be explained using theories of neurophysiology, neuroanatomy, and childhood development. The accepted neurophysiology was based on research conducted by the physiologist Sherrington.[4] The theory was based on the assumption that functional movement was under rigid hierarchical control within the nervous system. It was during this era that treatment approaches, such as proprioceptive neuromuscular facilitation (PNF)[5], as well as those developed by Bobath,[6] Rood,[7] Ayres,[8] Johnstone,[9] and Brunnstrom,[10] were established. The therapists who developed these various approaches had one thing in common—they all tried to explain their various treatment protocols using scientific theories of that time regarding how the nervous system was regulated. Those clinicians were very keen observers of movement, normal and abnormal. Although the basic science knowledge of the time was limited and in time the theories needed to change because of the evolution in understanding of motor control, motor learning, and neuroplasticity, the movements observed by therapists during that time are the same movements observed by therapists today. Theories will change as new research opens new avenues of science analysis, but keen visual observations of functional movements and limitations will always remain a critical skill for the PT and PTA. Many of the previously mentioned approaches are still used and retain similar treatment applications and interventions; however, the treatment rationale for each of the various approaches utilizes more current research and evidence to explain its validity. In the 1970s and 1980s, some therapists[11,12] were teaching integrated approaches based on a systems model and functional training versus a more traditional Sherringtonian/hierarchical[13] sequential model. Once physiologists and neuroanatomists began to analyze movement while the animals were awake, they realized that the Sherrington model was not as accurate as Bernstein's model[14,15] presented decades before. Since the latter part of the 20th century, therapists have changed the model used for CNS control and learning. All bodily systems influence how the CNS controls movement, and that ultimate control may be generated in a dynamic hierarchical fashion[16,17] in a top-down model[18] or using a dynamic multiple systems interactions model.[14,15] The complexity of the human body and the motor control needed to maintain functional control over striated and smooth muscle during normal activities cannot be denied. Yet, only within the past 20 years has the concept of neuroplasticity evolved and begun to play a critical role in decision making regarding how a patient should be evaluated and which interventions might best lead to optimal functional outcomes following CNS injury.[19]

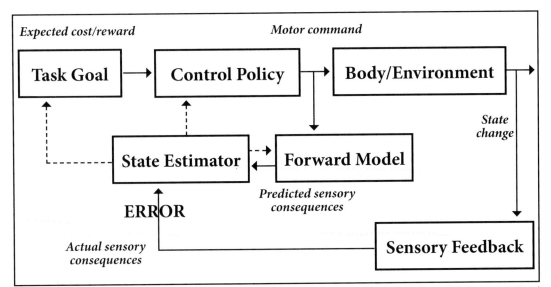

Figure 3-1. General schema for the control of movement. (Adapted from Shadmehr R, Krakauer JW. A computational neuroanatomy for motor control. *Exp Brain Res*. 2008;185[3]:359-381.)

MOTOR CONTROL

Motor control is the study of how the CNS regulates the musculoskeletal system and the environment in the generation of movements for the attainment of specific task goals. Three elements are crucial in motor control. It involves (1) a neural circuit—the cortex, brainstem, cerebellum, and spinal cord—that underlies the processing of inputs and outputs; (2) a motor plan (usually the limb), or the effector of the output of the neural circuit; and (3) the environment, in which movement takes place, shaping the interplay between the neural circuit and the motor plan. We shall see in the next paragraphs the interplay among these elements in the generation of movement.

Movement generation can be described as a sensorimotor loop[20] (ie, a series of transformations between sensory signals and motor commands, a chaining of one sensorimotor event to another). It has been said that learning has occurred when patients gain consistency and efficiency over the control of the elements needed to generate the movement. As Albert Einstein once said, nothing happens until something moves. To make something happen is the driving force of all the complex movements we humans have learned to do and be skillful at. Time and again humans have been able to master highly complex movements. And it is primarily because people are endowed with an amazing neural circuitry that underlies the processing of sensory inputs and motor outputs.

Many of the simple functional movements that humans carry out on a daily basis require complex control and networking among different areas of the CNS, the neural circuit. The control of movement, to some extent, can be likened to the coordinated action of each of the instrument players in a symphony orchestra. There are different instrument players, and one's performance affects others' performances. It is not enough to know how to play well; one must also know how to take signals from the conductor and be aware of the others' performances. The same thing occurs when the CNS generates body movements. Many CNS structures are involved, and each one effectively communicates with other CNS structures to deliver a smooth and well-coordinated movement (Figure 3-1).

Figure 3-1 illustrates the processes involved in movement generation.[21] Everyone's movements are goal oriented. Given a task goal (eg, reaching for a coffee mug off to the left side of one's body), the control system chooses a control policy. This is a mapping of the task goal to motor commands of turning the head toward the cup, lifting the arm, and grasping the coffee mug. This choice is made based on some criteria such as the expected cost (eg, the level of difficulty to get to the coffee mug) and reward (eg, drinking coffee). Then, the control system generates the motor command, which is a particular way of activating groups of muscles to move the hand in a certain trajectory from its starting location to where the coffee mug is. For this, the system has taken in some knowledge of the motor plan. This is the current body configuration (eg, arm posture) relative to the position of the coffee mug. The way one reaches for the cup will be different if the cup is nearby or at some distance to the left. For these reaches, different joint movements and muscle activation patterns are required, and, consequently, different biomechanical forces are generated. Lastly, the system has to take into consideration the environment in which reaching takes place (eg, on a cluttered desk or cleared table or in a dark room). The control of reaching is different when it takes place in a dark room because one cannot rely on visual feedback to guide one's movement, thus requiring one to rely on another sensory modality, such as proprioception. While sensory feedback is not necessary to perform some movements, the control system relies on sensory information of past movements to guide upcoming movement and online sensory feedback for ongoing movement. Thus, whether the coffee cup is on a cluttered or cleared table creates different perceptual challenges to the CNS, which has the potential to change the motor response. The motor command is also mapped to a set of predicted sensory outcomes, referred to as the *sensory forward model*. This refers to what a person expects to feel on accomplishing the task. Now, imagine a scenario when, on lifting up the coffee mug, the person overshoots the grip force by lifting an empty mug instead of a full one. The system had planned for a grip force appropriate for a mug filled with coffee and relied on a forward model that predicted sensory outcomes of lifting a full mug. Fortunately, most individuals' systems are able to take in the new information, calculate an error, and modify the movement plan so that the next time the cup is picked up, the right grip force should be generated. When the motor command leads to success in achieving the goal, it produces the expected change in the performer and/or the environment. When the motor command fails to do so, there is an error associated with the predicted sensory outcomes: "I expected my hand to reach the cup if I moved this way, but instead my hand ended in a completely different place." This task of comparing the predicted with the measured sensory consequences has been attributed to a state estimator. In the presence of error, modifications may take place in (1) the control policy (ie, changing the way one activates muscles), (2) the forward model (ie, changing the predicted sensory outcomes based on new sensory input), or (3) the task goal (ie, making new coffee or changing the weight of the fluid).

Perturbation studies give therapists a window into the nature of the controlled movement parameters and adaptive strategies. Numerous motor control studies have used perturbed arm-reaching (loads, visuomotor rotations), walking, and posture. An example of widely used perturbation in motor control studies is the application of force fields during reaching movements.[22,23] Subjects are asked to move a cursor to a target displayed on a screen by moving a robotic manipulandum. Hand trajectories during unperturbed reaching typically follow a straight path from the start hand position to the end target position. After performing some trials of unperturbed reaching, subjects are exposed to a force field. It is a velocity-dependent force whose direction is always perpendicular to the direction of hand movement. Figure 3-2 illustrates how hand trajectories change in the presence of unexpected perturbations. Early in adaptation, the subject's hand is pushed to the side and misses reaching the target. The hand trajectory shows a huge deviation from the intended straight trajectory (trajectory errors) to the target location (endpoint errors). With practice, the subject learns to compensate for the force field, as can be observed in the reduction in the trajectory and endpoint errors. Thus, motor errors like the initial trajectory errors and endpoint errors drive adaptation and the return to straight-hand trajectories. At this stage, the subject has learned to control movements predictively rather than through successive late feedback corrections.

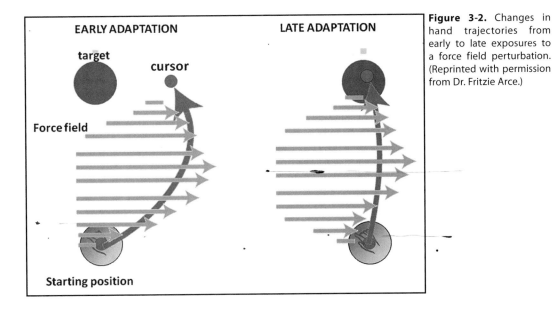

Figure 3-2. Changes in hand trajectories from early to late exposures to a force field perturbation. (Reprinted with permission from Dr. Fritzie Arce.)

These studies and others have shown that straightness of the hand trajectory and minimum endpoint variability are invariant features of arm-reaching movements. What happens if the subject has no access to error information (eg, because of a loss of sensation or brain injury leading to an inability to predict sensory states associated with a motor command)? How does the system control movements in such contexts? One way to simulate this in an experimental setup is to withdraw the sensory feedback on the cursor position so subjects are no longer able to see their trajectory and endpoint errors.[22] Subjects in both feedback conditions were able to correct their trajectory and endpoint errors. However, trajectories became straight with visual feedback but remained curved without it. The different trajectories suggest differences in the information conveyed by vision and proprioception. Other similar studies have demonstrated the interaction between sensory and motor processes and their role in motor control.[24,25]

It is not the PTA's responsibility to know what movement dysfunctions correlate with what types of lesions, the location of lesions, or the status of a lesion, but it is the responsibility of the PTA to recognize a change in the control of a pattern or functional skill and inform the PT. This can be a critical health issue when the change seems to be toward dysfunction versus function. One of the challenges in understanding motor control is realizing that the PT's or the PTA's motor control over his or her body affects feedback to the patient. The patient's ability to perform a task depends on his or her own inherent mechanisms, which may vary from the therapist's regardless of a CNS lesion.[26] One of the most obvious differences is probably anthropometric. The clinician's height, weight, flexibility, strength, endurance, etc, affect the motions that can be reinforced through feedback to the patient. In addition, these same body parameters affect how a patient can perform movement. The easiest example to articulate is observing how a short versus a tall person comes out of a chair. Observe your fellow classmates or clinicians and you will be surprised at the difference.

When analyzing motor control of a specific movement, such as walking, the therapist will look at many motor programs that are running simultaneously. These programs include the following: automatic walking, postural control of the head, axial muscles and trunk in open and closed chain environments, balance programs from heel strike to heel strike of both legs, arm swing and how it perturbs the patient, and the environment within which the patient is walking (eg, wood floor, shag rugs, cement walkway, grass on level ground versus up and down inclines). Each one of these programs is a movement sequence being controlled by the CNS. The CNS must control and modify all of these programs simultaneously in order for a clinician to observe normal walking within the environment specified. Some patients may lose one of the multitudes of programs, and therefore a PTA could be expected to help train the patient to run a complex program, such as walking. The activity may be performed under a variety of controlled environments, such as with a body weight bearing overhead suspension system, an exoskeleton, or another assistive device such as a cane or walker. The decision as to which mechanism to use with the patient may depend more on available tools and the environment within which the training is done. A body weight–support system and a treadmill reduce the individual's need to run adequate postural programs and reduce the variable power production used throughout the gait cycle. The frequency of stepping can be controlled externally while foot placement can be assisted by a PTA. As the patient gains control of posture, walking, balance power, stepping frequency, and symmetrical stride length, the amount of suspension can be reduced, which demands more motor control by the patient. Similarly, an exoskeleton can reduce the demands on the patient but is still a very expensive rehabilitation tool not found in every facility. In order for the patient to gain motor control, the environment must allow the patient to achieve the desired movement. Thus, control on a hard surface is easier than control on a compliant surface, such as grass or deep carpeting. Often removal of unneeded sensory stimuli, such as noise, excessive colors, and people moving within the environment, can allow the CNS to control movement such as walking. To say that control is independent, the therapist needs to reintroduce that sensory information while the patient is running the programs.

There are many aspects of CNS function that lead to motor control. Sensory processing is critical for motor learning and becomes vital if the program being run needs changing. Thus, not only systems considered motor (such as the basal ganglia, cerebellum, and frontal lobes) are necessary when a patient is performing functional activities. Perception of the environment plays a key role in determining what control is necessary to succeed in a task. If a patient has sensory or perceptual dysfunctions, the end result may be motor control problems, although the deficit may not be within the motor system. The PTA is not responsible for analyzing all these perceptual motor problems but should be able to evaluate whether a patient is failing at the task or becoming frustrated because of errors. The control of movement and posture is a complex interaction of many systems. Following CNS injury, the control over those systems can become compromised. It is up to the PT and the PTA to create the optimal environments for the patient to regain the control necessary for functional activities.

MOTOR LEARNING

Motor control and motor learning are basically 2 sides of the same coin. Learning how the brain learns is especially important when there is injury in the neural circuitry. The system often has to relearn motor skills. This is the scenario clinicians face in the rehabilitation setting. PTs and PTAs train patients to regain their function, initially assisting them and then taking them to optimal levels of performance. Therapists want functional skills gained or achieved in one session to be carried over to other practice environments and with longer periods in between practice.[26]

Motor learning is the study of how individuals acquire, modify, and retain motor memories so they can be used, reused, and modified during functional activities. Examples of functional motor memory patterns include rolling, postural control of the head and trunk in all planes of movement, coming to stand, toilet training, feeding, walking, running, skiing, mountain climbing, spelunking, playing group sports, or any other combination of simple to complex motor behaviors synthesized to allow for success at the motor task.

Principles of motor learning can be summarized in 4 major points: (1) learning is a process of acquiring the capability for skilled action; (2) learning results from experience or practice; (3) learning cannot be measured directly—instead, it is inferred based on behavior; and (4) learning produces relatively permanent changes in behavior; thus, short-term alterations are not thought of as motor learning.[12] Motor learning is a complex process reflecting the nervous system's response to a task-specific activity that emerges from an interaction between the need to perform the task and the environment within which the task is being performed.[26-29] The difference between a short-term change in behavior and motor learning can be demonstrated when a PTA is working with a patient on rolling from supine to side-lying. At the beginning of the treatment session, the patient may need both verbal and physical assistance to complete the task, yet, by the end of the session, is able to roll independently. The next day, the patient may not roll independently from supine to side-lying even with verbal cueing but is more quickly able to roll without assistance. This is an example of a short-term alteration in which permanent motor learning has not occurred. When the patient is consistently capable of rolling independently over time (a relatively permanent change in behavior), motor learning has occurred.

A variety of components affect motor learning; how movement is expressed is a result of the interaction of all the components. These components include the context within which a motor program is practiced, the schedule of practice, the stage of motor learning of the behavior, how feedback is applied, and the type of feedback applied. Each is discussed separately.

Practice Context

Practice context refers to the way a therapist chooses to teach the motor activity. There are 4 practice context categories: whole learning, pure-part learning, progressive/sequential-part learning, and whole to part to whole learning.

Whole Learning

Whole learning refers to practicing a behavior or task in its entirety. Simple and discrete motor tasks (activities that have a definite beginning and end), such as rolling over in bed, sit to stand, or scratching one's head, generally require whole learning. Asking an individual to stand up from a chair is a whole program. The PTA may break the activity into 4 steps by asking that same individual to scoot forward, place both feet 6 inches apart, shift weight over the feet, and then stand up. When breaking down the task, the patient may have more difficulty following the instructions than if he or she were asked to just stand up. Asking an individual to stand up requires one program that incorporates all the steps but is best practiced as a whole activity. When a specific impairment such as strength, range, or balance is identified, a PT may ask a PTA to treat the impairment or impairment train first (ie, strengthening, increasing range of motion, balance training under specific environments, etc), but then the activity must be practiced as a whole program for motor learning to occur. It is incorrect to assume that strengthening a muscle will automatically lead to an individual being able to perform a functional skill, such as standing up from a chair.

Pure-Part Learning

Pure-part learning is used for complex activities where the component parts are discrete motor programs in and of themselves. When learning a tennis serve, an individual needs to learn (1) how to throw the ball into the air vertically with a specific height expected and using the nondominant arm, and (2) how to traject the dominant arm while holding the racket in order for the face of the racket to hit the ball overhead with a specific angle and force. It does not matter whether the individual is taught first how to throw and second how to traject the racket. Ultimately, both need to be learned and then practiced together as a whole activity. Though it is not critical which part is taught first, they must come together in order for motor learning to occur. As a clinical example, a PT asks a PTA to teach an individual to stand up from and sit down onto a chair. The first part of the activity, to attain and stop at the vertical upright standing pattern, requires the strength, range, postural control, and balance needed to shift one's weight over one's feet; concentric contractions from sit to stand using posture, balance, and movement patterns; and knowledge of where vertical is in space. The second discrete part of this motor program requires going from stand to sit. Eccentric control over the same patterns is required; thus, the 2 movements are unique in their programming. At times, a PTA may assist the patient to standing and then practice one-quarter of both parts of the pattern (eg, sit down a little, say, onto a bar stool, and then rise to stand with control). Once the patient can easily do these movements, the PTA can increase the range within which the patient practices (2 unique programs). What determines the amount of range is the ease and fluidity of the patient's movements. Once the patient can lower to the height of a normal seat and return to standing, the PTA needs to have the patient sit down, relax, and then stand up. The ultimate goal is to have the patient practice the whole program once both parts are learned. This is an example of pure-part learning even though only one-quarter of both patterns are initially practiced. The decision to start in standing could be made because the patient was not able to generate enough force to come to stand or the force generated was excessive. There are many reasons why a patient might be asked to begin in standing. The PTA could collaborate with the PT to decide whether training the patient to independently come to standing is an appropriate approach for a specific patient. Starting in sitting or in standing will lead to independence of the patient in the sit to stand to sit program as a whole, but one way may be easier for the patient to learn, and this may reduce the time needed to learn the skill.

Progressive/Sequential-Part Learning

Progressive/sequential-part learning is employed when teaching intermediate skills and serial tasks (which are composed of several discrete tasks) that require many steps that must be performed in a specific sequence to be considered successful. When practiced, the learning always begins with the same initial step and follows in sequence with additional steps. Line dancing is an example of a sequential part task. If the components of the dance are taught to individuals as unique parts, different groups of people will put those parts together in different sequences, thus creating chaos on the dance floor. In a therapeutic environment, a PTA may want to teach a patient how to stand up from a wheelchair (w/c). This task consists of 3 activities: lock the brake on the w/c, pick up the foot pedal, and then come to stand. Although these 3 activities are separate parts of the whole, teaching the patient to perform them in a specific sequence or order will help the patient to learn not only the activity but also the sequential series within which it should be performed. This is especially true when patients have specific types of perceptual impairment. Again, collaboration with the PT will assist in determining whether this approach may be beneficial for a specific patient. Every PT and PTA has or will have a patient who stands up and then tries to either lock the brake or pick up the foot pedals. Often, the result is the practitioner writing up an incident report because the patient falls.

Whole to Part to Whole Learning

Whole to part to whole learning is the most frequently used in the clinical environment. An individual is first asked to perform the whole task; the clinician then breaks down the task into separate components and reconstitutes the entire program. The purpose is to have the patient execute the whole task so that a complete task analysis can be made. In a task analysis, the clinician needs to recognize what parts of the task are missing, what components of the movement are functioning, and what parts function intermittently and in limited ranges or positions in space. From this analysis, the results should help the PTA in determining what components need to be practiced when or in what sequence. Also, when some improvement is achieved by the patient, the PTA could determine if it is appropriate to practice the whole task. This type of practice generally incorporates impairment training, which needs to then be incorporated into the program as a whole.

If there is some uncertainty as to whether the task should be taught through whole, pure-part, progressive/sequential-part, or whole to part to whole learning, consulting and collaborating with the supervising PT is appropriate before beginning the intervention. If the PT has not learned to articulate this type of analysis into the clinical decision making, the PTA can help the PT by asking the clinician to verbally explain this analysis and resulting approach to intervention. If neither feels totally comfortable, then using a book similar to this one can help both clinicians analyze the situation and determine what is best for the patient. Whether PTs or PTAs, many clinicians make

---

Box 3-1
Summary of Practice Contexts

Whole Learning: Motor program is practice as a whole. Whole learning should be taught for simple programs, such as rolling over, coming to sit, coming to stand, and walking. If the program is not available to the patient, then the PTA must break it into usually sequential parts. For example: coming to stand from a chair. The patient is asked to come to stand in one fluid program. If the patient does not have enough power, then strengthening is appropriate. Once there is enough muscle power, again instruct the patient to come to stand incorporating the gained power.

Pure-Part Learning: Pure-part learning means that there are 2 or more parts to make up a program. Both parts are essential, but it is not important to teach one before the other. Cutting vegetables for a soup might be an example. It does not matter which vegetable is cut first, but all must be cut before cooking.

Progressive/Sequential-Part Learning: Progressive/sequential-part learning is based on the requirement that the sequence of motor programs needed to carry out the skill has a sequential nature. If that sequence is mixed up, the skill will either fail or the end result could cause a fall. Once a patient comes into the clinic in a w/c and needs to transfer onto the mat, there is a sequential process for that activity. Once the patient gets to the mat, he or she must first lock the brakes and pick up the foot rests before he or she stands, pivots, and sits down. Without using that sequence, the patient may stand, pivot, and fall either because the w/c moved or the foot pedals caused him or her to trip.

Whole to Part to Whole Learning: Most PTs/PTAs use this type of learning when teaching a motor skill. First the patient is asked to perform an activity as a whole (eg, coming to stand from the chair), then the therapist will identify what parts (impairments) need to be practiced or regained, and that will become part of the plan of care. As the patient regains control over the impairments, the activity is reintroduced and practiced as a whole activity. At times the clinician will also use sequential parts along with the activity to make sure the patient has corrected both the parts (impairments) and the sequence needed to be successful in the task.

---

decisions based on experience or gut feeling. Encouraging these individuals to clearly articulate their clinical decisions using accepted terminology helps reduce miscommunication and facilitate achievement of desired outcomes in an efficient manner. (Refer to Box 3-1 for a summary of these types of learning contexts.)

Practice Schedule

This motor learning component refers to the nature and frequency at which the patient practices the task. As practice is a critical element to motor learning, identifying which practice schedule best matches the task is important. There are 3 categories of practice schedule: mass, variable, and random practice.

Mass Practice

Mass practice is characterized by the individual practicing a particular skill in its entirety. This type of practice schedule is used to learn or relearn a skill that is essential for ADL. Regardless of how simple or complex the functional task, initially the individual needs to perform mass practice of the whole task. Thus, if parts of the task need to be learned as discrete components, they can be taught using pure-part, progressive/sequential-part, or whole to part to whole learning. However, to achieve permanent motor learning, the entire pattern/motor task must be practiced frequently enough for the CNS to learn the pattern as a whole. A PTA may need to guide or instruct the patient to practice any or all components of the whole task or the whole activity itself, but for the learner to initially retain the learning, mass practice is essential. In an inpatient rehabilitation level of care, a patient comes to the PT clinic 1, 2, or 3 times a day to practice the functional skills within a mass-practice clinical environment. A PT may need to determine the skill level at which the patient is performing to determine whether it is appropriate to delegate the intervention to a PTA. If the only way a patient can perform a task is with constant correction of error and constant manual contact, then the PTA needs to develop the skills necessary to initially guide the patient in the motor tasks or the task should remain within the scope of the PT. If, on the other hand, the patient needs to either practice with guidance in order to stay within the motor task or needs to work on specific components or impairments, these activities are well within the scope of practice of the PTA.

Mass practice, from a practical perspective, is the opportunity for the patient to repetitively practice a motor pattern or functional movement with few interruptions; this helps limit distractions that can hinder the CNS from remembering the motor task being taught. Normal motor development, as discussed in Chapter 2, is an excellent illustration of the role of mass practice in a child's development of functional movement. For example, a child may try to succeed at a movement task such as rolling over. Once the child experiences success, the child will practice this activity repeatedly. The parents may become very frustrated because the child may roll off a bed or will try to roll when being bathed or having a diaper changed. The child's CNS knows that, to learn that motor task, this type of practice is critical. Once the motor memory is consolidated, the individual will no longer need to mass practice unless the external environment changes. For example, if an individual learns through mass practice to walk on a hard, flat surface, that person should be able to automatically use that motor memory within that environment. If the person now wishes to walk on grass or up or down a hill, the environment for walking has changed, and mass practice will again be necessary in order to learn the variations of walking as an automatic adaptation. As an individual begins to automatically retrieve motor memories during ADL, the amount of practice needed is reduced. Similarly, the number of tasks the CNS might be asked to do, whether motor or cognitive, should increase between practicing the specific functional movements. Motor learning requires mass practice, but the PT must realize that if the individual stops practicing a task, then future performance of the skill may deteriorate.

Distributed Practice

Distributed practice is used when the patient has acquired a motor memory of the task, but impairment errors occur and practice is still needed to ensure long-term motor memory. With distributed practice there are intervals between practice that are equal to or greater than the time spent practicing. This type of practice is generally used in situations or environments when patients generally do not require a very high level of care or assistance in performing the activity. The specific frequency of intervention and practice should correlate with the needs of the patient and proceed from more frequent to less frequent as the patient progresses with independence. When practicing a large number of activities, with limited time to truly embed the learning of any motor task, the patient may not gain long-term independence in anything. Thus, selecting functional activities that gain the greatest independence for the patient is very important. Those programs or activities need to be valued by the patient to create the motivation to practice. The decision about what to practice may fall into the responsibility of the PT; the practice itself certainly is within the scope of practice of the PTA. There may be certain functional activities that the patient is mass practicing while others are on a distributed practice schedule. An example of distributed practice might be ambulating with a walker. Initially, the patient would need to spend a lot of time just practicing using the walker. Once on a distributed schedule, the patient may still need standby assistance but is not expected to practice every hour; instead, he or she practices sometime in the morning and afternoon but in between works on other functional activities.

Random Practice

Random practice refers to practice performed independently without a scheduled frequency or order to the practice. Random practice is, ultimately, the responsibility of the patient and/or caregiver. Once the patient can practice independently or with standby assistance, the activity must become part of that individual's daily-living life skill. Generally, neither the PT nor the PTA must be present during random practice; however, follow-up visits may be indicated to ensure that practice has been incorporated into the patient's lifestyle. The arrangement of a daily-living random practice schedule should be part of a home program, and the PTA may be given the responsibility of monitoring these ADL. For example, a patient may be independently coming out of the chair and walking to the bathroom or kitchen but be losing that ability over time because of lack of practice according to his spouse. Simultaneously, because of a medical condition, the man must drink a glass of water hourly. That water can be made accessible to the individual on a table by his chair or at the water source such as a sink. If the patient is told that he needs to get up and go to the kitchen or bathroom for a glass of water every hour, he will automatically practice sit to stand, walking a certain distance, and then returning to his chair and sitting back down. The patient is empowered to the responsibility of drinking the water, but the whole activity incorporates functional movements that are practiced automatically as part of the daily routine. If he misses getting up once or twice a day, it will not affect his motor learning because he is randomly practicing the activity independently.

Stages of Motor Learning

Many authors have described the critical junctures in the process where an individual learns a specific task, and they generally follow a 3-stage sequence. Learning a motor skill usually starts with an individual cognitively thinking and practicing the tasks frequently, with a considerable amount of errors in performance, improving to a point at which the activity is performed automatically and with very few, if any, errors (Box 3-2).

Stage 1: Cognitive Stage/Acquisition of a Motor Skill

Stage 1 is the phase at which the patient is learning a new skill or relearning an old one as a whole activity. At this stage, an individual needs to practice often and needs a lot of external feedback from the clinician in order to be successful. However, allowing the patient to practice and recognize errors in task performance and then self-correct during the subsequent practice are important during this initial stage. For example, if a patient is coming to stand and shifts weight to the lateral aspect of the foot, then there is a greater likelihood of falling; however, if he or she is allowed to recognize the error in weight bearing and then self-corrects the activity, then the boundaries of the activity are being practiced and learned. The patient would then be using both postural and balance programs to maintain control over the weight-bearing leg. Giving the patient time to self-correct before providing the external feedback is important. For example, allowing the patient to continue performing the task if he or she is not able to self-correct the movement results in the reinforcement of the wrong motor program. That is, if a PT asks a patient to stand, and as the patient executes the task, he or she starts to fall and is unable to self-correct, then performs the task again with the same result, the patient is no longer in the coming to stand pattern. He or she is then practicing falling! In this example, the appropriate thing to do is to then provide feedback to the patient as to the performance, determine a way for the patient to recognize the errors internally if appropriate and possible, and then allow the patient to perform the activity of coming to stand again with the appropriate amount of assistance. The PTA would need to prevent the individual from falling and help him or her stay within the coming to stand pattern.

There are many ways to encourage an individual to stay within the pattern. Teaching the patient to respond to inherent/intrinsic feedback from within the body is a critical component of this stage

---

Box 3-2

Stages of Motor Learning

Stage 1: Cognitive Stage/Acquisition of a Motor Skill
Stage 2: Associative Stage/Refinement
Stage 3: Autonomous Stage/Retention

---

of learning. When in the acquisition stage of motor learning, the environment used for practice should be consistent, and the type of practice is generally mass practice. In this stage, the motor skill is typically under conscious control; automaticity of the movement performance is not yet achieved. Once a patient begins to automatically respond to the demands of the external environment by the use of an appropriate control policy (eg, automatically stepping when the weight of the body is forward enough on the foot to trigger a stepping reaction), the patient executes movements in a feed-forward pattern. This feed-forward pattern means that the individual no longer needs feedback or sensory input for the CNS to know that walking is the appropriate response. As an example, the feed-forward mechanism is similar to that of a DVD player. Once the equipment is told to run the movie, the player will continue running the movie until it is told to stop. Likewise, when the motor system, because of either the external environment or internal environment of the individual (motivation, cognitive decision, etc), is told to walk, the person will walk until a change is required. That motor system will continue to walk the musculoskeletal system until some aspect of the CNS changes that decision. Feedback to the CNS is often the critical component of the CNS's decision to change a control policy. Thus, as a PTA begins to understand the stages of motor learning, consideration of feedback variables will need to be incorporated into these appropriate stages.

Stage 2: Associative Stage/Refinement

Stage 2 is the stage when a patient can execute movements within specific environmental constraints, decreases the number of errors during the activity, and applies less effort during performance. Generally, the environment used during performance is consistent, although variance in the specific components is present. For example, if a patient is able to sit on a hard surface as long as he or she does not reach and perturb him- or herself more than 20 degrees, then the task is learned but is limited in range, power, and/or balance when perturbed beyond range. He or she is in the refinement phase. A PTA may want to add an activity of reaching for objects in space slightly beyond the 20-degree mark. The PTA may want to retain the same environment (eg, a hard surface) while allowing the patient to refine the movement and self-correct. Then the patient may be asked to sit on a compliant surface but only move within the original 20 degrees. As the patient gains control reaching beyond the 20 degrees while on a compliant surface, the therapist can enlarge or refine the activity. At this stage, a patient is enlarging control within a specific environment.

Stage 3: Autonomous Stage/Retention

Stage 3 is the stage at which the patient moves to a variety of different environments and retains control of the whole task. Continuing the previous example, once the patient has learned to sit on a hard surface, the PTA may to move to a compliant surface, such as a gymnastic ball, and ask the patient to throw and catch an obstacle. The true hallmark of learning is the ability to retain the skill and transfer the skill into different settings and under different conditions and environmental and cognitive challenges.[29]

Feedback

There are 2 types of feedback: intrinsic and extrinsic. Feedback depends on sensory input. When patients have sensory loss, often feedback mechanisms are lost or inconsistent, and compensation through alternative sensory systems is indicated.[30-34]

Intrinsic Feedback

Intrinsic feedback is based on sensory responses inherent to the patient's body as part of the desired movement itself. For example, the muscles and joints tell the CNS where the trunk and limbs are in space and which limbs are in an open or closed chain. The vestibular system in the inner ear tells the CNS where the head is in space. Both sensory mechanisms are inherent and are the primary input for refinement and retention of posture and movement. This input is ongoing and the motor system may use a feed-forward mechanism. The PT should determine whether there is conflict or loss in inherent feedback. If deficits exist, the PT may delegate the specific activities that allow the patient to regain accurate sensory awareness during the activity or substitute another sensory system. For example, if in sitting the patient is unable to equally bear weight on both ischial tuberosities because of a decreased sense of pressure or proprioception, the PTA may place a mirror to allow the patient to self-correct using vision (assuming that the patient's visual perception is intact). If the lack of appropriate intrinsic feedback or an alternative compensatory input system is unavailable, then error in the movement cannot be corrected and may lead to failure in obtaining functional independence.

Extrinsic Feedback

Extrinsic feedback is based on an outside source providing feedback. There are many types of extrinsic feedback. Biofeedback, auditory feedback from a therapist's voice, use of a mirror, and touch, pressure, and proprioceptive input feedback that the therapist uses during handling techniques are a few of the many extrinsic feedback mechanisms PTs and PTAs use. This type of feedback can lead to better performance during a motor activity, but until the patient self-corrects using inherent feedback, independence is not obtained. There are 2 types of extrinsic feedback.[35-39] Knowledge of performance feedback uses a sensory system (such as the therapist's voice) to inform the patient as to whether the quality or efficiency of the movement pattern is achieved. This type of feedback is given as the person is performing the task and generally at critical times to ensure the individual accomplishes the task. A PTA may say, "You are doing fine, Mr. B, but you need to keep your balance over your feet," "you need to push down on your walker," or "put your foot farther forward." Knowledge of results feedback informs the patient as to whether the task is accomplished or how close the movement comes to accomplishing the task. The type of feedback is given at the end of the task and truly gives feedback as to the entire activity or task performed. The PTA may say, "Mrs. J, you came to standing without my help" or "you should not sit down without looking because you just sat on Mr. M." Both types of feedback give the learner information regarding error. Constant feedback leads to immediate behavioral performance, but the patient will learn to rely on external feedback and will not develop a need to process inherent information necessary to learn the task independently. As an example, a PTA verbally corrects many aspects of walking, and the patient does very well by the end of the morning session. In the afternoon, when the patient is asked to walk again, his or her performance is the same as the beginning of the morning and does not show the changes made by the end of the morning session. Obviously, the patient here is depending on external feedback from the PTA and not learning to perform the task independently. There is a very fine line between whether the patient is depending on the external feedback to functionally move or is using that feedback to develop an internal awareness.[40] The PTA can determine this difference by withdrawing the feedback and observing whether the patient can retain the motor skill both during treatment and at the following session.

Table 3-2
Summary of Motor Learning Concepts

Type of Learning	Practice Parameters	Feedback Schedule
Initial learning	Mass practice of motor program or functional skill. Reintroduction of corrections of impairments into the functional skill. Will begin with block design.	Needs knowledge of both performance and results. Initial reinforcement is immediate, thus showing high performance but lower retention.
Learning shows programming, but with large number of errors	Practice will go from mass to distributed as the patient begins to self-correct errors. Widening of the window of range within the program can increase. Design will move from block to random as program becomes more automatic. Mental practice can be used to encourage internal repetition.	May still use knowledge of performance during times when patient's error exceeds the range of the program, but knowledge of results will in time become the most important feedback. As PTA moves to variability of practice, the program will become more generalizable. Reinforcement becomes more intermittent with a higher degree of retention.
Learning shows motor program has been established	Practice schedule should go from distributed to random with the patient being motivated to run the correct procedure. Patient is self-motivated to perform the programs as part of daily living and social responsibilities.	Patient internally corrects using inherent mechanisms and no longer needs PTA to reinforce motor learning, except for social reasons. We all like to hear we are doing well.

External feedback can be provided in several different ways. Summary feedback is when the feedback is given after a set number of trials of the task (eg, after every other or every third trial). Faded feedback initially provides feedback after every trial, then decreases to every other trial, every third, every fourth, etc. During a delayed feedback the clinician withholds the feedback for a short time (ie, a 5-second delay) after the task has been performed.[41] When facilitating motor learning, faded feedback appears to be most effective as the feedback becomes increasingly intermittent throughout patient trials (practice), and therefore the patient has to rely more on internal feedback and self-correction to perform the task safely and efficiently. Delayed feedback also allows for improved motor learning by providing the patient time to self-assess performance. However, the specific feedback schedule depends on the patient and the task to be learned and practiced. This is another area in which the PT/PTA collaboration and communication are important in setting up optimal feedback and practice parameters. But, whether under the direct supervision of a PT or within an environment where the PTA has some autonomy, there is clear evidence to show that PT interventions following CNS damage does lead to motor learning and consequent improvement in an individual's ability to perform functional activities.[42] Those data clearly identify the need for physical therapy interventions in individuals following CNS damage. (Refer to Table 3-2 for a summary of types of practice and feedback needed to reinforce motor learning.)

Physical Therapist/Physical Therapist Assistant Collaboration in Relation to Motor Learning Activities

Approaches to facilitate learning or relearning of a motor skill is a critical component when providing interventions aimed at optimizing function. Remember that a complex motor activity may consist of a variety of motor programs. Following injury to the brain, the memory of each program may need to be evaluated by the PT. It is the PT's decision to run certain aspects of an entire program. Delegation of any of those activities can be given to the PTA. For example, an individual who has suffered a traumatic brain injury may need to relearn specific components of a task. The PT may ask the PTA to bring the patient to standing using the right lower extremity (LE). If both legs were used, then the left leg might go into a strong extensor pattern, such as hip extension and adduction, knee extension and ankle inversion, and plantarflexion. Thus, the right leg is ready to stand, but the left is not. The PTA may be instructed to bring the patient to stand, then bend the left LE at the knee and place the left knee on a stool. In this way, the right leg can practice all components of standing and the left leg can still practice postural control of the hip without going into a strong extensor pattern. This delegation to the PTA is appropriate, and many PTAs may also be given the responsibility to transition the patient to bilateral standing as long as the left leg has developed the necessary postural control to inhibit a total extensor synergy.

NEUROPLASTICITY

Neuroplasticity is defined as cellular adaptations in the CNS that allow an individual to learn novel skills or relearn functions previously lost because of cellular death by trauma or disease at any age. The changes occur in response to a variety of external and internal demands placed on the individual's CNS. Within an optimal treatment environment, the resultant behavior leads to functional recovery and allows the individual to regain or attain a higher quality of life. In reality, neuroplasticity occurs throughout life. Internal adaptations of the CNS to height, weight, endurance, normal and chronic disease, and cellular death over a lifetime allow all of us to maintain function as our bodies change. Similarly, external environments vary over a lifetime, such as climate, exercise level, dietary demands, and changes in habitat. The CNS has to adapt to these changes as well. When trauma or disease causes dramatic, observable changes in behavior, then everyone around becomes aware of those variances. Theory from the early- to mid-20th century led therapists to believe that once cellular death had occurred, there was nothing that could be done except to compensate for lost function. It was believed that plasticity within the CNS was not possible. Therapists working with patients with CNS disease or trauma could not reconcile the discrepancy between theory and patient recovery following disease or trauma. Therapists have always dealt with function and physicians with pathology. Often, the pathology, according to the physician or basic scientist, would indicate that function was impossible, yet therapists dealing with behavior found that patients often got better and regained lost motor function. In the past 2 decades, with the advent of better measurement tools and research on human models, scientists and researchers have discovered that the brain is much more plastic than previously thought. It has been found that, given an appropriate environment to learn in, the brain can learn or relearn despite cellular damage.[43–49]

Neuroplasticity provides an explanation at the basic science level for behavior that therapists have observed since the beginning of the profession. Previously, clinicians, especially master clinicians, had difficulty explaining or could not explain how patients regained function; however, they could observe and measure those behaviors. As a clinician and therapist, Umphred always believed that if a motor behavior looked right at her or other people, was easy and enjoyable for the patient, then somehow the intervention was creating change in the direction of normality and functional recovery no matter the theory. Neuroplasticity helps to explain why patients were regaining function even though the medical system of the time said they could not. This theory has helped guide therapists with intervention delineation. The CNS will always try to succeed at a task presented as long as the individual is motivated to succeed.[26] If the environment used to teach a task is too difficult, then a patient will find other ways to try to succeed at the task. For example, if a patient cannot flex the hip at push-off, he or she will circumduct the hip or use some alternative movement pattern to succeed at bringing the limb forward. These alternatives are easily identified and, if practiced, will become a new movement pattern for the patient; it will, however, require more energy because it is less efficient. It will affect synergy patterns, postural control, balance, and needed power throughout the range. Therefore, it would be better to try to trigger the patient's normal walking patterns before choosing some compensatory solution. The complex theory and its relationship to function often falls into the responsibility of the PT and not the PTA, but that does not mean that the PTA will not discover the movement patterns that lead to normal function. The PTA has sensory input to the eyes and ears and kinesthetic feelings from touch and pressure that can help lead to solutions to a patient's functional recovery. Thus, it is the PTA's job to become a keen observer of functional movement and report changes in those behaviors to the PT. A patient's movement or postural problems are usually answered by the patient's own motor responses and truly reflect the plasticity of the CNS.

Kleim and Jones[50] synthesized the pertinent research on neuroplasticity in a way that provides specific suggestions in the application of neuroplasticity in rehabilitation practice. For more information, the reader is encouraged to review this research article. The following principles have direct implications in PTA practice:

1. "Use it or lose it."[50] As mentioned earlier, the PTA has the responsibility of encouraging the patient to acquire and practice normal movements that improve functional performance. Movements and functional patterns that are not performed or practiced are lost, including the motor circuitry responsible for that movement in the CNS. For example, following a stroke, a patient may have a reduced ability to use an arm or leg. Without rehabilitation, over time, the patient will learn not to use the affected extremity, leading to the concept of learned nonuse. Because of this, the neuronal circuitry responsible for the movement occurring on the affected extremities also disappears. It is very difficult to overcome learned nonuse, but more recent research states that it is possible.

2. "Use it and improve it."[50] It is not sufficient to just encourage use of the affected extremity. Specific training to improve function on that limb consequently drives the changes in the brain that reinforce this improvement.

3. "Specificity."[50] The training to improve function has to be specific. This means that the PTA must choose activities that will directly improve the quality and efficiency of the desired movement. For example, if the goal is to strengthen the LEs to improve the performance of sit to stands, the PTA must practice the particular activity with the patient. Performing open-chain strengthening exercises for the LEs may improve strength but will not necessarily translate to an improved ability of the patient to stand up from the sitting position. In addition to specificity, the activity must be meaningful for the patient (see #5, Saliency Matters).

4. "Repetition and intensity matter."[50] The practice of a particular activity must include the appropriate amount of intensity to drive the needed neuroplastic changes to regain the movement or function. Most recent research on this topic clearly shows that the intensity of therapy that we currently provide the majority of our patients/clients is **not** sufficient to drive these changes. It is therefore important to maximize practice by optimizing the patient's adherence to his or her home program. Additional approaches to optimizing repetition in practice include the use of a patient contract and an activity log to document performance of a home program and activities to encourage or force the use of the more affected extremities.

5. "Saliency matters."[50] The chosen activity being practiced must be meaningful for the patient. This means that the patient perceives the importance of the movement or task and sees how practicing this task leads to the attainment of goals and functions that he or she desires.

CONCLUSION

If a patient has never learned normal motor patterns (eg, in the case of trauma at birth), the movement pattern must be mass practiced in an environment where success is possible, reinforcement accurate, and potential actualized. If the individual has already learned a movement strategy such as walking and suffers a traumatic incident such as traumatic head injury or stroke, the potential exists to regain a previously learned pattern or to learn a new one in the intervention environment of the therapist. An individual must first learn a pattern or task-specific program and then practice enough for the control over that program to become automatic, as in the feedforward motor program. A learned program is similar to a disc placed in a DVD player. The CNS determines the pattern and will run the program (or disc) until the CNS is told to change it. As an example, the therapist places the client in an environment where the patient's CNS determines that walking is the appropriate program to play. The type of walking observed tells the therapist what programs are interacting and being controlled by the patient. That person runs the motor control of walking until either the CNS tells it to do something else or the motor control of that individual cannot self-correct the error; thus, the environment forces a new pattern. A person falling because of a surface change for which the person cannot compensate is an example of external environmental change that forces a loss of motor control over walking. Understanding motor learning and what patterns the CNS can use to control the motor system's response to a required movement can give tremendous insight into the prognosis of a patient with movement dysfunction following insult to the CNS. How the map fits together will be influenced by the PT, the PTA, the patient, and the environments within which the patient can learn. The following case examples should help the PTA understand the theoretical principles presented in this chapter.

CASE STUDIES

The following specific case examples are patient examples similar to those discussed in later chapters. The PTA is not expected to be able to answer these clinical questions after reading this chapter. Instead, the PTA can use these cases to help integrate the information presented in this chapter with information presented in all the chapters that discuss specific clinical problems. It is recommended that the learner read this chapter, the case examples, and the questions to identify appropriate questions regarding motor learning, motor control, and neuroplasticity as they relate to patient care. After reading and analyzing any particular chapter dealing with a clinical problem, the PTA can return to this chapter, find an appropriate case, and then progress through the questions and answers to better integrate this material into decisions on clinical management.

CASE #1

The patient is a 6-month-old child diagnosed with spastic diplegia. She was born 8 weeks premature and was extremely flaccid at that time. The child's gestational age would be placed at 4 months, giving the child the 8 weeks she should have remained in utero. However, the tonal characteristics of the child are extensor dominant in the trunk and LEs. The child has more control over the arms than the legs but loses function of the arms when placed in positions that require a lot of trunk stability, such as sitting or pressure on the feet in standing. The child does not have adequate head control and is unable to roll over, come to sitting, or sit independently. The PT has asked the PTA to use a handling technique with rotation of the trunk initially in side-lying. The PTA should rotate the child's lower trunk on the upper trunk to facilitate rolling and have one of the patient's LEs lead with hip and knee flexion (without holding the ball of the foot). As the child begins to respond to rolling, the PTA encourages the child to assist with the movement itself. Second, the child should be placed on the PTA's bent knees with the head in vertical and, with small-degree changes of the trunk, the PTA should facilitate small movements of the head and thus assist the child in gaining head control. As the child responds with head movement that brings the head to face vertical, the PTA enlarges the degrees of motion. The PTA works from vertical toward horizontal (both toward prone and supine) and back to vertical. The PTA only goes as far as the child's postural responses to head control are observed. Thus, the PTA is given the responsibility of working on both rolling activities and development of head control.

QUESTIONS

1. Why has the PT asked the PTA to perform these activities? Why were those activities important in improving the child's movement abilities?

2. Is the request within the domain of the PTA?

3. At what stage of motor learning is the child?

4. What type of practice context would you choose? The response needs to relate to whole, pure-part, progressive/sequential-part, and whole to part to whole learning.

5. What type of practice schedule would you expect the PTA to use? When considering the practice schedule, what type of feedback would be used initially, and how would that feedback be changed as the patient improves?

6. Why would you expect change, and what might it look like? When or why would you ask the PT to change the interventions delegated?

CASE #2

The patient is a 5-year-old boy who suffered an anoxic event due to drowning. Before the injury, he was an active, healthy child in kindergarten and doing very well. The child was in a coma for 1 week and in a vegetative state for 3 weeks. He is now stable and has been sent to neurorehabilitation for physical therapy. The patient can roll and come to sitting although his trunk tone is low. He can be placed in sitting and remain there independently as long as he is not perturbed or asked to move. He cannot stand up from sitting and does not control going from sit toward horizontal. The PT has asked the PTA to work on sitting balance and strengthening of the postural extensors of the trunk and hips. The PTA has placed herself in kneeling behind the child, using her own leg to support the boy's trunk from behind. This brings the boy into a vertical postural pattern while sitting. The PTA then asks the child to reach for toys and hand them to his mother. Once the child begins to hold and respond with balance reactions, the PTA moves the child to sitting on a gymnastic ball and continues to work on sitting and balance control. Next, using the same gymnastic ball, the PTA rolls the child toward prone and then into a vertical kneeling posture, using the ball to help support the trunk extensors. Then, using toys and manipulating the ball, the PTA increases the demand on the child's motor system to maintain and/or regain upright posture during play.

QUESTIONS

1. Why has the PT asked the PTA to perform these activities? Why were those activities important in improving the child's movement abilities?

2. Is the request within the domain of the PTA?

3. At what stage of learning is the child?

4. What type of environmental context would you choose?

5. What type of feedback/reinforcement schedule would you expect the PTA to use?

6. Why would you expect change, and what might it look like? How would you as a PTA examine this child's motor control and determine that a change in intervention would be appropriate?

CASE #3

The patient is a 27-year-old man who suffered a traumatic brain injury following a head-on collision while driving his car without a seat belt. He has been in the intensive care unit for 4 days and has been transferred to the rehabilitation unit today. The PT has performed the initial evaluation of the patient. At this time, he is conscious but has extremely low tone. He is unable to come to sitting or standing independently, and he does not have enough tone to sit independently. The PT has asked the PTA to sit the patient on the side of the bed with the feet supported, first by raising the head of the bed, then guiding the patient into sitting. The PTA can either kneel behind the patient on the bed with a ball in the patient's lap and the patient's arms over the ball, or the PTA can sit in front of him and make sure his weight is forward over his pelvis with his arms on the PTA's shoulder. The goal is to increase the length of time the patient is able to sit semi-independently. As the patient gains control and strength, the PTA has him begin to reach for real targets, such as a cup or ball, while maintaining trunk and pelvic control. The goal is to gain independent sitting. This is accomplished through the patient being challenged by perturbation of his weight over his hips during reaching or regaining balance if shoved. The PTA is also asked to work on transfers between the bed and the w/c and back to reduce the total dependency he now has when performing transfers.

QUESTIONS

1. Why has the PT asked the PTA to perform these activities? Why were those activities important in improving the person's movement abilities?

2. Is the request within the domain of the PTA?

3. At what stage of learning is the patient concerning sitting?

4. Is the PTA working on new learning or relearning an old program?

5. What type of environmental context would you choose (quiet or noisy, hard or soft surface)?

6. What type of feedback/reinforcement schedule would you expect the PTA to use?

7. Why would you expect change, and what might it look like? When or why would you ask the PT to change the interventions delegated?

CASE #4

The patient is a 59-year-old man with the medical diagnosis of Parkinson's disease. He is able to perform all functional activities at a certain rate, but he has great difficulty regaining his balance if he trips and difficulty initiating changes such as sit to stand and stand to walk. He especially complains of problems turning (eg, turning into the bathroom or turning and walking back to the dining room with his food). First, the PT asks the PTA to teach the patient to use a partial rotation pattern when coming to sit versus the adult sitting pattern he is using. The PT also asks the PTA to have the patient practice going from sit to stand to sit on a variety of surfaces, with the chair or stool at a variety of levels. The PT delegates placing this patient on the treadmill, first at his normal gait pattern and then changing the settings to encourage fluctuation in walking speed and height of incline. The fourth task for the PTA is to create a maze for the patient to walk through that requires him to turn at each corner. Initially, he should be instructed to just walk, and then he should progress to walking through the maze facing a specific direction. Once he can do this independently, the activities will become his home exercise program, which he must practice in order to maintain function for as long as possible. Additionally, there are other activities the PT may delegate to the patient's significant other or caregiver because the patient still needs to continue practicing but does not need a PT or a PTA to help with these functions at this time.

QUESTIONS

1. Why has the PT asked the PTA to do these activities? Why were those activities important in improving the person's movement abilities?

2. Is the request within the domain of the PTA?

3. At what stage of learning is the adult in relation to concerning walking?

4. Is the PTA working on new learning or relearning an old program?

5. Why did the PT select the specific environmental context, and why should it work?

6. What type of reinforcement schedule would you expect the PTA to use?

7. Why would you expect change, and what might it look like? When or why would you ask the PT to change the interventions delegated?

CASE #5

The patient is a 71-year-old male with the medical diagnosis of a mild right cerebrovascular accident with resulting left hemiplegia. He can sit independently but does not have equal weight bearing on the left hip. With assistance, he can come to standing with the majority of weight on his right leg. The PT has delegated to the PTA the activity of weight shifting in sitting. Specifically, the PTA is to have the patient reach with his right arm over to the left side as far as possible and increase that range as the patient improves. If he can use the left arm to do the same, then the PTA is to also include that extremity. Second, the PTA is to assist the PT in placing the patient in a harness in order to do supported weight bearing on the treadmill. Once the patient is in the position and the PT determines the pace and degree of body weight support, the PTA will be assisting the patient with his left leg in order to practice walking.

QUESTIONS

1. Why has the PT asked the PTA to do these activities? Why were those activities important in improving the person's movement abilities?

2. Is the request within the domain of the PTA?

3. At what stage of learning is the adult concerning walking?

4. Is the PTA working on new learning or relearning an old program?

5. Why did the PT select the specific environmental context?

6. What type of reinforcement schedule would you expect the PTA to use?

7. Why would you expect change, and what might it look like? When or why would you ask the PT to change the interventions delegated?

REFERENCES

1. Galea MP. Physical modalities in the treatment of neurological dysfunction. *Clin Neurol Neurosurg.* 2012;114(5):483-488.

2. dos Santos Mendes FA, Pompeu JE, Modenesi Lobo A, et al. Motor learning, retention and transfer after virtual-reality-based training in Parkinson's disease—effect of motor and cognitive demands of games: a longitudinal, controlled clinical study. *Physiotherapy.* 2012;98(3):217-223.

3. Schenkman M, Hall DA, Barón AE, Schwartz RS, Mettler P, Kohrt WM. Exercise for people in early- or mid-stage Parkinson disease: a 16-month randomized controlled trial. *Phys Ther.* 2012; 92(11):1395-1410.

4. Liddell EG. Cajal and Sherrington. *Lect Sci Basis Med.* 1956–1958;6:100-115.

5. Knott M, Voss DE. *Proprioceptive Neuromuscular Facilitation.* New York, NY: Harper and Row; 1968.

6. Bobath B. *Abnormal Postural Reflex Activity Caused by Brain Lesions.* 3rd ed. Frederick, MD: Aspen Publications; 1985.

7. Rood M. The use of sensory receptors to activate, facilitate, and inhibit motor response, autonomic and somatic, in developmental sequence. In: Scattely C, ed. *Approaches to Treatment of Patients With Neuromuscular Dysfunction.* Third International Congress, World Federation of Occupational Therapists. Dubuque, IA: William Brown Group; 1962.

8. Ayres AJ. *The Development of Sensory Integration Theory and Practice.* Dubuque, IA: Kendall/Hunt Publishing; 1974.

9. Johnstone M. *Restoration of Normal Movement After Stroke.* New York, NY: Churchill Livingstone; 1995.

10. Brunnstrom S. *Movement Therapy in Hemiplegia.* 2nd ed. Philadelphia, PA: JB Lippincott; 1992.

11. Carr JH, Sheperd RB. *Movement Science: Foundations for Physical Therapy in Rehabilitation.* Frederick, MD: Aspen Publishers; 1987.

12. Umphred DA. *Neurological Rehabilitation.* St Louis, MO: CV Mosby; 1985.

13. Sherrington CS. *The Integrative Action of the Nervous System.* New York, NY: Cambridge University Press; 1947.

14. Bernstein N. *Coordination and Regulation of Movement.* New York, NY: Pergamon Press; 1967.

15. Tuller B, Turvey MT, Fitch HI. The Bernstein perspective II: the concept of muscle linkage or coordinative structure. In: Kelso JAS, ed. *Human Motor Behavior. An Introduction.* Hillsdale, NJ: Erlbaum; 1982.

16. Brooks VB. *The Neural Basis of Motor Control.* New York, NY: Oxford University Press; 1986.

17. Horak F. Assumptions underlying motor control for neurological rehabilitation. In: *Contemporary Management of Motor Control Problems: Proceedings of the II STEP Conference.* Alexandria, VA: Foundation for Physical Therapy; 1991.

18. Gordon J. A top-down model for neurologic rehabilitation. Presented at: III Step Conference: Linking Movement Science and Intervention; 2005, Salt Lake City, UT.

19. Cramer SC, Sur M, Dobkin BH, et al. Harnessing neuroplasticity for clinical applications. *Brain.* 2011;134(6): 1591-1609.

20. Ghahramani Z, Wolpert D, Jordan M. Computational models of sensorimotor integration. In: Morasso P, Sanguineti V, eds. *Self-Organization, Computational Maps, and Motor Control.* Amsterdam, The Netherlands: Elsevier; 1997:117-147.

21. Shadmehr R, Krakauer JW. A computational neuroanatomy for motor control. *Exp Brain Res.* 2008;185(3):359-381.

22. Arce F, Novick I, Shahar M, Link Y, Ghez C, Vaadia E. Differences in context and feedback result in different trajectories and adaptation strategies in reaching. *PLoS One.* 2009;4:e4214.

23. Shadmehr R, Mussa-Ivaldi FA. Adaptive representation of dynamics during learning of a motor task. *J Neurosci.* 1994;14(5 Pt 2):3208-3224.

24. Ebenbichler GR, Oddsson LI, Kollmitzer JO, Erim ZE. Sensory-motor control of the lower back: implications for rehabilitation. *Med Sci Sports Exerc.* 2001;33(11):1889-1898.

25. Gallese V, Lakoff G. The brain's concepts: the role of the sensory-motor system in conceptual knowledge. *Cogn Neuropsychol.* 2005;22(3):455-479.

26. Roller P, Lazaro R, Byl N, Umphred D. Motor control, motor learning and neuroplasticity. In: Umphred D, Lazaro R, Roller P, Burton G, eds. *Umphred's Neurological Rehabilitation.* 6th ed. St Louis, MO: Elsevier; 2012:69-97.

27. Shumway-Cook A, Wollacott M. *Motor Control: Translating Research Into Clinical Practice.* 4th ed. Philadelphia, PA: Lippincott Williams & Wilkins; 2011.

28. Candia V, Weinbruch C, Elbert T, Rockstroh B, Ray W. Effective behavioral treatment of focal hand dystonia in musicians alters somatosensory cortical organization. *Proc Natl Acad Sci USA.* 2003;100(13):7425-7427.

29. Goh HT, Sullivan KJ, Gordon J, Wulf G, Winstein CJ. Dual-task practice enhances motor learning: a preliminary investigation. *Exp Brain Res.* 2012;222(3):201-210.

30. Kuo AD. The relative roles of feedforward and feedback in the control of rhythmic movements. *Motor Control.* 2002;6(2):129-145.

31. Sullivan KJ, Knowlton BJ, Dobkin BH. Step training with body weight support: effect of treadmill speed and practice paradigms on poststroke locomotor recovery. *Arch Phys Med Rehabil.* 2002;83(5):683-691.

32. Winstein CJ. Knowledge of results and motor learning: implications for physical therapy. *Phys Ther.* 1991;71: 140-149.

33. Vahdat S, Darainy M, Milner TE, Ostry DJ. Functionally specific changes in resting-state sensorimotor networks after motor learning. *J Neurosci.* 2011;31(47):16907-16915.

34. Wong JD, Kistemaker DA, Chin A, Gribble PL. Can proprioceptive training improve motor learning? *J Neurophysiol.* 2012;108(12):3313-3321.

35. Schmidt RA, Lee TD. *Motor Control and Motor Learning: A Behavioral Emphasis.* 3rd ed. Champaign, IL: Human Kinetics; 1999.

36. Lehrer N, Attygalle S, Wolf SL, Rikakis T. Exploring the bases for a mixed reality stroke rehabilitation system, part I: a unified approach for representing action, quantitative evaluation, and interactive feedback. *J Neuroeng Rehabil.* 2011;8:51.

37. Lehrer N, Chen Y, Duff M, L Wolf S, Rikakis T. Exploring the bases for a mixed reality stroke rehabilitation system, Part II: design of interactive feedback for upper limb rehabilitation. *J Neuroeng Rehabil.* 2011;8:54.

38. Rikakis T. Utilizing media arts principles for developing effective interactive neurorehabilitation systems. *Conf Proc IEEE Eng Med Biol Soc.* 2011;2011:1391-1394.

39. Carr JH, Sheperd RB. *Neurological Rehabilitation: Optimizing Motor Performance.* Philadelphia, PA: Elsevier Limited; 1998.

40. Fairbrother JT, Laughlin DD, Nguyen TV. Self-controlled feedback facilitates motor learning in both high and low activity individuals. *Front Psychol.* 2012;3:323.

41. O'Sullivan SB, Schmitz TJ. *Physical Rehabilitation: Assessment and Treatment.* 5th ed. Philadelphia, PA: FA Davis; 2007.

42. Hollands KL, Pelton TA, Tyson SF, Hollands MA, van Vliet PM. Interventions for coordination of walking following stroke: systematic review. *Gait Posture.* 2012;35(3):349-359.

43. Nudo RJ. Functional and structural plasticity in motor cortex: implications for stroke recovery. *Phys Med Rehabil Clin N Am.* 2003;14(1 Suppl):S57-S76.

44. Ward NS, Brown MM, Thompson AJ, Frackowiak RS. Neural correlates of motor recovery after stroke: a longitudinal fMRI study. *Brain.* 2003;126(Pt 11):2476-2496.

45. Das A, Franca JG, Gattass R, et al. The brain decade in debate VI. Sensory and motor maps: dynamics and plasticity. *Braz J Med Biol Res.* 2001;34(12):1497-1508.

46. Hashino O. Neuronal bases of perceptual learning revealed by a synaptic balance scheme. *Neural Comput.* 2004;16(3):563-594.

47. Jackson PL, Lafleur MF, Malouin F, Richards C, Doyon J. Potential role of mental practice using motor imagery in neurological rehabilitation. *Arch Phys Med Rehabil.* 2001;82(8):1133-1141.

48. Kandel ER, Schwartz JH, Jessel TM, Siegelbaum SA, Hudspeth AJ. *Principles of Neural Science.* 5th ed. New York, NY: McGraw-Hill; 2012.

49. Arya KN, Verma R, Garg RK, Sharma VP, Agarwal M, Aggarwal GG. Meaningful task-specific training (MTST) for stroke rehabilitation: a randomized controlled trial. *Top Stroke Rehabil.* 2012;19(3):193-211.

50. Kleim JA, Jones TA. Principles of experience-dependent neural plasticity: implications for rehabilitation after brain damage. *J Speech Lang Hear Res.* 2008;51(1):S225-S239.

Please see accompanying Web site at

www.healio.com/books/neuroptavideos

4

Intervention Procedures

Sharon L. Gorman, PT, DPTSc, GCS
Darcy A. Umphred, PT, PhD, FAPTA

KEY WORDS

- Functional training
- Impairment training
- Motor programs
- Sensory retraining

CHAPTER OBJECTIVES

- Differentiate the categories of intervention into functional training, impairment training, hands-on guidance, and sensory or somatosensory retraining to gain or regain functional skill and participate in life.

- Identify when intervention is not improving stated goals.

- Identify when patient is successfully performing functional activity without assistance or guidance.

- Appreciate the importance of participation training in optimizing the patient's/client's quality of life.

INTRODUCTION

Intervention, as defined in the *Guide to Physical Therapist Practice*, is "purposeful and skilled interaction of the [physical therapist] PT with the patient/client."[1] Although the definition of intervention continues to define the role of the PT, intervention is intertwined in the role of the physical therapist assistant (PTA). To the PT, intervention incorporates the following: (1) coordination, communication, and documentation of services; (2) patient- or client-related instruction; and (3) direct patient intervention. Within these 3 categories, coordination of services is the only area

Umphred DA, Lazaro RT, eds.
Neurorehabilitation for the Physical Therapist Assistant,
Second Edition (pp 69-115).
© 2014 SLACK Incorporated.

that should never be delegated to the PTA. Therefore, the PTA needs to develop skills in communication with the PT, other health care practitioners, the patient, and caregivers. Documentation skills, when appropriately delegated, are a critical form of communication with other individuals on the patient's team and with outside organizations such as accreditation organizations and third-party payers. (Refer to Chapter 7 for additional materials on documentation.) Although portions of the reexamination could be part of the PTA's delegated responsibilities, it is not within the role of the PTA to interpret the examination results unless the PT has clearly identified a plan of care that incorporates change in relation to patient test results. The PTA begins practice with intervention and then may be asked to follow up with reexamination using the original tools or other methods of examination. It is within the PTA's scope of practice to teach patients and families functional skills, home programs, and discharge programs only if the PT has taken the responsibility of clearly identifying what those skills or programs are. Within the framework of PTA practice, intervention precedes examination. This book reflects that same model, and this chapter precedes the chapter on examination. The PTA should not be asked to perform an initial examination on the patient and interpret the result, to establish a treatment protocol, or to determine that the patient no longer needs service and write a discharge summary. Those are actions that are the PT's responsibility. If the PTA is asked to perform them, then it could place the patient (consumer of a product) at risk, and both the PT and the PTA can be held liable. Given the previous scenario, a PTA is being misused and the patient given an incorrect perception of the services being provided. This particular area and the problems it creates is becoming an area for claims denial, malpractice, and consumer fraud. It is the PTA's responsibility to identify his or her scope of practice and to recognize when the patient is at risk, even when components of intervention have been delegated. The primary role of the PTA within the therapeutic community is direct intervention with the patient. It is very appropriate to delegate treatment interventions to the PTA when the services of the PTA will positively affect patient progress and when the role of either PT or PTA would, similarly, enhance that progress.

Physical therapy interventions encompass a vast area of techniques that incorporate interactions with the cardiopulmonary, integumentary, musculoskeletal, and neuromuscular systems.[1] Although the specific pathology or disease identified by the physician may fall within one of these body systems, PTs and PTAs do not treat disease or pathology; they treat the impairments, activity limitations, and participation restrictions caused by those diseases or pathologies. For that reason, similar physical therapy techniques may be used for multiple medical diagnoses, or multiple physical therapy interventions may be incorporated into a patient's treatment plan although that individual has one specific disease. For the PTA to identify risk factors or contraindications and abnormal signs exhibited by the patient during a physical therapy session, knowledge of human anatomy, physiology, and disease processes are always a part of a PTA's education.

It is the primary responsibility of the PT, when delegating portions of the plan of care to the PTA, to have adequate knowledge of the patient's status and abilities, as well as the abilities of the PTA to whom patient care is being delegated. To assist PTs as well as PTAs in understanding the complex decision making required to make a determination that direct patient intervention can be delegated to a PTA, the American Physical Therapy Association has created a PTA Direction Algorithm (Figure 4-1). This algorithm can be used by PTAs to identify areas of change or uncertainty regarding the patient's status, ranging from the scope of PTA work, patient condition, specific outcomes to be addressed by direct PTA intervention, abilities/knowledge/skills of the PTA, liabilities and risk, and payers. Oftentimes, especially in people with neurological dysfunction, changes in the patient's presentation or medical status may be first noted by the PTA during an intervention. It is the PTA's responsibility to report to the PT any questionable behaviors of the patient at the beginning, during, or at the conclusion of an intervention. If the PTA has any question or concern regarding the health of the patient and/or appropriateness of the intervention itself, that PTA is bound by law and ethics to communicate that concern to the PT as quickly as possible. For that reason, the PTA is often asked to check heart rate, blood pressure, skin color,

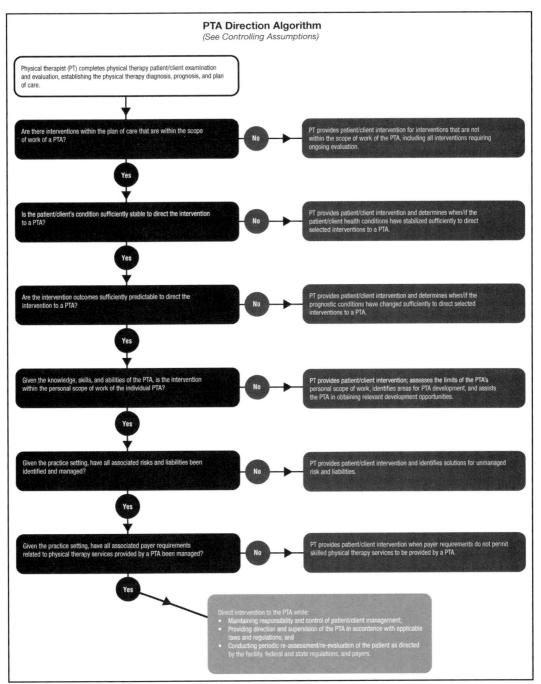

Figure 4-1. Algorithm used to determine whether an intervention should be delegated to the PTA. (Reprinted from www.apta.org/PTinMotion/2010/9/PTAsToday, with permission of the American Physical Therapy Association. Copyright © 2010 American Physical Therapy Association.)

pain levels, depth and rate of breathing, levels of consciousness, and cognitive response patterns of patients. These assessments become a part of ongoing intervention and are discussed in Chapter 5 on examination. Before the patient interventions are delegated, the PT has the legal responsibility to check all contraindications and risk factors to guarantee that the patient can safely receive treatment. Even though this check should make the PTA feel safe that a patient will not be harmed by intervention, monitoring patient signs is a critical component to maintain that safety parameter.

This text discusses patients and clients who have had some form of central nervous system (CNS) disease, pathology, or trauma with resultant motor dysfunction of a variety of types. The chapter on motor learning and motor control provides important background information on how individuals learn a motor skill and how therapeutic interventions can be optimized to facilitate return of function. Specific intervention recommendations for specific medical diagnoses can be found in Chapters 8 through 13 of this text. In addition, a chapter on cardiopulmonary impact on motor dysfunction will also lead the PTA to avenues of intervention interactions, strategies, and ways to enhance patient performance. (Refer to Chapter 14 for this discussion.) The concept of intervention through direct patient contact will be the focus of this chapter. In the last chapter of this book, additional discussions of alternative intervention strategies and approaches considered as complementary therapies are also presented to widen the PTA's understanding of possible intervention strategies. To gain skills in any of these complementary therapies, additional education is needed before application is appropriate.

Designing Successful Interventions: Things to Consider

The ultimate goal of any physical therapy intervention is to optimize activity and participation and help the patient achieve the highest quality of life possible. Interventions must be thoughtfully designed, carefully monitored, and assessed for effectiveness. Two important things the PT needs to consider when designing these interventions include the patient's cognitive understanding of the task and his or her attitude toward the activity. To maintain this quality of care, the PTA also needs to be able to understand the cognitive and the emotional level at which the patient interacts.

Cognitive Understanding of the Task

There are areas of CNS processing that are not considered motor but directly affect motor performance. Perception, levels of consciousness, and distractibility all affect motor control. The perceptual problems and residual movement dysfunction following CNS damage are huge. The PTA is not expected to evaluate or analyze these problems and their impact on movement, but rather to appreciate that they exist and how they affect the presented movement problems. For example, if a patient post-head injury overshoots a target and then self-corrects to the target, it is a perceptual problem (praxis) and falls into the area of cognitive problems. If instead the patient tries to self-correct the movement throughout a trajectory toward the target, it is a motor control problem (ataxia) and a sign of cerebellar involvement. The difference between these 2 movement problems needs to be recognized by the PTA, but interpretation of its consequences needs to be determined by the PT. The PTA needs to recognize when the patient changes behaviors or motor responses, and whether those responses seem better or worse than when first observed. Those changes need to be communicated to the PT. The causation of the changes could be perceptual learning and improvement, motor control itself, or some other problem, but that determination is not the responsibility of the PTA.

Attitude Toward the Activity

The patient's emotional system plays a key role in regulation of muscle tone, in adherence to performance of the activity, in the belief in the importance of the activity and in its relationship to life, and in his or her confidence toward the PTA as a health care provider. Similarly, the PTA must acknowledge that those 4 areas affect the motor responses and attitudes of the practitioner. Many individuals, patients, and practitioners radiate tension into their shoulders and necks throughout a stressful day, which can be recognized by a family member at the end of the day. A patient who has motor control problems to begin with will often exaggerate the problems when under pressure or upset. These behaviors are not triggered consciously; it is the emotional system's response to the interactions during the day, whether it is increased tension after a day of work or exaggerated movements following an interactive day. Similarly, when individuals are depressed, their motor system is also depressed, and movement is more difficult and tiring. The PTA needs to be aware of the emotional responses of individuals during therapy. Many times following CNS insults, patients have less control of their emotional reactions; thus, they may get angry more easily, cry more often, and laugh inappropriately. Many of these patients recognize the behaviors as inappropriate but cannot control the emotional system. It is very important that the PTA create environments within which the patient can develop motor control of the neuromuscular and the emotional environment. If lack of success in a task creates anger, then it may be important for the PTA to articulate and highlight what the patient did right and was successful in performing, rather than the mistakes that the patient made. Understanding the emotional reactions of a patient and the stimulus that triggered that response and determining whether it helps or hurts the learning is a skill that all clinicians need to develop. If, during a transfer, a therapist demands that a patient stand up, the patient may stand because he or she (1) feels angry, (2) feels disempowered or humiliated (that he or she is being treated like a child), or (3) just wants the activity to finish, so the therapist will go away. The patient's emotional reaction will create extensor tone, and that tone will help generate the force needed to stand, but teaching someone to stand on top of anger means that every time the individual wants to stand, he or she will need to be angry. By controlling the noise, distractions, and rate of success or failure, the PTA can allow the patient to practice the movement activities successfully without the influence of the emotional system. Once the motor programs are established, reintroducing emotional and perceptual challenges can be integrated into the functional activity as impairment training. The PTA is responsible for carrying out the established program designed by the PT. When the patient is ready or his or her CNS seems capable of handling additional stress, it should be recognized by the PTA and that information given to the PT. The decision to change the environment and make it more complex is the responsibility of the PT, unless the PTA has been given clear parameters to identify and document specific changes in behavior and the activity or components to be changed. Patients will go through phases of adjustment to their respective CNS disease or trauma. Similarly, families will be going through adjustments. There is no guarantee that the patient, the family, or the health care providers will be adjusting in a similar manner or time sequence. Thus, the PTA needs to have some understanding of how adjustments or emotional liability affects motor performance. Refer to Chapter 6 for additional information.

CATEGORIES OF INTERVENTION

Delegated intervention to a PTA will fall within 1 of 5 categories, each category having different focus: (1) functional activity training, (2) impairment training, (3) hands-on the therapist, (4) somatosensory retraining, and (5) participation training. The first categories primarily reflect function within the motor system and movement dysfunction of the patient, and the fourth category encompasses individuals with sensory or processing problems that result in motor dysfunction. The fifth area addresses life and those activities the individual values and wants to participate in as he or she transitions from rehabilitation back to life's demands and activities. If the goal of physical therapy treatment is purposeful and meaningful functional movement activities, then the ultimate goal of every treatment program should be empowering the patient to achieve independent functional control over movement within the respective environment whenever possible. The PTA should remember that it is just as much his or her responsibility to identify competencies in intervention procedures as it is for the PT to acknowledge those competencies when delegating intervention within the plan of care. If the PTA is unfamiliar or lacks the necessary skills to provide the identified interventions, then it is important to discuss that with the PT and ask for assistance/guidance within any specific area.

Functional Training

Functional training interventions focus on 3 areas: (1) activities of daily living (ADL), such as bed mobility or ambulation; (2) instrumental activities of daily living (IADL), which include activities that an individual does after waking up, dressing, and moving, such as shopping, using a computer or phone, cooking, and managing money or medications; and (3) participation and leisure time activities that are self-selected and considered to give a person quality of life, such as group activities (eg, attending worship services, going shopping), group sports (eg, basketball, baseball), individual sports (eg, golfing, swimming, running, fly-fishing), and group or individual physical enhancement activities (eg, martial arts training, water aerobics, treadmill, or elliptical training). All 3 of these areas fall within the category of functional training. When intervention focuses on specific activities, the patient needs repetitive practice of that activity to regain or maintain skill in the functional motor strategies needed to perform the activity (see Chapter 3). If the goals of the intervention include performance of any one of these skills, then the functional motor plan is already available to the patient, and only practice and variance within the environment is needed for perfection. In this case, a PT should definitely delegate this activity to the PTA. As the patient improves skill in these activities, delegation may be given to family members or caregivers, when those people are available and willing.

Functional training in ADL includes bed mobility, coming to sit and stand from various surfaces, transferring onto and from various chairs (eg, a wheelchair [w/c] or a toilet), transferring into and out of a shower or tub, ambulation on all types of surfaces with various types of visual environments (eg, normal lighting, darkened environment, or in a crowded street), dressing and undressing, and using ambulatory aids (eg, crutches, a cane, or a walker). In a home health environment, the PTA may be asked to performing additional functional training, such as teaching and practicing bathing, eating, and cooking; however, more often the occupational therapist and/or a certified occupational therapy assistant will be responsible for the patient's practice with these activities. The goal of functional activity training is not to guide the patient with the hands-on skill of the therapist, but rather to guarantee that the patient is performing these activities safely and with repetitive practice. Repetitive and random practice schedules will solidify responses to these activities as automatic, the patient no longer needing to think through the steps of the movement and, instead, performing the activity without effort in a feed-forward program. (See Chapter 3 for practice variations with regard to functional training.) Many times, patients will desire a high level of motor performance as their goal and become very frustrated that the treatment program focuses on activities that individuals assume they can do or should be able to do. For example, if an individual wants to return to fly-fishing at his cabin on a lake, determining how he will get from his cabin to the beach and whether he will sit or stand while fishing will help the therapist communicate to the patient why he is practicing sit to stand and ambulation activities. Once the patient understands that practice will lead to the ultimate goal of fly-fishing, the individual usually becomes a motivated and adherent patient. Functional training should be the ultimate goal of any sequential treatment plan. Understanding the components critical for any functional movement leads to the second category of intervention strategies.

When a PTA is practicing functional training, the entire movement may be broken down into smaller components with the easiest aspects practiced first to have the patient realize that the activity is possible and success within reach. For example, if independent sit to stand and back to sit is identified as a goal in the plan of care, the PTA has the option of how the patient will initially practice that activity. The activity could begin once the patient was assisted to stand by having him first begin to lower his body onto a bar stool or a chair or a high/low table/mat that has been raised up. This type of activity decreases the need for full power, postural integrity, and changing from relaxed sitting in flexion to standing with postural stability. Once the patient can lower onto the edge of the chair and reverse the motion and come to stand, 3 additional aspects of the activity can be changed. First, the object used as a chair can be lowered so additional range and power is required to accomplish the activity; second, the patient can be asked to lower to sit, relax on the edge, and then come back to stand; and third, the patient can be asked to lower to the seat, move back into sitting, and then come back to stand. Each of these activities creates additional demands on the motor system and enlarges the patient's ability to gain control over that specific movement pattern.

All functional activities need core body stability or postural stabilization to hold the body in space as the individual moves from one functional position to another, as well as maintaining the body against gravity when just sitting or standing. Thus, teaching the individual to move the trunk and lower limb or trunk and upper limb combines an extremity with the trunk, which provides the postural or core stabilization. Rolling requires head, upper body, and trunk as a pattern for rolling or one leg that goes into hip flexion and internal rotation along with knee flexion as the trunk and head follow the movement. These patterns teach bed mobility. Often the patient can begin normal functional movement in sitting before being independent in the category of bed mobility because of the tone problems in the supine position that arise after CNS deficits. For that reason, functional training may need to begin in vertical sitting. This position provides the greatest base of support (BOS) outside of horizontal and the least amount of power needed to maintain the trunk in an erect posture. Having the patient work on small postural adjustments off vertical while using an upper extremity (UE) to reach toward a target will strengthen the muscles being activated, incorporate balance activities when sitting, and require the integration of an upper limb with the trunk movement. Similar activities can be performed with the lower extremity (LE) by asking the patient to shift weight and begin to stand up. As a functional activity, the PTA should be observing movement that looks normal and integrated. The range of motion (ROM) can be enlarged as the patient runs and controls postural adjustment off midline until he or she is capable of going from sit to horizontal or sit to stand. If abnormal tone is triggered by these activities, then potential impairment training may be needed before the patient would be expected to control normal movement from one spatial position to another.

Progressing the Functional Training Activities: Rate of Movement and the Ability to Alter Rate

As individuals grow and learn to control the functional movements, they simultaneously learn to control the rate or speed of those movements. For example, as children learn to walk, they also learn to walk slower and faster. As the rate increases, the walking will turn into running. A PTA may be instructed to teach a patient walking using a walker. Initially, the patient will walk very slowly and should progress to better control and a faster progression. With CNS damage and relearning, often the patient is taught to walk while cognitively thinking about each aspect of the program: pick up the walker, step with the right foot, pick up the walker, and then step with the left foot. As the patient has never walked with a walker, this is a new motor program. The PTA needs to remember that the patient once had a rate of walking that was normal for that person. It may have been as slow as the movement when using the walker, but more often, it would have been faster. If the PTA needs to impairment train in this area, then the patient needs to practice the movement at various speeds. This impairment training can be accomplished by using a metronome or a forced stepping environment such as a treadmill, or by the PTA actually holding onto the walker and pulling the patient forward, triggering a stepping reaction to increase the rate of the walking.

Impairment Training

This category is associated with interventions that are system specific and that focus on a component of a movement that has resulted in dysfunction within the functional activity. There are many subcategories in this area of treatment. Impairments may be the direct result of musculoskeletal problems such as ROM limitations, muscle weakness due to disuse, biomechanical misalignment due to joint problems, or leg-length discrepancy. A plan of care that eliminates or minimizes these impairments certainly would be appropriate to delegate to a PTA.

Similarly, cardiopulmonary or peripheral vascular disease can create many types of pain, poor endurance to exercise, and even lightheadedness and confusion when the oxygen (O_2) levels drop. For that reason, the PTA will often be asked to monitor breathing, heart rate, blood pressure, and O_2 level using a finger gauge and pain scales regardless of the medical diagnosis of the patient. If PTAs ever have concerns about the cardiopulmonary/peripheral vascular system, they should be communicated to the PT of record. If that PT is unavailable, concerns should be shared with another PT, nurse, or physician.

Areas of integumentary problems encompass medical complications from ulcers, burns, or reddened areas, or any unusual reactions of the skin before, during, or following a therapeutic intervention. These impairments are especially important to understand if the patient is being asked to practice specific activities that entail movement across a surface (eg, rolling, coming to sit, or sitting for an extended period of time). Similarly, if a scar limits ROM and thus movement function itself, then interventions that mobilize the tissue using therapeutic modalities to increase tissue elasticity will be delegated to the PTA. The PTA must then be aware that those modalities can also burn the patient, especially if the skin or vascular system cannot accommodate the modality. Patients with long-term contractures following CNS injury often have skin integrity problems. The skin becomes very fragile and thin and thus splits easily if ROM over the joint creates too much stretch at too high a rate. If the skin splits at the joint, it will cause not only pain but also an open wound. The PTA will need to work slowly and pay constant attention to the skin reaction when treating most patients after neurological insults with contractures and limited skin mobility.

Interventions to Improve Joint Mobility (Range of Motion)

In many physical therapy clinics, exercises that improve joint ROM are delegated to a PTA. When the only limitation is musculoskeletal, the complexity and skill of performing ROM on a patient need not be difficult. However, when treating a patient with ROM limitation possibly secondary to a neurological dysfunction, a variety of parameters must be considered before delegation: (1) During the ROM, does the joint stay in a correct biomechanical position throughout the range? (2) Is the limitation of range due to hypertonicity around the joint? If so, what muscles are hypertonic and how are they interacting in patterns of movement? With introduction of a rotatory pattern, can the limb be moved into and out of the areas of limitation? (3) What rotatory patterns are limited? If rotation is incorporated into the ROM exercise, does the hypertonicity decrease? If so, does the patient have a stable joint, or are muscles around the joint hypotonic? These are questions the PT should consider before delegating this activity. Once the responsibility has been delegated, the PTA should continue to ask these questions. When the range increases and/or the tone around the joint changes, the PTA should report that change to the PT, and potential intervention strategies for impairment training may need modifying.

The PTA must always remember to stabilize the joint throughout the motion. The PTA must make sure the pattern of motion used by the patient to perform the activity is normal without substitutions of muscles not normally engaged during the specific motion. The PTA may be asked to instruct the patient to perform the activity within a certain degree of motion and to slowly increase that range as the patient demonstrates normal motor control. If the patient complains of pain, often the cause of pain is misalignment of the joint and can be corrected by moving the joint into a better biomechanical position. As long as the patient is able to correct the joint alignment, then the PTA is impairment training. Once the PTA does the correction for the patient, it is no longer impairment training but hands-on intervention. Fear of pain during ROM often causes muscle splinting, which leads to incorrect alignment of the joint(s). That fear is often associated with the memory of some other health care practitioner having moved the limb when the patient did not have any control; that movement might then create an initial pain response as well as the memory of the experience. The PTA needs to teach the patient that pain is not acceptable and that the patient needs to tell the practitioner when it hurts. The PTA must recognize a pain grimace response in addition to requesting verbal communication of pain. If the patient is being assisted through part of the range that may have pain, the patient must trust that the PTA will stop once pain is present. If not, the patient will continue splinting or guarding the joint. Gaining the patient's trust often results in eliminating splinting because of fear of pain and simultaneously causes a gain in ROM.

Interventions to Improve Neuromuscular System Impairments

Impairments within the neuromuscular system include activity states of the spinal motor generators (hyper- or hypotonicity and rigidity), stereotypic or reflexive patterns within functional movement (eg, flexion and extension synergies, reflexive response such as asymmetrical and symmetrical tonic neck reflexes, and positive [+] supporting reactions), balance problems (eg, sensory input and balance synergy problems), resting fluctuation in motor tonicity (nonintentional tremor), fluctuation in motor tonicity on purposeful activity (athetosis, ataxia), reaction time to perturbations, rate of movement (how fast or slow the CNS will run a program), cognitive understanding of the task (perception, levels of consciousness, and distractibility), and attitude toward the activity (motivation, levels of emotional stability, and ethnic bias). A brief description and some intervention suggestions will be included within each subsection of this practice pattern.

States of the Spinal Motor Generators (Hyper- or Hypotonicity and Rigidity)

A common impairment seen in patients with CNS damage is an altered state of the spinal motor generators. This altered state can create a variety of movement dysfunctions. When the motor generators are firing at too high a rate, the result will create muscle reactions that are hypertonic and/or reactive to stretch. Usually, when these generators are firing and causing hypertonicity, the response is not seen in an individual muscle but is seen in patterns of muscle interactions referred to as synergies. An agonist, or isolated muscle, is naturally linked to other muscles (agonistic synergy) that work closely with a particular muscle to perform specific functional movements. Similarly, if the generators are not firing adequately in a muscle group, then the behavioral response will often be hypotonicity within a pattern of movement. Except in specific peripheral nervous system injury or disease, behavior responses are more likely to be seen in patterns. At times, a limb many have a hypertonic agonistic synergy while the antagonistic synergy is hypotonic. If both the agonistic synergy and the antagonistic synergy are hypertonic, then movement in both directions is limited, and the person may exhibit rigidity. Hypertonicity is an abnormal state of the motor generators and usually follows hypotonicity within muscle groups and instability of the joint. Because of hypotonicity, the body will naturally try to maintain joint integrity and create additional tone in other muscles around the joint structure. Instructing the patient to perform slow, relaxing rotation away from the tight pattern along with deep breathing often lowers the state of the motor pool and decreases the hypertonicity. An example may be a patient with Parkinson's disease who demonstrates trunk rigidity. An appropriate intervention for this condition that can be performed by the PTA is having the patient in hook-lying position, then performing slow and gentle lower trunk rotations to decrease tone, in preparation for functional activities such as rolling, coming to sit, transfers, and ambulation.

The PTA must remember that decreasing hypertonicity does not guarantee stability of the joint or joints or volitional control over movement. Many times, decreasing hypertonicity forces the therapist into a hands-on approach to intervention versus impairment training because of the decreased state of the motor pool resulting in hypotonicity or weakness.

Stereotypic or Reflexive Patterns Within Functional Movement

Patients' movement responses following CNS injury often include stereotypic or reflexive patterns of movement (eg, flexion and extension synergies, reflexive response such as asymmetrical and symmetrical tonic neck reflexes, and supporting reactions). These programs are often the only patterns available to the patient's CNS when an external or peripheral stimulus demands or requires a motor response. Similarly, when neuronal loops within the CNS trigger involuntary motor response patterns, the motor system drives those available programs. Thus, individuals in lowered states of consciousness may exhibit hypertonic synergistic patterns of motor responses (eg, extension synergies incorporating hip and knee extension, internal rotation, adduction of the hip, plantarflexion, and pronation of the foot). Most synergies and reflexive patterns are inherent or preprogrammed within the CNS and have been incorporated and integrated within early motor development. These patterns reflect combinations of movement patterns in response to demands placed on the CNS from peripheral input systems and internal feedback loops. Specific reflex responses are identified in Chapter 5. Specific impairment training techniques that discourage repetitive practice of these stereotypic patterns can be found in Chapters 8 through 13. An easy concept to remember is that the opposite movement pattern from the involuntary pattern is often the solution to gaining or regaining motor control. Adding rotation away from either synergy pattern can lead to more functional movement. By activating the antagonistic synergy, the hypertonic synergy or reflex pattern will often automatically be dampened through the interaction of programs within the CNS. The PTA must be cautioned that by triggering the antagonistic synergy, what may happen is just a shift from one synergy to another. If the patient is able to independently run these antagonistic programs or components of these programs, then the therapeutic environment is considered impairment training. The patient's CNS must be able to control both agonistic and antagonistic synergy patterns and various combinations of muscle patterns within those synergies to move to functional training. If the patient's motor programming is stuck in one synergy or 2 stereotypic patterns, the patient will be very limited in responses to the demands of life. These stereotypic patterns often force the biomechanical position of joints to be misaligned, leading to secondary musculoskeletal impairments at a future time. A physical therapy goal will generally encompass reduction of hypertonicity and obligatory responses of stereotypic programs. The PTA needs to remember that the causation of hypertonicity synergies is often instability within joint structures. Similarly, the use of reflexive or stereotypic patterns is the CNS's response to environmental demands, which require gravitational postural responses. To empower the patient's CNS to gain or regain the fluid control over multiple patterns of movement, the environment must be modified so that the response can be appropriate to the demand within the environment. This may require environmental adaptation and/or hands-on guidance to guarantee the CNS is in control of the programs, regardless of how limiting that might be early in the therapeutic intervention process. Again, if by adapting or limiting the environment the patient is capable of initiating and maintaining a normal movement sequence, then the PTA is impairment training. Once the PTA adds hands-on control of the movement itself, the activity is no longer impairment training and then falls under the next section for Categories of Intervention.

Resting Fluctuation in Motor Tonicity (Nonintentional Tremor)

Patients with diseases within the basal ganglia or associated pathways often have resting tremors in the hands, tongue, and even the feet. Within the hands, the nonintentional movement is often referred to as a pin-rolling pattern. Whether the patterns are in the hands, feet, or tongue, these movements are involuntary and in a specific flowing movement pattern and illustrate a lack of control or inhibition by the CNS to some automatic motor programming. The tremors are often exaggerated when the patient has strong emotional reactions to the environment, but sometimes can be controlled upon intentional movement. Often, the tremors can be decreased with slow, deep breathing; visualization by the patient of a relaxing environment (eg, picturing a waterfall or watching the wave action of the ocean); and weight bearing of the extremities. Nonintentional tremors usually do not limit function. The patient must determine whether the movement is socially limiting. Refer to Chapter 13 for specific recommendations for intervention ideas for individuals with basal ganglia problems.

Fluctuation in Motor Tonicity Upon Purposeful Activity (Athetosis, Ataxia)

Patients who have cerebellar problems or motor control problems over certain motor programs may have fluctuation of motor tone when moving. If a patient lacks the postural programming to stabilize the joints during movement but has the power and range to generate the movement program, the patient will have problems controlling the rate or speed of the movement and the ability to slow down or reverse the movement during functional activities. Thus, the PTA will observe a lack of axial and trunk stabilization when the patient is moving, especially when the distal segment is non-weight bearing, such as the swing phase of gait. Movements often seem too powerful for the activity, and the patient often overshoots the target. The movements themselves are less exaggerated during weight-bearing activities because of the increase in proprioceptive input through approximation and the normal postural patterns required. For that reason, patients can practice movements with weighted vests or exercise tubing used as resistance and compression to a movement during reaching and the swing phase of gait. If the patients can don the weighted vest or belt themselves and the PTA is to observe and guard during the activity, this intervention would be impairment training. If the PTA needs to apply the resistance and/or compression during a movement, then it is hands-on intervention and not considered impairment training.

Interventions That Improve Balance and Postural Control

Balance is an important component of critical functional activities. Balance is required for the patient to control all programs needed to either maintain the body's BOS over its center of gravity (COG) or to replace the body's COG back under its BOS (Figures 4-2A and B). Balance can also be considered a component of a larger movement, such as the postural stability needed to reach an object, coming to standing, walking, sitting and eating, or dressing. Providing interventions that improve balance impairments could be delegated to PTAs.

Balance training can focus on maintaining or regaining balance once an anticipated or unexpected perturbation occurs. A perturbation occurs when a directional force causes the body to react to maintain or regain balance (COG) over a specific BOS. That BOS may be one foot, both feet, a foot and a knee (one-half kneel), both hips in the sitting position, or the entire body (the trunk, head, and hips) when a person is lying down and rolling from side to side. The ability to react to the perturbation is based on sensory input from the proprioceptive, vestibular, and visual systems and inherent balance synergy programs (ankle, hip, and stepping). In addition, when the patient is instructed in the use of a support system (eg, a cane, walker, or transfer bar), a therapist needs to consider the balance within the points of support used by the individual for ambulation or movement from one base to another. Generally, there is a balance aspect to all movement and, thus, a patient will incorporate balance programming as part of the functional activity while moving. Balance training includes creating environments in which the patients will (1) perturb themselves (eg, by weight shifting during reaching or walking), (2) perturb and replace their COG (eg, by stepping or protecting themselves with their arms when falling), and (3) regain balance when an external force, either anticipated (recognized that the perturbation will occur, such as a child running without looking toward you) or unanticipated (it just happens), perturbs them during a movement activity (eg, being bumped or shoved by someone else while walking). The PTA is often asked to encourage patients to automatically react to weight shifting during reaching, transferring, and ambulating. The only way those automatic reactions can be observed is when the PTA either distracts the patient's attention during a movement or perturbs the COG without notice.

Figure 4-2A. Balance: Maintaining COG within the existing base of support.

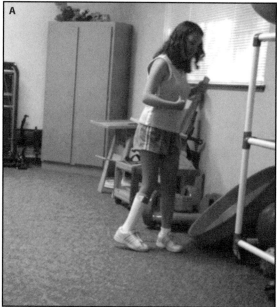

Figure 4-2B. Balance: Replacing the base of support back under the center of gravity, stepping.

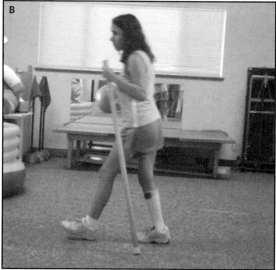

There are many ways to enhance balance reactions.[2] Incorporating the 3 sensory modalities of proprioceptive, vestibular, and vision will often help the patient to respond adequately to perturbations.[3] Obviously, balance reactions can be facilitated in sitting by asking the patient to reach toward objects in various directions. Similarly, the PTA can give gentle perturbations to the patient while sitting and see whether normal balance responses are present. If so, more forceful pushes can be given that will facilitate both balance and strengthening. By adding weight at the shoulders or hips, proprioception is enhanced and will add important sensory input to the CNS. The PTA must simultaneously be aware that adding weight means the patient will need additional power or strength to move. Similarly, increasing resistance to forward movement when walking by using an exercise band around the waist again increases the proprioceptive input. The therapist can increase and decrease that resistance, which changes the perturbation of the forward movement. Similarly, if the PTA shifts diagonally behind the patient, the specific perturbation changes.[4]

If the PT asks the patient to close his or her eyes and then perturbations are given, only proprioception and vestibular systems are available to the patient with regard to balance. The PTA can observe and see whether the patient's balance responses remain intact or diminish once vision is taken away. This determination is very important. If the patient does not have adequate balance with vision occluded, then walking or moving at night may become dangerous and place the patient at a high risk of falling. Recommendations that direct the family to place nightlights in hallways and any room that might be used by the patient are very important to help avoid falling at night.

Asking the patient to sit or stand on compliant surfaces such as foam (Figure 11-7) or rocker boards challenges the proprioceptive system and forces the patient to use vestibular and vision as the sensory input for balance. Practicing walking on these types of surfaces will determine whether the individual can safely walk on grass or outdoor surfaces that are uneven. If going to the park with grandchildren or playing with friends at the beach is important to the individual, then practicing on uneven and compliant surfaces needs to be incorporated into the plan of care. Also, going outside and practicing on the specific type of surface that the individual will be walking on, such as grass or sand, will further enhance the training and link the function to the environment in which the patient will perform once out of the therapy situation. An example of this link is illustrated in Box 4-1.

There are certain situations where balance impairments are caused by subsystem problems, and therefore working on that specific impairment may improve balance. For example, standing balance may be impaired by lack of ankle dorsiflexion mobility, either by dorsiflexor weakness or tight gastrocsoleus. In this case, strengthening the ankle dorsiflexors or stretching that gastrocsoleus (or both) could improve balance.

Vestibular Rehabilitation

A specialized aspect of balance training addresses interventions that improve the function of the vestibular system. The vestibular system's primary responsibility is to maintain clear vision during head movement. It also assists in orienting the head and trunk to vertical in relationship to gravity. As stated previously, the vestibular system is one of the sensory receptors responsible for balance and is located within the inner ear. Although the vestibular system is not the most important sensory modality for balance, when dysfunctional it can cause severe balance problems. The vestibular system is a highly sensitive end organ that reports head movement in all directions using the labyrinths of both inner ears along with the utricle and saccule, which identify the head position in space whether the person is lying down supine or prone, in side-lying, sitting, or standing. Individuals with vestibular problems often have signs of vertigo, dizziness, nausea, poor posture control, nystagmus (rapid movement) of the eyes, and complaints of falling.

Vestibular problems can be central or peripheral in origin. The most common peripheral vestibular problem is benign paroxysmal positional vertigo. In this condition, a calcium carbonate crystal (called *otoconia*) collects and lodges within the semicircular canals. When this happens, the sensory receptors in these canals send false signals to the brain, causing the symptoms mentioned above. A common PT intervention for this problem is called *canalith repositioning* to move the otoconia out of the way. This repositioning can reset the vestibular system and clear the semicircular canals of any obstructions, but that procedure is not delegated to the PTA because of the constant reassessment that needs to occur initially and throughout the procedure.

The vestibular and auditory systems both share the eighth cranial nerve to communicate with the CNS. The eighth cranial nerve enters the nervous system in the lower brainstem. Individuals with a medical disease referred to as Ménière's disease[5] will complain of ringing of the ears along with presenting vestibular signs, especially vertigo and nausea. Given ringing sounds (auditory) and vertigo (vestibular), the connection between the auditory and vestibular sensory systems through the eighth cranial nerve can be clearly shown. This particular disease would

---

Box 4-1

Case Example: Incorporating Normal Activities Into Balance and Strength Training

Umphred was called by a vice president of the university where she taught and asked to come to her home and help with her husband's continual rehabilitation. She explained that he had a stroke but did very well. He proceeded with inpatient rehabilitation for 3 weeks, then outpatient physical therapy for another 4 weeks, beginning with 3 times a week and tapering to once a week the last week. He then had home health care for 4 weeks, with the PT coming twice a week. He used a cane but had now gone back to the walker. He was able to function independently at the time the therapy was stopped. It had been a month and he was now having balance problems, was not safe walking independently around the house, and had stopped walking outside. He needed assistance getting out of his chair and spent the day reading. His wife came home at lunch to make sure he had food and to walk him to the bathroom. She was very concerned about his reduction in function and wondered whether he needed to be placed in a care facility or whether she should retire to take care of him.

The PT went to the home and observed the individual move. He was able to stand up independently but was unsteady, weak, and concerned he would fall. He was able to walk with the cane or walker but again was fearful of falling and complained that his leg muscles felt tired. The therapist noticed a water pitcher and glass by the chair and asked why that was there. The individual explained that he was a diabetic for more than 20 years and needed to drink a glass of water every hour to maintain control over his diabetes. The therapist asked him if he could walk the 35 feet to the kitchen sink and if so to demonstrate. He did so without any signs of falling. The therapist then recommended to the individual and the wife that she no longer leave a pitcher of water with him when she goes to work and that he should get up every hour and go to the sink to get his water. She also said she would be back in a couple of days to see how he was doing. Within the first week he was no longer having difficulty getting out of the chair, no longer had a fear of falling, and had given up the walker and was using a cane for balance assistance. By the end of the second week, he was actually going outside and walking around on the sidewalk. He began by walking 10 to 15 feet and turning around and then increased that distance as he felt stronger. By the end of the month, he was again going to the store with his wife and walking around, interacting with her and with life.

All the therapist did was change one thing in the environment that forced balance and strength training as part of daily living and used a motivator that he had already incorporated into his living style (getting a glass of water hourly). He did his own therapy without anyone identifying that he needed to keep practicing strength and balance activities as part of his daily living. Once they were incorporated into his life, he regained all of the function he had worked so hard to regain during rehabilitation.

---

be considered an external vestibular problem because the disease is located external to the CNS. Acute/chronic labyrinthitis and unilateral peripheral vestibular hypofunction[6] are other external vestibular problems that cause the patient to demonstrate similar clinical symptoms. To a PTA, the symptoms can be the same, and the greatest concern is the patient falling.[2]

The vestibular problem could also be central in origin. Individuals who have damage to the brainstem from meningitis, tumors, cerebellar damage, brainstem strokes, or spinal/head trauma will often demonstrate vestibular dysfunction. This may involve the vestibular nuclei, cerebellum, midbrain, and higher cortical centers. In central vestibular problems, interventions often include exercises that gradually habituate the vestibular system to the movements or situations that trigger the dizziness or disequilibrium response. It is necessary for the patient's CNS to learn to readapt

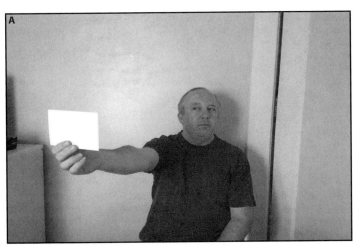

Figure 4-3A. VOR exercises. Both exercises may be progressed by increasing the speed of movement while the focus is maintained on the target. VOR X1: The card remains stationary and the person moves his head from side to side, keeping his eyes on the target on the card.

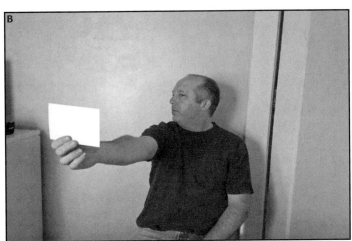

Figure 4-3B. VOR X2: The head and the card are moved in opposite directions at the same time, while the person keeps his eyes on the target on the card.

to vestibular stimulation. There are several interventions that could be delegated to the PTA in this situation; examples include VOR X1 and X2 exercises. In the VOR X1 exercise, the patient is positioned in the sitting position (then progressed to standing as able) and holds an index card with a printed "X" (the target) in the middle. The patient holds this card at eye level and is asked to move the head from side to side and told to keep the "X" in clear focus. If the patient is able to maintain a clear focus, then the patient is asked to increase the speed of the side-to-side movement. Next, the same exercise is performed, but this time the head is moved up and down. This exercise is performed in 1-minute bouts. As the patient improves, he or she can progress to the VOR X2 exercise. It is basically the same as the X1 exercise, but this time, the patient moves the head side to side while simultaneously moving the index card from side to side in the opposite direction as the movement of the head. Again, the patient is asked to keep a clear focus of the target. If the target becomes blurry or jumps around, the speed is decreased (Figures 4-3A and B).

Another goal of vestibular rehabilitation is to challenge the vestibular system during standing and gait. When the body seems to be in motion, one primary goal of the vestibular information is to determine whether the motion is caused by the body swaying on a hard surface (movement over one's BOS) or whether the surface itself is causing the perturbations (standing on a compliant surface such as a pillow or being shoved by something such as a dog). Thus, with vestibular rehabilitation, one primary goal is adaptation of the vestibular input so the patient can once again tolerate this information. Once that is achieved, then creating activities that help the CNS process vestibular input along with somatosensory and vision can become an objective. Introducing activities that encourage the person to walk through obstacle courses that have compliant and noncompliant surfaces, then adding throwing and catching balls or striking at objects such as balloons, can further enhance the use of all 3 sensory modalities to optimize balance. Any activity that encourages normal balance reactions can be used sequentially as part of vestibular rehabilitation and balance training. Various vestibular exercises can be found online and incorporated into a therapy session or set up for practice at home once the patient is capable of performing home exercises.[7,8] Interventions may be delegated to the PTA. An example of a patient with vestibular dysfunction can be found online under the examination section of Chapter 5.

Balance problems caused by the vestibular system can often be modified by using both vision and proprioception input to facilitate balance reactions. The patient can use electronic tools such as the Nintendo Wii Balance System or other electronic devices to increase the proprioceptive feedback as well as the visual recognition of successfully completing the task presented. These tools can be used to enhance proprioception and vision and modify the CNS's sensitivity to vestibular problems. Computerized environments such as virtual reality or immersive environments can also be successfully used as part of vestibular rehabilitation.[9] The use of these types of environments for training will become more common in the future, and the PTA may be delegated the training by the PT. (Refer to the section on technology later in this chapter.)

Dual Tasking as Part of Balance Training

One important aspect of balance training is dual tasking or performing 2 tasks simultaneously. This type of training forces the motor system to respond with adequate balance reaction while the patient is concentrating on a specific task. There are an infinite number of activities a PT can perform that are considered dual tasking. For example, if the patient is asked to walk and count backward by 3 starting at 100, the activity is considered dual tasking. Dual tasking just means that the patient's attention needs to be on some cognitive activity while the motor system is running a movement such as walking, eating, or brushing one's hair. Often therapists think a patient has adequate balance, but once the individual's attention is placed on something other than reacting to a perturbation, the patient will fall. If a patient is practicing a transfer while the television is on and something on the TV draws his or her attention, the question would be: "Does the patient stop the transfer and sit back down, fall during the transfer, or automatically continue with the motor activity while attending to what was on the TV?" This dual tasking is the only way a therapist can have confidence that the patient will respond adequately when perturbed during everyday life.[10–13] In many neuromuscular conditions, the ability of the patient to successfully dual task may be impaired. This is a very important skill to teach the patient to provide the opportunity to again participate in normal life activities, which require an individual to take on multiple tasks. For example, increasing cognitive load by asking the patient to walk and talk at the same time or by having the patient perform 2 motor tasks like walking while transporting a cup full of water are common interventions that may improve dual task performance.

In addition to dual tasking, the therapist can increase the difficulty of the activity itself. Asking the patient to walk down a hallway with no obstacles still requires balance. Asking the patient to walk through an obstacle course that has turns and a lot of visual distortions such as mirrors or toys to step over creates additional difficulties. Asking the patient to walk sideways through the same maze while singing "Happy Birthday" or listing the names of his or her closest friends increases the difficulty of the motor requirements and also is dual tasking. When the PTA has a group of individuals who need or would benefit from balance training and who have similar balance impairments, a group class can be created. Using stations and pairing the individuals as partners can create a fun and social experience. Examples of what might be performed at various stations for dual tasking and balance exercises are found in Box 4-2.

Box 4-2

Examples of Activities That Could Be Used in a Group Balance Class

---

Station 1: Have 2 individuals perform stand to sit while throwing a light ball back and forth. Increase the activity by either increasing the weight of the ball to cause greater perturbations or increase the distance between the 2 chairs.

Station 2: Have 2 individuals walk down a rug that has objects underneath such as tubes, foam, egg cartons, or balls. Increase the difficulty by having the patients either talk to each other while walking, walk while blindfolded, or walk carrying a tray initially with a glass only and then with a glass with water. If a patient has vestibular problems, do not use a blindfold for this activity because the individual will likely fall.

Station 3: Have each participant practice hitting a hanging ball with a plastic bat or a long cardboard tube. Increase the difficulty by having the hanging ball move.

Station 4: Have each patient walk up and over 2 steps or up and down a few steps. Increase the activity by having them talk to each other.

Station 5: Have each patient sit on a chair that has a compliant surface, such as a seat on a rocker or soft form, so his or her weight will not allow him or her to feel the horizontal surface. Have the patients throw and catch plastic balls. To increase the difficulty, make the balls smaller and heavier.

Station 6: Have a pair hit a balloon back and forth with their hands while standing. Increase the difficulty by having the pair increase the distance between each other.

The PT may recommend that the PTA record what is happening at each station. This can be performed by having the pair of individuals write down or check off how many times they completed the task as well as the difficulty level achieved. The participants can see their improvement when they are asked to record. The PTA can observe whether any patients are decreasing their accomplishments, which might mean a problem is developing (progressive deterioration, a new health issue, a depressed patient, or some other body system problem).

Reaction Time to Perturbations

Reaction time to a perturbation is based on 3 important aspects of the CNS. First, the brain must receive accurate and nonconflicting sensory information from proprioceptive, vestibular, and visual peripheral receptors. Second, the brain must process this information at various levels. Third, the CNS must select and control the correct motor programs to respond appropriately. Thus, the PTA may be instructed in the direction and force of perturbations within specific positions to impairment train this function. If the PTA is providing perturbations as a means of training the patient to improve balance reactions, the PTA must start with light perturbations, then progress to greater forces as the patient is able to successfully maintain balance following these activities. The PTA can then alter the direction of force (forward-backward, side to side, or diagonal, etc) and then also the rate of perturbations. This will improve not just anticipatory reactions, but also reactive control.

Hands-On Therapeutic Intervention or Augmented Treatment Intervention

In the therapeutic environment, there are often situations in which the therapist needs to provide additional assistance—whether using his or her hands or other devices— to allow the patient to more successfully succeed in the task being practiced. Although hands-on therapeutic intervention or augmented treatment intervention is not necessarily exclusive of functional or impairment training, it is presented as a separate category so the PTA will understand more clearly the various options available with regard to providing additional assistance that may allow for more successful outcomes.

The goals of using the therapist's hands during therapeutic interventions are as follows:

1. To guide or assist the patients during functional movements.

2. To control specific patterns of movement while preventing stereotypic patterns.

3. To give patients the sensory input as feedback for correct movement control.

4. To allow patients to experience the functional movements that will encourage them to move from one spatial position to another.

5. To create a limited environment where patients can succeed at the desired task.

6. To motivate patients by letting them experience some aspect of success and potential accomplishment toward a desired function.

The PTA may be instructed by the PT to teach the patient by verbally describing, visually demonstrating, or kinesthetically handling through a movement. The PT gives those instructions because the best way for the patient to learn has been identified. This is referred to as a learning style. If this has not been identified, the PTA can try instructing the patient using each style or a combination of the 3. It is very important that the PTA know his or her learning style because all of us tend to teach through the style with which we are most comfortable. The preferential style of the PTA may not be the best for the patient. It is the responsibility of all health care practitioners to create the optimal environment for learning, which means, initially, to teach through the style of the patient and then progress to less optimal styles to allow the patient to adapt to the external world.

Relaxation Techniques

There are many techniques the PTA can use to teach or encourage a patient to relax. The one approach that will not work, but is often used, is asking the patient to relax. This is especially true with patients who have increased tone or hypertonicity. The presence of hypertonicity points out the fact that the person is unable to decrease the tone voluntarily or the patient would.[14,15]

The use of slow, deep breathing encourages the patient to use the diaphragm, which will relax the autonomic system and generally relax tension and tone.[16,17] If the patient can follow commands, then having him or her practice this type of breathing will help relax the system and reduce tone. This can be practiced in supine, side-lying, sitting, or even standing positions. Asking the patient to participate in this type of breathing can empower the patient to a technique that will help reduce tension and tone when life or the internal or external environment triggers the motor response.[4]

The environment within which the patient is living, whether in a rehabilitation center, a skilled nursing facility (SNF), or at home, can often be used to decrease the tension or tone. Many types of music will relax individuals, and the PTA can determine the best music to use by asking the patient or the patient's family. Having calm, soft music in the background can help bring the emotional system into balance, and that system often creates tension or tone in muscles.[15] Similarly, lighting in the room can affect the tone of patients. Bright lighting or darkness can be very alerting and often will increase tone. Soft, natural lighting from the sun is the best, if available. Similarly, the PTA's voice can be a critical factor in teaching relaxation. If the PTA has a high-pitched voice, the voice itself can often increase tone, while a soft, monotone voice can lead to relaxation.[4]

When touching the patient, the PTA should use firm or constant pressure versus a light touch. Light touch is very alerting and often creates a protective response that, when a patient cannot control tone, will only increase that tone. Thus, when moving from one point on the body to another, do not let go of the first hold until the second spot on the skin/body has been touched. Once the initial touch is accepted and the patient relaxes, the PTA should not let go and retouch because the patient will again need to relax to the new touch. If the initial deep pressure touch is held as the new touch is applied, the patient often does not see the new touch as threatening and thus has no need to elicit a protective reaction. It is often recommended that the PTA also inform the patient before changing holds, allowing the patient's CNS time to adjust to the fact that new sensory information will be applied from the second touch. The PTA needs to use observational skill to identify the responses of the patient and how the patient responds to the touch.

Another way to help decrease tone or cause relaxation is a technique that can be used when the patient is supine. Take hold of the heel of a foot with one hand while placing the second hand under the back of the knee, placing the knee in slight flexion. If one of the patient's legs is more involved or has higher tone than another, start with the least involved leg. Then gently use a pushing motion up through the leg, causing slight compression and oscillations that travel up the leg into the spine and neck regions. The speed of the oscillations is patient dependent. Always begin with slow, gentle oscillations. Then, increase the speed and force slightly and see whether the patient's body shows more relaxation. The patient's response to the oscillations will tell the PTA the best amount of force and speed to use. This approach should never be very forceful or performed at a high speed. If the patient can follow commands, have him or her take slow, deep breaths as the PTA oscillates from the leg. This will combine the diaphragmatic breathing and the gentle oscillation, causing even more relaxation. This approach should never cause pain. The PTA may observe oscillations through the leg and lower spine and then, as the movement approaches the higher spinal segments, those segments may move as one unit. This may be an indication of tightness within the spine and should be reported to the PT to determine whether additional spinal treatments need to be applied. These restrictions may also be the site of pain in a patient because those segments move as one unit, are tight, and may be compressed. Again, discussion with the PT is appropriate.

When confronted with a patient who has very high extensor tone when supine, this technique is often very effective prior to having the patient roll. Once the tone begins to decrease, the PTA can easily flex the knee and hip with rotation, triggering a body-on-body righting reaction and thus beginning the motion of rolling. The patient can more easily take control of the movement once the hypertonicity has been reduced.

The same type of oscillations can be performed from the head, but the PTA is cautioned first to ask the PT whether it is appropriate, and then, if told to incorporate it into the plan of care, to begin very gently, holding the head with both hands. Make sure hands do not cover the ears because that will take away auditory sound and often causes the patient to become alert, which increases tone. The PTA needs to use observational skills as well as his or her own tactile and proprioceptive feedback to determine the speed and intensity of the oscillations. The patient's response to the gentle movements will determine the rate and amount of gentle compression. Again, the patient can be asked to breathe deeply while the oscillations are performed. Often, the PTA can observe specific areas of tightness once the patient begins to relax. The oscillations should cause gentle movement within the entire body of the patient. There may be joints, especially in the spine, that are restricted, and those joints will move as one unit. If the PTA finds something he or she does not understand, reporting and discussing those findings with the PT is appropriate. The PT can be asked for guidance to determine the best way to handle the restrictions. When oscillating from the head, the PTA should never try to trigger a neck-on-body right reaction because the weight of the body is too great. The PT may use this technique to begin head-on-body righting with a small child, but it takes tremendous skill and should not be performed by the PTA until those skills have been learned and the PT has given that aspect of intervention to the PTA. Relaxation can be part of using handling techniques but, again, high tone is often generated because of a lack of stability within the joints themselves so the PTA must exercise caution when handling after relaxation is triggered. Normalizing muscle tone using relaxation techniques is the goal, not taking away hypertonicity and replacing it with hypotonicity.

These gentle oscillations can be applied through the knee when the patient is in the sitting position to encourage postural extension of the trunk. Another way to facilitate the same postural extension is by having the patient sit on the side of the mat while the PTA is sitting on a therapy ball behind the patient. The ball can be placed against the trunk to provide stability and facilitate postural extension while the PTA slips 2 legs along the lateral aspects of both sides of the patient's trunk and under the arms. The PTA can slowly bring the patient's arms into abduction and slight external rotation of the shoulder by slowly rocking on the ball from side to side. This abduction and external rotation will also facilitate postural extension of the trunk. The PTA can slowly shift weight on the ball from side to side, which will cause the patient to laterally move from one hip to another. If capable, the patient can be asked to reach with one hand toward a target as the PTA shifts weight onto the hip that would naturally bear weight as the patient reaches toward the target. This technique will cause reduction or relaxation of high tone and facilitate balance reactions and postural extension of the trunk. These techniques can be combined as the patient begins to take control over the movement itself.[4] Examples of these relaxation techniques can be found on the video site that accompanies this text. It is recommended that the PTA practice these skills with another PTA. In that way, the PTA, acting as the patient, can provide feedback to the individual performing the techniques. Individuals with normal tone will still relax when these approaches are applied. The PTA can observe how different people react differently given the same relaxation techniques.

Handling Techniques

Techniques that are used to guide a movement from one position to another are considered handling techniques. There are many ways to guide or facilitate movement.[18-24] Techniques such as proprioceptive neuromuscular facilitation (PNF)[18] were initially designed to focus on various motor impairments within specific patterns of movement or various diagonal patterns. The focus of this approach is often strengthening muscle groups, increasing range within specific functional patterns, facilitating agonistic and antagonistic patterns to gain coactivation or stability around joints during both weight-bearing and nonweight-bearing activities (closed- and open-chain activities), and guiding the patient within patterns to move in horizontal (rolling), coming to sit, standing, and ambulating. A PTA may be introduced to these patterns during school, but developing a high level of skill requires additional training and many hours of practice. A section of this chapter specifically discusses PNF and its application to patients with CNS dysfunction.

The approach that originally used the term *handling techniques* was the Bobath approach,[19,20] an approach that, within the United States today, has evolved into a methodology known as Neuro-Developmental Treatment (NDT).[20] Although specific aspects of the approach have changed and the theoretical constructs behind the methodology have incorporated more current theories of motor control, motor learning, and neuroplasticity, many of the techniques remain the same. For specific information on NDT, please refer to a later section in this chapter.

In general, a PTA will need to learn how to "handle" or guide a patient in performing the following activities:

1. Rolling over or from side to side in bed.

2. Coming to sit from the horizontal position whether on the floor or in bed.

3. Moving over one's BOS in sitting to independently sit for reaching, feeding, donning clothes, etc.

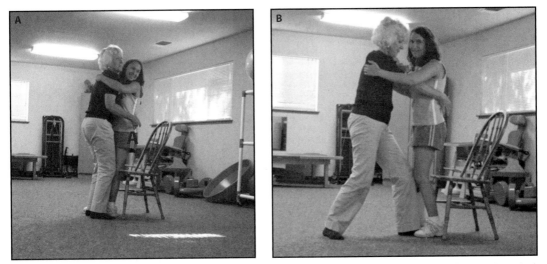

Figure 4-4. Handling a dependent patient when coming to stand for a transfer. (A) Incorrect: The therapist is vertical, and the patient is off vertical and falling backward. (B) Correct: The therapist is slightly off vertical, and the patient has the opportunity to feel vertical or upright posture.

4. Coming to stand from both a horizontal position when on the floor or bed (half-kneel to stand or squat to stand) or while rising from a chair (partial squat to stand) to reach or prior to initiating walking.

5. Inability of the patient to perform an activity because of abnormal muscle function (eg, weakness, hypertonicity, or fluctuation in the state of the motor pool).

6. Perceptual/cognitive problems create movement distortions or level of consciousness prevents interactions.

7. When the patient needs to participate in a successful movement response to realize potential within his or her motor control system.

Although entire textbooks[21,25,26] discuss specific handling techniques and patterns of movement to be used to assist patients following a CNS insult, the PTA is encouraged to watch individuals move, to shut one's eyes, and to feel the movement as the body rolls over, comes to sit, moves in sitting, rises to standing, and walks. If a therapist is guiding a patient through a movement, the therapist needs to differentiate feedback that relates to the therapist regarding where the clinician is in space from the feedback that tells the therapist where the patient's body is in space. For example, if a PTA is guiding a patient to standing from a w/c or chair and is guarding the patient by limiting flexion of the patient's knees, then the feet of the therapist and the patient will occupy space very close to each other. If the therapist is feeling totally stable and vertical, the patient's body cannot be in the same vertical position, and generally, the patient will be leaning backward and have a sense of falling. If, on the other hand, the therapist feels slightly off balance posterior, then the patient has an opportunity to stand erect. Once the patient is erect, there will be little need to grab the therapist, the patient's biomechanical system will be stacked optimally, the feedback to the patient will be accurate with regard to verticality, and the entire environment will often become more relaxed for both individuals (Figures 4-4A and B).

Handling techniques are often used to assist a patient to roll over. That patient may be at a low state of consciousness, may have flaccid or hypertonic extremities, may not be able to follow a command, or may not want to move. Generally, it is easiest to assist a patient to roll by handling a LE. If the patient is in supine (on the back) and needs to roll to the side (to relieve body pressure, to change sheets, to prepare to come to sit, or some other functional activity), the PTA will often handle from one LE. The extremity of choice will be the leg that needs to move to attain a

Figure 4-5A. Rolling the patient to the side using the leg or foot as the point of control. Initially handle leg into flexion, slight abduction, and external rotation.

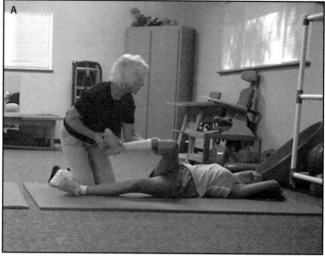

Figure 4-5B. Handle the rotation at the pelvis by maintaining flexion of the hip with slight abduction while guiding into internal rotation.

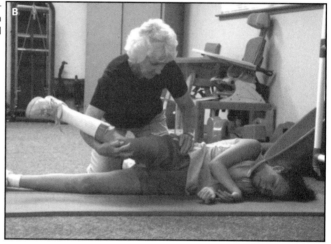

side-lying position. That is, if the patient needs to roll to the right, the left leg will need to flex, slightly abduct, and externally rotate initially, followed by flexion and internal rotation to guide the pelvis onto the right side. The opposite would be true if rolling to the left. The specific amount of flexion, abduction, and external rotation needed initially depends on the patient's muscle tone and ROM. The PTA should guide or control the pelvis at the hip, using the entire leg while moving the leg toward the desired side (Figures 4-5A and B). The trunk will follow the pelvis either through a body on head or a body on body on head righting reaction.

Handling an individual from side-lying to sit is easily performed by applying pressure to the patient's topside anterior iliac crest in a downward and posterior direction (Figure 4-6A). The PTA may need to assist the patient's upper body and head. This can be performed by supporting the patient from the back, under the bottom side arm (brachial plexus) and head (Figure 4-6B).

Once the patient is in a sitting position, a large variety of movement activities can be guided and practiced. The PTA can support the patient from the back while sitting on a ball (Figure 4-7A). In this position, the PTA can control both UEs as well as the trunk to assist in activities such as weight shifting and reaching. The PTA can work on similar activities while in the half-kneel position (Figure 4-7B). The leg that the therapist is using to kneel on can also be used to support the patient's trunk while the half-kneeling leg can be used to direct the patient's UE during reaching

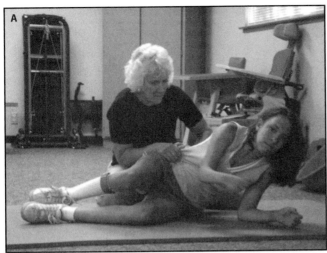

Figure 4-6A. Handling from side-lying to sitting. Pressure is placed in a downward and posterior direction on the topside anterior iliac crest to guide the topside hip into sitting.

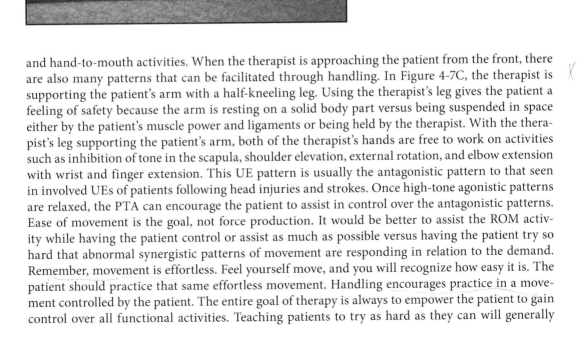

Figure 4-6B. The patient's upper body and head are guided to vertical by supporting the patient's trunk under the brachial plexus and head from the back on the bottom side.

and hand-to-mouth activities. When the therapist is approaching the patient from the front, there are also many patterns that can be facilitated through handling. In Figure 4-7C, the therapist is supporting the patient's arm with a half-kneeling leg. Using the therapist's leg gives the patient a feeling of safety because the arm is resting on a solid body part versus being suspended in space either by the patient's muscle power and ligaments or being held by the therapist. With the therapist's leg supporting the patient's arm, both of the therapist's hands are free to work on activities such as inhibition of tone in the scapula, shoulder elevation, external rotation, and elbow extension with wrist and finger extension. This UE pattern is usually the antagonistic pattern to that seen in involved UEs of patients following head injuries and strokes. Once high-tone agonistic patterns are relaxed, the PTA can encourage the patient to assist in control over the antagonistic patterns. Ease of movement is the goal, not force production. It would be better to assist the ROM activity while having the patient control or assist as much as possible versus having the patient try so hard that abnormal synergistic patterns of movement are responding in relation to the demand. Remember, movement is effortless. Feel yourself move, and you will recognize how easy it is. The patient should practice that same effortless movement. Handling encourages practice in a movement controlled by the patient. The entire goal of therapy is always to empower the patient to gain control over all functional activities. Teaching patients to try as hard as they can will generally

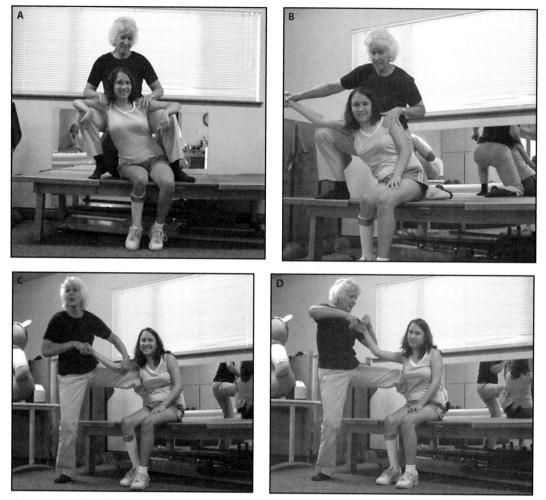

Figure 4-7. (A) Handling while in sitting. The therapist sits on a ball while supporting the trunk while placing the arms/shoulder girdle in flexion, abduction, external rotation, and scapular protraction. (B) The therapist supports the patient's trunk with the leg that is kneeling while using the half-kneeling leg to support a shoulder allowing the patient's arm to elevate; externally rotate with shoulder protraction. (C) While the patient is in sitting, the therapist supports the patient's involved upper extremity and slowly assists in shoulder elevation, external rotation, and shoulder pro- and retraction. (D) Handling from the front. The therapist handles the patient from the hand and posterior hip. These handling positions should be changed frequently enough to keep the patient from becoming dependent upon the therapist's hands.

create a large amount of hypertonicity and, thus, limit functional control. The PTA can handle the patient's pelvis and pelvic movement by handling the anterior hip through downward and posterior pressure on one side while applying downward and anterior pressure on the opposite posterior pelvic rim. This pressure will facilitate postural extension of the trunk and encourage the patient to sit up and weight shift (Figure 4-7D).

Patients can be brought to standing in many different ways. The patient can be guided to standing from sitting with the therapist guiding from one UE. Usually, the PTA should guide from the more involved UE (Figures 4-8A and B). If the patient needs maximal assistance to come to stand, then a ball and a high/low mat or table can be used effectively. First, bring the patient forward in the chair. Next, place his or her UEs over a medium-size ball, which can then be placed on the edge of the high/low mat. Next, bring the patient forward over the ball as the ball rolls onto the mat. The

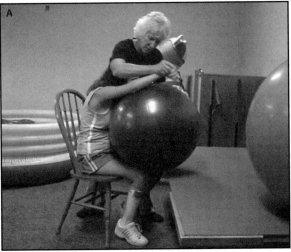

Figure 4-8A. Guiding to stand from the more involved side. The ball is positioned in front of the patient within the patient's lap.

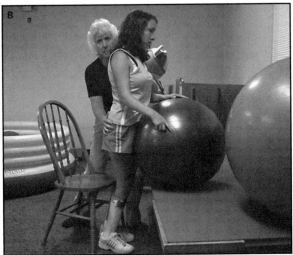

Figure 4-8B. The patient and the ball are guided in order to roll the patient's COG over her feet before bringing her to upright.

patient's COG should now be over the feet, with the hips flexed and the trunk supported by the ball. Next, the PTA can press on the high/low mat control device and begin to raise the mat/table. The table will bring the patient to stand in a relaxed manner with maximal support. The arms should remain relaxed in shoulder elevation and scapular protraction. Once the trunk is stacked into a biomechanical position, the PTA may need a counterforce in front of the ball to avoid the ball slipping away from the patient and therapist. Initially, the handling techniques will need to be from the side of the patient. As soon as the patient is relaxed with the trunk resting over the ball with the feet flat, the therapist can reposition his or her body to the rear of the patient. At that time, the therapist can reach under the patient's upper trunk and guide the upper body toward a vertical posture. Generally, the head will right after the shoulders, and the patient will be standing in a normal upright position. The patient will feel stabilized between the therapist and the ball. Weight shifting can be practiced to encourage body support over the feet. If the patient slowly rolls the ball from side to side, forward, and backward, he or she will be facilitating his or her own perturbations for balance and postural reactions. The PTA can also practice partial stand to squat by having the patient or therapist control the table mat's position as it goes up and down. Once the patient can go from stand to sit and back up again, he or she will usually have the sit to stand pattern within the

Figure 4-8C. The patient is guided onto a large ball. Slow rocking can be done in this position in order increase relaxation.

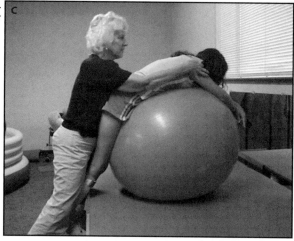

Figure 4-8D. Roll the patient onto her feet while relaxed in order to maintain normal postural extension without causing extensor hypertonicity.

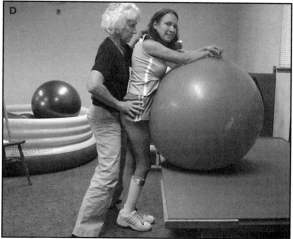

motor control of his or her CNS. Therapists often use this same approach on children, using a ball that is large enough to bring the child into standing off the ball (Figures 4-8C and D).

The PT may ask the PTA to begin ambulation training before the patient comes to standing independently. The PTA must remember that ambulation uses different combinations of motor programs than the sit to stand or stand to sit. The PTA may be asked to stabilize the ankle/knee interactions using an orthotic device. Similarly, the PT may want the PTA to instruct the patient in the use of either a walker or a cane to assist in balance and stability during gait. It is very important for the PTA to emphasize an erect posture of the patient's trunk and head. If the patient is encouraged to stand and walk on bent hips, the patient will need more power to hold him- or herself upright, will fatigue more quickly, and will limit the type of balance reactions available to the CNS. Additional recommendations for handling children, adolescents, and adults can be found in Chapters 8 through 13. A recording of handling techniques that illustrate rolling, coming to sit, sit to kneel, kneel to half-kneel, and half-kneel to stand can be found online to complement this text.

Use of Assistive Devices While Handling

A PTA may use pulleys, exercise tubing, bolsters, wedges, balls, foam, and taping to limit or encourage specific movement patterns while preventing others. For the patient to be considered functionally independent, the PTA and/or PT needs to remove the need by the patient for handling techniques and/or the need for therapeutic/adaptive equipment. The continued use of adaptive equipment may allow the patient to be functional without another person assisting, but that equipment often limits the environment within which the patient can function.

Body weight–supported treadmill training (BWSTT) is considered an augmented approach. The degree of augmentation may be as assistive as when the PT or PTA needs to control a motor response, such as placement of the foot during the swing phase or limited to only unloading some of the patient's body weight. This augmentation is performed to drive an appropriate motor response and, thus, keep the entire LE within an acceptable parameter of performance during gait.[27-30] Additional information regarding BWSTT can be found later in this chapter.

Using the Sensory System to Enhance/Reinforce or to Retrain Function

Following CNS insults, many patients have decreased sensory awareness and/or sensory processing problems.[31-35] It is the PT's responsibility to evaluate for these deficits, but delegation of training may be given to the PTA. Thus, the PTA needs to be aware of each sensory system and how intervention may increase or decrease input to any one of these systems. Similarly, some patients develop sensory processing problems because of overuse, as seen in dystonia. Understanding the sensory systems and their function is critical:

1. In order to use them appropriately as part of treatment in the clinical environment

2. For identifying when the patient is negatively reacting to that input

3. To understanding how sensory retraining can lead to functional ability as seen in patients with dystonia

The auditory system was already discussed in relation to the use of voice as a therapeutic tool. Similarly, when the PTA demonstrates to the patient, the patient's visual system is engaged in reception and interpretation of the visual array. At times, the environmental input of either or both auditory and visual sensory information may be overwhelming to the CNS and actually decrease function. Thus, the PTA may be asked to initially intervene in a quiet environment in a room where the walls are painted a solid color without pictures or windows. Once the patient begins to improve in motor function, the auditory and visual environments can become more complex and more demanding of the CNS to continue to run appropriate motor programs while the world bombards the brain with sensory information. The PTA also needs to remember that when working with the elderly, these systems may have changed over the lifetime, and an increase in the amount of specific input may be necessary to facilitate learning.[36,37]

Similarly, proprioception and vestibular information can be increased or decreased depending on the intervention environments created by the therapist. Often, having the patient supine in a quiet environment can lead to a high awareness of proprioceptive information at joints and muscles using assistive motions and joint compression and traction. Once the patient begins to feel those sensations, the PTA can move the patient to more physically demanding environments, such as sitting, and have the patient again be aware of the sensory input. These types of treatment environments would be considered sensory training or sensory processing training. They can often be performed during the patient's rest periods because they require relaxation and, when accompanied by deep breathing, will often decrease the state of the motor generators, thus dampening inappropriate proprioceptive information from the muscles and joints. Many philosophies and/or intervention suggestions[22,38–41] learned through readings and course attendance emphasize this type of sensory training.

Having patients differentiate sensory objects with vision shielded is a way to help them develop or relearn sensory discriminations. Initially, the patient may need to kinesthetically feel and see the object. Then, the object is shielded from sight and the patient is asked to recognize what is being felt. That recognition can be through verbal responses or pointing to pictures of similar objects. There is an endless number of ways patients can be taught to process sensory information. Some of those possibilities will be taught while in school, some taught by other therapists in the clinic, some taught in courses, and some discovered by the PTA. This process of learning will continue throughout a therapist's professional lifetime as long as the PTA remains open to learning new skills.

Obviously, the sensory systems are part of learning and are critical to relearning functional movement. When a sensory system itself is damaged, the function may be lost or diminished or even cause additional problems to the motor system. This damage can be due to a stroke, head injury, degeneration, or demanding repetitive activity over a long period of time. Dystonia is considered a problem in kinesthetic sensory processing. It is often considered a problem of overuse of a system that has led to dysfunction or inappropriate processing of that specific sensation.[42–50] Dystonia is often seen in individuals who repetitively and often use a specific motor pattern at a high speed. Musicians, typists, and computer users all repetitively use specific motor patterns as part of daily living. The result can lead to the somatosensory system no longer being able to differentiate slight differences in input, and the end result is a mass motor response to activity. When the individual wants to type specific letters on a computer, all fingers type simultaneously, thus causing tremendous error in the motor response. A musician who uses rapidly changing motor responses within a small ROM demands fine gradation and can overuse the system with the result that the somatosensory system can no longer differentiate those fine changes in input.[42,46,47] Dystonia can also be due to a genetic predisposition that develops as the person ages. No matter the causation, sensory retraining begins by having the individual practice some of the same patterns of movement but in different spatial positions, which trigger different sensory neurons both peripherally as well as on the primary and secondary sensory cortices.[40,42,49] There is a lot of research on dystonia, and the PTA needs to be aware that this problem can exist and that there are treatment protocols to help the individual retrain the sensory cortices.[42,43,48,49] The PTA will know that the treatment objectives are being met by the patient's success at doing the IADL or participation activity that has been set as the goal.

Participation Training

The World Health Organization's International Classification of Functioning, Disability and Health model, as discussed in Chapter 1, stresses that problems with functional activities often decrease an individual's ability to participate in life. Thus, prior to beginning intervention, it is very important to determine those activities that the individual values and hopes to return to once rehabilitation has been completed. An individual may want to go fly-fishing, bird watching, golfing, gold panning, or to religious services or participate in some other type of activity that he or she hopes to resume. Those activities fall under the category of "participation" and lead to improved quality of life. Any activity that might be considered a high level of motor function will most likely incorporate postural function, reciprocal limb movements, ambulation, and many other motor programs that blend together to create the activity the individual values. For that reason, the PTA should inquire into what the individual hopes to someday be able to accomplish. After the individual describes what is needed to perform that activity, the therapist needs to create an environment that will lead to accomplishment of that activity. For example, assume an individual wants to fly-fish but has had a stroke in the left hemisphere and thus shows signs of right hemiplegia. His sitting balance is poor, he has moderate use of this right UE, and his right LE has developed an extensor synergy typically seen post-stroke. The therapist should never tell the patient that his fly-fishing days are over because no one knows that. Instead, ask the patient what he has to do when he is fly-fishing. Assume initially that he is going to perform this activity while sitting. Ask him or a family member to bring in his fishing rod. The base of the rod can be placed in a weighted can that will hold the rod vertical. Then, have the patient sit on the side of a mat with a gym ball supporting his right shoulder. Use a Velcro (Velcro USA) glove to secure his right hand to the rod. Ask the patient to slowly move the rod back and forth similarly to part of the ROM he might use to cast the rod. The range can be enlarged as the shoulder function returns. This activity will automatically perturb his sitting balance, and neuroplasticity should help with regaining that function. The PTA can sit behind the patient on another gym ball or in the kneeling position and maintain the patient's trunk in postural extension while moving his right arm back and forth as if he were casting. The activity is not yet fly-fishing, but as a PTA you are providing the environment that will lead to participation in that activity. The specific activity (in this case, fly-fishing) is determined by the patient. It is the creativity of the PTA that encourages the patient to regain the motor function needed to maintain hope that the patient will again participate in those activities that were loved prior to the stroke. The PTA can use a variety of measures (as described in Chapter 5) to reassess the patient's gains in muscle strength, postural control, balance, and UE mobility, all of which are important attributes of performing the activity of fly-fishing. The same activity analysis needs to be performed with each activity the patient chooses. Do not select an activity that you as a PTA think would be good for this patient. Instead, empower the patient to those activities he or she wants to participate in. The internal motivation will lead to practice. Repetitive practice leads to motor learning and then to motor control. (Refer to Chapter 3.) Getting the emotional commitment from the patient is a key to being successful and obtaining positive outcomes following physical therapy. The PTA should always remember that if he or she feels uncomfortable or does not understand the goal or activity the patient is requesting, it is appropriate to discuss the activity with the PT. The PT may also be unfamiliar with the desired activity of the patient, but 2 professionals will be able to come up with many more components within the activity and thus break the task down into a sequential process of learning that can be used to guide the patient toward the desired motor skills.

Limiting Environmental Parameters and Using Adaptive Equipment to Enhance Training

The PT may ask the PTA to conduct a home visit to evaluate environmental factors that will limit functional independence. For example, a patient may be able to walk on a hard surface while in the rehabilitation center, but his or her home may have thick pile carpeting with soft foam support. These 2 environments are not compatible. Either the patient needs to learn to walk on compliant surfaces while under the care of physical therapy or the PT needs to recommend that the family pull up the carpet and replace the floor with something that is a noncompliant surface. If the patient needs to stand and take a step or 2 prior to transferring onto the toilet in his or her bathroom, then that pattern of movement of stepping, turning, and sitting needs to be emphasized as part of the intervention program versus transferring on and off a toilet to a chair.

Similarly, if a patient has difficulty rising from a 90-degree angle in sitting, such as from a toilet or lounge chair, a raised toilet seat or a chair that raises the patient to vertical can assist in making the individual more independent within his or her home environment. The use of adaptive equipment for feeding, long shoehorns for donning shoes, and Velcro for ties can give an individual more freedom in ADL. The reality is that even if a patient has the potential and neuroplasticity to regain total independence, priorities must be set by the PT and patient because of limitations in funding and caps on number of visits. Just because the patient is no longer eligible for physical therapy services does not mean he or she can no longer learn and regain function. It is the PT's and the PTA's job to empower that individual to hope. This does not mean unrealistic expectations. On the contrary, it means identifying steps that the patient needs to follow to regain functions that are important to that individual. That goal should be the long-term home program that turns into everyday life activities, not a lifelong physical therapy program.

The PTA needs to remember that every time a patient is reinforced by the therapist's voice, feedback is being given to the patient. The use of voice has many effects on the CNS of the patient. A loud voice, unless the patient is hard of hearing, can be perceived as yelling at or speaking down to the patient. High pitches can become irritating to a patient, whereas very low pitches can be relaxing. The PTA needs to learn how to modulate the voice to optimize the motor responses of the patient. As the patient regains motor control during intervention, the PTA needs to change the voice's volume and pitch to allow the patient's CNS to practice control under a variety of environmental circumstances.

One very important environmental adaptation for the patient is positioning between therapy sessions. The decision of correct positioning of the limbs and trunk should be a team decision so that consistency is practiced throughout the day. It is very important that the limbs do not hang passively against gravity. This is one of the primary reasons a flaccid shoulder will begin to sublux. The response of the CNS to subluxation is to create stability, and thus, hypertonicity generally develops. That hypertonicity is in patterns or synergistic programs, and those programs can continue to sublux the shoulder because of asymmetry across the shoulder girdle. Some subluxations of the shoulder can be prevented by placing pillows under the arm so that the pull of gravity is not vertical. The limb can be placed on a lapboard to support the shoulder. Tape can be used to maintain shoulder alignment. There are many ways to position limbs while sitting and lying down. Pillows, splints, or cones for the hand are often used between therapy sessions. If the PTA is not sure of correct positioning of the patient, it is appropriate to ask the PT for suggestions. The PTA needs to remember that no clinician has all the best answers to the best intervention for each patient. As a PTA, you may find something that works better for the patient. It is your job to show the PT. It is the PT's job to try to figure out why it works.

Equipment such as canes, w/cs, walkers, transfer boards, shower chairs, and raised toilet seats are often needed when teaching individuals ADL and IADL and are often used during interventions as part of a PTA's skills. Measuring the appropriate length of a quad-cane or a regular cane is within the scope of the PTA's practice, and whether the patient is safe to move from a quad-cane to a regular cane may be expected by the PT to be within the parameters of the function of a PTA. Even if the PTA does not feel comfortable making those decisions early in his or her clinical career and asks for guidance from the PT, with clinical experience many of these decisions will definitely be delegated to the PTA. In some SNF facilities, the PTA orders equipment for the patient to take home when discharged from the facility. Again, the PTA can determine the appropriate measurements of an adjustable shower chair, raised toilet seat, or walker. Which w/c to order can be much more complex, but today, the PT often uses the w/c distributor to help make those decisions. The distributor often has a variety of w/cs and will measure the patient's body dimensions prior to a therapist making any of those decisions. It may be in time that this responsibility will fall to the PTA's scope of practice, but again, the expertise of the distributor should always be available as well as the availability of the PT for recommendations.

SPECIAL FOCUS AREAS:
EMERGING EVIDENCE-BASED TREATMENT APPROACHES

Constraint-Induced Movement Therapy

Constraint-induced movement therapy (CIMT) has been developed as an intervention to improve individuals' functional ability. Most research and applications of CIMT are directed to the UEs, although the principles and techniques are being applied to the LEs as well. CIMT was developed based on several principles: learned nonuse, task-specific training, intense practice that drives neuroplasticity, and behavioral interventions that optimize compliance to a specific exercise regimen.[51–53] In its basic format, CIMT consists of restraining the less-involved extremity (for the UE through the use of a mitt, sling, or glove) for 90% of the day, thereby forcing the individual to use the affected arm in specific tasks. "Shaping" or adapted-task practice is task-oriented training that involves timed trials that ask the patient to perform a particular movement in successive repetitions. The intent of shaping is to drive specific neuroplastic changes in the cortex and to overcome learned nonuse. These timed trials could involve ten 30-second trials with the therapist providing encouragement and feedback during this portion of the training. The next component is called task practice, during which the patient performs functional, meaningful, and salient activities for 15 to 20 minutes at a time. The goal of this training is to perform functional activities that are challenging and important for the patient. The last component includes the behavioral strategies, which are aimed at optimizing practice of the home program. This includes the development of a behavioral contract, a daily exercise journal in which the patient documents the activities performed at home, and periodic assignments of skills to be performed at home. The training is usually performed in a rehabilitation environment where assistance is available and the restraint monitored, and practice is performed up to 6 times daily for at least 2 weeks. Because this type of therapy requires one functional upper limb and one upper limb that show deficits within the motor system, this type of therapy is generally used with individuals post-stroke.[54] A minimum criterion of motor function (10 degrees of finger and 20 degrees of wrist extension) has been shown to be necessary to gain functional control over the hand.[54] The literature is mixed when this type of treatment is initiated in patients soon after their stroke; for this reason, it is not recommended that the PT delegate this intervention if CIMT is used with a patient who is earlier than 3 months post-stroke.[55–59] In contrast, the literature supports CIMT for individuals who had their stroke 3 to 6 months prior to beginning this therapy.[54,60–64] Although most patients who receive this intervention are found within a rehabilitation environment, there is some literature to support this treatment approach with children within the home environment.[65,66]

Whether in inpatient acute rehabilitation or in rehabilitation training within SNFs, PTAs may be asked to perform components of this intervention. The PT should initiate the plan of care and then delegate appropriate tasks to the PTA. The shaping and task-practice components of the intervention could be supervised by the PTA. Initially the PTA may need to assist the extremity in the task-specific movement(s), but the patient is also expected to force the use of the involved extremity. The PTA may need to use handling to facilitate normal movement but should move to have the patient initiating and controlling the movement. The patient is expected to participate actively during each session, and each session should focus on intensive, repetitive task-specific training. This specific training should be identified by the PT of record in the plan of care.[52–54]

Integrating Technology Into Clinical Practice: Body Weight–Supported Treadmill Training, Exoskeletons, Robotics, and Virtual Reality Environments

Technology takes many forms today and will be used more often in the future. This topic covers the use of body weight–support systems, exoskeletons on either ULs or LEs, virtual reality visual adaptive environments, balance equipment, computer technology for cognitive and motor training, and training using interactive gaming programs. This technology has many uses during intervention activities, which a PTA might be expected to use.

The use of BWSTT is one way to decrease the demand for trunk and axial postural control while practicing ambulation (refer to Figures 8-12A and B, Figure 11-10, and Figure 12-7). The amount of power the patient needs for trunk or core postural function can be controlled through suspension while the treadmill simultaneously triggers normal walking patterns. There are various ways to unweight an individual. Some systems use a harness suspended over a treadmill, some are support systems that allow over-ground training ambulation, and others suspend a patient using air and an inflatable suit that the patient dons.[67] There are also suspension systems that can be placed on tracks within a home or physical therapy clinic to allow the individual to practice walking. As the core trunk or postural muscles gain power and endurance, the amount of body weight support can be reduced. Simultaneously, the therapist can demand the patient respond to different speeds and inclines of the treadmill itself. The goal certainly is walking without the need for suspension at all if this is a possibility. Some patients never gain that control, but exercising using BWSTT will keep other muscles strong and provide cardiopulmonary and circulatory function. Functional electrical stimulation could also be used to augment motor output and facilitate movement. Many of these systems can also allow therapists to work on both sitting and standing balance without requiring the patient to control full body weight. This encourages the patient to activate motor control to tolerance and triggers postural coactivation without eliciting abnormal tone.[67,68] (Refer to Chapters 8, 11, and 12 for illustrations on BWSTT.) BWSTT has been shown to be effective in various patient populations, including individuals who have been diagnosed with stroke,[69–73] cerebral palsy,[74,75] Parkinson's disease,[76] multiple sclerosis (MS),[77] and traumatic brain injury.[78,79]

The PTA must always remember that for a patient to become functionally independent, the individual will still need to gain internal postural stability, strength, range, and motor programs without the use of a support system such as an overhead harness. PTAs certainly could be expected to train individuals using BWSTT. These systems are also used by PTs to obtain reliable measures for establishment of specific plans of care. PTAs may be asked to use these same tools to measure ongoing gains following treatment as well as measures of outcomes following interventions.

The following is a specific example of the role of the PTA in this particular intervention approach. At times, the PT will delegate to the PTA a functional activity within which impairment training and control over specific aspects of a motor program are incorporated. An example of this type of combination would be using a body weight–support harness while having a client walk on a treadmill (refer to Figures 8-12A and B, Figure 11-10, and Figure 12-7). The functional activity practiced is walking, varying the rate and incline of the treadmill-walking track to accommodate impairment problems. The motion itself should trigger a stepping program; the PTA should not need to assist in the walking. The body weight–support system eliminates the need for full power and programming for posture and movement during the functional activity. By partially supporting the body weight, the patient is expected to control the entire feed-forward walking program and all its component programs within his or her capable limits. The PTA can change the rate of walking, the power needed to generate force during walking, the incline or decline of the movement, and other components of walking (eg, hard and soft surfaces of the shoe). All these aspects are considered impairment training because the patient is forced to self-correct the programming within the limits of the impairments. As soon as the PTA needs to guide the movement itself (eg, picking up the foot and placing it in its correct biomechanical position), the body-support intervention is not impairment training but would be considered within the third category of intervention. In this third area, considered hands-on guidance by therapists, the PT or PTA may need to use hands-on control to guide motor responses to keep the patient within an acceptable parameter of performance. At the beginning of training, the patient may need help using the involved LE in push-off, swing phase, and heel striking. With repetitive practice, the patient should regain control over that specific pattern of movement. Given the intervention example of body weight–supported walking, the PTA might be delegated both impairment and functional training within the patient's control parameters.

Another type of technology that a PTA may see in the clinic is the use of an exoskeleton. Exoskeletons provide joint stability and are used to assist individuals who have limb-specific stabilization problems, such as someone who has suffered a stroke. Many of these exoskeletons are very expensive and are being used for research. The exoskeleton has a computer program that is sensitive to the force, range, and task-specific movement needed by the patient during the activity. The UE exoskeletons are primarily used in patients post-stroke, whereas the LE technology has been used with individuals who have had a stroke, a spinal cord injury, MS, or Parkinson's disease.[67] Although exoskeletons are not commonly seen in physical therapy clinics, their use will become more frequent as the demand increases and the cost becomes more affordable. At that time, the PTA may be expected to train the individual using an exoskeleton. Many of these devices can be found on the Web as well as information regarding the manufacturer's recommendation of the exoskeleton's primary use.

Virtual reality and interactive gaming are quickly becoming intervention approaches used in stroke rehabilitation and other types of CNS involvement. Virtual reality creates a visual world that is representative of the environment within which the specific task is used and has been used effectively with individuals post-stroke,[80–83] individuals with MS[84] or traumatic brain injury,[85] children who have cerebral palsy,[86] and children who have developmental delays.[87] As an example of the use of a virtual reality environment for an adult, consider the PTA as working on teaching the IADL of grocery shopping using a cart while the patient is on a treadmill. The patient would hold onto a rail at the front of the treadmill. As the patient applies pressure on the support structure, which visually looks like the handle of a grocery cart, and starts walking within the virtual reality environment visually shown in front, she will perceive she is walking down an aisle in a grocery store. When the patient stops to determine whether she wants X versus Y items in the grocery aisle, the treadmill will also stop. The treadmill is driven by the movement of the patient as she starts walking. Using these types of environments, the patient can be monitored for balance, motor coordination, and any other motor impairment that might be a critical factor related to independence and fall risk. For a child, the virtual reality may be a playground or a fantasy world.

Gaming programs that require physical interactions are also quickly becoming a part of clinical practice and considered technology available within a physical therapy environment. The Nintendo Wii and the Sony PlayStation gaming programs that can facilitate balance, strength, and ROM along with other motor strategies have quickly become part of a PT's toolbox related to intervention ideas.[88–90] A patient can be supported using a harness to prevent any chance of falling while actively participating in the activity shown on a TV using one of the gaming programs. The patients can be bowling, skiing, sailing, playing golf, or practicing any other motor skill they value as quality of life participation activities that they plan to return to in the future. For patients of any age, these activities can be fun, competitive with other individuals, and social, and they provide immediate feedback as to success. The programs can store memory of the participant's successes from day to day and objectively show rates of improvement. For individuals whose recovery seems very slow, the patients often do not see these improvements, and this is one way to give concrete, positive feedback regarding their recovery.

Obviously, the use of technologies can be combined. The BWSTT can be used in a virtual environment. The gaming programs can be used as part of telecommunication from a distance.[91] Where technology will take therapy in the future is open to the imagination. The one thing that seems predictable is that PTAs will be using these technologies as part of their scope of practice within the near future.

Specific Intervention Techniques: Proprioceptive Neuromuscular Facilitation and Neuro-Developmental Treatment

This section will discuss 2 specific intervention approaches that have been used in populations with movement dysfunctions due to neurological problems. These 2 techniques involve all categories of intervention: functional training, impairment training, augmented (hands-on) intervention, and even somatosensory retraining. The pervasive use of these approaches in neurological rehabilitation necessitates the discussion of these approaches in detail.

Many critics of these approaches cite the lack of solid scientific evidence behind their use. While that may be currently true, many factors—such as the variability in the use and application of these techniques, the complexity of research methodologies that involve neurological intervention studies, and the lack of valid, reliable, sensitive, and specific tools to assess progress—are major considerations.

It is important to incorporate the principles of neuroplasticity when performing these interventions. This includes selecting activities that are salient, meaningful, and functional for the patient, taking into account the amount of repetitions and the context by which these interventions are used.

Proprioceptive Neuromuscular Facilitation

PNF is an intervention that uses movement patterns incorporating multiplanar, diagonal, functional movement with rotation and inhibition/facilitation principles to effect muscle coordination, strength, and/or length.[18,92] PNF has applications to orthopedic and neuromuscular populations because of its versatility as an intervention. PNF combines patterns, either for the limbs, the trunk, or the whole body, with techniques that can address passive, active-assisted, isometric, concentric, and/or eccentric muscle activity.[92] By combining the movement pattern with the appropriate technique, PNF can be used with multiple types of patient impairments ranging from difficulty initiating movement, movement timing, coordination, co-contraction, static holding, stretching, and strengthening.

PNF was developed based on the neurophysiological principles of muscles discovered by Sherrington in the 1900s and Sister Kenney's manual therapy techniques.[93] Herman Kabat, a neurophysiologist and physician, with Margaret Knott and Dorothy Voss, both PTs, worked in the 1950s to further develop PNF techniques and nomenclature at Kasier Vallejo in California. Knott and Voss published the first book describing PNF in the 1960s.[18] The initial population of patients who drove the development of this technique were individuals suffering from the motor impairments caused by polio. This disease attacked the alpha motor neuron, and this approach is especially effective when considering alpha motor neuron involvement. Polio did not affect upper motor neurons, so these individuals maintained their original motor learning and could draw on those programs to assist in regaining motor function. This approach is especially effective with individuals with orthopedic complications or spinal cord injury because those individuals exhibit impairments of sensory and motor neurons coming to and from the spinal column as well as the peripheral system itself. Today, Kasier Foundation Hospital in Vallejo, California, has an internationally recognized residency program for PTs wishing to intensively study PNF.

The most common PNF patterns are those addressing the limbs, pelvis, or scapulae (Table 4-1).[92,93] While the patient is moving through these patterns, a variety of sensory inputs are

	Table 4-1 **Proprioceptive Neuromuscular Facilitation Patterns for Extremities and Trunk**	
	Start Position	**End Position**
Upper Extremity		
D1 flexion	Shoulder: Extension-adduction-internal rotation Elbow: Extension Forearm: Pronation Wrist: Extension Fingers: Extension	Shoulder: Flexion-adduction-external rotation Elbow: Flexion Forearm: Supination Wrist: Flexion Fingers: Flexion
D1 extension	Shoulder: Flexion-adduction-external rotation Elbow: Flexion Forearm: Supination Wrist: Flexion Fingers: Flexion	Shoulder: Extension-adduction-internal rotation Elbow: Extension Forearm: Pronation Wrist: Extension Fingers: Extension
D2 flexion	Shoulder: Extension-adduction-internal rotation Elbow: Extension Wrist: Extension Finger: Extension	Shoulder: Flexion-abduction-external rotation Elbow: Flexion Wrist: Flexion Finger: Flexion
D2 extension	Shoulder: Flexion-adduction-external rotation Elbow: Flexion Wrist: Flexion Finger: Flexion	Shoulder: Extension-abduction-internal rotation Elbow: Extension Wrist: Extension Finger: Extension
Lower Extremity		
D1 flexion	Hip: Extension-adduction-internal rotation Knee: Extension Ankle: Plantarflexion	Hip: Flexion-adduction-external rotation Knee: Flexion Ankle: Dorsiflexion
D1 extension	Hip: Flexion-adduction-external rotation Knee: Flexion Ankle: Dorsiflexion	Hip: Extension-adduction-internal rotation Knee: Extension Ankle: Plantarflexion
D2 flexion	Hip: Extension-adduction-internal rotation Knee: Extension Ankle: Plantarflexion	Hip: Flexion-abduction-external rotation Knee: Flexion Ankle: Dorsiflexion
D2 extension	Hip: Flexion-abduction-external rotation Knee: Flexion Ankle: Dorsiflexion	Hip: Extension-adduction-internal rotation Knee: Extension Ankle: Plantarflexion

(continued)

Table 4-1 (continued)
Proprioceptive Neuromuscular Facilitation Patterns for Extremities and Trunk

	Start Position	End Position
Pelvis		
Anterior elevation	Pelvis: Depression-posterior rotation	Pelvis: Elevation-anterior rotation
Posterior depression	Pelvis: Elevation-anterior rotation	Pelvis: Depression-posterior rotation
Anterior depression	Pelvis: Elevation-posterior rotation	Pelvis: Depression-anterior rotation
Posterior elevation	Pelvis: Depression-anterior rotation	Pelvis: Elevation-posterior rotation
Scapula		
Anterior elevation	Scapula: Depression-downward rotation	Scapula: Elevation-upward rotation
Posterior depression	Scapula: Elevation-upward rotation	Scapula: Depression-downward rotation
Anterior depression	Scapula: Elevation-downward rotation	Scapula: Depression-upward rotation
Posterior elevation	Scapula: Depression-upward rotation	Scapula: Elevation-downward rotation

implemented by the therapist to facilitate movement. Verbal directions are given in a loud, encouraging voice with short commands such as "Push, now, harder." The therapist's manual contacts are very precise, with the hands over muscles he or she wishes to activate during the pattern using a supportive grip. These manual contacts can be used to provide resistance or support, as needed, depending on the goal of the PNF intervention and the patient's level of motor impairment. Additionally, the therapist can apply joint distraction to facilitate flexion or joint approximation to facilitate extension. To facilitate initiation of the movement, the therapist may deliver a quick stretch to the muscles performing the movement.

The therapist then combines the facilitation techniques and the movement pattern with different PNF techniques addressing how the muscles are contracting and the timing of movements; common PNF techniques are shown below[92]:

- **Rhythmic initiation:** Begins with the therapist moving the patient through the desired movement using passive ROM, followed by active-assistive ROM, active ROM, and finally providing resistance through the ROM.

- **Contract relax and hold relax:** Techniques used either for stretching or for short-duration change to abnormal muscle tone. By using either the Golgi tendon organs or reciprocal inhibition, the patient contracts selected muscles followed by a sustained passive stretch provided by the therapist (contract relax), or passive stretch provided by the therapist is followed by an isometric holding contraction by the patient (hold relax).

- **Rhythmic stabilization:** The patient holds a position while the therapist applies manual resistance. No motion should occur from the patient. The patient should simply resist the therapist's movements. The therapist holds this resistance, and then switches to the alternate pattern, again with the patient holding. Usually rhythmic stabilization is performed in the direction of rotation.

- **Alternating isometrics:** Similar to rhythmic stabilization, but the resistance is applied to both sides of the joint, usually not in the direction of rotation.

For example, the patient may have weakness of the right dorsiflexors due to a stroke. Because of this weakness, the patient demonstrates gait deviations such as shortened right step length, toe contact on the right during initial contact in stance phase, and a foot drop. PNF intervention may be used to strengthen the dorsiflexors while also working on timing and coordination of dorsiflexion in relation to the knee and hip joint. Intervention may start with a limb pattern ending in the right LE in hip flexion, knee flexion, and dorsiflexion. To start, rhythmic initiation may be used to acquaint the patient with the PNF pattern and to allow for passive and active-assisted dorsiflexion, depending on the extent of the patient's weakness. The therapist can increase the resistance to the dorsiflexors as the patient's strength increases to add more challenge. Initially the patient may be positioned in left side-lying and transition to supine, sitting, and standing as the ability to handle the extra resistance of gravity and the challenge of trunk control/balance increases. As the patient masters the PNF pattern motorically and strength improves, then other techniques such as rhythmic stabilization or alternating isometrics can be added or substituted. At an advanced level, the therapist can resist the pattern while the patient ambulates (in the parallel bars if extra stability and UE support is needed).

PNF interventions can also assist in retraining activities such as transfers and gait. Patients with poor trunk control, particularly poor ability to stabilize the trunk via co-contraction during other dynamic movements, such as sit-to-stand transfers, may benefit from PNF interventions. In sitting, the therapist can use rhythmic stabilization with manual contacts at the scapulae and anterior shoulder to work on maintaining an engaged co-contraction (coactivation) of the trunk and increase strength and endurance for maintaining an upright and midline trunk position. This can then be put into a functional task such as sit to stand by applying resistance to the upper trunk through the anterior lean needed at the beginning of the transfer and changing the resistance to more approximation through the shoulder girdle during the lift-off portion of the transfer. The approximation during lift-off will facilitate the patient's trunk and LE extensors, the muscle groups needed to successfully perform lift-off and achieve standing.

Pelvic PNF intervention is commonly employed in gait training. The pelvic PNF patterns can be used selectively to assist the patient with specific phases of gait. For example, should the patient demonstrate a posteriorly rotated pelvis during the swing phase, the pelvic anterior elevation pattern may be used as an intervention. Starting in the side-lying position, the pelvic anterior elevation pattern may be practiced with rhythmic initiation first to familiarize the patient with the pattern and allow the therapist to see what pelvic ROM the patient has, and then the therapist can apply resistance that the patient's strength can tolerate. The therapist can also adapt the resistance to have the patient work on either concentric or eccentric pelvic motor control. This can then be transitioned to gait, as the therapist applies the same resistance to the pelvis during the transition from stance to swing phase of gait.

Full body patterns, such as mass flexion, incorporate multiple PNF patterns and techniques into functional movements such as rolling, allowing for more complex movements and requiring more motor control from patients. Mass flexion is a PNF full body pattern that combines the pelvic anterior elevation pattern with the scapular anterior depression pattern, requiring the whole length of the trunk on one side to be active. Mass flexion pattern can be used as an intervention to help a patient with rolling from supine to side-lying. For example, your patient has had a stroke causing left-sided hemiparesis. PNF intervention may begin with the patient in the right side-lying position practicing the pelvic and scapular patterns individually.[18,94] Once the patient can perform each of these 2 patterns with sufficient control, they can be combined and performed simultaneously to produce the mass flexion pattern. To progress this intervention, the patient can be positioned in a quarter roll position and perform mass flexion with a rolling motion. As the patient gains competence, he or she can be positioned in supine and perform mass flexion with the complete rolling motion.

PNF is an intervention technique that is immensely flexible in application with patients.[92] Therapists can adapt the PNF patterns to work on only one joint to target isolated areas of deficits. Because the patterns and techniques can be interchanged to address specific patient goals and can be advanced within and across treatment sessions, PNF is a valuable intervention to work on a variety of motor system and motor control impairments. The PTA needs to be familiar with basic PNF patterns and techniques, as these may be part of the plan of care determined by the PT.

Neuro-Developmental Treatment

As stated earlier, NDT is an intervention approach, commonly used with people of all ages who have neurological dysfunction, that uses facilitation and inhibition techniques provided in a direct, hands-on approach.[19,25] NDT interventions are individualized based on the patient's impairments and activity limitations and are guided during sessions by the patient's response to treatment.[19] NDT is used in both physical therapy and occupational therapy treatment.

The NDT approach was developed by Berta (physiotherapist) and Karel Bobath (psychiatrist/neurophysiologist) in Germany in the mid-20th century and is sometimes still referred to as the *Bobath concept*.[19,95,96] Originally developed for adults with hemiplegia after stroke and children with cerebral palsy, today NDT is used for many neurological diagnoses. The early theoretical basis of NDT surrounded the restoration of normal postural reflexes progressing rigidly through the developmental sequence to normalize movement. The theoretical basis for NDT has progressed as our understanding of the CNS, motor learning and motor control, and neuroplasticity have evolved. Today, NDT aims to achieve the goal of developing optimal movement patterns through the use of orthotics and appropriate compensations, instead of aiming for completely "normal" movement patterns. The NDT approach is promoted through the Neuro-Developmental Treatment Association,[97] which also provides continuing education specific to NDT, including extensive courses of study for treatment of babies, children, and adults.

Concepts key to the NDT approach include patient handling techniques to facilitate and/or inhibit movement interfering with normal movement patterns using key points of control.[19,25] Handling, in the NDT approach, is therapeutic in nature and uses the therapist's hands and body to provide manual contact and directional cues to the patient's body. The touch used, as light as possible to encourage the best patient response and most movement possible from the patient, is specific to the impairments demonstrated by the patient. Although the touch is light in pressure, it is proprioceptive and does not elicit a light touch withdrawal. Patients with touch sensitivity need deeper touch to facilitate postural patterns and functional movement. The specific touch depends on the reaction of the patient and should be enough to cause appropriate facilitation or inhibition to the patient's muscles, while also providing cues as to the direction of movement.[25,95,96]

Therapists analyze postures and movements, looking for movement dysfunctions present when the individual is asked to move. The NDT approach requires active participation from the patient and the therapist, as the therapist must perform ongoing assessments of the success of the handling in normalizing the patient's movement while the patient must be actively performing the posture or movement.[25] Depending on the patient, rehabilitation goals may work to improve any or all of the following: postural control, coordination of movement sequences, movement initiation, body alignment or posture, abnormal muscle tone, or muscle weakness.

Handling should be provided using key points of control.[19,25] Any part of the patient's body may be a key point of control; this distinction is related to what joint or body segment is required for performance of the selected activity. For example, using the NDT approach to achieve midline trunk orientation in sitting may use key points of control at the patient's sides (above the hip bones), with the therapist keeping an open hand with the fingers spread wide apart. This key point of control allows the therapist manual contact with the abdominal muscles as well as the lower ribs and extensor muscles. As key points of control move farther away from the body segment initiating the movement, the response of the patient may be delayed. For example, the therapist may select the shoulder girdle region of the patient as a key point of control for midline trunk orientation, by placing a hand over the top of the shoulder, with the open hand contacting the clavicles and the scapular spines. This allows the therapist to facilitate left-right orientation, as well as anterior-posterior orientation. Because this point of control is farther away from the abdominal and back extensor muscles, the response seen in the patient may be delayed. The specific response will also require more motor control on the part of the patient, because the handling is more removed from the specific region of the lower trunk and abdominals.

The NDT approach uses many contact points and not just the hands/fingers to provide manual facilitation. One example commonly encountered in the neurological population involves the therapist using his or her tibia in contact with the patient's tibia to provide manual and directional cues for knee control during standing, transfers, and gait. This key point of control allows the therapist to simultaneously use both hands to provide input in other areas, while also providing important handling to the patient's LE.[95] Likewise, the therapist may use the forearm against other body segments of the patient while the hands are also providing handling. This adaptation is common to control the position of the UE in support during sitting. The therapist faces the patient and uses the forearm on the posterior region of the patient's elbow to provide input to keep the elbow extended and pushing into the surface, while the therapist's hand is on the patient's trunk to provide input about trunk control.

The NDT approach also stresses the importance of the trunk in the patient's ability to sustain postural control in a vertical position (such as sitting or standing) and for normal movement (such as walking).[96] Many NDT sessions will include portions that focus on the patient's ability to maintain upright postural trunk control in quiet vertical activities and during dynamic movement. Additionally, to address abnormal muscle tone, the NDT approach uses weight-bearing postures to facilitate coactivation around joints, which pulls in postural function. For patients with hypotonic limbs, weight bearing can also facilitate normal joint alignment, such as in the glenohumeral joint, while also facilitating the limb extensor muscles by way of joint approximation. Weight bearing can also facilitate more normal muscle tone in patients with hypertonicity and/or spasticity by using reciprocal inhibition.[19]

Conclusion

Intervention possibilities are numerous,[98] and many are yet to be discovered.[99] As stated previously, the ultimate goal of physical therapy intervention is the patient regaining all movement function as an effortless and enjoyable motor experience. This goal may often be unrealistic given the extent of the lesion, the potential of the patient, and the time available to the PT or PTA for treatment. As a result, decisions need to be made and goals established based on the specific needs of the patient and family given the environmental restraints of the home, the support systems, the number of visits, the motivation of the patient, and the total health of the individual. The PTA may be delegated many aspects of the intervention program, and the PT may retain certain components. It is the PT's responsibility to delegate appropriately. If the PTA is unsure of the delegated intervention strategies, then the PTA must ask for help. In that way, the PT will develop better communication strategies, and the PTA will develop better intervention skills.

This chapter presented 5 categories of intervention: functional training, impairment training, hands-on therapeutic or adaptive intervention, somatosensory retraining, and participation training. The ultimate physical therapy goal is functional motor recovery in all aspects of life activities. Although the intervention may need to begin with sensory training and hands-on intervention, the goal is to work toward independent functional motor control by the patient. During physical therapy treatment, often specific impairment training needs to be incorporated, such as increasing ROM, decreasing hypertonicity while increasing muscle strength, or increasing respiratory input and exhalation for better oxygenation of the muscle tissues and better endurance. Once a patient can independently run motor programs in a feed-forward fashion, the practice needs to become a life activity to retain the skill. At this time, practice needs to be delegated to family, friends, caregivers, and the patient. Transferring throughout the day, brushing teeth, washing hair, and getting from bed to living room to kitchen to outside are an adult's everyday expectations. Generally, if the patient is empowered to learn or relearn those functional skills, the patient will continue to move and practice these skills as part of daily life. If, on the other hand, those activities are thought of as therapy and something that has to be done to get out of the hospital or health care services, then the empowerment of those patients to their own motor potential has not been accomplished, and often, carry-over into life activities is not actualized. As soon as the patient stops practicing, skill can be lost and function decreased. A clinician may find the same patient returning to therapy because he or she has lost function, but in reality, the patient has lost or never obtained the motivation to continue what was learned during the initial physical therapy intervention period. There are many additional reasons why a patient may lose function over time. He may become ill and thus lose muscle endurance, and it becomes too hard to do those daily activities. She may have another insult to her CNS or have a progressive problem. None of those medical conditions is within the power of the PT or PTA to control, but helping to empower the patient to realistic possibilities is critical for motivation. It is not acceptable for the daily therapeutic program to be satisfying to the therapist without those feelings of accomplishment extending to the patient. Patients need the feeling of success to continue on a road of learning. Empowering the patient to his or her potential is a critical aspect of intervention and certainly part of the PTA's role during intervention. Life changes from day to day, but all of us want to feel that, no matter where we are on this path of learning, we have more potential to learn and grow each day. A patient is no different.

Case Studies

Case #1

Mrs. Jones is a 78-year-old woman who has a history of falling. She has a history of diabetes and knows she is to drink water once an hour. After magnetic resonance imaging scans, blood studies, and various other medical examinations, the physician could not make a definitive diagnosis regarding her falling. The patient was sent to physical therapy to determine whether interventions might help. At the initial visit, Mrs. Jones had a black eye and informed the PT that she had fallen into her closet when she tried to get a shoe. After a thorough balance assessment, the PT determined that Mrs. Jones had all balance strategies, adequate ROM, and knew when she was falling. She used to swim daily with her friends at her senior living facility inside pool but had stopped after an episode of pneumonia. During that episode, she stayed at her daughter's apartment next to hers. During that time, she remained in bed the majority of the day for slightly more than 4 weeks. She has become very inactive, lives in a small apartment, and goes out only when her daughter takes her to the doctor. She no longer drives, and her daughter does all her grocery shopping. She usually heats a microwave dinner in the evening and has cereal and fruit or cheese for her breakfast and lunch. Her daughter often brings a meal and eats with her. Mrs. Jones is weak, especially in her ankles, knees, and hips bilaterally. That weakness is especially true in her postural muscles in both legs and her back. She spends the majority of the day sitting in her rocking chair, watching TV or reading. She has a large pitcher of water by her chair, which allows her to have her hourly glass of water. She also speaks in short sentences. She fatigues quickly during physical activity and has a slowed reaction time to perturbations. The PT has delegated 5 interventions to the PTA before a reassessment. The PT gave the PTA the following instructions:

1. Have Mrs. Jones practice getting up and down from her chair at least one time an hour by telling her to go to the kitchen and get a glass of water instead of using a pitcher by her chair. Give the responsibility to Mrs. Jones because she is independent in this activity and has walls to stop her falling if she loses her balance.

2. Have Mrs. Jones practice reaching for her shoes and donning them:

   a. First, sitting from her chair: Session 1.

   b. Second, standing with a support arm holding onto a table, a chair, or some other stable piece of furniture: Sessions 2 and 3.

   c. Third, standing with a shoe directly within her BOS: Sessions 3 and 4.

   d. Fourth, standing, have her shoe sequentially farther and farther away from her limits of stability. Progress to reaching into the closet by Session 5: progress through this sequence as she increases her tolerance to moving over her COG without falling. She may progress faster or slower depending on her endurance and fear of falling.

3. Teach Mrs. Jones diaphragmatic breathing:

   a. First, while lying on her bed: Session 1.

   b. Second, when standing or walking. Session 2: count the number of syllables she uses in a sentence at the beginning of therapy and at the end. Document and report those numbers to the PT following each session.

4. After you, the PTA, can walk with Mrs. Jones a distance of 25 yards (distance to the mailbox and back), instruct the daughter to walk with her mother daily to the mailbox. The daughter should be told that the goal is to increase that distance on a weekly basis. She might walk with her mother to the pool, rest, and walk back. Once she can do that easily, have her mother begin swimming on a daily basis.

QUESTIONS

1. What clinical symptoms would the PTA want to immediately discuss with the PT?

2. Under which area of intervention does this program fall?

3. Are all activities appropriate to be delegated to the PTA?

CASE #2

Charley is an 8 year old who was diagnosed with cerebral palsy at 3 months of age. His family has been told he has spastic diplegia. He was in therapy as an outpatient in a developmental program until age 5 and now receives physical therapy 2 times per week while in school. Charley recently underwent heel cord lengthening. The child was placed initially in casts to maintain ROM and allow healing. The casts have now been bivalved and will be used as night splints. The child has now been referred to the outpatient clinic in order to regain functional use of his LEs for gait. The PT has delegated strengthening exercises of the gastrocsoleus muscles to the PTA. The PTA is instructed to do passive stretching to the ankles with a focus of gaining approximately 5 degrees beyond 90 degrees at each session with the goal of gaining and maintaining 110 degrees of ankle ROM for ambulatory activities. The PT also wants the PTA to do strengthening exercises in patterns that encourage the child to break up the extensor synergy (+ supporting reaction) while incorporating ankle function both in weight bearing and non-weight bearing. These activities can be encouraged in sit to stand, side-stepping, half-kneel to stand, and kicking a ball with one foot while maintaining balance and support.

QUESTIONS

1. Are these interventions within the scope of practice of the PTA?

2. Under which area of intervention does this program fall?

3. How would the PTA document change in range and power of the LEs, and how is that affecting functional behavior?

CASE #3

The patient is a 28-year-old man who suffered a head trauma following an auto accident 10 days previously. No orthopedic or integumentary problems exist. The patient has a tracheotomy and is intubated for feeding. He lost consciousness immediately, and the paramedics had to resuscitate him following a cardiac arrest. He was without O_2 for only 2 minutes, and the doctors do not anticipate any severe anoxic injury. The patient was in the intensive care unit for 2 days and has been transferred to a subacute rehabilitation unit. The patient is in a vegetative state, considered Level 3 on a Rancho scale. The PT is working with the patient on a ball in the vertical position sitting and kneeling to try to facilitate automatic postural trunk and head control. The PT has delegated ROM exercises to the PTA as well as horizontal rolling and bed mobility. The PT wants the PTA to encourage rolling by handling from the LEs. Initial handling should begin with the patient in the side-lying position and facilitate rolling toward prone and back toward supine. As the patient begins to automatically respond, the PTA is to increase the ROM of the rolling activity with the hopes that the patient will begin to roll. The PT has instructed the PTA to work in the patient's bed in the morning and on the mat in the physical therapy clinic in the afternoon. Following the PTA intervention, the PT will work on sitting and kneeling, with the PTA assisting by guarding the patient (controlling the roll of the ball) and encouraging interactions with the patient while in the patient's visual gaze.

QUESTIONS

1. Are these interventions within the scope of practice of the PTA?

2. What clinical signs would the PTA want to report immediately to the PT?

3. How would the PTA document change?

4. Under which area of intervention does this program fall?

CASE #4

The patient is a 58-year-old woman who suffered a left cerebrovascular accident 2 weeks ago. She is a chief executive officer of a large corporation and suffered her stroke following a 22-hour air flight. She was returning from a business trip to East Asia. She has minimal speech involvement and has functional motor use of her right UE and LE; however, she has significant loss in sensation. She has normal sensation in her face, trunk, shoulders, and hips but has poor proprioception in her right knee and ankle and no proprioception or tactile sensation in her right elbow, wrist, or hand. She is right-hand dominant. Because of the poor sensation, she is unable to use proprioception to anticipate a perturbation, which could cause a fall in standing or during ambulation. She uses her visual and vestibular system to compensate for poor proprioception, but when distracted in standing or during ambulation, she is slow to react and tends to fall. She has automatic protective extension in a feed-forward UE movement, but without vision, has little idea where her arm is in space or whether her hand is functionally doing anything. The PT has delegated to the PTA various UE sensory awareness exercises with the patient with and without vision. The PT has instructed the PTA to:

1. Have the patient hold various objects first in the left hand and then in the right. The patient is first asked to look at the object while it is in the left hand, manipulate it, and then visualize what it looks like.

2. Have the patient first find an object (spoon, marble, comb, sandpaper, cotton, etc) in sand and rice with visual assistance, then perform the same activity without vision. If she cannot perform this activity initially, the PTA will tell her what the object is, then have her look at it, shut her eyes, and visualize the form while manipulating it.

The PT was performing sensory awareness retraining first in the supine position, moving to sitting, and ending in standing to facilitate bilateral integration and better somatosensory cortical awareness. Once the patient had some awareness of the right LE, the PT delegated to the PTA bilateral LE weight-bearing activities in a body weight–supported harness over the treadmill. The PTA was instructed to:

1. Have the patient practice rocking on her feet, visualizing the symmetrical movement at both ankles.

2. Have the patient practice weight shifting onto and off the right LE, then shift to the same activity on the left.

3. Have the patient begin ambulation while in the harness on a treadmill while visualizing the movement in her right LE. Once she acknowledges that she feels her right LE and is able to ambulate on the treadmill with only 10% of her body weight supported, the PT should be told in order to begin gait training in various sensory environments without body support. The PT will use the virtual reality program to assist the patient in IADL. Once the patient is able to successfully complete the tasks using virtual reality, the PT will use the Nintendo Wii Balance Program to have the patient practice those motor activities she enjoyed doing prior to the stroke. The PTA will be responsible for guarding the patient once she begins using the Wii to guarantee that she does not fall.

QUESTIONS

1. Are these interventions appropriate to delegate to the PTA?

2. What clinical symptoms would the PTA want to immediately discuss with the PT?

3. How would the PTA document change in the areas of intervention?

4. Under which area of intervention does this program fall?

REFERENCES

1. *Guide to Physical Therapist Practice.* 2nd ed. Alexandria, VA: American Physical Therapy Association; 2001.

2. Allison L, Fuller K. Balance and vestibular dysfunction. In: Umphred D, Lazaro R, Roller M, Burton G, eds. *Umphred's Neurological Rehabilitation.* 6th ed. St Louis, MO: Elsevier; 2013.

3. Galea MP, Said CM, Remedios LJ. Feldenkrais Method balance classes are based on principles of motor learning and postural control retraining: a qualitative research study. *Physiotherapy.* 2010;96(4):324-336.

4. Umphred D, Lazaro R, Roller P, Byl N. Intervention techniques for clients with movement disorders. In: Umphred D, Lazaro R, Roller M, Burton G, eds. *Umphred's Neurological Rehabilitation.* 6th ed. St Louis, MO: Elsevier; 2013.

5. Arroll M, Dancey CP, Attree EA, Smith S, James T. People with symptoms of Ménière's disease: the relationship between illness intrusiveness, illness uncertainty, dizziness handicap, and depression. *Otol Neurotol.* 2012;33(5):816-823.

6. Brodovsky JR, Vnenchak MJ. Vestibular rehabilitation for unilateral peripheral vestibular dysfunction. *Phys Ther.* 2013;93(3):293-298.

7. Hain TC. Vestibular Rehabilitation Therapy (VRT). Chicago Dizziness and Hearing. www.dizziness-and-balance.com/treatment/rehab.html. Accessed February 6, 2013.

8. 4 Awesome Exercises for Balance and Leg Strength #64. RenegageHealth.com. www.youtube.com/watch?v=e6pnogAnKFU. Accessed February 6, 2013.

9. Gottshall KR, Sessoms PH, Bartlett JL. Vestibular physical therapy intervention: utilizing a computer assisted rehabilitation environment in lieu of traditional physical therapy. *Conf Proc IEEE Eng Med Biol Soc.* 2012;2012:6141-6144.

10. Crowner B, Kelly VE, Lee YA. Dual-task and context-dependent learning to modify functional motor performance, balance, and fall risk, Part 1: theoretical background and interpretive considerations. In: Combined Sections Meeting of the American Physical Therapy Association; January 21–24, 2013; San Diego, CA.

11. Doyle MS, Hershberg JA, Howard R, Osborn MB, Wagner JM. Dual-task and context-dependent learning to modify functional motor performance, balance, and fall risk, part 2: clinical implications and applied interventions. In: Combined Sections Meeting of the American Physical Therapy Association; January 21–24, 2013; San Diego, CA.

12. Fritz NE, Basso DM. Dual-task training for balance and mobility in a person with severe traumatic brain injury: a case study. *J Neurol Phys Ther.* 2013;37(1):37-43.

13. Yogev-Seligmann G, Giladi N, Gruendlinger L, Hausdorff JM. The contribution of postural control and bilateral coordination to the impact of dual tasking on gait. *Exp Brain Res.* 2013;226(1):81-93.

14. Park ER, Traeger L, Vranceanu AM, et al. The development of a patient-centered program based on the relaxation response: the Relaxation Response Resiliency Program (3RP). *Psychosomatics.* 2013;54(2):165-174.

15. Umphred D, Thompson MH, West TM. Limbic systems influence over motor control and learning. In: Umphred DA, Lazaro R, Roller M, Burton G, eds. *Umphred's Neurological Rehabilitation.* 6th ed. St Louis, MO: Elsevier; 2013.

16. Busch V, Magerl W, Kern U, Haas J, Hajak G, Eichhammer P. The effect of deep and slow breathing on pain perception, autonomic activity, and mood processing—an experimental study. *Pain Med.* 2012;13(2):215-228.

17. Iglesias SL, Azzara S, Argibay JC, et al. Psychological and physiological response of students to different types of stress management programs. *Am J Health Promot.* 2012;26(6):e149-e158.

18. Knott M, Voss DE. *Proprioceptive Neuromuscular Facilitation.* New York, NY: Harper and Row; 1968.

19. Bobath B. *Adult Hemiplegia: Evaluation and Treatment.* 2nd ed. London, England: William Heinemann Medical Books; 1978.

20. Bly L. A historical and current view of the basis of NDT. *Pediatric Phys Ther.* 1991;3:131-135.

21. Brunnstrom S. *Movement Therapy in Hemiplegia.* 2nd ed. Philadelphia, PA: JB Lippincott; 1992.

22. Feldenkrais M. *Awareness Through Movement.* New York, NY: Harper and Row; 1977.

23. Goff B. The application of recent advances in neurophysiology to Miss M Rood's concepts of neuromuscular facilitation. *Physiotherapy.* 1972;58(12):409-415.

24. Johnstone M. *Restoration of Normal Movement After Stroke.* New York, NY: Churchill Livingstone; 1995.

25. Bobath B. *Abnormal Postural Reflex Activity Caused by Brain Lesions.* 3rd ed. Frederick, MD: Aspen Publications; 1985.

26. Bly L. *Baby Treatment Based on NDT Principles.* San Antonio, TX: Therapy Skill Builders; 1999.

27. Barbeau H, Visintin M. Optimal outcomes obtained with body-weight support combined with treadmill training in stroke subjects. *Arch Phys Med Rehabil.* 2003;84(10):1458-1465.

28. Hesse S, Werner C. Partial body weight supported treadmill training for gait recovery following stroke. *Adv Neurol.* 2003;92:423-428.

29. Hicks AL, Adams MM, Martin GK, et al. Long-term body-weight-supported treadmill training and subsequent follow-up in persons with chronic SCI: effects on functional walking ability and measures of subjective well-being. *Spinal Cord.* 2005;43(5):291-298.

30. Stein J. Motor recovery strategies after stroke. *Top Stroke Rehabil.* 2004;11(2):12-22.

31. Carey LM, Matyas TA. Frequency of discriminative sensory loss in the hand after stroke in a rehabilitation setting. *J Rehabil Med.* 2011;43(3):257-263.

32. Chabok SY, Kapourchali SR, Saberi A, Mohtasham-Amiri Z. Operative and nonoperative linguistic outcomes in brain injury patients. *J Neurol Sci.* 2012;317(1–2):130-136.

33. Schabrun SM, Hillier S. Evidence for the retraining of sensation after stroke: a systematic review. *Clin Rehabil.* 2009;23(1):27-39.

34. Tyson SF, Hanley M, Chillala J, Selley AB, Tallis RC. Sensory loss in hospital-admitted people with stroke: characteristics, associated factors, and relationship with function. *Neurorehabil Neural Repair.* 2008;22(2):166-172.

35. Sinanović O, Mrkonjić Z, Zukić S, Vidović M, Imamović K. Post-stroke language disorders. *Acta Clin Croat.* 2011;50(1):79-94.

36. Goble DJ, Coxon JP, Wenderoth N, Van Impe A, Swinnen SP. Proprioceptive sensibility in the elderly: degeneration, functional consequences and plastic-adaptive processes. *Neurosci Biobehav Rev.* 2009;33(3):271-278.

37. Shaffer SW, Harrison AL. Aging of the somatosensory system: a translational perspective. *Phys Ther.* 2007;87(2):193-207.

38. Ayres A. *Sensory Integration and Praxis Test (SIPT) Manual.* Los Angeles, CA: Western Psychological Association; 1989.

39. Byl NN. Focal hand dystonia may result from aberrant neuroplasticity. *Adv Neurol.* 2004;94:19-28.

40. Byl N, Roderick J, Mohamed O, et al. Effectiveness of sensory and motor rehabilitation of the upper limb following the principles of neuroplasticity: patients stable poststroke. *Neurorehabil Neural Repair.* 2003;17(3):176-191.

41. Byl NN, Nagarajan SS, Merzenich MM, Roberts T, McKenzie A. Correlation of clinical neuromusculoskeletal and central somatosensory performance: variability in controls and patients with severe and mild focal hand dystonia. *Neural Plast.* 2002;9(3):177-203.

42. Altenmüller E, Jabusch HC. Focal dystonia in musicians: phenomenology, pathophysiology, triggering factors, and treatment. *Med Probl Perform Art.* 2010;25(1):3-9.

43. Byl NN. Diagnosis and management of focal hand dystonia in a rheumatology practice. *Curr Opin Rheumatol.* 2012;24(2):222-231.

44. Coq JO, Barr AE, Strata F, et al. Peripheral and central changes combine to induce motor behavioral deficits in a moderate repetition task. *Exp Neurol.* 2009;220(2):234-245.

45. Dolberg R, Hinkley LB, Honma S, et al. Amplitude and timing of somatosensory cortex activity in task-specific focal hand dystonia. *Clin Neurophysiol.* 2011;122(12):2441-2451.

46. Hinkley LB, Dolberg R, Honma S, Findlay A, Byl NN, Nagarajan SS. Aberrant oscillatory activity during simple movement in task-specific focal hand dystonia. *Front Neurol.* 2012;3:165.

47. McKenzie AL, Goldman S, Barrango C, Shrime M, Wong T, Byl N. Differences in physical characteristics and response to rehabilitation for patients with hand dystonia: musicians' cramp compared to writers' cramp. *J Hand Ther.* 2009;22(2):172-181.

48. Rosenkranz K, Butler K, Williamon A, Cordivari C, Lees AJ, Rothwell JC. Sensorimotor reorganization by proprioceptive training in musician's dystonia and writer's cramp. *Neurology.* 2008;70(4):304-315.

49. Rosenkranz K, Butler K, Williamon A, Rothwell JC. Regaining motor control in musician's dystonia by restoring sensorimotor organization. *J Neurosci.* 2009;29(46):14627-14636.

50. Steeves TD, Day L, Dykeman J, Jette N, Pringsheim T. The prevalence of primary dystonia: a systematic review and meta-analysis. *Mov Disord.* 2012;27(14):1789-1796.

51. Oujamaa L, Relave I, Froger J, Mottet D, Pelissier JY. Rehabilitation of arm function after stroke. Literature review [in English and French]. *Ann Phys Rehabil Med.* 2009;52(3):269-293.

52. Sunderland A, Tuke A. Neuroplasticity, learning and recovery after stroke: a critical evaluation of constraint-induced therapy. *Neuropsychol Rehabil.* 2005;15(2):81-96.

53. van der Lee JH. Constraint-induced movement therapy: some thoughts about theories and evidence. *J Rehabil Med.* 2003;(41 Suppl):41-45.

54. Wolf SL, Winstein CJ, Miller JP, et al. Effect of constraint-induced movement therapy on upper extremity function 3 to 9 months after stroke: the EXCITE randomized clinical trial. *JAMA.* 2006;296(17):2095-2104.

55. Boake C, Noser EA, Ro T, et al. Constraint-induced movement therapy during early stroke rehabilitation. *Neurorehabil Neural Repair.* 2007;21(1):14-24.

56. Dromerick AW, Edwards DF, Hahn M. Does the application of constraint-induced movement therapy during acute rehabilitation reduce arm impairment after ischemic stroke? *Stroke.* 2000;31(12):2984-2988.

57. Dromerick AW, Lang CE, Birkenmeier RL, et al. Very early constraint-induced movement during stroke rehabilitation (VECTORS): a single-center RCT. *Neurology.* 2009;73(3):195-201.

58. Humm JL, Kozlowski DA, James DC, Gotts JE, Schallert T. Use-dependent exacerbation of brain damage occurs during an early post-lesion vulnerable period. *Brain Res.* 1998;783(2):286-292.

59. Kozlowski DA, James DC, Schallert T. Use-dependent exaggeration of neuronal injury after unilateral sensorimotor cortex lesions. *J Neurosci.* 1996;16(15):4776-4786.

60. Lin KC, Wu CY, Wei TH, Lee CY, Liu JS. Effects of modified constraint-induced movement therapy on reach-to-grasp movements and functional performance after chronic stroke: a randomized controlled study. *Clin Rehabil.* 2007;21(12):1075-1086.

61. McIntyre A, Viana R, Janzen S, Mehta S, Pereira S, Teasell R. Systematic review and meta-analysis of constraint-induced movement therapy in the hemiparetic upper extremity more than six months post stroke. *Top Stroke Rehabil.* 2012;19(6):499-513.

62. Peurala SH, Kantanen MP, Sjögren T, Paltamaa J, Karhula M, Heinonen A. Effectiveness of constraint-induced movement therapy on activity and participation after stroke: a systematic review and meta-analysis of randomized controlled trials. *Clin Rehabil.* 2012;26(3):209-223.

63. Treger I, Aidinof L, Lehrer H, Kalichman L. Modified constraint-induced movement therapy improved upper limb function in subacute poststroke patients: a small-scale clinical trial. *Top Stroke Rehabil.* 2012;19(4):287-293.

64. Myint JM, Yuen GF, Yu TK, et al. A study of constraint-induced movement therapy in subacute stroke patient in Hong Kong. *Clin Rehabil.* 2008;22(2):112-124.

65. Chen CL, Kang LJ, Hong WH, Chen FC, Chen HC, Wu CY. Effect of therapist-based constraint-induced therapy at home on motor control, motor performance and daily function in children with cerebral palsy: a randomized controlled study. *Clin Rehabil.* 2013;27(3):236-245.

66. Lin KC, Wang TN, Wu CY, et al. Effects of home-based constraint-induced therapy versus dose-matched control intervention on functional outcomes and caregiver well-being in children with cerebral palsy. *Res Dev Disabil.* 2011;32(5):1483-1491.

67. Byl K, Bly N, Byl M, et al. Integrating technology into clinical practice in neurological rehabilitation. In: Umphred D, Lazaro R, Roller M, Burton G, eds. *Umphred's Neurological Rehabilitation.* 6th ed. St Louis, MO: Elsevier; 2013.

68. United States Department of Veterans Affairs. Journal of Rehabilitation Research and Development. www.rehab.research.va.gov/jour/11/484/hidler484.html. Accessed July 31, 2013.

69. Combs SA, Dugan EL, Ozimek EN, Curtis AB. Effects of body-weight supported treadmill training on kinetic symmetry in persons with chronic stroke. *Clin Biomech (Bristol, Avon).* 2012;27(9):887-892.

70. Duncan PW, Sullivan KJ, Behrman AL, et al. Body-weight-supported treadmill rehabilitation after stroke. *N Engl J Med.* 2011;364(21):2026-2036.

71. Fluet GG, Merians AS, Qiu Q, et al. Robots integrated with virtual reality simulations for customized motor training in a person with upper extremity hemiparesis: a case study. *J Neurol Phys Ther.* 2012;36(2):79-86.

72. Høyer E, Jahnsen R, Stanghelle JK, Strand LI. Body weight supported treadmill training versus traditional training in patients dependent on walking assistance after stroke: a randomized controlled trial. *Disabil Rehabil.* 2012;34(3):210-219.

73. Kelley CP, Childress J, Boake C, Noser EA. Over-ground and robotic-assisted locomotor training in adults with chronic stroke: a blinded randomized clinical trial. *Disabil Rehabil Assist Technol.* 2013;8(2):161-168.

74. DiBiasio PA, Lewis CL. Exercise training utilizing body weight-supported treadmill walking with a young adult with cerebral palsy who was non-ambulatory. *Physiother Theory Pract.* 2012;28(8):641-652.

75. Kurz MJ, Wilson TW, Corr B, Volkman KG. Neuromagnetic activity of the somatosensory cortices associated with body weight-supported treadmill training in children with cerebral palsy. *J Neurol Phys Ther.* 2012;36(4):166-172.

76. Rose MH, Løkkegaard A, Sonne-Holm S, Jensen BR. Improved clinical status, quality of life, and walking capacity in Parkinson's disease after body weight-supported high-intensity locomotor training. *Arch Phys Med Rehabil.* 2013;94(4)687-692.

77. Swinnen E, Beckwée D, Pinte D, Meeusen R, Baeyens JP, Kerckhofs E. Treadmill training in multiple sclerosis: can body weight support or robot assistance provide added value? A systematic review. *Mult Scler Int.* 2012;2012:240274.

78. Esquenazi A, Lee S, Packel AT, Braitman L. A randomized comparative study of manually assisted versus robotic-assisted body weight supported treadmill training in persons with a traumatic brain injury. *PM R.* 2013;5(4)280-290.

79. Moriello G, Frear M, Seaburg K. The recovery of running ability in an adolescent male after traumatic brain injury: a case study. *J Neurol Phys Ther.* 2009;33(2):111-120.

80. Bergmann J, Krewer C, Müller F, Koenig A, Riener R. Virtual reality to control active participation in a subacute stroke patient during robot-assisted gait training. *IEEE Int Conf Rehabil Robot.* 2011;2011:5975407.

81. Laver KE, George S, Thomas S, Deutsch JE, Crotty M. Virtual reality for stroke rehabilitation. *Cochrane Database Syst Rev.* 2011;(9):CD008349.

82. Lucca LF. Virtual reality and motor rehabilitation of the upper limb after stroke: a generation of progress? *J Rehabil Med.* 2009;41(12):1003-1100.

83. Piron L, Turolla A, Agostini M, et al. Exercises for paretic upper limb after stroke: a combined virtual-reality and telemedicine approach. *J Rehabil Med.* 2009;41(12):1016-1102.

84. Fulk GD. Locomotor training and virtual reality-based balance training for an individual with multiple sclerosis: a case report. *J Neurol Phys Ther.* 2005;29(1):34-42.

85. Mumford N, Duckworth J, Thomas PR, Shum D, Williams G, Wilson PH. Upper-limb virtual rehabilitation for traumatic brain injury: a preliminary within-group evaluation of the elements system. *Brain Inj.* 2012;26(2):166-176.

86. Green D, Wilson PH. Use of virtual reality in rehabilitation of movement in children with hemiplegia—a multiple case study evaluation. *Disabil Rehabil.* 2012;34(7):593-604.

87. Salem Y, Gropack SJ, Coffin D, Godwin EM. Effectiveness of a low-cost virtual reality system for children with developmental delay: a preliminary randomised single-blind controlled trial. *Physiotherapy.* 2012;98(3):189-195.

88. Deutsch JE, Borbely M, Filler J, K, Huhn K, Guarrera-Bowlby P. Use of a low-cost, commercially available gaming console (Wii) for rehabilitation of an adolescent with cerebral palsy. *Phys Ther.* 2008;88(10):1196-1207.

89. Saposnik G, Teasell R, Mamdani M, et al. Effectiveness of virtual reality using Wii gaming technology in stroke rehabilitation: a pilot randomized clinical trial and proof of principle. *Stroke.* 2010;41(7):1477-1484.

90. Flynn S, Palma P, Bender A. Feasibility of using the Sony PlayStation 2 gaming platform for an individual post-stroke: a case report. *J Neurol Phys Ther.* 2007;31(4):180-189.

91. Lewis JA, Deutsch JE, Burdea G. Usability of the remote console for virtual reality telerehabilitation: formative evaluation. *Cyberpsychol Behav.* 2006;9(2):142-147.

92. Voss DE, Ionta MK, Myers BJ. *Proprioceptive Neuromuscular Facilitation: Patterns and Techniques.* 3rd ed. Philadelphia, PA: Lippincott Williams & Wilkins; 1985.

93. International Proprioceptive Neuromuscular Facilitation Association. PNF History. http://www.ipnfa.org/index.php?id=113. Updated January 10, 2013. Accessed January 15, 2013.

94. Baum N. Proprioceptive neuromuscular facilitation shoulder progression for patients with spinal cord injury resulting in quadriplegia. *Phys Ther Case Reports.* 1998;1(6):296-300.

95. Smedal T, Lygren H, Myhr K-M, et al. Balance and gait improved in patients with MS after physiotherapy based on the Bobath concept. *Physiother Res Int.* 2006;11(2):104-116.

96. Lennon, S. Gait re-education based on the Bobath concept in two patients with hemiplegia following stroke. *Phys Ther.* 2001;81(3):924-935.

97. Neuro-Developmental Treatment Association. www.ndta.org. Accessed July 31, 2013.

98. Umphred DA, Lazaro R, Roller M, Burton G, eds. *Neurological Rehabilitation.* 6th ed. St Louis, MO: Elsevier; 2013.

99. III STEP: symposium on translating evidence into practice. University of Utah, July 15–22, 2005. *Special Editions: Phys Ther.* 2006;86(4,5,6).

Please see accompanying Web site at
www.healio.com/books/neuroptavideos

5

Examination Procedures

Patricia Harris, PT, MS
Lisa Ferrin, PTA, AS

KEY WORDS

- Balance testing
- Examination
- Functional testing
- Impairment testing
- Neuromuscular examination
- Pain assessment
- Participation
- Sensory testing

CHAPTER OBJECTIVES

- Discuss the purposes of a neuromuscular examination.

- Identify the responses expected from specific neuromuscular examinations.

- Identify and discuss the role of the physical therapist assistant (PTA) in assessing patients with central nervous system movement problems by using follow-up tests and measures.

- Identify and discuss what assessment tools a PTA should be competent to administer in relation to the established plan of care and physical therapy prognosis.

- Clarify and discuss when and why it is appropriate for the PTA to perform the neuromuscular follow-up examination and when the test procedures should be performed by the physical therapist.

INTRODUCTION

Examination is defined by the *Guide to Physical Therapist Practice* (the *Guide*) as "a comprehensive screening and specific testing process leading to diagnostic classification or, as appropriate, to a referral to another practitioner."[1] Evaluation is defined as "a dynamic process in which the physical therapist (PT) makes clinical judgments based on data gathered during the examination."[1] "The initial examination is required prior to the initial intervention and is performed for

Umphred DA, Lazaro RT, eds.
Neurorehabilitation for the Physical Therapist Assistant,
Second Edition (pp 117-150).
© 2014 SLACK Incorporated.

all patients/clients."[1] "Reexamination is the process of performing selected tests and measures after the initial examination to evaluate progress and to modify or redirect interventions."[1] The physical therapist assistant (PTA) may identify when a reexamination is indicated based on "new clinical findings or failure to respond to physical therapy interventions."[1] This chapter follows the chapter on intervention to be consistent with the process used by a PTA. Within the PT's frame of reference, examination along with evaluation precede development of a plan of care and the intervention process. Within the paradigm of the PTA, reexamination follows initiation of intervention strategies identified within the plan of care. Thus, the order of the first section of this book is aligned closely with the professional role of the PTA. There are typically 3 types of formal examinations and evaluations used by a PT when a patient receives physical therapy: (1) an initial examination/evaluation, (2) a reexamination/evaluation, and (3) a discharge examination/evaluation. Not all components of an examination are repeated for the second 2 types of examinations. Based on the findings, the PT establishes a physical therapy movement diagnosis, which "indicates the primary dysfunctions toward which the PT directs interventions."[1] Based on the physical therapy diagnosis, the PT develops a prognosis that is "the determination of the predicted optimal level of improvement in function and the amount of time needed to reach that level."[1] The PT then establishes the plan of care, which is the "culmination of the examination, diagnostic, and prognostic processes."[1] The plan of care includes short-/long-term goals, physical therapy interventions including duration and frequency, prognosis, and discharge plans.[1] A complete examination allows the identification of movement problems that can be appropriately managed through physical therapy intervention. Refer to Figure 1-3 for clarification of this model. In addition, the examination/evaluation enhances the patient's achievement of optimal health and well-being by identifying the interactions of various body systems as they relate to the patient's signs and symptoms and progress with rehabilitation. This examination/evaluation process also protects the patient by identifying potential life-threatening or emergency conditions and/or the need to refer to other individuals who will be able to better manage aspects of the patient's care. The PTA uses the information obtained by the PT to guide delivery of patient intervention. The one examination tool a PTA must use each time the patient is seen is a review of body systems and identification of any change in those systems. This is a critical aspect of patient care and can be a life-threatening situation if a problem develops and is not identified during any treatment session.

This chapter will focus on the initial examination process performed by the PT and include a discussion of the role of the PTA in the reexamination and discharge examinations. Following the *Guide*,[1] the neuromuscular examination should consist of the patient or client history, a review of systems, and tests and measures appropriate to the medical diagnosis and movement dysfunctions identified by the PT.

It is important for the PTA to be familiar with the components of the neuromuscular examination. An understanding of the components of the neuromuscular examination guides delivery of the interventions included in the PT's treatment plan. The physical therapy examination begins with the patient history.

PATIENT HISTORY

The patient's history is the starting point for the PT's initial examination. The patient's history is obtained through the patient's medical record, intake forms, questionnaire, and interview (which may include the patient's interpretation of why he or she requires the services of a PT and the patient's goals for therapy). According to the *Guide*,[1] the patient history should include many if not all of the components found in Box 5-1.

The interview of the patient is performed in a private area to protect the patient's privacy and allow the patient to feel comfortable and open when answering questions. The PT gathers the initial patient history. Additional information pertinent to the medical history may become evident

---

Box 5-1
Categories to Be Included in the Patient History

- General demographics: age, sex, race/ethnicity, primary language, education
- Social history: cultural beliefs and behaviors, family and caregiver resources, social interactions, social activities, and support systems
- Employment/work (job/school/play)
- Developmental history
- Living environment: devices and equipment, living environment and community characteristics, projected discharge destination
- General health status
- Social/health habits (past and current)
- Family history
- Medical/surgical history
- Current conditions/chief complaints that led the patient/client to seek the services of a physical therapist
- Functional status and activity level
- Medications: over the counter and prescriptions
- Results of other clinical tests: laboratory and diagnostic tests

---

during subsequent visits with the PTA, who would then report and document the new findings to the supervising PT. Refer to Chapter 7 for additional identification of documentation responsibilities of the PTA.

BODILY SYSTEMS REVIEW

The next portion of the patient examination is the review of systems. The systems review examines the influence of bodily systems on the patient's complaint.[1] A brief examination of the status of the systems the PT needs to consider can be found in Box 5-2.

The purpose of the systems review is to determine whether there is a need for medical referral and the influence of the status of the systems on the patient's prognosis and plan of care. If the PTA is the individual providing intervention, then a brief systems review prior to beginning any treatment may be the first time early identification of a system problem becomes evident. Thus, the PTA needs to understand not only why the PT performed the systems review initially but also how to review these systems before beginning any intervention to identify when a patient needs to be seen by a medical provider or other health professional.

TESTS AND MEASURES

Tests of Body Functions and Structures

There are tests and measures specific to each of the areas of the physical therapy examination. These tests and measures assist the PT in interpreting the patient's status. According to the *Guide*,[1] tests and measures are used to identify signs and symptoms, to determine the physical therapy

---

Box 5-2
List of Bodily Systems Screened by the Physical Therapist and Physical Therapist Assistant

- Cardiovascular
- Pulmonary
- Integumentary
- Gastrointestinal
- Endocrine
- Musculoskeletal
- Neuromuscular
- Vision
- Ear/nose/throat
- Urogenital
- Hematologic/lymphatic
- Psychological

---

diagnosis and prognosis, to establish the plan of care, to determine changes in the patient's status, and to identify the progression toward or the achievement of goals. Certain portions of the tests that were performed by the PT during the initial examination may be assigned to the PTA for reexamination during the course of treatment. If the PTA identifies additional clinical signs and symptoms, she or he should communicate these findings to the PT. The PT will determine whether additional tests are needed.

Vital Signs

Monitoring vital signs is essential for safe patient treatment. There are 5 vital signs[2]: heart rate, respiration rate, blood pressure, temperature, and pain. Vital signs screen for potential medical complications and establish the ability of the patient to tolerate physical therapy intervention. Vital signs need to be assessed before each treatment and, depending on the patient's medical status, during the treatment session to determine the patient's ability to tolerate therapy. In addition, oxygen saturation rates may be taken via pulse oximetry to determine the patient's blood oxygenation level.[3]

Pain Assessment

Assessment of pain can be particularly problematic in a patient with a neurological problem. According to the Commission on Accreditation in Physical Therapy Education (CAPTE), the PTA should be able to "administer standardized questionnaires, graphs, behavioral scales, or visual analog scales for pain" as well as recognize "activities, positioning, and postures that aggravate or relieve pain or altered sensations."[4]

The following are commonly used pain scales:

- The Numerical Rating Scale[5]: The patient is asked to rate his or her pain from 0 (no pain) to 10 (worst pain possible).

- Visual analog pain scale (VAS)[5]: The VAS is a 10-cm line with the left-hand side representing no pain and the right-hand side indicating the worst imaginable pain. The patient marks a point along the line to indicate the level of pain (Figure 5-1). This scale has been found to be unreliable for individuals with impaired abstract reasoning skills.[6]

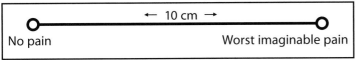

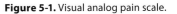

Figure 5-1. Visual analog pain scale.

- Wong-Baker FACES Pain Rating Scale[7]: The Wong-Baker FACES Pain Rating Scale is a series of 6 faces ranging from a smiley face for 0 or no hurt to a distraught face for 10 or worse hurt. This scale requires little instruction and does not require verbal instruction. The reader can view the Pain Rating Scale at www.WongBakerFaces.org.

- Checklist of Nonverbal Pain Indicators (CNPI)[8]: The CNPI is a list of 6 pain indicators (verbal complains, facial grimaces and winces, bracing, restlessness, rubbing, and vocal complaints) that are scored as 0 if the behavior is not observed and 1 if the behavior is observed even briefly. The CNPI is reliable and valid for older adults with acute or chronic pain, patients in critical care units, and patients with dementia.

- Pain Assessment in Advanced Dementia (PAINAD)[9]: The PAINAD assesses 4 pain indicators (breathing, negative vocalization, facial expression, and consolability). Each item is scored from 0 to 2, with 0 indicating no pain and 2 indicating considerable discomfort.

- Pediatric pain scales[10]:

  - CRIES (Crying Requires Increased Vital Signs Expression Sleeplessness): Appropriate for use with neonatal infants in the first month of life. The CRIES assesses 5 variables: crying, oxygen requirements, facial expression, vital signs, and sleeping pattern. The variables are scored from 0 to 2, with a maximum possible score of 10. Higher pain expression is indicated by a higher score.

  - Neonatal Infant Pain Scale (NIPS): Appropriate for use with infants, NIPS assesses 6 variables (facial expression, crying, breathing pattern, arms, legs, and state of arousal) that are scored in 1-minute intervals before, during, and after a painful intervention. The variables are scored from 0 (no pain) to 2 (pain).

  - FLACC: (Face, Legs, Activity, Crying, Consolability Scale): The FLACC is used to measure post-procedural pain intensity in young children. The FLACC ranks 5 indicators (face, legs, activity, crying, and consolability) on a 3-point severity scale (0 to 2), with a maximum total score of 10.

Facial expression scales, such as the Wong-Baker FACES Pain Rating Scale described above, are commonly used with children age 5 or older when children are able to rate pain intensity.[10]

Observation

Observation occurs continually throughout the examination and treatment of each patient by the PT and the PTA. Observation involves using the senses of vision, hearing, and smell to identify potential abnormalities. Some of the areas the PTA should observe are the patient's appearance, general movement patterns, posture, areas of swelling/edema, facial expression, breathing pattern, body odors, and ability to communicate. Observation of any of these abnormalities, especially if they have changed, can guide the PTA and the PT in the need for further examination.[11]

Mental Status

Mental status includes consciousness and arousal, orientation, attention, and higher cognitive functions. Understanding the patient's mental status is important in determining the patient's ability to function in the physical therapy setting. According to CAPTE,[4] the PTA should be able to recognize "changes in the direction and magnitude of patient's state of arousal, mentation, and cognition." Understanding the patient's mental status allows the PTA to appropriately deliver physical therapy interventions and to accurately document the patient's response to treatment.

Table 5-1
States of Altered Consciousness
Coma	A state of unresponsiveness from which the patient cannot be aroused even with strong stimuli. The patient's eyes are closed.[12]
Stupor	Arousable only by continuous, vigorous stimuli.[12]
Obtunded	Slower psychological response to stimulation with an increased need for sleep. Difficult to arouse from sleeping. Confusion and drowsiness is noted when awake.[12]
Vegetative state	Cycling of arousal states with periods of eye opening in an unresponsive patient.[12] Regular sleep-wake cycles and normal respiratory patterns are also present.[13] If the vegetative state lasts longer than 30 days, the term *persistent vegetative state* is used.[12]
Minimally conscious state	Severely impaired consciousness in which there is behavioral evidence of minimal but definite presence of self- or environmental awareness.[12] Evidence may include the ability to follow simple commands, the presence of gestural or verbal yes/no responses, intelligible speech, and nonreflexive movements or affective behaviors.[13]
Syncope	Fainting; a temporary loss of consciousness frequently as a result of a drop in blood pressure.[13]
Delirium	Not oriented to time, place, and people in the environment but still oriented to self. Delusions or hallucinations may be present.[12]

(Adapted from Lundy-Ekman L. *Neuroscience: Fundamentals of Rehabilitation*. St Louis, MO: Elsevier Inc: 2013 and Posner JB, Saper CB, Schiff N, Plum F. *Plum and Posner's Diagnosis of Stupor and Coma*. New York, NY: Oxford University Press; 2007.)

Consciousness and Arousal

Arousal is the patient's responsiveness to stimulation and indicates readiness for activity.[1] Arousal is an important component in identifying the state of consciousness. Terms used to describe levels of consciousness are listed in Table 5-1. A change in arousal, attention, and/or cognition must be communicated to the PT or appropriate medical professionals.

Orientation

Orientation is the ability of an individual to cognitively adapt within an unfamiliar environment, allowing for accurate awareness of person, place, time, and situation. The individual is assessed according to either 3 domains (orientation to person, place, and time), abbreviated as "oriented × 3/3" or 4 domains (orientation to person, place, time, and situation), abbreviated as "oriented × 4/4". When a patient is not oriented to one or more domains, it is documented with the domains that were correctly identified listed within parentheses (eg, "oriented × 2/4 [person, place]").[14]

Attention

Attention is the patient's ability to stay focused on a task. There are several categories of attention: selective attention, sustained attention, alternating attention, and divided attention.[14] These categories are defined in Box 5-3.

A common test that is used to examine several aspects of arousal, attention, and cognition is the Mini-Mental State Exam (MMSE).[15] The MMSE is a proprietary test[16] composed of 8 sections:

Box 5-3
Definitions of Types of Attention

- Selective attention: The patient's ability to concentrate on a task while screening out unnecessary information. One method of testing selective attention is the Digit Span Test, in which the therapist gives the patient a short list of numbers to recall either forward or backward.
- Sustained attention (vigilance): The patient's ability to maintain time on task. Sustained attention is tested by observing the patient's ability to remain on task, documenting the type of task and the amount of time the patient was able to sustain attention to the task.
- Alternating attention (attention flexibility): The patient's ability to shift attention between multiple tasks. Alternating attention is tested by examining the patient's ability to shift between different tasks.
- Divided attention: The patient's ability to perform 2 tasks simultaneously (eg, examining the patient's ability to walk and talk at the same time [Walkie-Talkie Test]).

(Adapted from O'Sullivan SB. Examination of motor function: motor control and motor learning. In: O'Sullivan SB, Schmitz TJ, eds. *Physical Rehabilitation*. Philadelphia, PA: FA Davis; 2007:230-231.)

- Orientation
- Immediate recall
- Attention
- Delayed verbal recall
- Naming
- Three-stage command
- Reading
- Writing

Results of the MMSE are important when planning interventions. Patients who demonstrate deficits in immediate recall may have difficulty following directions. The patient who has difficulty with 3-stage commands may have difficulty learning the proper technique for wheelchair (w/c) transfers. Instructing the patient to "position the w/c next to the bed, apply the locks, scoot forward, lean forward, and transfer" would contain too many commands for the patient with sequencing problems to follow. If the patient has delayed verbal recall, he or she may have difficulty listing total hip precautions.

The Cognitive Abilities Screening Instrument (CASI)[17] is a nonproprietary test that examines 6 key cognitive abilities: digit span **or** other mental tracking; verbal fluency; reasoning/judgment; expressive language; visual construction; immediate free verbal recall **or** delayed free verbal recall **or** cued verbal recall.

Sensation

A patient's sensory status provides valuable information to the PT and PTA. First, specific patterns of sensory impairment indicate possible damage from any number of areas in the central nervous system (CNS).[18] For example, patients with radial nerve impairment will experience sensory loss along the radial side of the dorsal aspect of the hand while patients with median nerve impairment will experience sensory loss along the radial side of the palmar surface of the hand.

Second, impaired sensation may result in specific movement impairments, such as a wide base of support (BOS) when walking secondary to impaired sensation in the feet for individuals with peripheral neuropathies. Finally, impaired sensation may predispose patients to injuries such as sprained ankles or damage such as Charcot joints.

Sensation can be divided into 3 major categories.[19] *Exteroceptive* (superficial sensation) refers to receptors located in the skin and the mucous membranes. Exteroceptive sensation includes tactile or touch sensation, pain sensation, and temperature sensation. *Proprioceptive sensation* (deep sensation) refers to receptors located in muscles, tendons, ligaments, and joints. Proprioceptive sensation includes proprioception (joint position sense), vibratory sense, and kinesthesia (movement sense). *Combined cortical sensory function*, which requires interpretation in the brain, includes stereognosis, graphesthesia, 2-point discrimination, touch localization, and double simultaneous stimulation.

Sensation can also be divided into 5 categories[13]:

1. Discriminative touch (primary sensation), which includes location of touch and tactile thresholds.

2. Discriminative touch (cortical sensation), which includes 2-point discrimination, bilateral simultaneous touch, and graphesthesia.

3. Conscious proprioception, which includes joint movement, joint position, and vibration, discriminative touch, and stereognosis.

4. Fast pain (lateral pain system), which is sharp, prickling pain.

5. Discriminative temperature, which is heat or cold.

Sensory Testing

There are several principles that apply to sensory testing[19]:

- It should be determined whether the patient is able to understand the testing procedure.

- The patient needs to be positioned comfortably and the areas to be tested should be accessible.

- The testing procedure should be explained prior to testing.

- The patient's vision should be obscured during the examination.

- The examination begins with the areas where sensation is unimpaired to be used as reference points and to make sure that the patient understands the test. The examiner then completes the rest of the examination in areas of suspected impairment.

- Sensation is documented as normal (100% accuracy), impaired (more than 50% but less than 100% accuracy) or absent (less than 50% accuracy). A diagram of the dermatomes or sensory distribution of the peripheral nerves may be used to illustrate the pattern of sensory impairment.[17] Figures 5-2A and B illustrate the dermatome level of innervation on the left and identification of the specific peripheral nerves on the right.

Discriminative Touch (Primary Sensation)

- **Light touch**[20]: A wisp of cotton is used for testing light touch (Figure 5-3). A wisp is obtained by pulling a cotton ball apart or by pulling off the end of a cotton swab. The wisp is touched to the skin without swiping and the patient is asked to identify when the stimulus is felt. Swiping the cotton wisps across the skin may give an inaccurate response, as swiping may stimulate the hair follicles or be interpreted as tickling.

- **Location of touch**[13]: The examiner lightly touches the patient with the fingertips or a wisp of cotton. The patient is asked to point to the area or tell the examiner where he or she feels the stimuli.

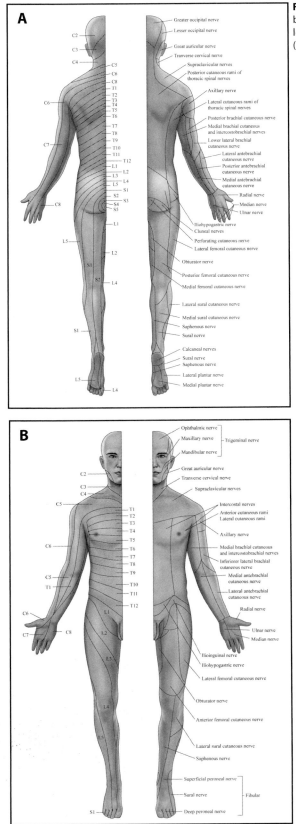

Figure 5-2. Example of pattern of sensory distribution (dermatome) or level of innervation on the left with the peripheral nerve name on the right. (A) Posterior view. (B) Anterior view.

Figure 5-3. Using a cotton wisp to test light touch.

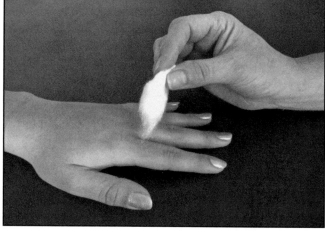

Figure 5-4. Using Semmes Weinstein monofilaments to test tactile thresholds.

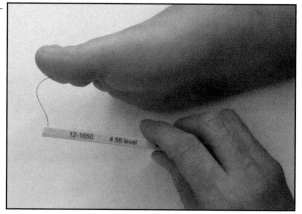

- **Tactile thresholds**[13]: Semmes Weinstein monofilaments may be used to test tactile thresholds and provide specific information about the degree of sensory loss (Figure 5-4). The monofilament is applied perpendicularly to the skin. Adequate pressure is applied to cause the filament to bend. The patient indicates whether he or she feels the touch. A patient with normal sensation of the foot can feel the 6-g filament everywhere on the foot. The inability to respond to a 10-g or greater filament may indicate a loss of protective sensation. This is particularly important for patients with peripheral neuropathies, often associated with diabetes, who may have decreased protective sensation. Loss of protective sensation places the patient at greater risk for formation of a pressure ulcer.

Discriminative Touch (Cortical Sensation)[13]

- **Two-point discrimination**: A 2-point discriminator is used (Figure 5-5) and set at distances appropriate for the area being tested, with the 2 points being moved closer and closer together until the subject is unable to distinguish the 2 points as separate.
- **Bilateral simultaneous touch**: Usually the forearms and shins are tested. The tester asks the subject to identify whether the tester is lightly touching one limb, the opposite limb, or both sides of the body at the same time. This test determines whether a person can attend to information coming from 2 areas at the same time.

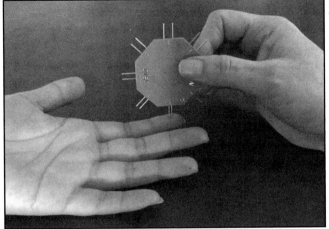

Figure 5-5. Using a 2-point discriminator to test for 2-point discrimination.

- **Graphesthesia**: The subject is positioned with his or her palm facing the examiner and fingers pointed upward. The examiner uses the eraser end of a pencil or similar object to trace a letter on the palm of the subject's hand. The subject is then asked to identify the letter.

Conscious Proprioception[13]

- **Joint movement (kinesthesia)**: The examiner, using a fingertip grip, grasps the lateral surfaces of the subject's limb. The joint is passively moved in small increments. The subject is instructed to tell the examiner whether the joint is being "bent" or "straightened." Errors would indicate that the subject does not reliably know when a joint is moving, which is significant during movement activities.

- **Joint position (proprioception)**: The examiner, using a fingertip grip, grasps the lateral surfaces of the subject's limb. The examiner moves the joint and holds it in a static position. The subject is asked to either replicate the position with the opposite limb or describe the position of the joint. Errors would indicate that the subject does not know where the limb is in space, which can have great significance during functional activities.

- **Vibration**: The examiner uses as tuning fork that vibrates at 128 Hz. The tuning fork is struck to create a vibration. The end of the vibrating tuning fork is then placed on a bony prominence. The subject is asked to report whether he or she feels the vibration or to indicate when the vibration stops.

- **Stereognosis**: The examiner places a common object, such as a paperclip or key, in the subject's hand. The subject is allowed to manipulate the object and then is asked to identify it. Errors would indicate that the subject with diminished vision would have difficulty selecting objects.

Fast Pain (Lateral Pain System)

A clean, unused safety pin is used to test pain sensation and to differentiate between sharp and dull. To test sharp, the sharp end of the safety pin is placed against the patient's skin, and enough pressure is applied to indent but not puncture the skin (Figure 5-6). Sliding the examiner's fingers down the pin ensures the correct amount of pressure. The rounded end of the safety pin is used to provide dull stimuli, which is alternated randomly with the sharp stimulus. The examiner then asks the patient to identify whether the sensation feels sharp or dull.[21] To map an area of impaired sensation, a pinwheel may be used. The handle of the pinwheel is held lightly between the examiner's thumb and index finger, and the pinwheel is rolled lightly across the subject's skin, circling the circumference of the limb. Specific patterns of sensory loss may indicate lesions in specific peripheral nerves.[13]

Figure 5-6. Using a pin to test pain sensation.

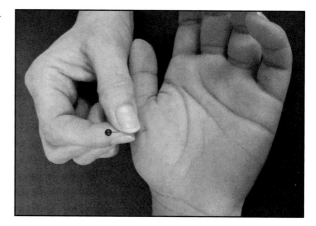

Box 5-4

Motor Examination Components

- Examination of range of motion
- Examination of muscular tone
- Examination of strength
- Examination of phasic stretch reflexes
- Examination of synergy

Discriminative Temperature (Heat or Cold)[13]

Two test tubes are used, one filled with hot water (the temperature should not exceed 45°C to avoid the possibility of a burn) and the other filled with crushed ice and water. The examiner touches the subject's skin with the test tubes in a random fashion and asks the subject to identify whether the test tube is hot or cold. Note that pain sensation and temperature sensation are carried in the same pathway in the spinal cord, so testing of both sensations may not be necessary, although loss of temperature sensation may precede the loss of pain sensation.

Motor Examination

The motor examination involves several components as identified in Box 5-4.

Examination of Range of Motion

Range of motion (ROM) refers to the available movement of the joints. Generally, goniometric measurements are used to indicate the available ROM of a joint. Note that accurate range of motion measurement may be difficult to obtain if the patient has cognitive impairments or abnormal muscle tone. Limited ROM will adversely affect the patient's postural alignment and ability to move in a biomechanically correct manner. For example, lack of adequate ankle dorsiflexion may cause the patient's knee to hyperextend during the stance phase of gait. A patient who lacks adequate hip flexion will have difficulty maintaining a sitting position. A patient with decreased shoulder flexion may have difficulty dressing.

	Table 5-2
	Terms Used for Motor Examination

Term	Definition and Comments
Muscle tone	The tension in the muscle fibers of a resting muscle. Muscle tone is tested by passively moving the limb through its range of motion and feeling for the amount of tension that is present. Muscle tone is not directly correlated with patient's the ability to move. Once the rigidity is relaxed, the muscles are often simultaneously weak and thus may show a decreased response to a quick stretch.
Spasticity	Velocity-dependent resistance to movement as a result of neuromuscular overactivity with resistance to movement increasing as the speed and amplitude of the movement increases.
Hyperreflexia	Excessive reflex response to muscle stretch. Hyperreflexia usually does not interfere with active movement. Often identified during testing of deep tendon reflexes.
Hypertonia	Excessive resistance to active or passive stretch.
Rigidity	A state of severe hypertonia. Both the agonist and antagonist are hyperactive, causing rigidity around the joint, although there is not necessarily an increase in response of the muscle to quick stretch.
Hypotonia	Decrease resistance to active and passive stretch. Hypotonia can be an insult in various parts of the brain but indicates that the lower motor neuron is not functioning adequately to create normal muscle tone. Hypotonia can also be the result of disuse of a muscle over a period of time, which is a severe problem with patients who have been bedridden or inactive.
Motor paralysis	Impaired ability to generate muscular force. This can be due to a problem within the muscle, the motor neuron leading to the muscle, or an insult at a higher level than the spinal cord.
Flaccidity	Absence of muscle tone. This also can be due to a problem within the muscle, the motor neuron leading to the muscle, or an insult at a higher level than the spinal cord, although flaccidity is considered more severe than paralysis.

(Adapted from Lundy-Ekman L. *The Motor System: Motor Neurons Neuroscience: Fundamentals for Rehabilitation.* 4th ed. St Louis, MO: Elsevier Inc; 2013.)

Examination of Muscular Tone

Many different terms are used for motor examination, as can be seen in Table 5-2.

There are several tests used to examine muscle tone. The Tardieu Rating Scale[22] and Modified Ashworth Scale[23] test the patient's degree of spasticity. When using the Tardieu Rating Scale, the patient is placed in the supine position, and the limb that is being tested is moved at different velocities. The amount of resistance is scored on a scale of 0 to 5, with 0 indicating that there was no resistance to passive movement and 5 indicating that the joint was immovable. When using the Ashworth Scale (Table 5-3), the limb is moved passively and the amount of resistance is scored on a scale of 0 to 4, with 0 indicating no increase in muscle tone and 4 indicating the limb was rigid. The type of muscle tone varies with the area of injury to the nervous system. For example, injury to a peripheral nerve results in low or no tone in the muscle (hypotonia), while injury to the spinal

	Table 5-3
	Modified Ashworth Scale

0	No increase in muscle tone.
1	Slight increase in muscle tone, manifested by a catch and release or minimal resistance at the end of the ROM when the affected part is moved in flexion or extension.
1+	Slight increase in muscle tone, manifested by a catch followed by minimal resistance throughout the remainder (less than half) of the ROM.
2	More marked increase in muscle tone through most of the ROM but affected part easily moved.
3	Considerable increase in muscle tone; passive movement difficult.
4	Affected parts rigid in flexion and extension.

(Reprinted from Bohannon RW, Smith MB. Interrater reliability of a modified Ashworth scale of muscle spasticity. *Phys Ther.* 1987;67[2]:206-207, with permission of the American Physical Therapy Association. This material is copyrighted, and any further reproduction or distribution is prohibited.)

cord usually results in hypertonia below the level of the lesion and damage to the basal ganglia, as seen in individuals with Parkinson's disease, results in rigidity.

Examination of Muscle Strength

Weakness can occur from damage to many areas of the CNS. Damage at the neuromuscular junction, where the nerve connects to the muscle, can result in weakness in disorders such as myasthenia gravis. Damage to the lower motor neurons (peripheral nerves), which connect the CNS to the muscles, can result in weakness from compressive injuries such as carpal tunnel syndrome or diseases including diabetes mellitus; viruses that attack the nerve tissues, including herpes varicella zoster (shingles) or Epstein-Barr; and an acute inflammatory demyelinating neuropathy, Guillain-Barré syndrome, which damages motor, sensory, and autonomic nerve fibers. Damage to an upper motor neuron (the brain or within the spinal cord) may also result in weakness depending on the area and extent of damage in the brain or spinal cord. Finally, lack of activity during the recovery process may lead to disuse weakness.[11]

There are several methods of examining muscle strength: formal manual muscle testing, dynamometry, and functional testing. There are several grading systems used for manual muscle testing. Daniels and Worthingham use a scale from 0 to 5, with 1 and 2 indicating the patient's ability to move with gravity minimized and 3 to 5 indicating the patient's ability to move against gravity with increasing amounts of manual resistance.[24] Kendall et al[25] use a scale of 0 to 10, with 1 to 3 indicating the patient's ability to move with gravity minimized and 4 to 10 indicating the patient's ability to move against gravity with increasing amounts of manual resistance indicating the patient's ability to move against gravity or with gravity minimized. A hand-held dynamometer,[26] which measures the force applied at the point of application, can also be used to measure grip strength. Performing a manual muscle test with a patient recovering from a neurological disorder can be difficult, and, in general, the interrater reliability of manual muscle testing against gravity with manual resistance is variable. When formal muscle testing is not possible, the patient's functional movements can be observed for signs of weakness, such as difficulty transitioning from supine to sit positions, the inability to rise from a seated position without pushing with the arms, or difficulty stepping up a curb. A specific pattern of weakness may indicate the area of damage within the CNS. For example, lower motor neuron (peripheral nerve) damage, such as the deep peroneal nerve, would result in difficulty with ankle dorsiflexion and toe extension. This lower

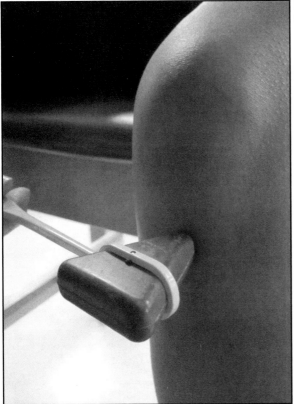

Figure 5-7. Using a reflex hammer to test phasic stretch reflex.

motor neuron damage would prevent an individual from dorsiflexing the foot while stepping up onto a curb or dorsiflexing the foot during the swing phase of the gait cycle. Damage to the nerve root (L4-5, S1) that supplies the deep peroneal nerve would also create weakness in the muscles innervated by the tibial nerve and the superficial peroneal, which also originate at nerve roots L4-5, S1. Damage at the spinal cord level of L4-5, S1 could result in bilateral weakness of the muscles innervated by L4-5, S1.

Examination of Phasic Stretch Reflexes

A phasic stretch reflex is a reflexive muscle contraction in response to a quick stretch.[12] Myotatic reflex, muscle stretch reflex, and deep tendon reflex are interchangeable with the term *phasic stretch reflex*. Presence of a phasic stretch reflex indicates that the monosynaptic reflex arc from the tendon through the spinal cord to the muscle is intact. Phasic stretch reflexes are tested by striking the tendon with a reflex hammer (Figure 5-7) and are graded as follows[14]:

0 = No response; always abnormal

1+ = A slight but definitely present response; may or may not be normal

2+ = A brisk response; normal

3+ = A very brisk response; may or may not be normal

4+ = A tap elicits a repeating reflex (clonus); always abnormal

An involuntary repetitive flexion and extension of the joint in response to a phasic stretch is known as clonus.[27] A clonus is examined by applying a quick stretch stimulus and then maintaining the stretch. A clonus that fades after a few beats is known as an unsustained clonus, whereas a clonus that continues is known as a sustained clonus. The presence of a sustained clonus is never normal.

Figure 5-8. Normal results of testing phasic stretch reflexes.

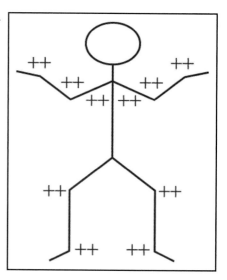

	Table 5-4 **Synergy Patterns of the Extremities**	
Limbs	*Flexion Synergy Components*	*Extension Synergy Components*
Upper	Scapular retraction, elevation, or hyperextension	Scapular protraction
	Shoulder abduction, external rotation	Shoulder adduction, internal rotation
	Elbow flexion	Elbow extension
	Forearm supination	Forearm pronation
	Wrist and finger flexion	Wrist and finger flexion
Lower	Hip flexion, abduction, external rotation	Hip extension, adduction, internal rotation
	Knee flexion	Knee extension
	Ankle dorsiflexion, inversion	Ankle plantarflexion, inversion
	Toe dorsiflexion	Toe plantarflexion

(Reprinted with permission from O'Sullivan SB. Assessment of motor function. In: O'Sullivan SB, Schmitz TJ, eds. *Physical Rehabilitation: Assessment and Treatment.* 4th ed. Philadelphia, PA: FA Davis Co; 2001.)

The results are frequently documented on a stick figure (Figure 5-8) with the number of "+"s corresponding to the grade of the reflexive response.

Examination of Synergy

Muscles that normally work together to produce a movement are known as synergists.[28] An abnormal synergy occurs when there is stereotypic coactivation of muscles that results in an abnormal coupling of movements at adjacent joints.[13] Refer to Table 5-4, which identifies the various synergies commonly seen in patients with CNS insults.

For example, during a lower extremity flexor synergy, the affected limb will tend to move into a combination of hip flexion, abduction external ration with knee flexion, and ankle dorsiflexion/

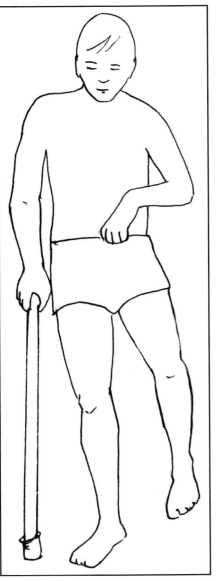

Figure 5-9. Patient attempting to ambulate with a lower extremity flexor synergy.

inversion. A flexion synergy during gait may lead to the inability of a patient to place the foot on the ground at initial contact, resulting in a fall (Figure 5-9).

One method of assessing synergies is the motor function section of the Fugl-Meyer Assessment of Motor Recovery After Stroke.[29] The patient is first asked to demonstrate a complete synergy by demonstrating active hip flexion, abduction external rotation with knee flexion, and ankle dorsiflexion/inversion of the affected leg. The patient is then asked to demonstrate movements out of synergy. For example, while standing, the patient is asked to place the affected lower extremity in 90 degrees of knee flexion with the hip in 0 degrees of extension and the ankle in dorsiflexion. Each component of the movement is scored based on how the movement component is performed.

Examination of Developmental Reflexes

A developmental reflex is a stereotypic response to a stimulus. Specific reflexes appear at specific ages so that developmental reflexes can be used to determine the child's level of development.

Figure 5-10. Nose-finger-nose coordination test.

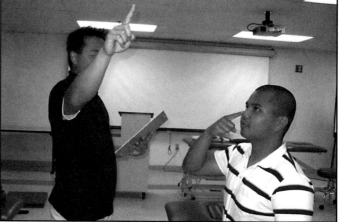

Except for righting, protective, and equilibrium reactions that are present in normal individuals throughout life, most developmental reflexes are not dominant past early childhood. Early developmental reflexes may appear when an adult is tired or under stress. Decreased inhibition of the reflexes may also occur when there is CNS damage. The developmental reflexes and testing are described in Table 5-5. The PTA must be able to identify the influence of developmental reflexes because the abnormal presence or absence of developmental reflexes may interfere with movement. For example, the patient may have difficulty rolling if there is a strong asymmetrical tonic neck present or the lack of equilibrium reactions may cause impairment of sitting balance.

Coordination

Coordination involves the sequencing, timing, and grading of multiple muscle groups, resulting in movement that is smooth, efficient, and accurate with the activation of multiple joints and muscles at the correct time with the correct amount of force.[30] Impaired coordination results in multiple disorders. The following are common tests used to examine coordination:

- Nose-finger-nose (Figure 5-10) is a test for dysmetria (the inability to make a movement of the appropriate distance). Dysmetria is tested by asking the patient to use the index finger to touch the nose then the therapist's finger. The therapist observes whether the patient is accurate or undershoots the target (hypometria) or overshoots the target (hypermetria).[30]

- Rapid alternating movements is a test for dysdiadochokinesia (the inability to make rapid alternating movements). Dysdiadochokinesia is tested by examining the patient's ability to produce rapid forearm supination-pronation or heel-toe movement smoothly with the correct force.[13]

- Heel to shin is a test for ataxia (a decreased coordination of muscle movements). The patient is placed in the supine position and requested to run the heel of one leg down the shin of the opposite leg.[30]

- Fregly-Graybiel Ataxia Test Battery[31] is a combination test for both coordination and balance. The test is composed of the following components: sharpened Romberg (standing heel to toe) with the eyes closed, walk 5 steps on a rail with the eyes open, stand on rail with eyes open, stand on a rail with eyes closed, stand on right leg with eyes closed, stand on left leg with eyes closed, and walk on the floor with eyes closed.

- Running and skipping may be used to identify impaired coordination in high-functioning patients who are ambulating without apparent deficits.

Table 5-5
Developmental Reflexes and Reaction Assessment

Reflex	Testing Position and Stimulus	Response
Flexor withdrawal	Supine or sitting position. Noxious stimulus (pinprick) to sole of foot.	Toes extend, foot dorsiflexes, entire leg flexes uncontrollably.
Crossed extension	Supine position. One leg fixed in extension. Noxious stimulus to ball of foot of the leg fixed in extension.	Opposite leg flexes, then adducts and extends.
Traction	Start in supine position. Grasp forearm and pull up from supine into sitting position.	Flexion of the shoulders, elbows, wrists, and fingers.
Moro	Sitting position. Sudden change in position of head in relation to trunk. Drop patient backward from sitting position.	Extension, abduction of arms, hand opening, and crying followed by flexion, adduction of arms across chest.
Startle	Any position. Sudden loud or harsh noise.	Sudden extension or abduction of arms. Crying.
Palmar grasp	Any position. Maintained pressure to palm of hand.	Maintained flexion of fingers.
Plantar grasp	Supine or sitting position. Maintained pressure to ball of foot under toes.	Maintained flexion of toes.
Asymmetrical tonic neck	Any position (commonly tested in supine). Rotation of the head to one side.	Flexion of arms and legs on skull side, extension of arms and legs on chin side ("bow and arrow" or "fencing posture"). Response may be stronger in the arms than legs.
Symmetrical tonic neck	Any position (commonly tested in supine). Flexion or extension of the head.	With head flexion: flexion of arms, extension of legs. With head extension: extension of arms, flexion of legs.
Symmetrical tonic labyrinthine	Prone or supine position.	With prone position: increased flexor tone or flexion of all limbs. With supine position: increased tone or extension of all limbs.
Positive supporting	Upright standing position. Contact to the ball of the foot.	Rigid extension (co-contraction) of the legs.
Associated movements or reactions	Any position. Resisted voluntary movement in any part of the body.	Involuntary movement in a resting extremity or increase in tonic muscle tension.
Neck righting acting on the body	Supine position. Passively turn head to one side.	Body rotates as a whole (logrolls) to align the body with the head.
Body righting acting on the body	Supine position. Passively rotate upper or lower trunk segment.	Body segment not rotated follows to align the body segments.

(continued)

	Table 5-5 (continued) **Developmental Reflexes and Reaction Assessment**		

Reflex	Testing Position and Stimulus	Response
Labyrinthine head righting	Upright position (standing or sitting). Blindfold eyes; alter body position by tipping body in all directions.	Head orients to vertical position with mouth horizontal.
Optical righting	Upright position (standing or sitting). Alter body position by tipping body in all directions.	Head orients to vertical position with mouth horizontal.
Upper extremities Protective extension forward, sideward, and backward	Sitting, kneeling, or standing position. Displace the center of gravity outside of the base of support.	*Forward:* Fingers and elbows extend, shoulders flex to support and to protect the body from falling. *Sideward:* Fingers and elbows extend, shoulders abduct. *Backward:* Fingers and elbows and shoulders extend.
Lower extremities Protective staggering forward, backward, and sideward	Standing. Displace the center of gravity outside of the base of support.	*Forward:* Subject steps forward when balance displaced forward. *Backward:* Subject steps backward when balance displaced backward.
Equilibrium reactions: Tilting	Supine, sitting, or standing position on a movable object such as a balance board or ball. Displace the center of gravity by tilting or moving the support surface.	Curvature of the trunk toward the upward side along with extension and abduction of the extremities on that side; protective extension on the downward side.
Equilibrium reactions: Postural fixation	Sitting or standing position. Displace the center of gravity in relation to the base of support but not outside of base of support. Can also be observed during voluntary activity.	*Sideward force:* Curvature of the trunk toward the external force with extension and abduction of the extremities on the side to which the force was applied. *Backward force:* Trunk flexion, extension of elbows with flexion of shoulders, and in standing plantarflexion of ankles. *Forward force:* Trunk extension, extension of arms, and in standing, dorsiflexion of ankles.

(Adapted from Barnes MR. *The Neurophysiological Basis of Patient Treatment. Vol II: Reflexes in Motor Development.* Atlanta, GA: Stokesville Publishing; 1978.)

Cranial Nerve Examination

Cranial nerves are peripheral nerves that originate from different structures in the brain.[13] There are 12 cranial nerves that are designated using Roman numerals I through XII. Cranial nerve I is the olfactory nerve and originates in the telencephalon. Cranial nerve II is the optic nerve and originates in the diencephalon. Cranial nerve III (oculomotor) and IV (trochlear) originate in the midbrain. Cranial nerves V (trigeminal), VI (abducens), and VII (facial) arise from the pons. The remaining cranial nerves, VIII (vestibulocochlear), IX (glossopharyngeal), X (vagus), XI (accessory), and XII (hypoglossal), arise from the medulla. The cranial nerves have 4 major functions[13]:

1. Innervation of the muscles of the face, eyes, tongue, tongue, jaw, and 2 neck muscles: the sternocleidomastoid and the trapezius.

2. Transmittal of somatosensory information from the skin and muscles of the face and temporal mandibular joint.

3. Transmittal of special sensory information related to vision, hearing vestibular, taste, smell, and visceral sensation.

4. Parasympathetic regulation of heart rate, blood pressure, breathing, digestion, and control of pupil size and the curvature of the lens of the eye.

Examining the cranial nerves provides information about the integrity of the parts of the brain where the nerves originate and about the functional loss caused by damage to the nerves.[13]

- Cranial nerve I (olfactory) controls the sense of smell and is tested by presenting familiar, nonirritating odors such as citrus, coffee, or cloves to each nostril. Damage to cranial nerve I may result in the inability to identify the substance (anosmia), a heightened sense of smell (hyperosmia), an altered sense of smell (parosmia), or the perception that a normal smell is unpleasant (carosmia).

- Cranial nerve II (optic) controls vision and is tested by examining the patient's visual acuity and the ability to perceive objects in different areas of vision (visual fields), acuity of vision, and pupillary response, in conjunction with cranial nerve III, to a bright light. Damage to cranial nerve II may result in complete loss of vision (anopsia), loss of half the field of vision of both eyes (hemianopsia), or loss of a quarter of the field of vision (quadranopsia).

- Cranial III (oculomotor) controls several of the muscles of the eyes and is tested by examining the patient's ability to look up, down, inward toward the nose (adduction), and combined up and in (a diagonal movement). Damage to cranial nerve III results in difficulty performing those specified eye movements.

- Cranial nerve IV controls the inferior oblique muscle, which causes the eyes to move down and in (adduction) and is tested by examining the patient's ability to move the eye combined down and in (a diagonal movement). Damage to cranial nerve IV results in difficulty performing the specified eye movements.

- Cranial nerve V (trigeminal nerve) controls facial sensation and the muscles of mastication (masseter, temporal, pterygoid, mylohyoid, and digastric) and is tested by using a pinprick to examine sensation of the face and manual muscle testing of the muscles of mastication. Damage to cranial nerve V results in impaired sensation to the face, weakness of the muscle of mastication, and impaired ability to chew.

- Cranial nerve VI (abducens nerve) innervates the lateral rectus muscle of the eye, which controls eye abduction and is tested by having the patient move the eye laterally. Damage to cranial nerve VI results in the inability to move the eye laterally.

- Cranial nerve VII (facial nerve) innervates the muscles of facial expression (eg, the orbicularis oris, nasalis, orbicularis occuli) and is tested by manually muscle testing the muscles of facial expression. Damage to cranial nerve VII results in paralysis of the muscles of facial expression.

- Cranial nerve VIII (vestibulocochlear) controls hearing and vestibular function (balance). The hearing component of the vestibulocochlear nerve is examined by formal auditory testing or having the examiner rub his or her fingers close to the patient's ear, then determining whether the patient is able to hear the sound. The vestibular component is tested through formal vestibular testing or a basic screening test for balance. Damage to cranial nerve VIII results in impaired hearing and/or balance.

- Cranial nerve IX (glossopharyngeal nerve) controls swallowing and, in conjunction with cranial nerve X, the sensation on the posterior third of the tongue, pharynx, and gag reflex. Cranial nerve IX is examined by testing the gag reflex by touching a tongue depressor to the posterior portion of the tongue or pharynx to determine whether a gag reflex is elicited. Damage to cranial nerve IX may adversely affect the patient's ability to swallow.

- Cranial nerve X (vagus nerve) provides innervation of the larynx (in conjunction with cranial nerve IX), pharynx, and viscera. Cranial nerve X is tested by looking for symmetrical elevation of the soft palate while the patient says, "Ahhh." Damage to cranial nerve X affects the patient's ability to swallow and speak. Digestive functions may also be adversely affected, and patients may stop eating because of the fear of choking.

- Cranial nerve XI (accessory nerve) innervates the trapezius and the sternocleidomastoid muscles and is tested by manually muscle testing the trapezius and sternocleidomastoid muscles. Damage to cranial nerve XI results in ipsilateral paralysis of the affected muscles.

- Cranial nerve XII (hypoglossal nerve) innervates the intrinsic muscles of the tongue. Cranial nerve XII is examined by having the patient protrude the tongue and observing the tongue for deviation or atrophy. The patient may also be requested to push the tongue into the cheek. The examiner tests the strength of the tongue by pushing against the tongue from the outside of the cheek. Damage to cranial nerve XII results in deviation of the tongue to the side of the lesion and may affect speech and swallowing.

Examinations for Balance

Balance is based on input from the somatosensory, visual, and vestibular systems and includes several important components:

- Center of gravity (COG): "The place in a system or body where the weight is evenly dispersed and all sides are in balance."[32]

- BOS: "The area of the body that is in contact with the support surface."[30] The BOS may include the contact area of an assistive device such as a walker or crutches.

- Equilibrium: Allows the body as a whole to adapt to changes or perturbations in the relationship of the COG over the BOS.[33]

- Protective reactions (parachute reactions): Extensor responses in the extremities, which occur when the COG is moved beyond the BOS as protection during a fall by either placing the hand out to regain equilibrium or stepping with the leg opposite to the perturbation.[34]

- Limits of stability: How far an individual in the upright position can lean in any direction without external support, such as taking a step, reaching with the arm(s), or falling.[35] The specific limits of stability vary depending on height, weight, and body composition such as leg length, foot size, and range of motion of the hips, knees, ankles, and forefoot of the individual being tested.

Examination of balance includes the examination of automatic postural responses to both fast and slow perturbations, anticipatory postural responses and volitional postural response as seen in normal activities of daily living (ADL) such as rising from a chair or walking on uneven surfaces. The major automatic postural responses (Figure 5-11) include the ankle, hip, stepping, and suspensory strategies, also known as *balance synergies*.[35]

- The ankle strategy/synergy occurs to counteract small displacements from the COG. The body moves as a unit over the feet, with the muscles contracting from distal to proximal. The

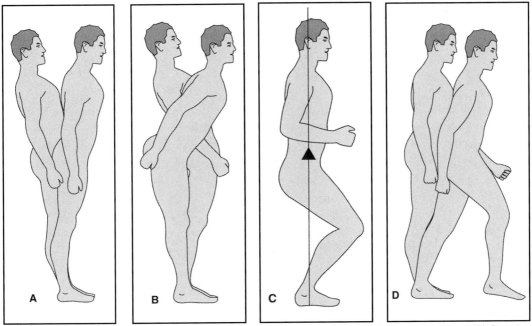

Figure 5-11. Automatic postural strategies. (A) Ankle strategy. (B) Hip strategy. (C) Suspensory strategy. (D). Stepping strategy. (Adapted with permission from Umphred DA, Lazaro RT, Roller ML, Burton GU, eds. *Umphred's Neurological Rehabilitation.* 6th ed. Allison L, Fuller K. Balance and vestibular dysfunction, 658, Copyright Elsevier [2103].)

head and hips move in the same direction, at the same time, as a unit. This synergy elicits muscle response at the ankles first.

- The hip strategy/synergy is used in specific situations such as a narrow surface or the edge of a surface where the individual does not want to step forward. The hip strategy is more complex than the ankle strategy because the head and hips move in opposite directions, occurring when sway is large, fast, and nearing the limits of stability. The hip strategy elicits muscle contractions from proximal to distal.

- The suspensory strategy/synergy also occurs in response to large displacements and results in a squatting response to lower the COG.

- The stepping strategy/synergy occurs in response to large displacements and results in the realignment of the BOS under the center of mass. Normal walking is an example of the use of the stepping strategy or synergy as the individual moves forward beyond the normal BOS and then replaces the foot back under the BOS at heel strike.

There are 2 tests for examining automatic postural responses. The first test is the Sensory Organization Test (SOT), in which the patient is positioned on a computerized movable forceplate with a movable visual surround[35] (Figure 5-12). The forceplate tests the somatosensory component of balance and body sway, and the movable surround and blindfold test the visual component of balance. The forceplate and the visual surround are changed to alter the surface and visual environment. By combining different configurations of the forceplate, movable surround, and blindfold, the examiner is able to isolate different components of the balance system. The test is divided into 6 conditions. In condition 1, the patient is receiving correct information from all 3 senses (vision, vestibular, and somatosensory); this acts as a baseline test. In condition 2, the eyes are obscured with a blindfold so that the patient is not receiving visual input and only somatosensory and vestibular input remain. In condition 3, the visual surround moves in conjunction with the patient's sway, providing inaccurate visual input that the patient must ignore. Somatosensory

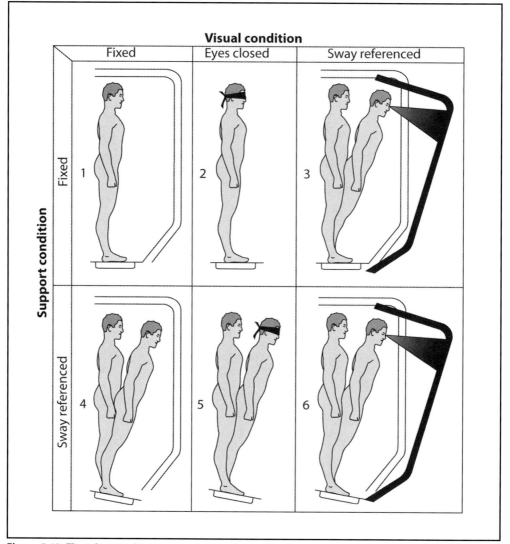

Figure 5-12. The 6 Sensory Organization Test conditions. The Sensory Organization Test determines the relative reliance on visual, vestibular, and somatosensory inputs for postural control using computerized dynamic posturography. (Adapted with permission from Umphred DA, Lazaro RT, Roller ML, Burton GU, eds. *Umphred's Neurological Rehabilitation.* 6th ed. Allison L, Fuller K. Balance and vestibular dysfunction, 658, Copyright Elsevier [2103].)

and vestibular inputs remain available. In condition 4, the support surface adjusts to the patient's sway, giving inaccurate somatosensory input while visual and vestibular inputs are still available. In condition 5, vision is absent and the support surface is sway referenced, resulting in no visual input and inaccurate somatosensory input. Only vestibular input is available. In condition 6, the forceplate and visual surround are sway referenced, and again the only accurate input is vestibular input.

The SOT examines which inputs are available to the patient and whether the patient can compensate for missing or distorted input. For example, if the patient demonstrates difficulty with condition 2, in which vision is obscured but somatosensory and vestibular inputs are unaffected, the patient might have difficulty in low-light situations, such as going to the bathroom at night. If the patient demonstrates difficulty with condition 4, in which somatosensory input is distorted by the sway-referenced forceplate but visual and vestibular input are not affected, the patient may have difficulty walking on compliant surfaces, such as thick carpeting. Input may also be distorted

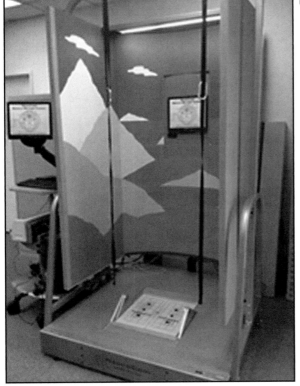

Figure 5-13. Neurocom SMART Balance System.

by physiologic or body system issues that have little to do with the neurological medical diagnosis in CNS insults. Examples might be impaired vision from diabetes, cataracts, macular degeneration, or Ménière's disease or decreased sensation as found in peripheral neuropathies. Computer-based equipment, such as the Neurocom SMART Balance System[36] (Figure 5-13) and the Biodex Balance System[37] (Figure 5-14), are used for examining and treating balance deficits and incorporate many of these factors into the programming.

The Clinical Test for Sensory Integration on Balance (CTSIB) was developed for use in the clinic and does not rely on computerized technology.[35] The CTSIB mimics the conditions of the SOT by using dense foam to replicate the movable forceplate, a blindfold to obscure vision, and a modified Japanese lantern to replicate the movable surround (Figure 5-15). Note that research has not supported the use of the modified Japanese lantern as an adequate substitute for the sway-referenced, movable surround.

Balance is divided into 2 major categories: static balance and dynamic balance. Static balance refers to the patient's ability to maintain an upright position. Although the word "static" is used to describe this component of balance, "quiet" may be a more accurate term, as there is nothing static about the static balance response. Although the patient seems not to be moving, there are continual slight postural adjustments over the COG. The balance system is being set to anticipate movement. Static balance could also be described as postural balance because the systems are working together to maintain the upright position. Dynamic balance is the ability to maintain upright posture while the body is in motion and might be better described as active balance.[35]

Quiet (static) balance is tested by observing the patient's ability to maintain a sitting and standing position.[35] To test active (dynamic) balance, the patient's ability to maintain an upright position while moving the COG within or outside of the BOS is evaluated. A commonly used grading system for balance is found in Table 5-6.

Figure 5-14. Biodex Balance System.

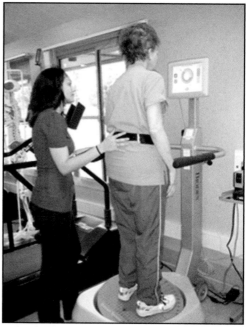

Figure 5-15. The Clinical Test for Sensory Integration on Balance using dense foam to mimic condition 4 of the Sensory Organization Test.

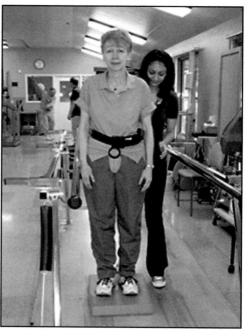

Functional Activities

Functional activities refer to the client's ability to perform various functional skills and ADL. The therapist first identifies the functional activities that the patient is able and not able to do, hypothesizes the possible impairments causing the limitations, and then tests the body systems and subsystems to identify the nature and extent of the impairment. What can the patient do and how? What can the patient not do and why? The approach is proactive and collaborative,

Table 5-6
Functional Balance Grades

Normal	Quiet/Static: The patient maintains steady balance without hand-hold support. Active/Dynamic: The patient accepts maximal challenge and easily shifts his or her weight (full range of motion in all directions).
Good	Quiet/Static: The patient maintains balance without hand-hold support, and there is limited postural sway. Active/Dynamic: The patient accepts moderate challenge, and he or she maintains balance when picking up an item from the floor.
Fair	Quiet/Static: The patient maintains balance with hand-hold support; however, he or she may need minimal assistance occasionally. Active/Dynamic: The patient accepts minimal challenge, and he or she maintains balance when turning his or her head or trunk.
Poor	Quiet/Static: The patient needs hand-hold support plus moderate to maximal assistance to maintain his or her position. Active/Dynamic: The patient cannot accept challenge or move without losing his or her balance.

(Adapted from O'Sullivan SB, Schmitz TJ. *Physical Rehabilitation: Assessment and Treatment*. 5th ed. Philadelphia, PA: FA Davis; 2007 and Allison LK, Fuller K. Balance and vestibular dysfunction. In: *Umphred's Neurological Rehabilitation*. 6th ed. St Louis, MO: Elsevier; 2013.)

capitalizing on the patient's potential and goals and promoting the therapist-patient partnership. It is important for the PT or PTA examining the patient's functional activity status to be receptive to the patient's view of his or her own functional abilities. It is useful to initially examine tasks where the patient may fail, as this can demonstrate an unexpected ability for the patient to perform the task successfully. However, there is no need to examine a functional skill repeatedly if there is a high likelihood of failure for the patient. This is extremely important because asking the patient to fail over and over is discouraging, decreases motivation to continue trying, and can create a negative treatment environment. On the other hand, when the PTA has a patient who thinks he or she is able to perform a task, it is important to let him or her realize the limitations. The patient's awareness of his or her inability to perform a task may act to motivate the patient's participation in physical therapy to work toward performing the task with less assistance and decreased risk of injury.

Multiple functional activities are assessed during the examination. These activities may include the patient's ability to roll, perform supine to sit, transfer (to bed, chair, car, etc), perform sit to stand, and walk or propel a w/c. In pediatric patients, developmental positions such as prone on elbows, quadruped, kneeling, and half-kneeling are examined.[11]

Accurate documentation of patient functional ability must include the amount of assistance, if any, required to perform a skill or task, as well as the amount of time required for completion of that task. Table 5-7 lists the terminology derived from the Functional Independence Measure (FIM) (Uniform Data System for Medical Rehabilitation)[38] describing assistance levels required by the patient. When selecting the appropriate descriptive term for the amount of assistance that the patient requires, it is important that the clinician accurately assesses the amount of effort put forth by the patient for the task as opposed to the amount of effort put forth by the clinician to select the most accurate assistance term.

Standardized tests have been developed to provide an objective assessment of a patient's impairments or functional performance. Understanding the components of these tests is essential for the

Table 5-7
Terminology and Definitions of Assistance Levels

Term	Definition
Independent	Patient consistently performs the skill safely with no one present and in a timely manner. If an assistive device is needed, include the name of the device.
Supervision or setup	Patient performs 100% of the task but requires verbal cueing, someone standing by, or someone must set up needed items.
Contact guarding	Patient performs 100% of the task but person assisting gives full attention to patient and has hands on patient for possible assistance or possible loss of balance.
Minimal assistance	Patient expends 75% or more of the effort for the task.
Moderate assistance	Patient expends 50% to 75% of the effort for the task.
Maximum assistance	Patient expends 25% to 50% of the effort for the task.
Dependent	Patient expends less than 25% of the effort for the task.

(Adapted from *Guide for the Uniform Data System for Medical Rehabilitation (Adult FIM)*. Version 4.0. Buffalo, NY: State University of New York at Buffalo; 1993.)

PTA to understand as he or she executes and progresses patient interventions. Components of the tests may be retested during interventions, revealing information regarding a patient's functional improvement and progression toward goals to be communicated to the patient and PT. There are many tests available to the physical therapy community, and it is important for the PT to identify those tests that are appropriate, valid, and reliable based on the patient's diagnosis and presentation. Examples of these tests are discussed next. Many of the tests discussed are available for personal use at the Rehabilitation Measures Database Web site.[38,39]

Standardized Impairment and Functional Tests

Berg Balance Scale

The Berg Balance Scale[40] (BBS) measures static and dynamic balance abilities. The test takes 15 to 20 minutes to complete. This test involves 14 tasks, including sitting to standing, standing unsupported, reaching forward with outstretched arm while standing, retrieving an object from the floor, and turning 360 degrees. The patient is rated on the ability to perform these tasks and given a score of 0, 1, 2, 3, or 4. The higher the score on a measure indicates greater independence. The total possible score is 56. A score of less than 45 indicates an increased risk of falling. A modified version of the BBS includes only the advanced balance items (items 6 through 14) and is used for testing higher functioning individuals. (Refer to the video for Chapter 5, which shows an individual performing the Berg Balance Test.)

Functional Reach

The Functional Reach Test[41] was developed as a quick screening for balance deficits in older individuals. The Functional Reach Test measures a patient's ability to reach forward beyond arm's length while standing without falling and maintaining a fixed BOS. A Modified Functional Reach Test was developed for patients who are unable to stand and is performed sitting. Newton developed the Multidirectional Reach Test. In addition to forward reach, the Multidirectional Reach Test also examines the patient's ability to reach sideways and backward. Normative values have been determined and are affected by age and height. This test takes approximately 5 minutes to complete.

Table 5-8
Timed Up and Go Cut-Off Scores

	Cut-Off Score(s)	Sensitivity (% Fallers)	Specificity (% Nonfallers)	Overall Prediction	Predicted Probability
TUG	≥ 13.5	80%	100%	90%	.77
TUG$_{manual}$	≥ 14.5	86.7%	93.3%	90%	.5
TUG$_{cognitive}$	≥ 15	80%	93.3%	86.7%	.5

(Reprinted from Shumway-Cook A, Brauer S, Woollacott M. Predicting the probability for falls in community-dwelling older adults using the Timed Up and Go Test. *Phys Ther.* 2000;80[9]:896-903 with permission from the American Physical Therapy Association. Copyright © 2000 American Physical Therapy Association.)

Performance-Oriented Mobility Assessment

The Performance-Oriented Mobility Assessment test[42] (the Tinetti Assessment Tool) was developed for use with an elderly population. The test is composed of 2 sections. The first section assesses balance and is composed of 9 items, including coming to standing, initial standing balance, and turning. The second section assesses gait and is composed of 7 items, including initiating gait, step symmetry, and sway of trunk during gait. A score of 0 to 2 is used in most categories, with a maximum score of 16 for balance and 12 for gait and a maximum combined score of 28. A score of less than 18 out of 28 indicates a high risk for falling. The test takes 10 to 15 minutes to complete.

Timed Up and Go

The Timed Up and Go (TUG)[43] measures the time it takes for an individual seated in a firm chair with arms and a back rest to stand up, walk 3 meters, turn around, and return to the chair. Cut-off scores indicating increased fall risk are available in Table 5-8.[44] The test typically takes 5 minutes or less to complete. There are variations of the TUG, which include the addition of cognitive and motor challenges. The addition of cognitive and motor challenges was found to increase the time for completion of the TUG, but there was no effect on the ability to predict fall risk. (Refer to the videotape of Chapter 5, which shows an individual performing the TUG.)

Motor Assessment Scale

The Motor Assessment Scale[45] assesses motor recovery over time. The scale is composed of 8 items examining motor function (supine to side-lying, supine to sit, sit to stand, balanced sitting, walking, upper-arm function, hand movements, and advanced hand function) and one item examining muscle tone. The items are scored on a scale of 0 to 10, with 0 indicating that the patient is unable to perform the task and 6 indicating optimal performance. The item examining muscle tone is difficult to use because of a lack of concise criteria for scoring, and as a result this item may be omitted.[46,47]

The Barthel Index

The Barthel Index[48] assesses the amount of assistance needed by a patient. The scale is composed of 10 items (feeding, bathing, personal toilet, dressing, bowel, bladder, toilet transfers, transfers to chair and bed, ambulation, and stair climbing). Each item is scored as 0, 5, 10, or 15, with 0 indicating that the patient is unable to perform the task, and higher scores, which vary from 5 to 15 depending on the item, indicating that the patient is independent. The total score will indicate the patient's dependence, level of care, and number of hours of assistance needed.

Functional Independence Measure

The FIM[39,48] is used to supply data to the Uniform Data System for Medical Rehabilitation from participating facilities. The data are used to develop summary reports for the facility. The FIM consists of 18 items in 3 domains that are examined at admission and discharge. Self-care examines the patient's ability in eating, grooming, bathing, dressing upper and lower extremities, and toileting. Sphincter control examines bladder and bowel control. The transfer section examines the patient's ability to perform bed/chair/w/c transfers and toilet/shower transfers. The locomotion section examines the patient's ability to walk or propel a w/c and manage stairs. The communication section examines the patient's comprehension and expression. Finally, the social comprehension section examines the patient's social interaction, problem solving, and memory. The items are scored on a scale of 1 through 7, with 1 indicating total assistance or not testable and 7 indicating complete independence. The FIM is a proprietary scale, and the examiner should be certified in the FIM System before entering the results into the medical record.

Participation

Participation in the International Classification of Function, Disability and Health terminology as developed by the World Health Organization is defined as an individual's involvement in a life situation.[49] Some examples of aspects of participation that can be examined for each individual include domestic life, interpersonal relationships, and community, social, and civic life. The term used to denote problems that individuals may experience in involvement in life situations is *participation restriction*. It is always important to obtain the patient's perception of how his or her medical condition, impairments, and activity limitations affect involvement in life and community. Many of the tests for participation and self-efficacy available for the PT to administer are in self-report format. Examples of tests used to collect data about participation are the Activities-Specific Balance Confidence Scale (ABC),[50] Short Form 36 (SF-36),[51] and Dizziness Handicap Confidence Inventory (DHI).[52]

CONCLUSION

The American Physical Therapy Association (APTA) has developed a model (Figure 5-16), based on a series of assumptions (Table 5-9), for supervision of the PTA by the PT.

After the initial examination, establishment of goals, and plan of care established by the PT, the PTA algorithm identified in Figure 5-16 should help the PTA determine progression within the plan of care, when a repeat of the initial tests and measures are needed, and/or when the patient's functional behavior needs to be discussed with the PT. The PTA needs to always remember that drawing conclusions from the tests and measures that change the plan of care is the responsibility of the PT and should not be placed within the scope of practice of the PTA.

This chapter provides an overview of the physical therapy examination process initially performed by the PT during the evaluation of the neurologically impaired patient, including the protocols for administration of more common tests and measures. The PTA must have an understanding of the reasoning behind the examination and administered tools specific to the patient diagnosis and presentation. This knowledge, including the use of standard tests, assists the PTA in contributing to the measurement of "the patient's progress with gait, locomotion, balance, and mobility."[53] The PTA serves a key role in functioning as the clinician who, during patient encounters and administration of interventions, measures progress and adjusts interventions within the plan of care based on reexamination of the test and measure outcomes

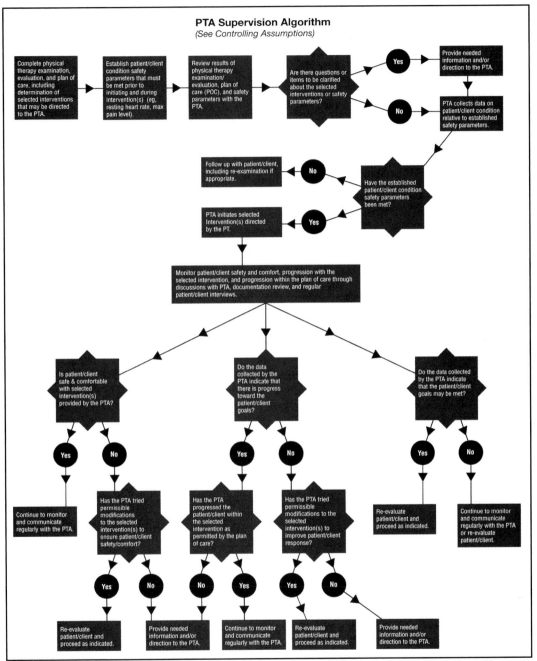

Figure 5-16. PTA Supervision Algorithm. (Reprinted from www.apta.org/PTinMotion/2010/9/PTAsToday, with permission of the American Physical Therapy Association. Copyright © 2010 American Physical Therapy Association.)

obtained during the initial PT's evaluation. This information further enhances the decision-making process between the PT and the PTA, which allows for the optimal level of care and improved outcomes. As the PTA's educational level increases and the roles and responsibilities change, examination skills and analytical reasoning will become an even more critical aspect of the responsibilities of the PTA.

Table 5-9
Controlling Assumptions for   **Physical Therapist Assistant Supervision**
The physical therapist (PT) integrates the 5 elements of patient/client management—examination, evaluation, diagnosis, prognosis, and intervention—in a manner designed to optimize outcomes. Responsibility for completion of the examination, evaluation, diagnosis, and prognosis is borne solely by the PT. The PT's plan of care may involve the physical therapist assistant (PTA) assisting with selected interventions.
The PTA has the knowledge, skills, and value-based behaviors needed to help the PT provide selected interventions as described in the plan of care. PTAs are clinical problem solvers who ensure patient/client safety and comfort and complete interventions selected to achieve desired outcomes. Other than PTs, PTAs are the only valid providers of physical therapy services.
The PT directs and supervises the PTA consistent with APTA House of Delegates positions, including Direction and Supervision of the Physical Therapist Assistant; APTA core documents, including Standards of Ethical Conduct for the Physical Therapist Assistant; federal and state legal practice standards; and institutional regulations.
All selected interventions are directed and supervised by the PT. The PTA does not perform interventions that require immediate and continuous examination and evaluation throughout, as described in APTA House of Delegates position Procedural Interventions Exclusively Performed by Physical Therapists. Procedural interventions within the scope of physical therapy practice that are performed exclusively by the PT include, but are not limited to, spinal and peripheral joint mobilization/manipulation (which are components of manual therapy) and sharp selective débridement (which is a component of wound management). The PT is also responsible for ensuring the PTA has the knowledge and skills required to safely and effectively complete the intervention.
The PT remains responsible for physical therapy services provided when the PT's plan of care involves the PTA assisting with selected interventions.
Selected intervention(s) include the procedural intervention, associated data collection, and communication—including written documentation associated with the safe, effective, and efficient completion of the task.
The algorithm may represent decision processes employed for either a patient/client interaction or an episode of care.
Communication between the PT and PTA regarding patient/client care is ongoing. The algorithm does not intend to imply a limitation or restriction on communication between the PT and PTA.

(Adapted from Controlling Assumptions APTA Web site. http://www.apta.org/PTA/PatientCare. Accessed January 12, 2013.)

ACKNOWLEDGMENTS

The authors of this chapter want to thank Rolando T. Lazaro, PT, PhD, DPT, MS, GCS, for his contributions to this chapter in the First Edition and his guidance in the development of this chapter.

REFERENCES

1. *Guide to Physical Therapist Practice*. 2nd ed. Alexandria, VA: American Physical Therapy Association; 2001.

2. Vital signs. Wikipedia. http://en.wikipedia.org/wiki/Vital_signs. Accessed January 5, 2013.

3. Schmitz, T. Vital signs. In: O'Sullivan SB, Schmitz TJ, eds. *Physical Rehabilitation*. Philadelphia, PA: FA Davis; 2007.

4. Commission on Accreditation in Physical Therapy Education. Evaluative Criteria PTA Programs. http://www.apta.org/search.aspx?q=Evaluative%20criteria%20PTA%20programs. Accessed January 13, 2013.

5. Williamson A, Hoggart B. Pain: a review of three commonly used pain rating scales. *J Clin Nurs*. 2005;14(7): 798-804.

6. Scherder EJ, Bouma A. Visual analogue scales for pain assessment in Alzheimer's disease. *Gerontology*. 2000;46(1):47-53.

7. Wong D, Baker C. Wong-Baker FACES Pain Rating Scale. http://www.wongbakerfaces.org/. Accessed January 5, 2013.

8. Feldt KS. The Checklist of Nonverbal Pain Indicators (CNPI). *Pain Manag Nurs*. 2000;1(1):13-21.

9. Warden V, Hurley A, Volicer L. Development and psychometric evaluation of the Pain Assessment in Advanced Dementia (PAINAD) scale. *J Am Med Dir Assoc*. 2003;4(1):9-15.

10. Srouji R, Ratnapalan S, Schneeweiss S. Pain in children: assessment and nonpharmacological management. *Int J Pediatr*. 2010;2010:pii:474838.

11. Lazaro RT. Examination procedures. In: Umphred D, Carlson C, eds. *Neurorehabilitation for the Physical Therapist Assistant*. Thorofare, NJ: SLACK Incorporated; 2006.

12. Posner JB, Saper CB, Schiff N, Plum F. *Plum and Posner's Diagnosis of Stupor and Coma*. New York, NY: Oxford University Press; 2007.

13. Lundy-Ekman L. *Neuroscience: Fundamentals for Rehabilitation*. 4th ed. St Louis, MO: Saunders/Elsevier; 2013.

14. O'Sullivan SB. Examination of motor function: motor control and motor learning. In: O'Sullivan SB, Schmitz TJ, eds. *Physical Rehabilitation*. Philadelphia, PA: FA Davis; 2007.

15. Folstein M. Mini-Mental State: a practical method for grading the cognitive state of patients for the clinician. *J Psychiatr Res*. 1975;12(3):189-198.

16. Mini-Mental State Examination. 2nd ed. http://www4.parinc.com/Products/Product.aspx?ProductID=MMSE-2. Accessed January 12, 2013.

17. Cullen B, O'Neill B, Evans J, Coen R, Lawlor B. A review of screening tests for cognitive impairment. *J Neurol Neurosurg Psychiatry*. 2007;78(8):790-799.

18. Bigley GK. Sensation. In: Walker HK, Hall WD, Hurst JW, eds. *Clinical Methods: The History, Physical, and Laboratory Examinations*. 3rd ed. Boston, MA: Butterworths; 1990. http://www.ncbi.nlm.nih.gov/books/NBK390/. Accessed January 6, 2013.

19. Schmitz TJ. Examination of sensory function. In: O'Sullivan SB, Schmitz TJ, eds. *Physical Rehabilitation*. Philadelphia, PA: FA Davis; 2007.

20. Reese NB. *Muscle and Sensory Testing*. 3rd ed. St Louis, MO: Saunders; 2012.

21. Gilman S, Newman SW. *Manter and Gatz's Essentials of Clinical Neuroanatomy and Neurophysiology*. 10th ed. Philadelphia, PA: FA Davis; 2003.

22. Haugh AB, Pandyan, AD, Johnson GR. A systematic review of the Tardieu Scale for the measurement of spasticity. *Disabil Rehabil*. 2006;28(15);899-907.

23. Bohannon RW, Smith MB. Interrater reliability of a modified Ashworth Scale of Muscle Spasticity. *Phys Ther*. 1987;67(2):206-207.

24. Hislop HJ, Montgomery J. *Daniels and Worthingham's Muscle Testing: Techniques of Manual Examination*. 8th ed. Philadelphia, PA: WB Saunders; 2007.

25. Kendall FP, McCreary EK, Provance PG, Rodgers MM, Romani WA. *Muscles: Testing and Function, with Posture and Pain*. 5th ed. Philadelphia, PA: Lippincott Williams & Wilkins; 2005.

26. White DJ. Musculoskeletal examination. In: O'Sullivan SB, Schmitz TJ, eds. *Physical Rehabilitation*. Philadelphia, PA: FA Davis; 2007.

27. Campbell WW, DeJong RN. *DeJong's The Neurologic Examination*. 7th ed. Philadelphia, PA: Lippincott Williams & Wilkins; 2013.

28. Lippert LS. *Clinical Kinesiology and Anatomy (Clinical Kinesiology for Physical Therapist Assistants)*. 5th ed. Philadelphia, PA: FA Davis; 2011.

29. Gladstone DJ, Danells CJ, Black SE. The Fugl-Meyer Assessment of Motor Recovery after stroke: a critical review of its measurement properties. *Neurorehabil Neural Repair*. 2002;16(3):232-240.

30. Shumway-Cook A, Woollacott MH. *Motor Control: Translating Research into Clinical Practice*. 4th ed. Philadelphia, PA: Lippincott Williams & Wilkins; 2012:162.

31. Graybiel A, Fregly AR. A new quantitative ataxia test battery. *Acta Otolaryngol*. 1966;61(4):292-312.

32. Center of gravity. Your Dictionary: The Dictionary You Can Understand. http://www.yourdictionary.com/center-of-gravity. Accessed January 6, 2013.

33. Martin ST, Kessler M. *Neurologic Interventions for Physical Therapy*. St Louis, MO: Saunders; 2000.

34. Ryerson SD. Movement dysfunction associated with hemiplegia. In: *Umphred's Neurological Rehabilitation*. 6th ed. St Louis, MO: Elsevier; 2013.

35. Allison LK, Fuller K. Balance and vestibular dysfunction. In: *Umphred's Neurological Rehabilitation*. 6th ed. St Louis, MO: Elsevier; 2013.

36. Setting the Standard in Balance and Mobility. http://resourcesonbalance.com/neurocom/products/SMARTBalanceMaster.aspx. Accessed January 12, 2013.

37. Biodex. http://www.biodex.com/. Accessed January 12, 2013.

38. *Guide for the Uniform Data Set for Medical Rehabilitation (Adult FIM)*. Version 4.0. Buffalo, NY: State University of New York at Buffalo; 1993.

39. Rehabilitation Measures Database. http://www.rehabmeasures.org/default.aspx. Accessed January 12, 2013.

40. Berg K, Wood-Dauphinee S, Williams JI, Gayton D. Measuring balance in the elderly: preliminary development of an instrument. *Physiother Can*. 1989;41:304.

41. Duncan PW, Weiner DK, Chandler J, Studenski S. Function reach: a new clinical measure of balance. *J Gerontol*. 1990:45(6):M192-M197.

42. Tinetti ME. Performance-oriented assessment of mobility problems in the elderly. *J Am Geriatr Soc*. 1986;34(2):119-126.

43. Podsiadlo D, Richardson S. The timed "Up & Go": a test of basic functional mobility for frail elderly persons. *J Am Geriatr Soc*. 1991;39(2):142-148.

44. Shumway-Cook A, Brauer S, Woollacott M. Predicting the probability for falls in community-dwelling older adults using the Timed Up & Go Test. *Phys Ther*. 2000;80(9):896-903.

45. Carr JH, Shepherd RB, Nordholm L, Lynne D. Investigation of a new motor assessment scale for stroke patients. *Phys Ther*. 1985;65(2):175-180.

46. Loewen SC, Anderson BA. Predictors of stroke outcome using objective measurement scales. *Stroke*. 1990:21(1):78-81.

47. Malouin, F, Pichard, L, Bonneau C, Durant A, Corriveau D. Evaluating motor recovery early after stroke: comparison of the Fugl-Meyer Assessment and the Motor Assessment Scale. *Arch Phys Med Rehabil*. 1994;75(11):1206-1212.

48. Guccione AA, Scalzitti, DA. Examination of functional status and activity level. In: O'Sullivan SB, Schmitz TJ, eds. *Physical Rehabilitation*. Philadelphia, PA: FA Davis; 2007.

49. Lazaro RT, Roller ML, Umphred DA. Differential diagnosis phase 2: examination and evaluation of functional movement activities, body functions and structures, and participation. In: *Umphred's Neurological Rehabilitation*. 6th ed. St Louis, MO: Elsevier; 2013.

50. Powell LE, Myers AM. The Activities-Specific Balance Confidence (ABC) Scale. *J Gerontol A Biol Sci Med Sci*. 1995:50A(1):M28-M34.

51. Anderson C, Laubscher S, Burns R. Validation of the Short Form 36 (SF-36) health survey questionnaire among stroke patients. *Stroke*. 1996;27(10):1812-1816.

52. Jacobson GP, Newman CW. The development of the Dizziness Handicap Inventory. *Arch Otolaryngol Head Neck Surg*. 1990;116(4):424-427.

53. American Physical Therapy Association. Minimum required skills of physical therapist assistant graduates at entry-level. http://www.apta.org/uploadedFiles/APTAorg/About_Us/Policies/BOD/Education/MinReqSkillsPTAGrad.pdf#search=%22minimum%20required%20skills%20physical%20therapist%20assistant%22. Accessed January 12, 2013.

Please see accompanying Web site at

www.healio.com/books/neuroptavideos

6

Psychosocial and Cognitive Issues Affecting Therapy

Gordon U. Burton, OT/L, PhD

KEY WORDS

- Adjustment
- Anger
- Anxiety
- Denial
- Depression
- Disengagement
- Engagement
- Hope
- Hostility
- Maladaptive
- Shock
- Spiritual/spirituality

CHAPTER OBJECTIVES

- Identify 6 stages of adjustment.
- Identify the difference between engagement and disengagement.
- Develop an understanding of the flexible stages of adjustment.
- Realize that all people are in a state of adjustment, not just clients.
- Recognize that each client is unique and needs to have individualized treatment.

INTRODUCTION

Why do any of us do the things we do? Why do we get up and go through the everyday trials and tribulations that we go through each day? How do we deal with our bodies changing from year to year or decade to decade? How do we deal with the fact that we will all die someday? How do we

Umphred DA, Lazaro RT, eds.
Neurorehabilitation for the Physical Therapist Assistant,
Second Edition (pp 151-163).
© 2014 SLACK Incorporated.

deal with all of the changes in our lives? How do we deal with functional limitations? How do we deal with disease and pathology?

These are some of the questions that clients may be dealing with on a daily basis, but with a bit of a different slant on the questions. In life, we are all trying to discover our unique purposes and how we are to identify and play roles that match this uniqueness and offer the highest quality in life. Clients try to adjust to life just like therapists. Clients have challenges; some of the challenges are unexpected, and some they are not prepared for. Most of us do not think about having an accident and severing our spinal cord, losing some of our brain functions, developing a tumor, or all of the above, but when it happens to us, we have to deal with its reality. "Dealing with it" will be called *adjusting* or *adapting* to a disability in this chapter. Some people (clients) adjust or adapt well while others do not, although most people adjust well enough to get by in society. In this chapter, we will discuss some of the highlights of this process, what it means to therapy, and your role as the physical therapist assistant (PTA).

Adjustment is an ongoing process for all of us. We are not suddenly adjusted to something. Adjustment is a fluid process that does not flow in just one direction. Family and loved ones often do not go through this process at the same speed or in the same way. Thus, the therapist must always be aware of where each client and each support person is at all times within this adjustment process to create the best environment and to provide the best intervention. The PTA's role in this process is to make the therapy process progress as smoothly and efficiently as possible.

Each day, you must adjust to successes, failures, accomplishments, and inadequacies; some are consistent failures, and some are consistent accomplishments. A client is no different. Adjustment and adaptation are how one gets through life. We all have limitations that we must adjust to—you will probably never be that ballerina or football star that you would like to be—but we will adjust, adapt, and move on with the process of living and aging. You may have had friends that never did adjust to not being what they wanted to be and are now angry or dysfunctional because of it. If we do not adapt to life, we become dysfunctional even if we have more life or therapeutic skill potential than others around us do. This may explain why some successful people in high school did not stay successful later in life. They did not adapt to changing life demands.

Some of the keys to facilitating adaptation in the client are to know how that client is unique and to learn what each client's adaptation process is. Do not try to make each client the same as every other client, and do not force your ways of coping on them. Two case studies in this chapter will help the reader develop both sensitivity to and the cognitive understanding of this adjustment process and how it changes as the client goes through life. One case involves a person who is growing up with a disability, and the other involves a person who acquired the disability after reaching adulthood.

In this chapter, Sally is a client who was born with cerebral palsy. She has had to adjust to being "different" all her life, and her "different" is normal for her. She has had to adjust to a society that often does not identify a role for her or has either a negative or an overly positive role that her medical diagnosis has forced on her. Sally can be emotionally damaged by either overly positive or overly negative stereotypes. An example of how an overly positive stereotype may cause problems is when a person is told he or she must give to society because of a gift of great intelligence. The person may have no need to be overly productive and is criticized or rejected because this potential is not being actualized to society's satisfaction. A negative stereotype may have the same damaging effect by limiting the person's concept of what could be accomplished, thus preventing that individual from growing and adapting to "be all that they could be." Sally must find her place and use her talents to accomplish what she would like to in life. This goal is difficult for every individual to accomplish, but for a client such as Sally, it may be even harder because she will have some perceived and real motor limitations that may prevent her from accomplishing this goal. Sally may have functional limitations in her upper and lower limbs even with the best therapy. She has to find ways to accommodate for these limitations to prevent them from hampering her love of life. Sally needs to learn how to deal with others and to deal with her physical body in a way that will allow her to adapt to what is needed physically, emotionally, and spiritually. Sally's case study is mentioned throughout this chapter to apply components of adjustment and adaptation to her life process.

The second case study used in this chapter involves a young adult male, Fred. Fred acquired a spinal cord injury (SCI) in his 20s. As an adult, he is in the process of adapting his goals and dreams to fit with his new capabilities and limitations following the traumatic injury. A therapist must always be aware of the attitudes of clients toward life activities following and preceding an insult. This event is not all negative because Fred was not goal directed or focused in his life before the accident. In that respect, Fred may benefit from the structure and guidance he will receive as part of this rehabilitation. He now must deal with the stereotypes and prejudices of others as well as some of the stereotypes and prejudices that he had regarding individuals he considered disabled before he was injured. He will have to discard some of his old goals or ways of dealing with life activities and challenges but will have an opportunity to focus on what he values as important in his life. This focus can lead to a better life for Fred. Some clients have said that they did not like who they were before their accident or where they were going with their lives and that the disability was a "godsend" to them. (It should be noted that these words were never spoken from a client with a new acute injury but from clients years after their injury.) Similarly, clients have communicated that "I had 10,000 opportunities before my injury and I only have 5000 now, but in either case I could only accomplish 1000 of them."

Roles are the patterns of operating that we go through each day without even thinking. They are how people go through most of life. There are roles for a child, a spouse or partner, a worker, a student, or any other stage or component of life. These roles allow adults to respond as if they were still children interacting with parents. Roles allow each of us to function as a sibling in one situation and a parent in another. Individuals are not cognizant of these roles, but these roles control individual behavior unless each person thinks about her or his behaviors and decides to change them. Roles are very useful in life because, as individuals, none of us has the time or energy to treat each situation in life as a new and novel one. In the case of a new body system problem, functional limitations, and the inability to participate in life activities that we valued before the insult or disease, all of our roles must be rethought and reexamined. This process takes time, energy, and a lot of emotional turmoil. Often, the person does not know what the problem is.

In the case of a person with an early or congenital body system problem and resultant functional limitations, as in our case study of Sally, that person must reexamine the current roles and beliefs in light of changes in function following therapy, deterioration of movement function following a surgery, or simply because role expectations were wrong in the first place. With an acquired disability, such as in the case study of Fred, the person is forced to reexamine all standard roles and change them where appropriate. He not only has to face body system problems that affect his functional skills, but he is also forced to deal with complex and primarily social phenomena. If a person does not yet know her or his own new abilities and limitations, that person may have a challenge finding and developing appropriate new roles. The PTA must be aware of how hard it is for Fred and Sally to reexamine all that they hold as true and, at the same time, deal with the cognitive and physical demands of the medical system and rehabilitation. If Sally were improving in therapy, she may wonder why this therapy was not offered earlier and wonder how many ways her life would have been improved if this had happened when she was younger. She may also feel threatened by her newfound abilities since she may have always used the lack of these abilities as a reason for not engaging in other threatening activities or roles (eg, dating, interacting socially with friends, or assuming gainful employment).

Fred may be experiencing similar emotional reactions as Sally but from another perspective. He may feel that all his abilities are slipping away. He may feel that all he has sacrificed for or delayed gratification for in his life has been wasted. Individuals who have delayed having sex may feel that following an accident such as a spinal injury, they will never know this aspect of life and feel angry about this great loss. Fred may need help in the redirection of his life roles and goals.

Performance is the main goal of therapy and is the main way that a person demonstrates capability. When performance or participation is impaired, the person may be threatened emotionally. When emotionally threatened, performance may be impaired. This is why it is important for the physical therapist (PT) and PTA to always be aware of the client and the client's support system's unique perspectives on the ramifications of the functional loss and the body systems creating that loss. The emotional system can assist or hinder therapy. Interaction with the staff may be the key to facilitating growth and development of the client with regard to emotional stability and security. The following are some key points for the reader to keep in mind.

GROWTH AND ADAPTATION

The therapist must keep in mind the context from which the client is coming. Just days ago, the client may have been walking around with no major problems and has now suddenly entered the physical therapy setting. The trauma may be multifaceted: (1) the physical trauma that may have occurred to the client, (2) the emotional trauma occurring to the client and the client's support system, and (3) the trauma of each of these bodily systems trying to protect the others. The interaction of these multifaceted components with one's life may lead to post-traumatic stress syndrome. This syndrome usually occurs within the first 6 months following the injury. This syndrome is observed more often in women,[1-3] but because of cultural barriers, can be hidden with men. The client may blame others, try to protect others, or be so self-absorbed that little else in the world is seen or heard. It may be helpful to get psychological aid for the client early in therapy if this is preventing optimal outcomes or creating obstacles in therapy.[4-8] It is the PTA's job to develop a trusting relationship with the client. Through this relationship, the client can be helped to focus on the goals of therapy and work on a positive perspective. One error of the medical system is focusing on the disability and pathology and not on the person and the positive capabilities still within the client's grasp.[9] This focus on the negative may cause the client to see only the injury, disease, or pathology and nothing else. In a Veterans Administration hospital, spouses of people with SCIs formed a group focusing on why the partners were married in the first place and never looked at the disability as disabling. After a short while, people concluded that they did not marry their spouses for their legs, and the fact that the legs no longer worked was not a major issue after all. This started the decentering from the medical disability model and the focus began being placed on the people and their future, which is the International Classification of Functioning, Disability and Health model today. If we can help clients focus on their function and not their dysfunction, the effect of therapy following treatment will be much better. More work needs to be performed to help clients realize their existing potential and to live their lives with the highest quality.[10-16] Focusing on how to live, move, and function is one of the keys to helping the client and the family work toward the future.[17,18] The PTA, under the direction of the PT, must help the client focus on the direction of treatment objectives and demonstrate how therapy translates into meeting the client's goals.[9] To discover the client's true goals, the therapist must gain the trust of the client and establish sound lines of communication. Distrusting health professionals may obstruct the adjustment process and lead to negative consequences.[19-22] Whenever possible, the client's support system should be enlisted to help establish realistic support for the client and establish goals. It has been found that if the client trusts the health professional, the client will be more compliant and will seek assistance when it is needed.[23,24]

In the case of Sally, the PT and PTA may work with Sally and her family to see what future goals would be realistic and within the domain of physical therapy. In the case of Fred, the goals may include the accomplishment of previous goals, if they are realistic, or may involve modifying his previous goals with adaptations. This is an issue in therapy for many reasons, but most crucially, when people feel unworthy or disempowered, they tend to perform poorly and have problems with compliance. This reaction may slow or stop the progress of therapy. Helping the client to adapt to the new body will help achieve the goals in therapy. Helping clients realize what they can accomplish and empowering them with the concept that they can find a way around many barriers and negative situations is a critical aspect of every therapeutic intervention.

Body Image

Body image is an all-encompassing concept that involves how the person and, to some extent, the support system views the person and roles that are expected to be assumed by that person. Many clients experience negative feelings about their bodies and generally negative psychological experiences after injury.[25–28] Even when clients do not have disfigurements that are readily observable, they often still report changes in body image and negative feelings of self-worth. One issue that may arise relating to body image is sexuality. This concept may take many behavioral forms: flirting, harassment, questions about fertility, or questions regarding whether the client is capable of performing the sex act at all. Flirting may be a sign that clients have had an assault on their femininity or masculinity. By flirting, clients are often trying to determine if they are still seen as a sensual being. In this case, a PTA may let clients down lightly by explaining that dating or flirting with clients is not allowed. This is to ensure that clients do not think that the turn-off is about their body system problems, functional limitations, and inability to participate. Sensitivity should be used because a client could think, "If a medical person finds me repulsive, then no one will ever see me as attractive." It is important for the therapist to try to ascertain the intent behind the behavior. Usually, this can be accomplished by evaluating feelings about the interaction. It is not within the scope of a PTA's duties to determine the stage of adjustment that may be directing client behavior. However, it is within the scope of a PTA's duties to develop caring sensitivity and be able to report to the PT or other health care professionals what has been observed in the client's behavior. If you, as the PTA, do not feel threatened or demeaned when the client is flirting, you still must report this to the PT of record. If you feel defensive, demeaned, or very uncomfortable, then you may be experiencing harassment. You should never be harassed on the job, and this client's behavior should be stopped immediately; you must tell the client that the behavior is making you feel uncomfortable and that it should stop now. Again, you should mention this behavior to your supervisor and/or team. If the behavior is considered chronic by the staff, a treatment plan should be designed to stop this behavior. This plan is not the responsibility of the PTA, but carrying out appropriate responsive behaviors to the patient's inappropriate actions is within that scope. It is important, however, to remember that sexual health should not be a neglected area of client treatment. It may take time for the client to ask the appropriate questions.[29,30]

Questions about any physical performance are within the domain of physical therapy. If the client is asking for information regarding positioning during sex, then this may be brought to the attention of a therapist. If the questions are regarding fertility, these should also be referred to an appropriate medical person. None of these questions should be discouraged or neglected because this area is important for your client's motivation and sexual health.[31–35] It is important for the PTA to know that in SCI, fertility will generally not be impaired for women, but issues of lubrication before sex should be addressed by the appropriate person. Men may have erection problems and ejaculation issues, but this can also be addressed by the appropriate person. It is now thought that male fertility issues resulting from an SCI may be dealt with and should not be ruled out.[36–40]

Sally may need to work on body image problems that have resulted from the misperceptions she gained from other people and the media. She may also have learned not to enjoy her body and to deny positive sensations because she has been clinically touched most of her life without regard to her need for privacy.

Fred, on the other hand, may need to talk to other people who have been disabled for a while to explore acquired misconceptions and negative stereotypes regarding the impact of disabilities and, specifically, his functional limitations. He may also benefit from practical information that people with similar medical diagnoses can provide.

Family and Client Adjustment

The role of the family must never be forgotten. Although earlier literature hinted that partner relationships may be negatively affected by a member being disabled, this is being questioned in regard to some disabilities, such as adult-onset SCI.[41] However, pediatric SCI and other disabilities may result in relationship problems.[42–45] It has been shown that adjustment and quality of life can be adversely affected by an inadequate physical environment, thus making the person more dependent. The result of the dependence appears to be poor relationships.[46–50] This can also be seen with the families in which a member has had a brain injury.[51] In studies on muscular dystrophy, it was found that physical dependence is not the only variable that needs to be considered; psychological issues need to be identified and considered as part of intervention.[52,53] According to Turner and Cox, the client and the family need help to work on a number of elements: "to develop new views of vulnerability and strength, make changes in relationships, and facilitate philosophical, physical and spiritual growth."[53] Turner and Cox also felt that the medical staff could facilitate the following: "recognizing the worth of each individual, helping them to envision a future that is full of promise and potential, actively involving each person in their own care trajectory, and celebrating changes to each person's sense of self."[53] Man observed that each family copes differently in relation to a brain-injured family member and that the family's structure should be explored to develop intervention guidelines.[54] It has also been noted that health care professionals should view the situation from the family's perspective to approach and support the family's adaptation.[55] This should be performed to help the client and the family accept the disability but, at the same time, to help them keep the negative views of society in perspective.[56] In general, it has also been found that family support is a significant factor in the client's subjective functioning[57] and that social engagement is productive.[58]

When dealing with children, it is important to realize that they often feel responsible for almost anything that happens in life (eg, divorce, siblings getting hurt, or general arguments between parents). It is important that the therapist helps the client and the siblings realize that they are not responsible for the client's condition. Part of this magical thinking that often appears is the concept that bad things happen to bad people; thus, the child is bad because a bad thing has happened. It is important to be sensitive to this ideation and help dispel this maladaptive thought pattern since it is not true or productive for the client or the siblings and may cause further adjustment problems later in treatment. Siblings of the client should be helped to see their roles as good siblings and should not be placed in the role of caretakers of the sibling with body system and functional limitations. In this way, all children can grow naturally without any one of the children being overly focused on. At the same time, it is a fact of life that the child with functional limitations will probably need physical assistance, therapy, increased medical care, and thus, more time devoted to her or him; this is just a fact of life.

It should always be noted by the medical establishment that having body system and functional problems is expensive in ways in which they are often not aware. There are the obvious medical costs of therapy, surgery, a wheelchair (w/c), or orthoses, but there are other costs such as the possibility of extra transportation, catheters for urination, w/c maintenance, adaptive clothing, and other ongoing costs not covered by most insurance plans. These costs add up and contribute to the emotional costs and demands on the family. Significant others may feel the need to work more to earn the money to cover such expenses, but then that person will not be around to help. This is only one of the many dilemmas that must be dealt with for the support system of the person confronted with body system and functional problems. The family may be encouraged to contact such groups as the Family Caregiver Support Network (www.caregiversupportnetwork.org) to get information and assistance with diverse topics such as being a caregiver, legal and financial aid, and communications (this group tends to focus on the adult but may still be a wonderful aid). Such groups will give information to all who need it and help to empower the family. This takes the focus off the medical condition and may help the family to gain a better and more balanced perspective on the condition.

Sally may have to work on skills that will encourage assertiveness and better decision making. She may need to help her family allow her to be more independent and become more of a risk taker in all aspects of her life.

Fred may need to work on coping skills and strategies that will help him deal with crises. He may have preconceived ideas of the limitations of someone with his medical diagnosis that will need to be changed.

Stress, Crisis, Loss, and Grief

The adaptation process is one that has been theorized about and speculated on, and it would appear that the human being is so complex that no 2 of us react just the same. This is a comforting fact because it means each of us is a truly unique individual. This also means that when you deal with clients, each is unique and is not a diagnosis or a routine entity. To do a good job, you have to listen to their stories, know the context of their lives, know their values, and understand their goals. This is a major undertaking in the context of a treatment session, but it should be your ideal goal for each client. This section will examine some thoughts on how clients adapt to a disability.

After an injury or disabling condition that limits function, the client and the family may go through an episode of depression that may interfere with the progress of therapy.[59-62] Depression and other inadequate coping modes will impede progress of therapy and decrease levels of life satisfaction for all involved.[2,63] Attempting to help the client and the family avoid depression by keeping them involved in functional and meaningful therapeutic activities is the challenge.[52] The longer the client is in a forced helplessness situation, the more likely it is that the client will feel depressed. Focusing on a positive goal that is relevant to the client and the family may help to keep the client directed toward the future and away from the negative aspects of the situation. If focusing on the client's goals is not enough, other treatment may be needed, and psychiatric assistance may be called for.[33,64,65] Acceptance of the disability without surrendering to the condition has been found to be associated with less anger, less hostility, and higher self-efficacy in the individual.[66,67] Denial may work for the very early stages of the disability, but if it lasts, it will hamper the client's progress. A client once explained that when he could not do anything, denial was very helpful, but as soon as he could start doing things for himself and others, denial was not at all helpful. Thus, the therapist's job is to help the client defocus from the medical impairment and handicap by focusing on function and the client's goals. If this is performed and the focus is on adaptive activities that have meaning to the client, the client will not experience the role of helplessness and dependence, and quality of life will be maximized.[68-73]

Livneh and Antonak presented a primer for counselors that can be adapted to assist the therapist in dealing with clients' adjustment to disability.[74] It should always be kept in mind that there is no normal or right way for a person to go through the adjustment process, and often, we will not see clients long enough to observe all of the stages of adjustment. Remember, there is not a static state of "adjustment" that the person reaches and there remains. We are all in various states of adjustment to life, and clients are no different.

Some of the observed mechanisms that have been noted are shock, anxiety, denial, depression, anger/hostility, and adjustment. All of these can be seen at some point in the client's life. These aspects of adjustment may be seen at any point of rehabilitation. Although the client may appear adjusted to one aspect of the functional limitations, the same client may be greeted with some new aspect of those limitations that he or she may not have experienced before. The client may then go into shock and start adjusting to this aspect of the problem anew. Adjustment is a process, not a place. Clients who have been adjusted to their disability for many years will lose or even gain function over time and must adjust to these changes. This is not a static process.

One aspect that the therapist must watch out for is a form of coping called *disengagement*—this may be denial or avoidance behavior, which can take many forms. It can result in substance abuse, blame, or refusal to interact. Research regarding people with head injuries has demonstrated that if a premorbid coping style for a person was to drink or use other drugs, the client may revert to these same styles of coping, which can result in poor rehabilitation outcomes.[75–78] It is important to help the client out of this quagmire. The skills of a therapist may not be enough to perform this in the short time that the client is in treatment, so a referral to social work or psychiatry may be in order. It is still the therapist's job to help promote engagement activities—these behaviors are goal oriented, problem solving, information seeking, and doing things to positively "beat the condition" and demonstrate independence.

Livneh and Antonak promote a number of activities for the health professional:

- Assisting clients to explore the personal meaning of the disability. "Training clients to attain a sense of mastery over their emotional experiences."[74] A way of doing this would be to help the client not demonstrate emotional outbursts or to look at her or his emotions and put them into perspective.[74]

- "Providing clients with relevant medical information. These strategies emphasize imparting accurate information to clients on their medical condition, including its present status, prognosis, anticipated future functional limitations, and when applicable, vocational implications."[38] This may be performed by helping the client and family access resources such as PubMed (pubmedcentral.nih.gov) online or helping them find medical references in the library.[38]

- "Providing clients with supportive family and group experiences. These strategies permit clients (usually with similar disabilities or common life experiences) and, if applicable, their family members or significant others, to share common fears, concerns, needs, and wishes."[38] This can be performed in rather unobtrusive ways: scheduling clients with the same disability at the same time so that they meet in the waiting room or while conducting group mat activities or hiring disabled individuals who are health care professionals that can discuss and model positive behaviors and answer relevant questions from the client's perspective. Remember that all clients are potential teachers for you as well as other clients.[38]

- Teaching clients adaptive coping skills for successful community functioning. "These skills include assertiveness, interpersonal relations, decision making, problem solving, stigma management, and time management skills."[74] This would entail role-playing situations: for example, an able-bodied person asking why the client is in a w/c, that person preaching to the w/c user because he must have offended God in some way, otherwise he would not be in a w/c, or telling the client that it is such a shame that she is disabled because she is so good looking and could have found a man if it were not for the disability. Role-playing can also be used to help a person deal with the possibly awkward experience of going to bed with a new partner and having to explain how to be undressed, what those tubes coming out of the body are for, or what positions are best for someone with this condition.[74]

Sally may work on role-playing to develop the skill to ask someone out for a date or to learn to be assertive at the bank or store. Fred may need to work on how to ask for assistance without feeling dependent or how to physically defend himself in the w/c.

Hope and Spiritual Aspects

The process of hope can be a generalized and positive force to reduce depression, the sense of powerlessness, and grief.[79–82] Clients need a realistic sense of hope. The question of what is realistic is always open to interpretation. A client with quadriplegia who was a deer hunter swore he would go to the mountains in the fall and shoot a deer. All of the staff knew that he was not being realistic, but he came in with venison in the fall from the deer he shot. Another client with quadriplegia lived on the East Coast and said that when he left the hospital, he would drive to the West Coast to live. The staff laughed about this, but sure enough, he was discharged and drove to the West Coast to live. It is hope that keeps most of us going in life. Hope is not always realistic. How many people really believe that they will win the lottery, if not this time, then maybe the next? Sometimes it is this hope that saves us from being overwhelmed by the other realities of life. Try not to take all of the client's hope away. He or she may win the lottery, shoot a deer, or drive to another part of the country.

Spirituality is something that provides hope, connection with others, and the reason for or meaning of existence for many (if not most) people. It is amazing that the medical community has been very slow to accept the power of spirituality since this area gives meaning to so many people's lives. Spirituality has been linked to health perception, a sense of connection with others, and well-being.[83-88] Anything that helps the client put the disability into perspective and move on with life in a healthy way is good. The Western medical system is based on pathology and focuses on that. Physical therapy focuses on doing and behavioral change that is productive. One of the dangers of the medical system is the entrapment in pathology to the point that the client may not see anything but pathology. Spirituality may help the client and the family to see that there is more to life than pathology, stimulate interaction with others, put the disability in perspective, give meaning to life (and the disability), and give the person hope and a sense of well-being.[89] This is what we all want for the client and the family.

Sally may benefit from talking to other people with cerebral palsy who have families, are chief executive officers of businesses, or are doing whatever they would like to do.

Fred may tap into what his new goals and dreams really are to see ways to accomplish those dreams.

Cultural Aspects

The culture, subculture, and beliefs of the client's family are aspects of the client to which the therapist must attend.[90-94] This concept includes beliefs about the world and maybe a belief about the cause of the disability or at least how the client is viewing the disability. Asking "Why do you think this happened to you?" can lead to a very enlightening experience. "Causes" may range from: "God is punishing me," "I deserved it," or "life is against me." The answer may frame the way that treatment is presented to the client. Using the client's frame of reference may promote trust, mutual acceptance of values, greater compliance with treatment, and a broadening of the therapist's view of the world. One of the great things about therapy is that clients teach us so much about life. Recognizing why a client does something that looks different to us may lead to a key to what that client may need in treatment. It may also help the PTA to see the world from a different perspective. Do not hesitate to let the client know that he or she helped you. Helping others is empowering to the client as well as the therapist.

One example of how the client's perspective can be very different from the therapist's is if, during treatment, a client says that she is going to die. When presented with the fact that she is in rehabilitation, is not going to die, and is about to be discharged, she falls silent. It is not until the client gets home that the therapist realizes the client was going back to an inner-city situation and that the client's fears of death have merit. Someone who is elderly and very disabled in this area of town is in a life-threatening situation, and she probably **is** going to die (other arrangements are quickly made for her discharge). If the therapist had listened better and knew the client's subculture, this incident could have been avoided. It should be noted that the therapist did try to find out what the client meant. The client thought that it was so obvious (in the client's world) that the therapist's lack of knowledge was a lack of caring for the client's welfare. We should try to avoid this kind of interaction at all costs.

Beliefs and values of cultures and families can play a profound role in the course of treatment. Such things as physical difficulties that can be seen are usually better accepted than problems that cannot be seen, such as brain damage that changes an individual's personality.[95-97] A person with a back injury may be seen as lazy, whereas a person with a double amputation will be perceived as needing help. At the same time, a person who has lost a body part may be seen as "not all there" in some cultures and is avoided socially. Thus, being attuned to the culture and beliefs of the client is imperative in therapy.

Sally will have some of her beliefs challenged. She will need to examine how she thinks about her possible future roles. She may want to examine whether she would like to have children, be a professional woman, or both. She will have to develop skills that will promote her goals, and she may look to role models who can demonstrate the positive behaviors that are necessary to accomplish these goals.

Fred was very unfocused in his life before the injury and will need help clarifying some of the behaviors that did not work for him before. In doing so, he will have to dispel some of the myths about the disabled that he was taught in his culture. With help, he may be able to see this event as a new beginning that will help him clean up his act.

Adjustment to disability opens a person to a unique situation and allows him or her to adapt to a changing environment in a productive way. If the person is not able to alter *maladaptive* behaviors and grow in a productive way, the best physical therapy in the world will not be able to make significant progress. We may get a client to perform all of the correct exercises and movement patterns but not to be a productive person who enjoys life. The PTA is a significant member of the team who needs to be aware of ways to promote productive behavior that results in a more functional person. It is not the PTA's job to be a psychologist, an occupational therapist, or a social worker, but it is important to assist the team and to promote productive behavior and function. The role of psychosocial function is intricately linked to quality-of-life issues. Movement not only expresses the motor system but is the only avenue that a client can use to express emotions, interact with other individuals, be empowered to bodily functions, and feel good about one's self. PTAs, as team members and colleagues who are delegated the responsibility of physical therapy interventions, need to identify their own personal beliefs, safety issues, biases, and learning styles and have respect for each patient's uniqueness. With this comprehension incorporated into the behavior of a PTA, that PTA will become a much better therapist, have better compliance from patients, and feel more satisfied as a provider of health care.

REFERENCES

1. Kennedy P, Evans MJ. Evaluation of post traumatic distress in the first 6 months following SCI. *Spinal Cord.* 2001;39(7):381-386.
2. Bruffaerts R, Vilagut G, Demyttenaere K, et al. Role of common mental and physical disorders in partial disability around the world. *Br J Psychiatry.* 2012;200(6):454-461.
3. Richards T, Garvert DW, McDade E, Carlson E, Curtin C. Chronic psychological and functional sequelae after emergent hand surgery. *J Hand Surg Am.* 2011;36(10):1663-1668.
4. Kennedy P, Rogers BA. Anxiety and depression after spinal cord injury: a longitudinal analysis. *Arch Phys Med Rehabil.* 2000;81(7):932-937.
5. Hannah SD. Psychosocial issues after a traumatic hand injury: facilitating adjustment. *J Hand Ther.* 2011;24(2):95-102.
6. Brewin CR, Garnett R, Andrews B. Trauma, identity and mental health in UK military veterans. *Psychol Med.* 2011;41(8):1733-1740.
7. Haagsma JA, Polinder S, Toet H, et al. Beyond the neglect of psychological consequences: post-traumatic stress disorder increases the non-fatal burden of injury by more than 50%. *Inj Prev.* 2011;17(1):21-26.
8. Freedy JR, Magruder KM, Mainous AG, Frueh BC, Geesey ME, Carnemolla M. Gender differences in traumatic event exposure and mental health among veteran primary care patients. *Mil Med.* 2010;175(10):750-758.
9. Mazaux JM, Croze P, Quintard B, et al. Satisfaction of life and late psycho-social outcome after severe brain injury: a nine-year follow-up study in Aquitaine. *Acta Neurochir Suppl.* 2002;79:49-51.
10. Ayyangar R. Health maintenance and management in childhood disability. *Phys Med Rehabil Clin N Am.* 2002;13(4):793-821.

11. Fusco O, Ferrini A, Santoro M, Lo Monaco MR, Gambassi G, Cesari M. Physical function and perceived quality of life in older persons. *Aging Clin Exp Res.* 2012;24(1):68-73.

12. King J, Yourman L, Ahalt C, et al. Quality of life in late-life disability: "I don't feel bitter because I am in a wheelchair". *J Am Geriatr Soc.* 2012;60(3):569-576.

13. Dahan-Oliel N, Shikako-Thomas K, Majnemer A. Quality of life and leisure participation in children with neurodevelopmental disabilities: a thematic analysis of the literature. *Qual Life Res.* 2012;21(3):427-439.

14. Rosenbaum P, Gorter JW. The 'F-words' in childhood disability: I swear this is how we should think! *Child Care Health Dev.* 2012;38(4):457-463.

15. Kim SJ, Kang KA. Meaning of life for adolescents with a physical disability in Korea. *J Adv Nurs.* 2003;43(2):145-155; discussion 155-157.

16. Stewart DA, Law MC, Rosenbaum P, Willms DG. A qualitative study of the transition to adulthood for youth with physical disabilities. *Phys Occup Ther Pediatr.* 2001;21(4):3-21.

17. Putzke JD, Richards JS, Hicken BL, DeVivo MJ. Predictors of life satisfaction: a spinal cord injury cohort study. *Arch Phys Med Rehabil.* 2002;83(4):555-561.

18. Jalayondeja C, Kaewkungwal J, Sullivan PE, Nidhinandana S, Pichaiyongwongdee S, Jareinpituk S. Factors related to community participation by stroke victims six month post-stroke. *Southeast Asian J Trop Med Public Health.* 2011;42(4):1005-1013.

19. Gullacksen AC, Lidbeck J. The life adjustment process in chronic pain: psychosocial assessment and clinical implications. *Pain Res Manag.* 2004;9(3):145-153.

20. Pinto RZ, Ferreira ML, Oliveira VC, et al. Patient-centred communication is associated with positive therapeutic alliance: a systematic review. *J Physiother.* 2012;58(2):77-87.

21. Lee YY, Lin JL. How much does trust really matter? A study of the longitudinal effects of trust and decision-making preferences on diabetic patient outcomes. *Patient Educ Couns.* 2011;85(3):406-412.

22. Sloots M, Dekker JH, Pont M, Bartels EA, Geertzen JH, Dekker J. Reasons of drop-out from rehabilitation in patients of Turkish and Moroccan origin with chronic low back pain in The Netherlands: a qualitative study. *J Rehabil Med.* 2010;42(6):566-573.

23. Trachtenberg F, Dugan E, Hall MA. How patients' trust relates to their involvement in medical care. *J Fam Pract.* 2005;54(4):344-352.

24. Kuipers K, Rassafiani M, Ashburner J, et al. Do clients with acquired brain injury use the splints prescribed by occupational therapists? A descriptive study. *NeuroRehabilitation.* 2009;24(4):365-375.

25. Taleporos G, McCabe MP. Body image and physical disability: personal perspectives. *Soc Sci Med.* 2002;54(6): 971-980.

26. Deans S, Burns D, McGarry A, Murray K, Mutrie N. Motivations and barriers to prosthesis users participation in physical activity, exercise and sport: a review of the literature. *Prosthet Orthot Int.* 2012;36(3):260-269.

27. Bombardier CH, Fann JR, Tate DG, et al. An exploration of modifiable risk factors for depression after spinal cord injury: which factors should we target? *Arch Phys Med Rehabil.* 2012;93(5):775-781.

28. Sylliaas H, Thingstad P, Wyller TB, Helbostad J, Sletvold O, Bergland A. Prognostic factors for self-rated function and perceived health in patient living at home three months after a hip fracture. *Disabil Rehabil.* 2012;34(14):1225-1231.

29. Fisher TL, Laud PW, Byfield MG, Brown TT, Hayat MJ, Fiedler IG. Sexual health after spinal cord injury: a longitudinal study. *Arch Phys Med Rehabil.* 2002;83(8):1043-1051.

30. Sander AM, Maestas KL, Pappadis MR, et al. Sexual functioning 1 year after traumatic brain injury: findings from a prospective traumatic brain injury model systems collaborative study. *Arch Phys Med Rehabil.* 2012;93(8): 1331-1337.

31. Phelps J, Albo M, Dunn K, Joseph A. Spinal cord injury and sexuality in married or partnered men: activities, function, needs, and predictors of sexual adjustment. *Arch Sex Behav.* 2001;30(6):591-602.

32. Kreuter M, Taft C, Siösteen A, Biering-Sørensen F. Women's sexual functioning and sex life after spinal cord injury. *Spinal Cord.* 2011;49(1):154-160.

33. Nortvedt MW, Riise T, Myhr KM, Landtblom AM, Bakke A, Nyland HI. Reduced quality of life among multiple sclerosis patients with sexual disturbance and bladder dysfunction. *Mult Scler.* 2001;7(4):231-235.

34. Cardoso FL, Savall AC, Mendes AK. Self-awareness of the male sexual response after spinal cord injury. *Int J Rehabil Res.* 2009;32(4):294-300.

35. Alriksson-Schmidt AI, Armour BS, Thibadeau JK. Are adolescent girls with a physical disability at increased risk for sexual violence? *J Sch Health.* 2010;80(7):361-367.

36. Brackett NL, Nash MS, Lynne CM. Male fertility following spinal cord injury: facts and fiction. *Phys Ther.* 1996;76(11):1221-1231.

37. Iremashvili V, Brackett NL, Ibrahim E, Aballa TC, Lynne CM. Semen quality remains stable during the chronic phase of spinal cord injury: a longitudinal study. *J Urol.* 2010;184(5):2073-2077.

38. Hirsch IH. Optimizing fertility potential in spinal cord injured men. *Can J Urol.* 2012;19(5):6437.

39. Monga M, Dunn K, Rajasekaran M. Characterization of ultrastructural and metabolic abnormalities in semen from men with spinal cord injury. *J Spinal Cord Med.* 2001;24(1):41-46.

40. Sønksen J, Ohl DA. Penile vibratory stimulation and electroejaculation in the treatment of ejaculatory dysfunction. *Int J Androl.* 2002;25(6):324-332.

41. Kreuter M. Spinal cord injury and partner relationships. *Spinal Cord.* 2000;38(1):2-6.

42. Vogel LC, Krajci KA, Anderson CJ. Adults with pediatric-onset spinal cord injuries, part 3: impact of medical complications. *J Spinal Cord Med.* 2002;25(4):297-305.

43. Majnemer A, Shevell M, Law M, Poulin C, Rosenbaum P. Indicators of distress in families of children with cerebral palsy. *Disabil Rehabil.* 2012;34(14):1202-1207.

44. Evans SA, Airey MC, Chell SM, Connelly JB, Rigby AS, Tennant A. Disability in young adults following major trauma: 5 year follow up of survivors. *BMC Public Health.* 2003;3(1):8.

45. Roscigno CI, Swanson KM. Parents' experiences following children's moderate to severe traumatic brain injury: a clash of cultures. *Qual Health Res.* 2011;21(10):1413-1426.

46. Seki M, Takenaka A, Nakazawa M, Takahashi H, Chino N. Examination of living environment upon return to home for patients with cervical spinal cord injury: report of a case [in Japanese]. *Gan To Kagaku Ryoho.* 2002;3(29 Suppl 3):522-525.

47. Jaracz K, Grabowska-Fudala B, Kozubski W. Caregiver burden after stroke: towards a structural model. *Neurol Neurochir Pol.* 2012;46(3):224-232.

48. Carod-Artal FJ, Egido JA. Quality of life after stroke: the importance of a good recovery. *Cerebrovasc Dis.* 2009;27(Suppl 1):204-214.

49. Raina P, O'Donnell M, Rosenbaum P, et al. The health and well-being of caregivers of children with cerebral palsy. *Pediatrics.* 2005;115(6):e626-e636.

50. Whiteneck G, Meade MA, Dijkers M, Tate DG, Bushnik T, Forchheimer MB. Environmental factors and their role in participation and life satisfaction after spinal cord injury. *Arch Phys Med Rehabil.* 2004;85(11):1793-1803.

51. Kneafsey R, Gawthorpe D. Head injury: long-term consequences for patients and families and implications for nurses. *J Clin Nurs.* 2004;13(5):601-608.

52. Natterlund B, Ahlstrom G. Activities of daily living and quality of life in persons with muscular dystrophy. *J Rehabil Med.* 2001;33(5):206-211.

53. Turner de S, Cox H. Facilitating post traumatic growth. *Health Qual Life Outcomes.* 2004;2(1):34.

54. Man DW. Hong Kong family caregivers' stress and coping for people with brain injury. *Int J Rehabil Res.* 2002;25(4):287-295.

55. Taanila A, Syrjala L, Kokkonen J, Jarvelin MR. Child: coping of parents with physically and/or intellectually disabled children. *Care Health Dev.* 2002;28(1):73-86.

56. de Klerk HM, Ampousah L. The physically disabled woman's experience of self. *Disabil Rehabil.* 2003;25(19):1132-1139.

57. Koukouli S, Vlachonikolis IG, Philalithis A. Socio-demographic factors and self-reported functional status: the significance of social support. *Health Serv Res.* 2002;2(1):20.

58. Mendes de Leon CF, Glass TA, Berkman LF. Social engagement and disability in a community population of older adults. *Am J Epidemiol.* 2003;157(7):633-642.

59. Martz E, Livneh H, Priebe M, Wuermser LA, Ottomanelli L. Predictors of psychosocial adaptation among people with spinal cord injury or disorder. *Arch Phys Med Rehabil.* 2005;86(6):1182-1192.

60. Pakenham KI, Cox S. Test of a model of the effects of parental illness on youth and family functioning. *Health Psychol.* 2012;31(5):580-590.

61. Bombardier CH, Richards JS, Krause JS, Tulsky D, Tate DG. Symptoms of major depression in people with spinal cord injury: implications for screening. *Arch Phys Med Rehabil.* 2004;85(11):1749-1756.

62. Pakenham KI, Cox S. Test of a model of the effects of parental illness on youth and family functioning. *Health Psychol.* 2012;31(5):580-590.

63. Chan RC. Stress and coping in spouses of persons with spinal cord injuries. *Clin Rehabil.* 2000;14(2):137-144.

64. Kishi Y, Robinson RG, Kosier JT. Suicidal ideation among patients during the rehabilitation period after life-threatening physical illness. *J Nerv Ment Dis.* 2001;189(9):623-628.

65. Andelic N, Sigurdardottir S, Schanke AK, Sandvik L, Sveen U, Roe C. Disability, physical health and mental health 1 year after traumatic brain injury. *Disabil Rehabil.* 2010;32(13):1122-1131.

66. Treharne GJ, Lyons AC, Booth DA, Mason SR, Kitas GD. Reactions to disability in patients with early versus established rheumatoid arthritis. *Scand J Rheumatol.* 2004;33(1):30-38.

67. Hoffman M. Bodies completed: on the physical rehabilitation of lower limb amputees. *Health (London).* 2013;17(3)229-245.

68. Holmbeck GN, Westhoven VC, Phillips WS, et al. A multimethod, multi-informant, and multidimensional perspective on psychosocial adjustment in preadolescents with spina bifida. *J Consult Clin Psychol.* 2003;71(4):782-796.

69. Sofi F, Molino Lova R, Nucida V, et al. Adaptive physical activity and back pain: a non-randomised community-based intervention trial. *Eur J Phys Rehabil Med.* 2011;47(4):543-549.

70. Voll R. Aspects of the quality of life of chronically ill and handicapped children and adolescents in outpatient and inpatient rehabilitation. *Int J Rehabil Res.* 2001;24(1):43-49.

71. Chiarello LA, Palisano RJ, Bartlett DJ, McCoy SW. A multivariate model of determinants of change in gross-motor abilities and engagement in self-care and play of young children with cerebral palsy. *Phys Occup Ther Pediatr.* 2011;31(2):150-168.

72. Ville I, Ravaud JF, Tetrafigap Group. Subjective well-being and severe motor impairments: the Tetrafigap survey on the long-term outcome of tetraplegic spinal cord injured persons. *Soc Sci Med.* 2001;52(3):369-384.

73. Majnemer A, Shevell M, Law M, Poulin C, Rosenbaum P. Level of motivation in mastering challenging tasks in children with cerebral palsy. *Dev Med Child Neurol.* 2010;52(12):1120-1126.

74. Livneh H, Antonak RF. Psychosocial adaptation to chronic illness and disability: a primer for counselors. *J Couns Dev.* 2005;83(1):12-20.

75. MacMillan PJ, Hart RP, Martelli MF, Zasler ND. Pre-injury status and adaptation following traumatic brain injury. *Brain Inj.* 2002;16(1):41-49.

76. Center for Substance Abuse Treatment. SAMHSA/CSAT Treatment Improvement Protocols. Substance Use Disorder Treatment for People With Physical and Cognitive Disabilities. Rockville, MD: US Substance Abuse and Mental Health Services Administration; 1998. Report No: (SMA) 98-3249.

77. West SL. Substance use among persons with traumatic brain injury: a review. *NeuroRehabilitation.* 2011;29(1):1-8.

78. DeLambo DA, Chandras KV, Homa D, Chandras SV. Spinal cord injury and substance abuse: implications for rehabilitation professionals. http://counselingoutfitters.com/vistas/vistas10/Article_83.pdf. Accessed September 5, 2013.

79. Lohne V. Hope in patients with spinal cord injury: a literature review related to nursing. *J Neurosci Nurs.* 2001;33(6):317-325.

80. Shiri S, Wexler ID, Feintuch U, Meiner Z, Schwartz I. Post-polio syndrome: impact of hope on quality of life. *Disabil Rehabil.* 2012;34(10):824-30.

81. Nunnerley J, Hay-Smith E, Dean S. Leaving a spinal unit and returning to the wider community: an interpretative phenomenological analysis [published online ahead of print October 5, 2012]. *Disabil Rehabil.*

82. Kortte KB, Stevenson JE, Hosey MM, Castillo R, Wegener ST. Hope predicts positive functional role outcomes in acute rehabilitation populations. *Rehabil Psychol.* 2012;57(3):248-255.

83. Delgado C. A discussion of the concept of spirituality. *Nurs Sci Q.* 2005;18(2):157-162.

84. Maggi L, Ferrara PE, Aprile I, et al. Role of spiritual beliefs on disability and health-related quality of life in acute inpatient rehabilitation unit. *Eur J Phys Rehabil Med.* 2012;48(3)467-473.

85. Lucchetti G, Lucchetti AG, Badan-Neto AM, et al. Religiousness affects mental health, pain and quality of life in older people in an outpatient rehabilitation setting. *J Rehabil Med.* 2011;43(4):316-322.

86. Potter ML, Zauszniewski JA. Spirituality, resourcefulness, and arthritis impact on health perception of elders with rheumatoid arthritis. *J Holist Nurs.* 2000;18(4):311-331; discussions 332-336.

87. Svalina SS, Webb JR. Forgiveness and health among people in outpatient physical therapy. *Disabil Rehabil.* 2012;34(5):383-392.

88. Waldron-Perrine B, Rapport LJ, Hanks RA, Lumley M, Meachen SJ, Hubbarth P. Religion and spirituality in rehabilitation outcomes among individuals with traumatic brain injury. *Rehabil Psychol.* 2011;56(2):107-116.

89. Treloar LL. Disability, spiritual beliefs, and the church: the experiences of adults with disabilities and family members. *J Adv Nurs.* 2002;40(5):594-603.

90. Saravanan B, Manigandan C, Macaden A, Tharion G, Bhattacharji S. Re-examining the psychology of spinal cord injury: a meaning centered approach from a cultural perspective. *Spinal Cord.* 2001;39(6):323-326.

91. Jull JE, Giles AR. Health equity, aboriginal peoples and occupational therapy. *Can J Occup Ther.* 2012;79(2):70-76.

92. Look MA, Kaholokula JK, Carvhalo A, Seto T, de Silva M. Developing a culturally based cardiac rehabilitation program: the HELA study. *Prog Community Health Partnersh.* 2012;6(1):103-110.

93. Kwong K, Chung H, Cheal K, Chou JC, Chen T. Disability beliefs and help-seeking behavior of depressed Chinese-American patients in a primary care setting. *J Soc Work Disabil Rehabil.* 2012;11(2):81-99.

94. Liu F, Williams RM, Liu HE, Chien NH. The lived experience of persons with lower extremity amputation. *J Clin Nurs.* 2010;19(15-16):2152-2161.

95. Brown SA, McCauley SR, Levin HS, Contant C, Boake C. Perception of health and quality of life in minorities after mild-to-moderate traumatic brain injury. *Appl Neuropsychol.* 2004;11(1):54-64.

96. Lindsay S, King G, Klassen AF, Esses V, Stachel M. Working with immigrant families raising a child with a disability: challenges and recommendations for healthcare and community service providers. *Disabil Rehabil.* 2012;34(23):2007-2017.

97. Clarke P, Smith J. Aging in a cultural context: cross-national differences in disability and the moderating role of personal control among older adults in the United States and England. *J Gerontol B Psychol Sci Soc Sci.* 2011;66(4):457-467.

Please see accompanying Web site at

www.healio.com/books/neuroptavideos

7

Documentation in Neurorehabilitation

Shannon Ryals, PTA

KEY WORDS

- Documentation
- Electronic health records
- Patient/client management

CHAPTER OBJECTIVES

- Discuss documentation guidelines that are pertinent to the physical therapist assistant (PTA).
- Identify important points when documenting tests and measures and interventions from the PTA standpoint.
- Discuss the relationship of documentation to payment for services and list reasons why payment for services is denied because of deficiencies in documentation.
- Discuss documentation formats commonly encountered by physical therapists and PTAs, including electronic health records.

INTRODUCTION

Documentation is one of the most important responsibilities a physical therapist assistant (PTA) will have. In the health care arena, documentation functions as a legal record of the services provided to the patient, a method to facilitate communication among health care providers, the basis for most reimbursement, and a potential source of data for evidence-based research.[1]

Documentation of physical therapy services spans the entire continuum of care. Documentation of the patient's care begins at the time of initial examination, evaluation, and development of the plan of care; continues for each subsequent visit and/or periodic summaries of the patient's care, including reassessments of progress following intervention; and terminates with the patient's discharge or discontinuation of physical therapy services. Who is responsible for all of this documentation? Physical therapists (PTs) as well as PTAs have roles in documentation. The American Physical Therapy Association's (APTA) position is that the PT should document and

Umphred DA, Lazaro RT, eds.
*Neurorehabilitation for the Physical Therapist Assistant,
Second Edition* (pp 165-176).
© 2014 SLACK Incorporated.

verify (by signature) the examination, evaluation, diagnosis, and development of the plan of care. Interventions provided by the PT or PTA should be documented and verified (through signature) by the PT, PTA, or both.[2]

In this text, the patient/client management model will be used as the framework for identifying and describing documentation of the patient/client with movement disorders secondary to neurological conditions (refer to Figure 1-3). The *Guide to Physical Therapist Practice*[3] outlines the key elements for providing physical therapy services. The 5 key elements of the patient/client management model are (1) examination, (2) evaluation, (3) diagnosis, (4) prognosis, and (5) interventions. In terms of documentation, it is important to identify the responsibilities of the PTA within the context of this model. As mentioned in Chapter 1, within this model, the PTAs are primarily involved in the element of interventions. However, it is also possible, even likely, that a PTA will be delegated tasks that fall within the examination element. Specifically, the PTA will likely be delegated tasks related to data collection of tests and measures. Consider the following example to illustrate when and how a PTA may be involved in data collection of tests and measures within the context of a patient being treated for neurological condition. A patient is referred to physical therapy following a diagnosis of a right cerebrovascular accident. The patient/client is initially examined and evaluated by the PT, and a plan of care is developed. The PT then delegates treatment of the patient to the PTA. The PT and PTA discuss the goals and expectations for the patient, including the need for the PTA to perform several delegated tests and measures periodically to determine the patient's progress. After 2 weeks, the PTA measures the patient's active and passive range of motion (ROM) and administers the Berg Balance Test to provide insight into the progress made in the patient's balance and the 2-point discrimination sensation test of the left lower extremity (LE) to determine changes in or progress with sensation. Documenting the results of the tests and measures, the interventions provided to the patient, and the progress of the patient during the interventions has become the responsibility of the PTA.

GUIDELINES FOR DOCUMENTATION

In its *Guidelines for Physical Therapy Documentation of Patient/Client Management*, the APTA has provided a set of generalized guidelines for documentation that is meant to span many practice settings.[2] These guidelines are not meant to be all inclusive but to serve as a basis on which documentation could be built. Be aware that individual facilities as well as payer sources may also have specific guidelines to follow for documentation. The following is a list of the APTA's guidelines[2]:

1. Documentation is required for every patient visit.

2. All documentation must comply with the applicable jurisdictional/regulatory requirements.

3. Handwritten entries should be made in ink and will include original signatures. Electronic entries are to be made with appropriate security and confidentiality provisions.

4. Errors should be corrected by drawing a single line through the error and initialing and dating the entry or through an appropriate mechanism for electronic documentation that clearly indicates that a change was made without deletion of the original record.

5. All documentation must include adequate identification of the patient/client and the physical therapist and/or physical therapist assistant.

    a. The patient's/client's full name and identification number, if applicable, must be included on all official documents.

    b. All entries should be dated and authenticated with the provider's full name and appropriate designation:

    i. Documentation of the examination, evaluation, diagnosis, prognosis, plan of care, and discharge summary must be authenticated by the physical therapist who provided the service.

    ii. Documentation of the interventions in visit/encounter notes must be authenticated by the physical therapist or physical therapist assistant who provided the service.

    iii. Documentation by physical therapist or physical therapist assistant graduates or other physical therapists and physical therapist assistants pending receipt of an unrestricted license should be authenticated by a licensed physical therapist, or, when permissible by law, documentation by physical therapist assistant graduates may be authenticated by a physical therapist assistant.

    iv. Documentation by students (SPT/SPTA) in physical therapist or physical therapist assistant programs must be additionally authenticated by the physical therapist or, when permissible by law, documentation by physical therapist assistant students may be authenticated by a physical therapist assistant.

  c. Documentation should include the referral mechanism by which the physical therapy services are initiated. Examples are:

    i. Self-referral/direct access

    ii. Request for consultation by another practitioner

  d. Documentation should include indications of "no shows" or cancellations.

WHAT TO DOCUMENT

Examination Element: Tests and Measures

PTAs are often delegated the duty of collecting data related to the tests and measures initially assessed by the PT at the time of the initial examination and evaluation. Tests and measures are reproducible objective assessments that initially provide the baseline against which all future assessments are compared to determine the patient's response to the physical therapy interventions. The objective data obtained during the assessment of these tests and measures also assist the PT in clinical decision making. Documenting objective tests and measures using quantitative techniques (scores, grades, ratings, etc) generally does not provide sufficient information about the abilities or impairments. Qualitative descriptions should also be included to provide the readers of the documentation further insight as to the quality of the patient's performance. In documenting the results of the tests and measures, it is essential to document how the specific tests or measurements relate to the patient's functional ability. In many cases, reimbursement is directly related to improvement in function. It is important to remember that neither the patient nor the payers care about ROM measurements such as how many degrees the patient can elevate the shoulder; they are more interested in how the patient's ability to elevate the shoulder will help in getting dressed. Clear, concise, and organized documentation of objective tests should communicate the link between the improvements made in specific impairments and the improvements noted in the patient's functional skills.

Organizing Tests and Measuring Data

In handwritten documentation, there is no specific standard rule on organizing the data. The data should be organized in a consistent sequence to provide the reader a clear picture of the patient's problems and abilities. The PTA should refer to the PT's initial evaluation to determine the organization of documenting the data. Objective data are often best documented in tables and columns to make quick and easy comparisons and for simplicity in following the information. Electronic physical therapy documentation programs have a predetermined structure in terms of where the tests and measures are documented within the program interface.

Common Suggestions for Documenting Tests and Measures

1. *Be consistent*: Perform and document tests and measures using the same method that the PT used in the initial evaluation. For example, in assessing dynamic standing balance of a patient who suffered a traumatic head injury, the PT may document using grades (good, fair, poor, etc) or by describing the patient's performance in terms of how much assistance is required (minimum assistance, moderate assistance, etc). Objective measurement such as a number on a specific assessment tool is always more accurate than a subjective result such as poor sitting balance. There can be a huge gap between the terms fair and good while the results on a balance scale such as the Berg is more objective and identifies a number as the patient moves from fair to good.

2. *Write from the patient's perspective*: Always document the performance of the patient. Take care to write from the perspective of accomplishments of the patient and not what was performed by the PTA. For example, in documenting the gait, the PTA should write: "The patient performed gait training with a hemi walker, 100,' on level surfaces with moderate assist × 1," not "The PTA performed gait training with the patient using a hemi walker for 100,' on level surfaces with moderate assist × 1."

3. *Be detailed but concise*: Full sentences are not a requirement; however, the PTA should include all necessary information in documenting each test. This allows another similarly trained PT or PTA to reproduce the test. It may not be necessary to include all details of standard testing procedures each time the test is reassessed, although, if there are any variations to the standard procedure, these details will need to be clearly written. For example, the PTA performs manual muscle testing (MMT) using alternative positioning because the patient is unable to maintain the standard position.

4. *Use action words* like *performed, demonstrated, completed*, etc, to indicate the patient's performance.

In providing physical therapy services to a patient/client who has a neurologically based diagnosis, the PTA can be expected to be delegated many tests and measures to reassess during the patient's rehabilitation process. The focus of the PTA when reassessing tests and measures is to collect the data (qualitative and quantitative) and provide that data to the evaluating PT for interpretation. Although not inclusive, the following are examples of tests and measures that may be assessed by the PTA:

1. *Vital signs*

   a. Heart rate: Note the location of the measurement (eg, brachial, radial, carotid, etc), quality, and rate.

   b. Respiratory rate: Note rate, depth, and regularity.

   c. Blood pressure: Note side of the body measured, patient's position, and reading.

Sample entry for vital signs:

Heart rate: (L) radial pulse = 72 beats per minute, strong and regular
Respiratory rate: 16 beats per minute, deep and regular
Blood pressure: sitting, (L) upper extremity = 120/80 mm Hg

---

2. *Pain*: Note the description, location, and severity of the pain. (Refer to Chapter 5 for additional information.) Remember, pain descriptions and severity are subjective assessments because the perception of pain will vary among individuals, and they should be documented in the subjective portion on the documentation form. In neurorehabilitation, it is also necessary to note the patient's nonverbal response to painful stimuli.

3. *Consciousness/cognitive function*

   a. Glasgow Coma Scale (GCS): The GCS is a standardized test used to determine the level of consciousness and degree of brain injury. The GCS is divided into 3 parts: eye opening, verbal responses, and motor responses. The patient's response is compared with the criteria for each part of the test and a resulting score is calculated. Each response is then rated using a scale ranging from 3 to 6 points. (For additional discussion, refer to Chapter 11.)

   b. Rancho Los Amigos Scale: PTAs asked to reassess the Ranchos Los Amigos Scale of cognitive function should observe the patient's performance and behavior and provide the rating of Rancho levels I through VIII based on their observation. (Refer to Chapter 11 for a thorough discussion of this scale.)

4. *Orientation* (to person, place, time, circumstances): PTAs assessing orientation are attempting to gain insights into the patient's level of cognitive ability. This may not require ongoing assessment; however, the PTA should reassess and report, especially if there is a noted change in the patient's behavior. Orientation is assessed by asking the patient some questions (interviewing) and taking note of the answers. Sample questions that could be used to assess orientation include the following:

   • What is your name? (person)

   • Do you know who I am? (person)

   • Where are we now? (place)

   • What happened to you? (circumstance)

   • What year is this? (time)

   The patient's responses to these questions can provide the PTA with important information about the patient's level of cognitive impairment and help in determining the methods used in teaching and communicating with the patient.

5. *Palpation*

   Muscle tone: Note the position of the patient during the assessment and the quality of muscle tone, using descriptors such as flaccid, hypotonic, normal muscle tone, hypertonic, and rigid. However, the PTA should use the same assessment techniques, assessment tools, and/or descriptions used by the PT during the initial examination and evaluation.

6. *Reflex testing*: In reflex testing the PTA should take care to reassess the delegated reflex(es) in the same manner that the PT initially assessed them. The PTA should record the presence or absence of the reflex and grade of intensity, if applicable.

   a. Deep tendon reflexes (biceps, triceps, knee jerk, etc).

   b. Superficial: Generally documented as present (+) or absent (–). May also include qualitative comments to further describe the reflex activity (eg, "gag reflex is present but is weak").

   c. Pathological: Normally documented as present (+) or absent (–).

7. *ROM measurements*: Note the specific side (left or right), the specific joint motion (shoulder flexion, shoulder external rotation, hip hyperextension), the range measurement from beginning to end (eg, if measuring left shoulder flexion ROM, the range should be documented

0 degrees to 160 degrees rather than 160 degrees), and any specific deviation from the standard testing procedures (such as alternative positioning). Other considerations include grouping the measurements in a logical sequence and by anatomical region. This will help to not only organize the documentation but also to avoid excessive positioning changes with the patient.

A sample entry for assessing ROM measurement:

A ROM (L) shoulder:
- Flexion = 0 degrees to 120 degrees
- Hyperextension = 0 degrees to 35 degrees
- Abduction = 0 degrees to 130 degrees
- External rotation = 0 degrees to 70 degrees
- Internal rotation = 0 degrees to 70 degrees

---

8. *Muscle strength*

   a. MMT: Traditional MMT cannot be used in assessing patients who have upper motor neuron lesions with tone abnormalities that often accompany such conditions. Examples of upper motor neuron lesions include cerebral palsy, cerebrovascular accident, spinal cord injury, and traumatic brain injury and are further discussed in specific chapters. However, MMT may be used to assess patients with selected peripheral nerve lesions. For the PTA documenting MMT, note which side of the body is being tested, the muscle group (knee extensors) or specific muscles (gluteus medius), and the muscle strength grade (2/5, 3+/5); group anatomic regions together to assist in organizing information, and take note of any modification from the standard techniques.

   b. Functional muscle testing is widely accepted for muscle strength testing in the neurologically impaired patient. This type of muscle testing involves close observation of the patient performing specific movements and/or functional activities. The PTA should note the patient's abilities to perform the movements and activities and include any qualitative descriptions that will further depict the patient's abilities.

9. *Posture*: The PTA should note the patient's position during the assessment, static versus dynamic movements, and description of abnormalities or malalignments observed while comparing one side with the other or comparing with standardized landmarks.

10. *Functional mobility*: When documenting functional mobility of the client, similar data should be captured for the various aspects of function. Again, the PTA is reminded to assess functional mobility using the same techniques used by the PT during the initial examination. The data recorded and documented for each form of functional mobility are described below:

   a. Bed mobility: Take note of the specific movements used by the patient when moving in bed (eg, rolling toward the right, rolling toward the left, supine to prone, supine to sit). Are assistive or adaptive devices used during the activities? How much assistance is required by the patient to complete the task? How many people are needed for assistance (moderate assist × 1)? What are the instructions, cues, and guidance provided to the patient? Describe the patient's safety in completing the task.

   b. Transfers: Note the patient's movements from one surface to the other (eg, bed to wheelchair, wheelchair to commode). Note each transfer as a separate action and avoid grouping all as transfers, especially if the patient's ability to complete each is different. Are assistive or adaptive devices used during the transfer? How much assistance does the patient require to complete the tasks? How many people are needed for assistance (moderate assist × 1)? What are the instructions, cues, and guidance provided to the patient? Describe the patient's safety in completing the task.

c. Balance: Take note to distinguish between static versus dynamic balance activities. Is the patient working on sitting or standing balance? What assistive or adaptive devices were used during the activities? How much assistance does the patient require to complete the task (some PTs may use a grading scale of *good, fair, poor*, etc, for assessing balance)? How many people are needed for assistance (moderate assist × 1)? What are the instructions, cues, and guidance provided to the patient? Describe the patient's safety in completing the task.

d. Gait: Note the distance traversed by the patient. Describe the type surface (level, unlevel, gravel, inclined, etc) the patient is walking on. What assistive or adaptive devices were used during the gait activities (wheeled walker, cane, ankle-foot orthosis [AFO], etc)? How much assistance does the patient require (minimum assist, moderate assist, etc)? How many people are needed for assistance (moderate assist × 1)? What are the instructions, cues, and guidance provided to the patient (eg, verbal instruction needed for sequencing with the cane)? Describe the patient's safety in completing the task.

e. Wheelchair management: Note the distance traversed by the patient. Describe the type of surface(s) (level, unlevel, carpet, tile, inclined, etc) the patient negotiated during the activity. How much assistance did the patient require to propel the chair and navigate obstacles such doors and elevators (minimum assist, moderate assist, etc)? What are the instructions, cues, and guidance provided to the patient (eg, verbal instruction needed navigating inward opening doors)? Describe the patient's safety in completing the task.

Sample entry for gait:

Patient performed gait training using a hemi walker and AFO on the (L) LE for 50′ on a level surface with minimum assist × 1 and verbal instructions for sequencing and placement of the hemi walker. Patient has a tendency to place hemi walker too far medially, causing a stumbling hazard.

In addition to the common areas of assessment described in the previous section, the PT may also use any number of standardized questionnaires or assessment tools. (Refer to Chapter 5 for a thorough discussion of examination tools a PTA might use.) The PTA should reassess the client with central nervous system deficits using the same questionnaire or assessment tool used in the initial evaluation. The PTA should follow the procedures of that tool as outlined, mirroring as closely as possible the same technique of assessment used by the PT during the initial evaluation.

Intervention Element

The intervention element is the PTA's greatest role in the patient/client management model. After the PT completes the initial examination and evaluation of the patient, the PT may delegate all or part of the patient's subsequent visits to the PTA. Documentation of the intervention allows the PTA to communicate what took place during each visit and the specific accomplishments of the patient. The APTA's *Guidelines for Physical Therapy Documentation of Patient/Client Management*[2] lists this information that should be documented for each client visit:

- *Patient's self-report*: This is the subjective part of the documentation. This information is gathered during the interview part of the session and may include information from those closest to the patient, such as a spouse, children, significant other, or caregiver. The PTA must become a skilled listener to identify red flags. Learning when to probe deeper into the patient's self-report by asking specific questions to obtain more details about the patient's condition is a skill that is necessary for accurate documentation. The PTA must also be able to distinguish between relevant and nonrelevant data. For example, the fact of the patient attending a card game with friends may not be relative to his condition, but his report of having difficulty getting into and out of the car is relevant to his functional status. Examples of information extracted from the patient/client/family member/caregiver report could include:
  - Perception of the patient's progress. For example, the patient may state, "I'm not having a good day today; I just don't feel as strong as yesterday."
  - Pain—Include the exact description, quoting the patient when possible. Note the location and intensity of the pain. For example, "The pain in my right thigh feels like thousands of ants biting me; it's a 10 out of 10!"
  - Changes in the patient's function. For example, "I was able to get my leg into the bed by myself."
  - Reports of the patient's response to the treatment sessions. For example, the patient's spouse states, "He was so tired from therapy that he slept through dinner" or "He transferred without my help for the first time today."
  - Statements that describe effectiveness of interventions. For example, "Using the walker helps me get to the bathroom easier; the nurse didn't have to help as much."
- *Identification of specific interventions provided during the session*, including details of frequency, intensity, and duration as appropriate, such as these examples:
  - Therapeutic exercises—Include the type of exercise; the anatomical motion; the muscle being exercised or name of the exercise; the sets, repetitions, and amount of time the exercise is performed, if applicable; and the equipment used (eg, 10# ankle weight).
  - Functional mobility—As noted previously in this chapter, information to include in this section describes how and what the patient performed during the therapy session. The following examples demonstrate functional mobility:
    - Specific movements and activities (gait training, wheelchair mobility, transfers, etc)
    - Assistive or adaptive devices used (wheeled walker, cane, AFO, etc)
    - How much assistance the patient requires and the number of people needed for assisting (moderate assist × 2, minimum assist × 1)
    - Instructions, cues, and guidance provided to the patient ("verbal reminders for the patient to push up from the arms of the wheelchair")
  - Equipment provided—Description of the equipment needs of the patient.
- *Changes in the patient's impairment, limitation, or disability status* related to the plan of care: The PTA should take care to note significant changes in the patient's status that may affect the plan of care previously established by the evaluating PT. Remember, it is not the PTA's role to determine whether changes need to be made in that plan of care and what those changes should be, although the PT may ask the PTA to make recommendations. The PTA's role is to report the change(s) to the evaluating PT.
- *Response to interventions*, including adverse reactions, if any: The PTA must develop a correlation between the tests and measures assessed and the interventions provided. This includes statements that note changes in the patient's impairments and/or functional status. For

example, the PTA may look at the objective data regarding the patient's functional strength in the affected LE and the patient's functional mobility status. The PTA may be able to comment that the interventions have been effective in increasing the strength in the LE, therefore improving the patient's ability to move from the supine position to sit or transfer from bed to chair. The PTA should avoid using ambiguous phrases such as "patient tolerated treatment well" or "patient is making progress toward the goals."[4] This type of vague statement does not provide quality evidence of any particular response to interventions provided to the patient.

- *Factors that modify the frequency or intensity of the intervention and progression toward physical therapy goals, including patient's adherence to the instructions*: This is the section of the note where the PTA must have a strong knowledge of the physical therapy goals set by the evaluating PT. Although the PTA may not address each and every physical therapy goal at each session, the patient's performance should be assessed and compared with the physical therapy goals on a regular basis. Data from the assessment of tests and measures and the objective data related to the patient's functional abilities provide the evidence for statements made about the patient's progress toward the goals. Documented information regarding the patient's progress toward the physical therapy goals includes the following:

  ○ A statement of whether the goal has been attained

  ○ Progress or no progress toward the goal

  ○ A decline in the patient's status related to the PT goals

---

Sample entry

Patient is making improvements in gait, transfers, and functional strength. The patient has met goals 1 and 2 and is making consistent progress toward goals 3 and 4.

- *Communication/consultation with providers/patient/client/family/significant other, etc*: The PTA should document ongoing communication and consultation with the evaluating PT regarding the progress of the patient, the need for reassessment/reevaluation, and/or recommendations for changes in the plan of care. This documentation of communication from the PTA to the PT provides evidence of PT/PTA teamwork and collaboration. For example, the PTA may indicate "will consult with the evaluating PT about a trial of electrical stimulation to address the patient's drop foot on the left LE." Efficiency and effectiveness of the physical therapy care of the patient depends greatly on the working relationship, and more specifically on strong communication, between the PT and PTA team.[5] Consultation with other providers may also be required at times. For example, the PTA may ask the social worker about the patient's discharge plans or the insurance coverage for a particular piece of equipment the patient will need. Additionally, the PTA should document consultation with family and caregivers for the purposes of providing education and instruction. For example, a patient with discharge plans back to home with caregiver support may require family training and instruction on proper transfer techniques and assisting the patient with gait. The PTA should document the date of the scheduled family training, the individuals present, and the type(s) of training that took place and comment on the family/caregiver learning during the training session(s).

- *Documentation to plan for ongoing provision of services for subsequent visits, which include but are not limited to:*
  - ○ Upcoming interventions with objectives
  - ○ Progression parameters
  - ○ Precautions

The PTA should document the plans and changes to be implemented in the subsequent patient visits. This part of the documentation outlines progression of the treatment plan (within the PT's established plan of care) or identifies specific interventions or areas of focus for subsequent visits (eg, "will progress to stair training on next visit" or "will focus on inhibition techniques for the hypertonicity in the patient's LE").

The following is a list of guidelines for writing this part of the note:

- Future tense: Because this part of the documentation refers to a future event, the PTA should use future tense terminology: "will focus…, will update…, will consult…," etc.

- Justify necessity of treatment: If making recommendations for changes within the established plan of care, the PTA should include a sound justification of the needed change and communicate that justification to the PT of record.

REIMBURSEMENT

As mentioned previously in the chapter, physical therapy documentation serves as the basis or justification for many types of reimbursement. The APTA defines reimbursement as "payment by the patient (first-party) or insurer (third-party), to the health care provider, for services rendered."[6] Physical therapy departments and clinics receive their reimbursements according to whether the patient has insurance and the type of insurance coverage the patient has. There are many rules and guidelines controlling the amount of reimbursement that is received, and the rules differ depending on the types of insurance policies, coverage, and payers. The success and sustainability of any physical therapy practice depends directly on the reimbursement payments received from the patient and/or the insurers. With physical therapy documentation being a key piece of information used in approving or denying payments, it is of the utmost importance that PTs and PTAs meet the payer's requirements. Thorough, clear documentation that communicates the patient's functional progress and need for continued skilled physical therapy treatments will help to ensure reimbursement is received.[7] The APTA also offers some insights in its *Defensible Documentation for Patient/Client Management*[8] on reasons for reimbursement denials:

- Poor legibility of handwriting
- Incomplete documentation
- No date of treatment sessions
- Abbreviations—too many used, reader unable to understand
- Documentation does not support the billing (coding)
- Does not demonstrate skilled care provided to the patient
- Does not support medical necessity of therapy services
- Does not demonstrate progress within the plan of care
- Repetitious daily notes showing no change in patient status
- Interventions with no clarification of time, frequency, or duration

More than just a record of the care and services provided to the patient, physical therapy documentation and its link to reimbursement and payment for the services provided is crucial for the viability of the physical therapy practice. PTAs must continually educate themselves on the ever-changing requirements of the various payers and regulatory institutions and seek to improve their documentation skills.

DOCUMENTATION FORMATS

Traditionally, physical therapy documentation has taken place in a variety of forms. Many of the forms used were, and in some cases still are, driven by the payer's requirements. The many formats of documentation are also aligned with federal and state guidelines, type of rehabilitation setting, type of reimbursement, and types of patients treated.

Traditional formats of physical therapy documentation include narrative forms; subjective, objective, assessment, and plan (SOAP) notes; check-off forms; fillable forms; and exercise logs. However, recent health care reform measures have been introduced to propel the health care industry to adopting electronic medical records (EMR). In 2009, the American Recovery and Reinvestment Act was signed into law. One of the measures of this act aims to require adoption of electronic health records by primary health care providers by 2014.[9] While PTs and PTAs have not been mandated to adopt the EMR as of this time, health care providers referring patients to them will expect they will use a compatible electronic health records system. Many of these health records systems are software packages that have the ability to link to the provider's scheduling and billing systems. The software packages typically contain templates for the components of documentation required of PTs and PTAs: initial evaluation, reevaluations, discharge summaries, daily notes, and progress notes. These templates are designed with an overarching objective: efficient use of time. Software developers have incorporated a variety of different data input methods, such as check boxes, toggle buttons, drop-down menus, standard terminology selection, and open boxes for narrative comments. The following are advantages of using EMR:

- Improved readability; it essentially negates the issue of illegible handwriting

- The ability to generate printed evaluations, reports, and progress notes

- The ability to generate letters to physicians or other health care providers based on the information entered

- More accurate tracking of billing

There are also several disadvantages of using an EMR system:

- Cost: The initial investment in the hardware (laptops, computer stations, tablets, etc) and the software package

- Maintenance: Regularly scheduled upgrades to hardware and software, regularly scheduled system backups to prevent lost data

- More difficulty in maintaining patient data security and confidentiality and meeting the standards of the Health Insurance Portability and Accountability Act,[10] which sets federal guidelines on how health information should be handled in electronic transmission

The following list includes examples of the aforementioned electronic documentation software packages specific to physical therapy practice:

- Casamba (www.casamba.net)

- ReDoc (www.redocsoftware.com)

- TheraOffice (www.rehabsoftware.com)

- WebPT (www.webpt.com)

- APTA Connect (www.apta.org/connect): In conjunction with Cedaron Medical Inc, the APTA has created its own electronic documentation platform

The documentation format influences the look and feel, functionality, navigation, and ease of data entry. However, it is the PTA's responsibility to ensure, regardless of the format, accurate and timely documentation occurs. The same rules and principles of documentation apply to electronic documentation as to more traditional handwritten forms of documentation. The electronic format incorporates an additional skill of learning to properly navigate the particular system used in the facility.

CONCLUSION

Documentation of physical therapy services is a very important duty of the PTs and PTAs who are providing care to the patients/clients. Within the patient/client management model of physical therapy care, the PTA's primary role is to deliver the interventions established within the PT's plan of care, which may sometimes include delegation of reassessment of selected tests and measures. This means PTAs must possess and use sound clinical problem solving and judgment to determine whether the patient is capable of performing the planned interventions and of responding appropriately to those interventions. The PTA must also decide the appropriate time to consult with the evaluating PT to report changes in the patient's status and progress within the set plan of care. Not only are PTAs responsible for documenting the care delivered and the results of the tests and measures assessed, they should take care to provide effective documentation of the communication and collaboration of the PT/PTA team. No matter what format is used, efficient and effective documentation is crucial to ensuring that efficient, effective, and safe care is delivered to the patient.

REFERENCES

1. Bircher W. *Lukan's Documentation for Physical Therapist Assistants*. Philadelphia, PA: FA Davis; 2008.
2. American Physical Therapy Association. *Guidelines: Physical Therapy Documentation of Patient/ Client Management*. http://www.apta.org/uploadedFiles/APTAorg/About_Us/Policies/BOD/Practice/DocumentationPatientClientMgmt.pdf. Accessed January 3, 2013.
3. American Physical Therapy Association. *Guide to Physical Therapist Practice*. guidetoptpractice.apta.org. Accessed January 3, 2013.
4. Clifton DW. "Tolerated treatment well" may no longer be tolerated. *PT: Magazine of Physical Therapy*. 1995;3(10):24-27.
5. Holcomb S. Recipe for effective teamwork: why some PT/PTA pairings thrive, to patient's ultimate benefit. *PT: Magazine of Physical Therapy*. http://www.apta.org/PTinMotion/2009/2/PTAViewpoint. Accessed January 15, 2013.
6. American Physical Therapy Association. 2011 glossary of payment terms. http://www.apta.org/Payment/Glossary. Accessed August 27, 2013.
7. Staples S. Thorough documentation can win reimbursement. *Adv Phys Ther Rehab Med*. 2005;16(20):68.
8. American Physical Therapy Association. Defensible documentation for patient/client management. http://www.apta.org/Documentation/DefensibleDocumentation/. Accessed January 16, 2013.
9. US Department of Health and Human Services. Health Resource and Service Administration. Health information technology. http://www.hrsa.gov/ruralhealth/resources/healthit/index.html. Accessed January 17, 2013.
10. US Department of Health and Human Services. Health information privacy. http://www.hhs.gov/ocr/privacy/. Accessed January 17, 2013.

Please see accompanying Web site at
www.healio.com/books/neuroptavideos

Children With
Central Nervous System Insult

Kristine N. Corn, PT, MS, DPT
Cynthia J. Hogan, PTA

KEY WORDS

- Anoxic brain injury
- Athetosis
- Cerebral palsy
- Diplegia
- Facilitation
- Handling techniques
- Hemiplegia
- Hypoxic brain injury
- Inhibition
- Quadriplegia
- Triplegia

CHAPTER OBJECTIVES

- Introduce the more frequently treated pediatric neurological diagnoses from insults that occur in utero, at birth, or shortly after birth.

- Differentiate between trauma to the central nervous system in the neonate and acquired trauma after 2 years of age that primarily affects the motor system.

- Present some of the more common characteristics observed in the pediatric neurological patient with the medical diagnosis of cerebral palsy.

- Introduce handling and treatment ideas for the neurologically impaired child.

Umphred DA, Lazaro RT, eds.
Neurorehabilitation for the Physical Therapist Assistant,
Second Edition (pp 177-210).
© 2014 SLACK Incorporated.

INTRODUCTION

Physical therapist assistants (PTAs) working in the pediatric neurological clinic or hospital will treat a wide and varied population of children who will continually challenge their critical thinking and creativity. When a child's central nervous system (CNS) is damaged, there can be one or more systems affected, depending on the location and cause of the insult. Physical therapists (PTs) and PTAs treat children with movement dysfunction and/or sensory processing disorders to prevent skeletal deformities and encourage normal development of motor skills and milestones. Often, insults to the CNS affect postural tone as well as distal muscle tone, strength, and sensory processing. The postural tone and motor control will influence and be influenced by feedback and feed-forward information from all the sensory systems (see Chapter 3). Some of the more common CNS diagnoses treated in a pediatric physical therapy department are cerebral palsy (CP), genetic disorders, autism spectrum disorders, sensory processing dysfunction, anoxic/hypoxic, and traumatic brain injury (TBI).

For some of these disorders, the causation is clear, whereas in other CNS dysfunctions, the causation is not well understood or is unknown. It is always helpful to have a clear medical diagnosis, but this is not always possible. In either case, the patient's clinical signs and symptoms (functional limitations) will help the PT determine the appropriate treatment program for each individual. The PT will then determine what portion of the treatment program will be delegated to the PTA and whether it is appropriate for the PTA to perform follow-up examinations that identify whether the intervention is meeting expected goals. In some of these medical diagnoses, such as CP and TBI, the specific therapy diagnosis and movement disorder depends on the muscle tone and the areas of involvement.

Although physical therapy always considers the medical diagnosis, the PT's function is to treat movement disorders associated with the medical diagnosis (Table 8-1). The classification of muscle tone is beneficial when evaluating and analyzing motor dysfunction and determining appropriate treatment (see Table 8-1).

Table 8-2 describes the area or areas of the body involved in motor dysfunction.

CEREBRAL PALSY

CP is the most common physical disability of childhood. Children with CP are generally seen as having motor control problems; however, they may demonstrate multiple sensory deficits that affect the CNS's normal maturation of motor control and ultimately their general development and function. The individual with CP incurred damage to the CNS during gestation (prenatal), at the time of birth (natal), or within the first few weeks of life (postnatal). Basic patterns of motor behavior have not been established at the time of the insult. These basic components of movement are essential in developing normal postural alignment, equilibrium, and protective responses. More automatic behaviors or stereotypical motor behaviors are repetitively demonstrated and elicited by sensory input or intention. These motor behaviors may become the dominant movement patterns as the child develops because of the limitations in available motor control. These patterns are considered abnormal and interfere with normal skill acquisition and motor control and ultimately limit their motor learning. (Refer to Chapter 3 for more information regarding motor function.) Depending on the child's age when the insult occurred and the extent of the involvement, a wide variety of dysfunction in postural control and skill development will be observed.

With or without a formal medical diagnosis of CP, a neonate who has suffered a CNS insult will, within the first few weeks of life, present with far more subtle motor involvement, unless the damage has been fairly severe. The infant's tone may be initially hypotonic, causing decreased head and trunk control. Reflexive movement patterns are present and may be appropriate based

Table 8-1
Areas of Motor Involvement

Area of Central Nervous System Involvement Due to Bleeds or Anoxia

Area of Insult	Cause	Involvement
Periventricular	Central bleed	Diplegic
Parietal lobe	Hemispheric bleed	Hemiplegic
Frontal motor	Global ischemia	Quadriplegic
Distal cortical		Spastic/multisystem
Cerebellar	Anoxia	Quadriplegic athetoid
Diencephalon	Total asphyxia	Ataxic

Classification by Muscle Tone

Pathology	Tone Quality	Impairment
Hypertonic	High tone	Decreased joint mobility and motor control problems
Hypotonic	Low tone	Increased joint mobility and motor control problems
Mixed programming	Low to high tone	Increased joint mobility of trunk and neck Decreased joint mobility of the extremities and motor control problems
Fluctuating programming	Athetoid	Decreased grading of strength/joint range of motion, poor stabilization, often normal mobility
Regulatory inconsistencies	Ataxic	Trunk instability, increased joint mobility, and gait
In programming		Disturbances in force, rate, timing

Table 8-2
Classification by Areas of Involvement

Medical Classification	Movement Dysfunction
Hemiplegic	The trunk and either both right extremities or both left extremities
Diplegic	The trunk and lower extremities have greater involvement than the upper extremities
Triplegic	The trunk and 3 extremities
Quadriplegic	The trunk and all 4 extremities

on the infant's age or corrected age for those born prematurely. It is essential for the PT to be well appraised of normal neonatal development. It is more common that a child of 12 months or older who is diagnosed with CP is referred for physical therapy because the child has not achieved the normal milestones and appropriate developmental skills (eg, coming to sit or sitting if placed in

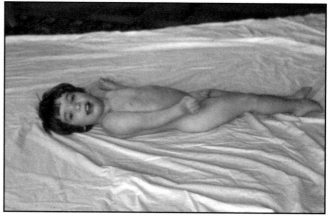

Figure 8-1. A child with severe tonal abnormality will often demonstrate involvement in all 4 extremities. This child would be considered to have spastic quadriplegia.

that position and moving independently from the sitting position). Children who are 12 months old should be crawling, pulling to stand, practicing standing balance, or even beginning to take their first steps.[1] (Refer to Chapter 2 for additional information on child development.) Once the PT has evaluated the child and determined what abnormal motor patterns should be eliminated, what normal motor behaviors need to be practiced, what sensory systems need to be heightened, and which ones require dampening, a plan of care can be established. This plan of care often incorporates the need to eliminate reflexive patterns that are limiting the development of normal movement while integrating protective responses, postural control, and improving motor responses that will lead to better motor control. From that plan of care, the PT should be able to delegate to the PTA the activities that are within the competencies of the PTA.

The older child, between 18 months and 4 years, may have developed compensatory patterns of movement that the PTA will be able to recognize as abnormal movement patterns that limit functional movement and the child's progression in motor control. The movement may be labored as the child attempts to overcome hypertonicity, asymmetric muscle tone, and decreased postural stability. Repetitive abnormal posturing that accompanies increased muscle tone will eventually cause contractual deformities of the soft tissues and can create more permanent joint deformities. When this occurs there is poor alignment of the joints in relation to each other, interfering with positioning, handling, and care.

Generally, these musculoskeletal problems are first observed in the more involved extremities (Figure 8-1). Without therapy and parental involvement, these soft tissue deformities may cause bony changes, skeletal deformities, and eventual dislocations. Although the hypotonic child does not have to work against increased muscle tone, the child needs to develop sufficient muscle strength and postural control to overcome gravity and be able to come to sit and stand. The hypotonic child generally presents with poor to fair head and trunk control (Figures 8-2 and 8-3). Low tone often causes deformities of the spine due to lack of sufficient symmetric postural control. With either hyper- or hypotonia, there is a complex interaction that interferes with selective motor control.[2] Selective motor control is defined as the ability to independently move a joint voluntarily. The inability to isolate a movement without activating or using other parts of a limb is thought to be correlated with the severity of the CNS lesion. Selective motor control is important for the motor control needed for normal functional activities. The PT will differentiate these motor dysfunctions as part of the initial assessment and should continue to evaluate the interventions used and the progress made during each treatment session. The PTA may be the primary professional responsible for that intervention, but the PT should always be informed about changes in the child, including positive and negative responses to that intervention. The delegation of intervention to the PTA depends on the stability of the child's CNS, the degree of movement dysfunction, the involvement of the body systems of the child, and the skill level of the PTA.

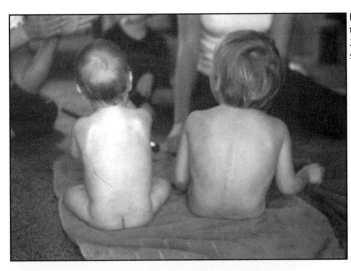

Figure 8-2. Comparison of sitting postures of a normal 6-month-old child to his 2-year-old brother with the diagnosis of spastic athetosis: Posterior view.

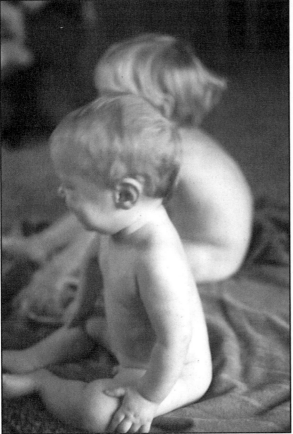

Figure 8-3. Comparison of sitting postures of a normal 6-month-old child to his 2-year-old brother with the diagnosis of spastic athetosis: Lateral view.

The severity of the insult has a significant role in determining the results of habilitation and is extremely important in prescribing the intensity, duration, and type of therapeutic intervention. Children diagnosed with CP are often classified as mild, moderate, or severe. Generally, with appropriate, intensive treatment initiated by 4 to 6 months of age, a mildly involved child will develop sufficient motor control to allow for normal movement patterns, and a moderately involved child will have mild deficits in movement development after physical therapy. A severely involved child can often change, becoming a child with moderate to moderately severe involvement. Although the medical diagnosis of CP is static, the growing and maturing CNS has plasticity (refer to Chapter 3), and the motor system will express these motor changes by increased fluidity of movement and skill development if the environment nurtures those movements. In turn, the opposite can occur without appropriate and intensive treatment at an early age. The mildly involved child often develops moderate disabilities, the moderate child develops severe disabilities, and the child who was initially severe often becomes even more involved.

TRAUMATIC AND ANOXIC/HYPOXIC INJURY

This medical diagnosis is generally applied to children over the age of 2 years. Children with TBI and near-drowning have one aspect of their CNS involvement in common: Both patients have sustained trauma to a nervous system that has already established normal patterns of movement and postural control. Thus, the child will have some knowledge of how to move based on motor memory and motor learning or control up to the age of the insult. This prior learning is often helpful in treatment, as opposed to the child with CP, who has had minimal to no experience developing normal patterns of movement and postural control.

CNS contusions and lacerations of the patient with a TBI can occur with or without skull fracture. Damage can affect any area of the brain, or laceration of the blood vessels supplying the brain can reduce the supply of oxygen to the area of brain. Cranial nerves may be injured, and diffuse axonal injury is the most common cause of primary lesions.[2,3] These injuries may result in coma or a persistent vegetative state secondary to damage as the result of lack of oxygen. These lesions can cause (1) increased intracranial pressure, (2) cerebral hypoxia or ischemia, (3) intracranial hemorrhage, (4) electrolyte imbalance from swelling, (5) secondary infection, and (6) seizures.[4] There are often physiological, cognitive, and behavioral changes along with movement dysfunction after a brain injury. As the child's CNS is adjusting to the insult and changes, the family and their CNSs are also reacting to changes to their family member. The family's input to the child with CNS damage can dramatically affect the outcome of therapy.

MEDICAL PROGNOSIS AND OUTCOME

Many of the treatment interventions used for children with CP can be applied to the patient with either contusions or anoxia; however, the outcome may be different based on the neural plasticity and/or prior learning. Although many authors have found that patients younger than age 20 usually recover,[5] this is not always the case. Van der Naalt et al[5] report a positive correlation between outcomes of patients with mild to moderate brain injury, lesions seen on computed tomography, and patients with cerebral edema. The Glasgow Coma Scale[6] is a consistent outcome predictor that is used with head trauma and near-drowning. (Refer to Chapter 11 for the specific rating scale and additional information.)

Outcomes for children with CP will vary based on the area of insult, severity, and when treatment is initiated.[7] Hoon et al[8] studied sensory motor deficits in CP children born preterm and used diffusion tensor imaging studies to determine that the fibers in the corticospinal and posterior thalamic tracks were significantly lower than those in children in the control groups. With early intervention, it is generally possible to improve the functional outcome in mildly and moderately involved children. The child with severe disabilities may become less severe and even able to achieve some functional goals. In all cases, physical therapy can make a significant difference in the lives of a child and his or her family, even if the functional outcomes are limited.

EVALUATION OF THE CHILD WITH NEUROLOGICAL IMPAIRMENT

Many tests and assessments can be used to determine a child's functional status. Some are used to determine the developmental age, others to establish motor control and function, and still others to determine the child's neurological status. Some evaluations are administered by neurologists, whereas others are performed in the clinic by the PT and occupational therapist. The PTA may be asked to perform and record some of the data collection, but the PT will interpret the findings.

Initially, the PT takes a thorough history of the pregnancy, labor, and delivery and the child's medical history. It is essential to assess impairments of all systems. These would include musculoskeletal, cardiopulmonary, neurological, and integumentary systems. Specifically, the PT should assess muscle tone, muscle strength, joint range of motion (ROM), tonic neck reflexes, sensory processing of the different sensory organs, patterns of posture and movement, and functional activities of daily living (ADL) of the child based on age-appropriate skills. General cognitive and social skills must be noted and considered when assessing the child's overall development.

When evaluating a very young child, it is important for the PT to recognize how rapidly the immature nervous system changes. These children must be reevaluated on an ongoing basis. The PT may ask the PTA to identify changes to determine when reassessment is required, irrespective of who does the examination. Handling and positioning of the child, effectively or ineffectively performed, can dramatically affect the child's sensory/motor system and positively or negatively alter his or her motor abilities and skills. Consequently, the PTA must be able to identify the effects of handling, positioning, sensory processing, and other interventions during a treatment session and report to the PT. Feedback from the PTA is essential in determining and identifying the necessary changes needed in the treatment program. Thus, the PTA must be able to differentiate changes in muscle tone and ROM, the quality and quantity of the movement being facilitated, the state of the sensory systems,[2] and identify the development of functional skills during a treatment session.

During assessment of an older child, the PT must examine the same systems as with the infant; however, contractures, deformities, and diminished motor development will affect motor function at a more complex level of development. From motor control theory,[3] it is important to determine whether (1) the basic motor patterns are available and appropriately used, (2) the appropriate synergies are selected or modified, (3) anticipatory reactions are present if feedback is to be used correctly, (4) sensory systems are able to perceive information from the environment and respond appropriately, and (5) the patient is able to use a variety of motor patterns that match appropriate performance and desired outcomes. (Refer to Chapter 3 for additional information.)

A large variety of tests are commonly used by therapists to evaluate the motor development and functional skills of children with CP (please see the Suggested Readings at the end of this chapter). The instruments the PT selects to evaluate the child with CP have differences. The PTA needs to be aware of what the results of the exam means in relation to the plan of care. The PTA will not be the one to initially evaluate the child or choose the instrument to be used, but follow-up examinations may fall into the practice of the PTA. If the PTA is unfamiliar with the instrument selected by the PT and is asked to perform follow-up examinations, it is the PTA's responsibility to either make sure the PT teaches the PTA how to use the examination tool and then cross-checks for reliability of the test result between the PT and the PTA, or to obtain additional education to administer the specific test with reliability. No instrument tells the therapist everything regarding what body systems have deficits and how that affects functional movement. Specific tests that examine specific systems like reflex testing do not tell the therapist how those results affect the child's ability to functionally move in all spatial positions, nor will a functional test inform the therapist of specific body systems that are causing the movement problems. For that reason, it is the therapist's responsibility to interpret the results and analyze the relationships between body system problems and how they affect functional movement and thus limit the child's developmental progression. Some therapists have a difficult time making those analyses, and some find it very easy. Similarly, some PTAs quickly see the links between specific system tests like balance, muscle power, and reflexes and how the results of those tests affect movement. For these reasons, it is very important that the PT and PTA communicate their thoughts and that both, as professionals, help each other grow, learn, and become better clinicians.

TREATMENT OF THE NEUROLOGICALLY IMPAIRED CHILD

Children with neurological impairment from birth trauma, TBI, or near-drowning have or may develop abnormal postural tone that can lead to the development of musculoskeletal complications. The long-term effect of inappropriate movement patterns can lead to catastrophic orthopedic problems in the future. These musculoskeletal impairments generally mean that the sensory/motor system should be assessed and treated early in the child's development. Whatever the cause, children with CNS insults will present with postural tone that is outside the range of normal, either too high (hypertonic) or too low (hypotonic). Tone can also be mixed or fluctuating (athetoid) or ataxic depending on the area of involvement within the CNS.

Postural tone and control is established by the CNS and responds to the environment of the child (see Chapters 2 and 3). The postural tone controlled from the CNS is influenced by the sensory/motor feedback from the various sensory organs and receptors. The environment in which a child is treated will also influence a treatment session. For example, if a child has high extensor muscle tone, often due to poor postural muscle control or joint stability, and the therapy treatment area is noisy and distracting, the sensory input itself will often increase that tone. Given that increase in tone, the child's CNS will have greater difficulty regulating muscle function and postural control. This problem can often be eliminated by decreasing the sensory input to the child that is coming from the environment. Eliminating the excessive noise, dimming the lights, lowering the therapist's voice, and making sure the touch itself is deep pressure versus light touch are all aspects of the intervention strategies that can be beneficial to the child. Reintroducing those types of inputs at a later date are important aspects of the plan of care to ensure the child has control of the motor system in spite of the environmental influences. In the case of generalized low tone, it may be beneficial to have a more stimulating environment to arouse the CNS. The sensory systems are often not given sufficient importance when treating children and need to be better regulated by the therapist and recognized for the impact they can have on treatment.[7] The same is also true for the respiratory and oral motor components that are often overlooked and undertreated in this population of children. Therapists may not realize the significant impact breathing and oral motor function have on specific motor behaviors, the general motor control system, and ultimately the development of the child.

Gravity cannot be eliminated from life, but the influence can be reduced by the child's position. By placing a child in side-lying as opposed to prone or supine positions, the influence of the cervical reflexes is reduced. In side-lying, slow, rhythmical, rotational movement of the trunk can further decrease hypertonicity of the extensor muscles both functioning for postural control through coactivation as well as general movement. It is important to note that using rotation through the body axis will alter the tone in abnormal synergy patterns that limit the child's function. This activity can be delegated to a PTA. As tone is decreased, it is then possible to work toward passive ROM of the trunk as well as the extremities to maintain functional range to support normal movement development. Sitting or standing vertical positions can also help eliminate gravitational effects on the postural system and decrease the coactivation demands placed on the motor control system, and often fall within the child's initial functional control. When the skeletal structures are vertical and properly aligned, this posture promotes appropriate muscle firing, generally causing a decrease in high muscle tone in the hypertonic muscles and an increase in muscle tone in the low-toned child through the CNS's normal postural responses. The reason for this change is that a vertical posture requires less muscle power to hold a head or trunk upright when the center of gravity (COG) is over the base of support (BOS) than when the child is off vertical and the COG is outside the BOS. Gravitational pull and biomechanics are the causation of these differences. Once there is sufficient increase in strength or normal muscle power, this technique may be used effectively by moving the COG slightly outside or beyond the established BOS, activating the firing of desired muscle synergies and facilitating the development of greater postural strength and control.

In this pediatric CP population, stereotypical posturing and repetitive patterns of movement can be observed in the trunk and extremities. These patterns are often due to hypertonicity that is accompanied by weakness and the lack of normal postural patterns or motor programs. Initially, the child may present with general hypotonus (referred to as a *floppy baby*), but commonly hyper-tonus develops, particularly in the extremities, as gravity demands stabilization of the joints to develop ways to respond to the activity. In a normally developing newborn, flexor tone has already developed during normal fetal maturation. This child at birth begins to increase the firing of the extensor muscles as well as the ROM, but after contraction the child will rebound back into a more flexed posture. In a premature infant or a child suffering an insult at birth, generalized low tone predominates without this flexor bias. Extensor tone is generally the first to develop in these children, partially influenced by the CNS and partially by environmental demands, such as gravity, positioning, and motivation. If the extensor muscles prevail without the balance of the flexor muscles, the child will be unable to establish midline head control and will become asymmetric, causing shortening of cervical and thoracic spine on one side (see Figure 8-1). This ipsilateral asymmetry generally occurs on the side of the body with higher tone. The child with increased extension will usually present with the lower extremities (LEs) in extension, adduction, and eventually internal rotation with the feet in plantarflexion. The upper extremities (UEs) are more variable in their posturing but are generally dominated by flexion at the shoulder, elbow, wrist, and hand along with ulnar deviation. These patterns of movement are seen in all postures and often intensify as the child works and is motivated to stabilize the body against gravity. As children repetitively use these patterns for postural control and movement, the patterns become stronger, and it is then more difficult to alter or normalize function. These behaviors are consistent with present theories of motor learning and control (see Chapter 3). Older children not receiving early intervention will have practiced and learned stereotypic patterns of movement, making it more difficult to intervene and promote or facilitate normal movement and good postural control.

In the hypotonic child, weakness and/or lack of postural control may also provoke posturing into abnormal patterns to provide stability. This helps the child stabilize vision but can dramati-cally affect normal development of the motor system. Without intervention, these children will most likely develop contractures and deformities of the joints as well as spinal curves.[9]

TREATMENT STRATEGIES

Treatment must be designed to improve functional movement and postural control over the proximal (trunk and axial joints of shoulders and hips) and distal joints, minimize and/or prevent contractures and deformities, maintain or improve the respiratory function, improve oral motor function for feeding and pre-speech activities, organize and integrate the sensory systems, develop attachment to caregivers, and promote social interaction and appropriate responses. No therapist can cognitively think through all these components as the child is being treated, so recognizing normal responses to handling the child is the best way to summarize whether all these components are being integrated. The more the movement looks and feels normal, the more the therapist can

Figure 8-4. Normal postural development of a 3- to 4-month-old child.

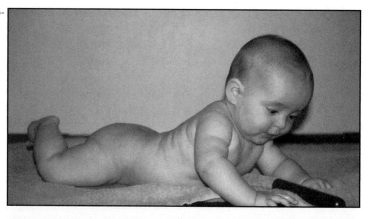

Figure 8-5. Normal development and tonal characteristics of the supine posture of a 3- to 4-month-old child.

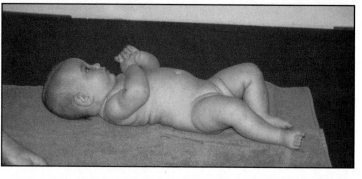

Figure 8-6. A child presented with extreme hypotonia at 6 months old. Although all 4 extremities were hypotonic at this age, he later developed and was diagnosed as a child with spastic diplegia.

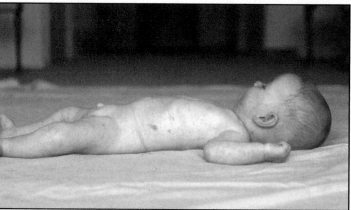

assume the child is integrating many of these aspects of normal sensory and motor development. To achieve higher functional levels of motor skills, a child must develop levels of competency working against gravity. In the initial stages of normal development, the child works on head control and shoulder girdle development while prone (Figure 8-4) or supine (Figure 8-5), bringing head, hands, and trunk to midline and thereby establishing the basis for postural control against gravity in sitting, standing, and ambulation. When this does not occur and there is insufficient tone (Figure 8-6) or increased tone (Figure 8-7), then normal development does not occur. As normal trunk and hip strength increase, the child can be placed in the sitting position (at approximately 6 months old). The infant without insult should sit with an erect spine, gradually gaining strength and stability for postural control and balance (Figure 8-8). The normal infant will spend a lot of waking hours practicing the development of postural control and balance while increasing

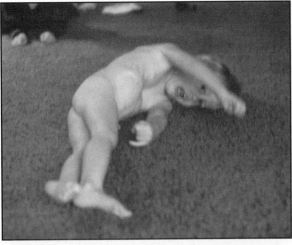

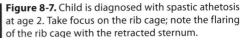

Figure 8-7. Child is diagnosed with spastic athetosis at age 2. Take focus on the rib cage; note the flaring of the rib cage with the retracted sternum.

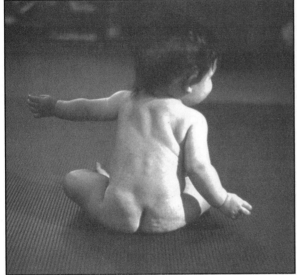

Figure 8-8. Child with normal development by age 7 to 8 months has adequate postural coactivation to allow for balance while her body is in motion. Function requires control of posture, equilibrium, protective responses, rotational forces, and perturbations against gravity while in motion.

in strength, endurance, range, and confidence over the various motor programs. This progressive development allows the child to control and practice more difficult programs and challenges presented within the environment. A child with CP will also spend that time trying to control the motor system to gain greater independence in function. Unfortunately, the programs available are often stereotypic and limit the child's control over the environment.

Between 7 and 8 months of age, the able-bodied child develops sufficient strength in the lower trunk musculature and pelvic girdle to allow coming to all fours (Figure 8-9); eventually, he or she will develop the ability to weight shift and crawl. Ultimately, the goal for all children is the ability to ambulate with a good to normal gait pattern, use both hands for playing and learning, and have the postural stability of the trunk, neck, and back of the tongue to communicate verbally. Because of the need for the motor system to control walking, balance, and posture simultaneously, early ambulation requires the child to often use one UE to assist (Figures 8-10A and B). Once those programs become more automatic and the variance within all of them under more control by the CNS, the child will shift to 2 points of support, leaving the UEs free to explore during ambulation. Children with normal functioning motor systems achieve these motor milestones, and these milestones are the basis for establishing developmental norms or developmental tests. These normally

Figure 8-9. Child is 7 to 8 months old. The child has the motor skill to come to all fours and remain in that position. Note that the hands are fists, which is normal when children first get up into this posture. In time, the hands will open and weight bear through the palmar surface with fingers and wrist extended.

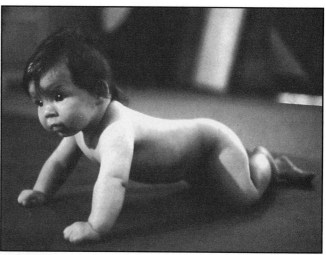

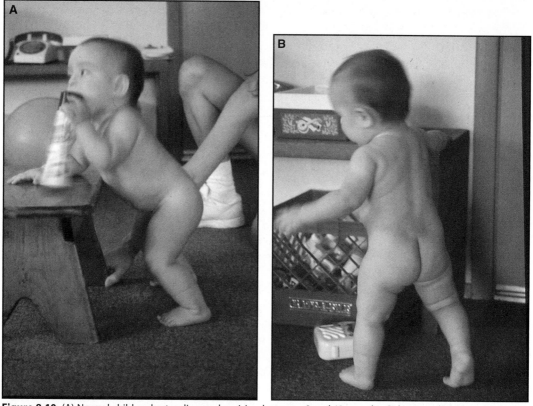

Figure 8-10. (A) Normal child early standing and cruising between 9 and 12 months. Side view: Child standing using a hip synergy center of gravity forward requiring upper body support. (B) Posterior view: Same child with weight distributed bet-ween lower limbs, but balance strategies still require upper body support: early cruising.

developing children have had adequate normal sensory input that gives the CNS the opportunity to organize and integrate the information. This in turn gives these children the ability to produce normal, appropriate responses, such as correcting their balance and/or catching themselves with protective responses. Unfortunately, in children with CP, many of these functional abilities are not possible. The severity and area of trauma to the CNS will be an important factor in the child's motor and cognitive abilities. It has been found, however, that by initiating treatment early, before abnormal patterns of posture and movement become well established and the skeletal system has been adversely affected, children can gain functional control. Treatment can be effective through handling and positioning, eliminating gravity, increasing or decreasing sensory perception, and changing postural tone while teaching new patterns of postural control and movement. The following are some basic concepts that can help promote improved postural control and movement.

- Positioning: to promote symmetry and midline control throughout the body while preventing neck hyperextension, elevated shoulders with adducted scapulae, trunk hyperextension, anterior pelvic tilt, and LE adduction with internal rotation.

- Therapeutic handling: to improve tactile, vestibular, proprioceptive, visual, and auditory processing[3,4,10-12]; assist in normalizing postural tone; develop righting and protective responses; and integrate sensory processing. When using handling techniques, it is extremely important to use appropriate therapist hand placement to stimulate and facilitate the intended sensory motor responses. These handling techniques allow the child to practice normal programming and correction of error while the therapist prevents the child from running stereotypic or abnormal patterns. The vestibular system may very likely be the most dominant sensory stimuli and, when used effectively, can either dampen the effects of hypertonus or heighten tone in the depressed postural system.

- Inhibition and facilitation: to promote more normal postural tone and encourage better ROM. Generally, the movement will first be inhibitory, followed by facilitation into normal patterns of function and movement.

- Water therapy: to alter muscle tone abnormalities, decrease the gravitational demands on postural muscles, and decrease resistance of movement of the extremities (eg, bathtub or pool).

- Oral motor therapy: to alter the muscle tone (hyper or hypo) of the oral motor structures to promote use of the cheek, lips, and tongue for feeding skills and pre-speech and speech function.

- Home exercise program: to augment clinic-based therapy and empower the family, caregivers, and/or patient. Home programs are used to encourage repetitive practice of normal movement patterns to further guarantee motor learning and encourage neuroplasticity. As discussed in Chapter 3, the child needs this repetitive practice to gain permanent motor control. Because the PT or PTA cannot spend the needed time with the child to guarantee function, active participation by caregivers needs to be integrated into the plan of care.

No matter what a child's functional level, it is critical to teach movement that can lead to function. Thus, it becomes important to know and understand normal movement patterns and how they develop. The PT and PTA are responsible for helping the child to produce normal movement to gain or regain functional control over the demands of life. Life is about movement. There is great joy in being able to move and, ultimately, to move effortlessly, effectively, and efficiently. During treatment, it is important that the PT and PTA strive to reach functional goals. To attain a functional goal, facilitation techniques may be used to promote more normal movement and function for ADL. Refer to Bly's book[13] for examples of how to assist a child in rolling, crawling, and coming to sit or stand and for a discussion of the importance of the therapist's handling skills, as it is beyond the scope of this chapter to discuss all these movement patterns. Also refer to the videos that accompany this book to visually recognize how a therapist might facilitate normal movement, whether that movement is elicited in an infant, child, or adult. As the child matures, adjunct therapies, such as horseback riding (hippotherapy), swimming, skiing, and dancing are wonderful activities that will help transfer therapy into function along with creating a normal, healthy environment that is fun and encourages social activities.

Treatment Strategies That May Be Delegated to a Physical Therapy Assistant

As stated earlier, children with CNS motor dysfunction have postural tone that is either too high or too low, creating functional limitations in the child's ability to control his or her environment. To maximize therapeutic techniques, it is important to first dampen or heighten the postural tone to bring it closer to normal, ultimately leading to coactivation around joints of the body important to the specific movement. These techniques should maximize the effects of the interventions on functional motor control over appropriate environmental activities. The following are the recommended treatment techniques or positions used by the PT or PTA.

Decreasing Postural Tone

- Side-lying, sitting, or standing postures. Encourage some internal postural tone or control without a demand that causes the CNS to compensate with abnormal tone.

- Slow, gentle rocking with rotation while in side-lying, sitting, kneeling, or standing and with specific emphasis on rotation within the trunk axis. Rapid spinning in short bursts and changing directions can decrease spasticity with the understanding that one must be aware of the response needed for the individual child.

- Rhythmic bouncing on the therapist's knee or using a ball.

- Slow movement in anterior-posterior, horizontal, vertical, and inverted postures. The child may be suspended in the PTA's arms while swinging or using a hammock, swing, or scooter board.

- Firm, consistent touch, avoiding intermittent touch. Firm or maintained touch causes the CNS to adapt, whereas intermittent/light touch provokes a withdrawal or a protective reaction.

- Deep pressure through joint structures (especially the axial trunk). This pressure has a calming effect on the CNS and develops postural tone or coactivation. This can be performed manually, using a Neoprene vest, or using a weighted blanket. It is very important when using deep pressure through joint structures that the joints themselves are in proper alignment. If the PTA is unsure of that alignment, the PT should be consulted.

- Inhibition of abnormal patterns of posture using antagonist pattern with rotation. If the child holds the arm in internal rotation, shoulder and elbow flexion with forearm pronation, wrist flexion, and finger flexion, then the pattern that would inhibit that static posture would be shoulder abduction with external rotation, elbow extension, and forearm supination with wrist and finger extension. The rotation (external versus internal, supination versus pronation) is a pivotal component of the child's CNS motor function and release of the abnormal posture. The therapist should never try to elicit a release through a quick motion or by use of extreme force because the quick motion elicits a stretch reaction and facilitates the abnormal pattern. In addition, a quick or powerful force elicited by the therapist has the potential of injuring and tearing the child's striated muscle fibers. The PTA always needs to remember that just static positioning of a child outside of abnormal patterns will not teach the child's CNS how to move in and out of that pattern. Thus, facilitating active motion should always be a focus of intervention.

- Facilitation of normal patterns of movement in all spatial postures once postural tone is closer to normal. These movement patterns must be easy for the child to assist if the therapeutic goal is to have the child's CNS gain control over the movement. It is essential to develop sufficient trunk strength for postural control during both quiet coactivation sitting and standing and dynamic movement in all planes. Initially, the child should be placed in and out of positions that ask the trunk to maintain postural control off vertical. The intervention might begin within a small (approximately 5 to 10 degrees off vertical in all directions) ROM that the child's CNS can function with control, and then increase the range as the responses become more automatic. If the child begins to lose control, the intervention should be changed. The cause for the loss of control may be fatigue, lack of endurance, or boredom. Regardless of the cause, if the response continues to elicit an inappropriate movement pattern, the specific activity needs to be changed. Once the child can control postural function in vertical, moving to more horizontal postural patterns can be introduced, such as on elbows or a 4-point (hands and knees) position.

- Using rotation to decrease tone within the trunk muscles. Placing a child in side-lying and working on rotation within the body axis will often decrease the strong extensor tone within the trunk itself. It is recommended that the PTA use one LE to begin the movement pattern by flexing and externally rotating the hip with knee flexion. Once the child's motor system begins to respond with a body-on-body rotation on head rotation pattern, the abnormal extensor tone will become more normal and the PTA should feel an effortless response by the child.

Increasing Extensor Tone and Strengthening Muscles for Postural Control

- Rapid movement using anterior-posterior, horizontal, or angular movement while in prone. The PTA can hold the child in his or her arms, over a ball, in a hammock swing, or on a scooter board using a slight incline to facilitate automatic postural extension of the head, trunk, and extremities. Again, it is important to remember that any movement performed quickly and creating a change in direction must be monitored and appropriate to the child's motor skills. As mentioned above, the therapist must make sure the child has adequate control in the neck muscles to respond to the weight of the head and avoid a whiplash injury.

- Facilitation of a biomechanically aligned, upright posture. Accomplished by increasing proprioception input through joint compression down through the trunk with small perturbations. Emphasis must be placed on accurate alignment of the trunk. If the alignment is abnormal, the child will learn that pattern, which has the potential of creating lordosis, kyphosis, or scoliosis in the future. These spinal curvatures are often seen in children with CP and create secondary problems in the coronary and pulmonary systems.

- Rapid and irregular bouncing and movement. While holding the child in your arms, on your lap, on a ball, or in a hammock swing, the PTA can quickly bounce the child and elicit postural or extensor responses while the child feels safe and secure, thus facilitating normal movement responses without creating fear.

- Weight shifting of the child. Initially weight-shift the child on a noncompliant surface, such as a hardwood or linoleum floor, while sitting or standing.

- Weight shift in sitting or standing on a compliant surface (eg, dense foam or tilt board). This intervention enhances visual and vestibular balance reactions along with postural control. These surfaces take away the normal proprioceptive input from the legs and trunk and force the child's CNS to interrupt the visual and vestibular sensory information to respond appropriately to the perturbation. In that way, the therapist is demanding the CNS to respond with normal movement given less sensory information or with some conflict between sensory input from visual/vestibular and proprioception.

- Spinning. This rapid acceleration increases vestibular stimulation and improves postural control. It can be performed by using a hammock or net swing, regular swing, or Sit 'N Spin

(Playskool). **Caution**: Overstimulating a child's system may cause autonomic responses, such as vomiting and headaches. Thus, the intervention needs to be highly monitored and the rate/speed of the spinning gauged to the child's responses.

- Intervention must be balanced with sufficient flexor tone. After increasing postural extensor tone (short extensor muscles of the trunk and axial joints) and muscle strength in a treatment session, flexor tone must be balance to provide stability around the joints and promote movement that is smooth, fluid, and controlled.

Increasing Trunk Flexor Tone and Muscle Strength for Postural Control and Mobility

- In supine: Bring child's hands to midline or bring child's hands to knees and/or feet into flexion. Initially, the child may need assistance, especially when taking shoulder protraction to neutral and the humerus into external rotation. This flexor pattern encourages development of flexor tone within a spatial position that biases the extensor muscles because of gravity's pull on the vestibular mechanism within the ears and the tactile input to the extensor surface of the skin. The child can be rocked back and forth while in this position, which will decrease hypertonicity of the extensor muscles while encouraging flexor bias.

- Breast- or bottle-feeding: With the child having proper alignment, work toward midline head control with hands to midline.

- Rolling: Facilitate from supine to side-lying to prone, with an emphasis on trunk rotation and head control. As the neck begins to flex and rotate, the arm on the nonweight-bearing side may retract influenced by the asymmetrical tonic neck reflex. If the therapist assists the arm into protraction as the neck rotates, often the child will demonstrate some functional reach and/or protective extension.

- Crawling: Reciprocal hands and knees or hands and feet, making sure the trunk flexors are active. The child may be placed on a scooter board to take away a proportion of demands on the postural system while encouraging reciprocal movement of limb patterns.

- Bouncing the child on the PTA's knee or on a ball with the child's trunk slightly off vertical in a posterior direction. This encourages head righting toward vertical while facilitating neck flexion. Taking the child's trunk slightly off vertical in an anterior direction or toward the therapist will encourage neck extension. Working back and forth over vertical increases ROM of the neck and helps to establish fluid coactivation of neck flexors and extensors. This head control is critical as the child moves in and out of more complex functional patterns during development of motor control. Without that normal head control, the child will compensate with abnormal tonal patterns to try to establish stability.[9]

- Swinging: Maintain flexion and extension for postural control with movement (coactivation) using a hammock or regular swing. Once the child has the ability to functionally control the trunk through postural coactivation of both flexors and extensors, play activities become fun, and the child will often laugh and smile. It will also decrease the frustration often seen in children who lack that postural coactivation.

- Spinning: Use postures in greater flexion while maintaining extension for postural control (coactivation) (eg, swing, Sit 'N Spin, rotating chair, in PTA's arms). Again, it must be stressed that the child should respond positively with motor reactions. If the child is scared, then reduce the speed and observe the reactions; as the child tolerates the movement, again increase the speed using the child's reactions to determine the rate of the movement.

INHIBITION AND FACILITATION TECHNIQUES

Inhibition and facilitation techniques are specific movements or positioning of the child, performed by the therapist, to decrease or increase the child's sensory motor system's responses to gravity, position in space, and movement. These treatment approaches may be used with the techniques described above. When there is an increase in muscle tone, in either a synergy pattern pulling in multiple muscles or a specific muscle response, treatment techniques that decrease tone will be required. Before presenting a discussion of intervention techniques for a child with the medical diagnosis of either quadriplegia or diplegia, a description of typical postures of the trunk, UEs, and LEs are described. During therapy, these children will present with many of the following postures, but each child presents variations based on the insult and the influences of his or her environment.

Typical Patterns Seen in Cerebral Palsy Children With Diplegia or Quadriplegia

Upper Thorax and Upper Extremities

The upper thoracic spine is often extended, causing the scapulae to adduct. The shoulder girdle is elevated and protracted, the humerus adducted and internally rotated, the elbow flexed, the forearm pronated, the wrist flexed with ulnar deviation, and the fingers flexed.

Lower Thorax and Lower Extremities

The lower thoracic and lumbar spine is often extended with the pelvis rotated forward; hips are extended, adducted, and internally rotated; knees are extended; and feet are plantarflexed.

Techniques to Correct These Typical Postures

- Place child in side-lying and gently rock forward and backward, adding passive rotation around the axis of the trunk. Be sure to do this activity to the right and the left side.

- When in the supine position, tone permitting, bring the LEs into flexion and the UEs into extension and hold until there is further decrease in tone. Then, begin to add small weight shifts, working toward postural control and balance in midline.

- Gradually bring the child into the supine position with the neck and trunk in flexion and the LEs flexed and abducted, and bring the arms into adduction to abduct the scapulae.

- The LEs are in hip flexion and may be brought out into some abduction and external rotation.

- Once the child is able to more easily attain these positions and hold them with less assistance, then it may be possible to gradually facilitate movement toward sitting, over into prone, or into postures requiring the head to come up with support on the forearms (on-elbows). It is always important to make sure the therapist is not preventing the child from using normal movement. The child may be able to control part of the range while needing help with other parts. During the time the child can control, that control should be allowed. When an abnormal tonal response begins to develop, then the therapist should inhibit that response and help facilitate the child's CNS ability to dampen the abnormal and use or run the normal motor pattern.

Presenting the many inhibition and facilitation techniques are far beyond the scope of this chapter. For a more thorough discussion of specific techniques, refer to Bly.[12]

The PTA and PT must always remember that many specific techniques will be taught while in a clinical setting or at continued education courses. Colleagues will find solutions to problems. The therapist needs to be open to listening and watching other therapists who are using techniques that are working. Observation can be a wonderful way to gain additional skills. The answer to every patient problem can be found within the patient. The PTA will inadvertently find solutions to problems, as will the PT. The key is communication with each other. The patient wants only to be empowered to regain the quality of life taken away by some pathology or accident. The role of the PT and PTA is to help the patient along that path of learning and not become the obstacle to the patient. With the help of the PT/PTA, the child will have a much better opportunity to develop normal movement responses to the demands of the environment and more independent motor control to participate in life.

Therapeutic Use of Toys

Play and the interaction of toys serve many purposes during therapy. Play is an important and integral part of physical therapy and needs to be an important aspect of a PTA's repertoire of clinical skills. Play promotes development of motor, cognitive, and social skills through fun and function, and may help distract the child during a therapy session to accomplish the necessary therapy. Toys are a key element to the success or failure of play during a treatment session.

Consider the following when selecting toys to be used during therapy or when suggesting toys to facilitate therapy at home:

- The child's capabilities
- The child's needs
- The cost of the toy
- Using toys/equipment that can be inexpensively replicated
- Evaluating what skills the toy can develop or expand

Children with gross motor delays may benefit from toys or activities requiring sitting balance to build postural tone. Examples of toys that encourage the use of these specific motor programs are exercise balls, Bilibo, Sit 'N Spin, or ride-on push toys. For fine motor delays, choose toys that encourage movement and are repetitive, such as shape sorters, peg boards, simple puzzles, and blocks. Chose mediums within which a toy can be hidden that encourage exploration and nonspecific results, such as corn meal, beans, and modeling compound. Playing with cars, trucks, or any rolling toy while prone, 4-point, sitting, or in another spatial position can encourage the development of trunk stability as well as UE mobility and gross grasp patterns. Using a toy, such as an airplane that is flying in space puts even greater demand on the limb holding the toy, requiring more stability of the trunk and axial joint.

Children like to explore new textures and objects. Containers with everyday household items, such as wooden spoons, measuring cups, plastic scrubbers, and measuring spoons, can motivate the child to play and imitate caregivers' normal activities. Activities that encourage manipulation help to build strength and endurance. Throwing and catching balls of different sizes, throwing balls into baskets, bowling a ball toward a target, using a bat and t-ball, playing musical instruments, and encouraging various arts and crafts are all play activities that can have meaning to the child. As long as the child is enjoying the activity and is successful at the task, these various toys can augment any therapeutic environment.

For children to work on fine motor skills and problem solving, consider puzzles, blocks of different weights and sizes, nesting blocks, and textured blocks that can help with tactile sensitivities and are fun. When children get a little older and toys are not necessarily the answer, telling stories and making up games with counting or rhyming are often sufficient to keep the child engaged and working with you.

Children with reduced or limited lung capacity along with low-tone facial muscles can be encouraged to blow using as deep a breath as possible. Initially, the PTA should have the child blowing items that require minimum effort, such as cotton balls, ping pong balls, and whistles. Later, the PTA can encourage blowing against greater resistance, such as playing musical instruments. How the therapist presents any of these items and interacts with the child in play will determine to some extent the child's willingness to make play his or her occupation.

Technology Today and in the Future

Today, the use of various types of technology has become common practice within the clinical setting of a PT. Computer gaming systems, such as the Nintendo Wii (Figures 8-11A through C) provide the PT and the PTA a tool to motivate children and adults to engage in specific interactive activities that can enhance balance, strength, endurance, and functional body movement as well as challenge their memory and problem-solving skills in a fun and functional way. These types of interactive activities are becoming more easily available and cost effective and can be used within the home environment as part of a home program.[14]

Similarly, the use of robotic technolog,y either as an exoskeleton or as a body weight–support system, is found in many physical therapy clinics. A variety of systems is available that assist the patient to move UEs or LEs. Because of the cost, robotic exoskeletons have not yet been adapted for use with children and are seldom being used outside of the clinical and research environment. The available body weight–support systems provide 2 variations in how to decrease body weight. A few systems decrease the weight of the body by inflating a large lower trunk and body suit that the client is fitted into. Once the air inflates and the suit begins to fill, the therapist can determine just how much of the body weight needs to be reduced. These systems can be placed above a treadmill so the therapist can elicit walking once the treadmill is turned on. The second type of body weight–support system uses a harness. The legs fit though the harness and then the harness is fitted to a suspension arm that lifts the body vertically to decrease the individual's body weight. The therapist can adjust the harness system to align the trunk vertically. Again, many of these systems are suspended over a treadmill. Once the treadmill is turned on and the patient's body weight is reduced, the PT/PTA team can trigger a forward-stepping reaction in both legs. If those reactions cannot be elicited, then one or both LEs can be moved by therapy team members to try to facilitate learning or relearning of normal walking. As is true of all motor learning, repetition of practice is needed for learning of the motor program and for providing an opportunity for the CNS to gain motor control. Many times the program is present but the power needed to walk is insufficient, so using body weight–supported treadmill training (BWSTT) allows the patient to build up strength while practicing walking.[14]

Many of the body weight–support systems have not yet been adapted for use with children. One system that has been designed and used effectively with children is the LiteGait (Mobility Research).[15] This system can be used in initial learning or retraining for adults as well as children. BWSTT has been shown to cause activation on the somatosensory cortices of children with CP and thus increase the potential for normal interaction between sensory and motor function.[16] Similar to all BWSTTs, the LiteGait provides the PT and PTA the possibility of promoting improved weight bearing and gait patterns by controlling postural alignment through an adjustable harness that supports the trunk and the amount of body weight the child's motor system needs to control the movement. Obviously, with the ability to unload the LEs, the opportunity to facilitate improved patterns of movement is possible. The PT or the PTA is able to manually assist limb placement and improve the motor programs while working to increase strength and endurance. As the patient improves, the PT needs to determine when the patient should attempt greater weight bearing into the LEs while maintaining proper alignment and control. A patient may be placed initially on a treadmill for consistence of surface and repetition of practice. Once the child can run the programs of gait, the plan of care should move to practicing walking on uneven or compliant surfaces. The LiteGait (Figures 8-12A and B), similar to other BWSTT systems, can be adapted to over-ground walking depending on the needs of the child. When placing a pediatric patient on a treadmill, it is often necessary to reduce the treadmill speed to 0.5 miles per hour or less. Many of these patients do not have the ability to reciprocally move at greater speeds. Unfortunately, this

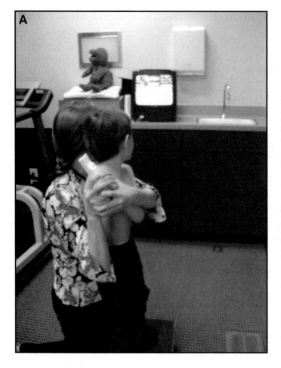

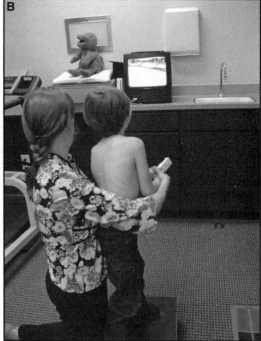

Figure 8-11. Use of the Nintendo Wii as a therapeutic tool. (A) Initiating swing using controller as if he was swinging at target on Wii. (B) Midswing at target on Wii. (C) Ending swing.

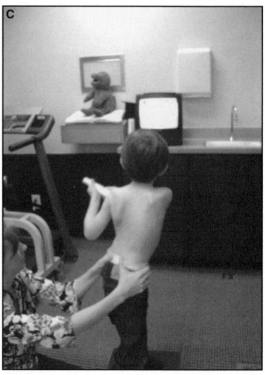

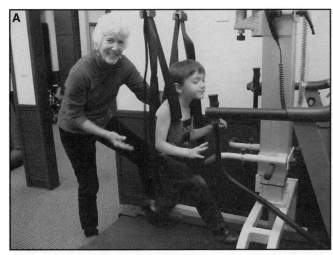

Figure 8-12A. Use of a body weight–support system. Ambulation on the LiteGait.

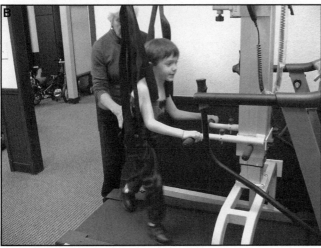

Figure 8-12B. Running on the LiteGait.

piece of equipment may be too costly for small, independent pediatric therapy clinics to afford. Very few families have the funds available to purchase a piece of equipment that provides this type of practice in a home program setting, but this may change as the demand for these types of products increases and production becomes more automated.

Therapeutic Horseback Riding (Hippotherapy)

Individuals have enjoyed riding horses as far back as humans were aware of horses. Horses have provided a means of expedited travel as well as assisting in the labor of transportation and farming. It has been only within the past few decades that horses have provided a new role. They have become a therapeutic tool used by PTs and occupational therapists when working with individuals with movement disorders. The major focus of the research in this area has been on hippotherapy with children.[17–22] Not all horses can assist in this type of service, just as not all therapists can work effectively with children, especially children with CNS damage. Horses used in hippotherapy must have a calm personality and a keen awareness of the children placed on their backs. Horses are able to provide smooth and rhythmic movement while walking and thus allow the child to respond with postural reactions and upright control of the head and trunk and to respond to mild perturbations as the horse is walking (Figure 8-13). For the safety of the child, walkers are often

Figure 8-13. One child (on the left) reacting to normal perturbations of the horse when back riding, while another child (on right) receives therapy during forward movement.

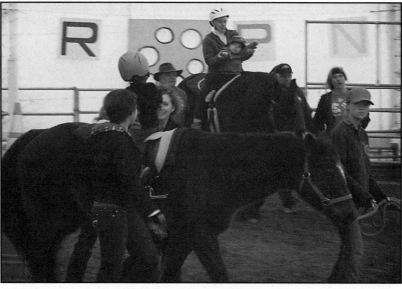

Figure 8-14A. Child forward riding with automatic postural adjustments while completing an activity of touching the assistant's hand.

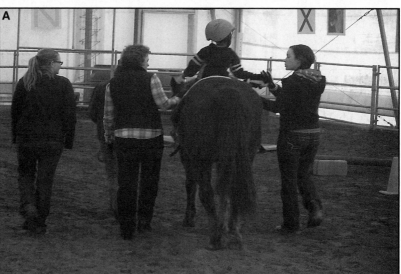

used on either side of the horse to assist in the child maintaining the COG over the BOS of the hips. Depending on the postural reactions that the child needs to practice, the child can be placed on the horse prone, supine, in forward upright sitting, backward upright sitting, hands and knees, knee standing, and, when appropriate, standing (Figures 8-14A through D). Many children begin hippotherapy without the necessary head and trunk control to maintain postural alignment and thus require a rider to sit behind them on the horse to help provide the needed postural stability and/or perform intervention (Figure 8-15). Once a child can ride without assistance, games can be used to take attention off the riding and onto a cognitive/motor task (Figure 8-16). Different types of perturbations can be introduced by having the horse step over obstacles or walk up and down a ramp.

The key to the therapeutic effectiveness of this type of intervention is, most importantly, safety while providing enjoyment and repetition of practice of specific movements so the child can automatically respond to the natural perturbation from the horse. There is evidence that this type of intervention does not benefit the cardiovascular system but is an exercise that allows the child to participate in an activity even if a problem of cardiovascular endurance is present.[23] Thus,

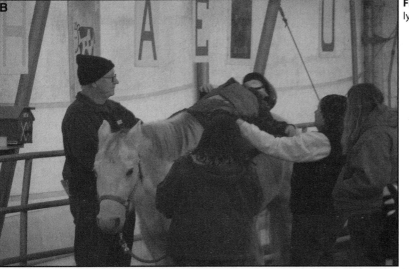

Figure 8-14B. Child riding lying supine.

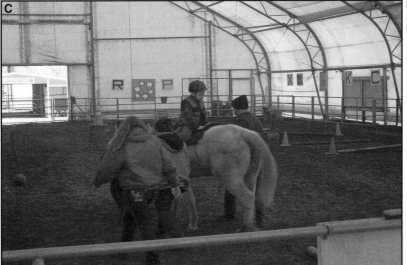

Figure 8-14C. Child back riding on the horse while the horse moves forward.

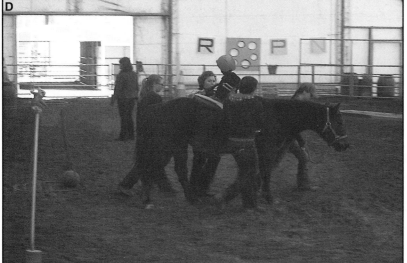

Figure 8-14D. Child side riding while the horse moves forward.

Figure 8-15. Child receiving physical therapy during the riding session.

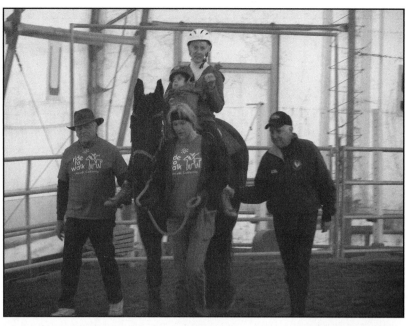

Figure 8-16. Child attending to throwing the bean bag into the target while automatically responding to the horse's shifting weight while standing.

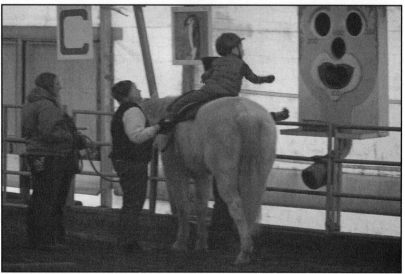

reactions of the child are involved in motor responses and allow for practice of postural reactions while the child enjoys a functional and recreational activity that other children enjoy in society. Three systematic reviews[17,18,22] of approaches and therapies that target lower limb function in children with CP identified evidence showing that hippotherapy as an intervention can be very beneficial to children with CP. Snider et al[20] showed evidence that hippotherapy was effective in treating postural symmetry and reactions within the trunk and hips and improving gross motor function. Zadnikar and Kastrin[22] reviewed 77 studies, placing strict criteria for inclusion in the review, and again found that therapeutic horseback riding clearly demonstrated improvement in postural control and balance in children with CP. Whalen and Case-Smith[21] also found that hippotherapy had a positive effect on gross motor function in children with CP. A variation on hippotherapy was the use of an electric horse to trigger normal postural control and balance in sitting.

Statistically significant results were identified within a population of children with the diagnosis of spastic diplegia.[19]

Hippotherapy is not limited to the treatment of children and has been found to be very effective in treating adults with a variety of medical diagnoses resulting in CNS damage.[24-27] More recently, hippotherapy is being used to treat veterans with head trauma, amputations, and post-traumatic stress disorders. This type of therapeutic intervention can be directly correlated to the International Classification of Functioning, Disability and Health model and its focus on normal activities and active participation in life. There are certainly major costs to this type of intervention, such as the boarding and medical costs of maintaining these animals. The horses that provide the best interventions are often older and calmer and thus will face normal aging as do all animals, including humans. But, to most therapists, the benefit provided to children with CP far outweighs any cost that it might take to maintain the health and longevity of these animals. For additional information regarding hippotherapy, go to www.ridetowalk.org.

CONCLUSION

Today, most of the children who were traumatized in utero or at birth or who had an insult early in their life will reach adulthood and progress into aging. Doing a Medline search or searching the Web, information regarding chronic problems within this population of individuals can be found under the heading "adults with development disabilities." Many of these individuals have or will develop new movement problems or associated organ system dysfunction as they age due to the stress and abnormality of movement and its force on the bones, muscles, nerves, peripheral vascular system, and internal organs. How the PT will approach these new challenges and what will be delegated to the PTA is not known today but will certainly be part of the future when discussing the roles of the PT and PTA in the health care delivery system.

A Physical Therapist Assistant's Perspective

I love kids and decided that working in pediatric physical therapy would be great. I asked to have my final rotation of clinical affiliations in a pediatric setting. The moment I walked into the clinic, I realized I was ill prepared for working in pediatrics. Everything my clinical instructor told me felt like new and overwhelming information. By the end of my 6-week clinical, I knew that this was where I was meant to be. I had never been so physically and mentally challenged and yet had such a sense of satisfaction and purpose. I am so grateful for a generous instructor who patiently taught me how to have a critical eye, listen to my hands, and use my hands to give the correct information and guide children in gaining motor control and confidence.

I think back to when I first started and how overwhelmed I felt. There is so much to learn, and what I have come to comprehend is that this journey will be a lifelong process of learning. Each child is unique. What works with the child one day might not work as well the next time you see the child. I have learned to be flexible, with lots of ideas for activities to accomplish the desired result. I have learned that if the child is not responding appropriately, it is because I am not giving the right input; it is not the child's fault. I have learned to be patient because the functional gains of the child can take more time than I like. I have gained confidence in my skills as a therapist but I also know my limitations. I do not hesitate to go to my PT for advice and assistance. This is what makes me an effective therapist.

Children can be very challenging clients. You are not just working with the child but with the whole family—and you need to earn the trust of both. Understanding each child and his or her situation makes you a better therapist. Children know when you are fully engaged or just going through the motions. You need to make therapy fun and functional so the child is fully engaged in therapy and gets the most from each session. From my experience as a clinical instructor and watching many students come through the clinic, I realize pediatrics is not for everyone. I suggest requesting a clinical rotation in a pediatric setting to give yourself a chance to see if this is the right specialty for you.

CASE STUDIES

CASE #1

TC was born 2 months premature. During labor, his mother experienced a drop in blood pressure. At birth, he was diagnosed with kidney dysfunction, and at 9 months of age, he underwent surgery to correct the problem. At 16 months of age, he was diagnosed with CP, only after his mother repeatedly asked the pediatrician about her concerns. He was first diagnosed with diplegia; however, the PT determined that this child's motor deficits included his trunk, both legs, and one arm (triplegia). At 18 months of age, he began physical therapy. At the time of evaluation, he lacked adequate head control, had no trunk control, and could not bear weight on his LEs. When placed in the standing position, his LEs pushed into the support surface, which stimulated the positive support reflex, thereby producing extension, adduction, and internal rotation of the LEs with the feet plantarflexed and inverted. The left UE was held in flexion, and the neck was hyper-extended. Following 6 months of treatment, once weekly and a home exercise program performed daily, he was able to be placed in sitting and maintain this position independently while perturbing his COG during play. He began rolling over in both directions, creeping on all fours, pulling up onto his knees, and attempting to pull to stand. When he began therapy, there were minimal vocalizations. Following 6 months of intervention, he had multiple vocalizations and a vocabulary of 30 words because of improved posture and motor control that directly affected respiration, phonation, and articulation.

Physical therapy interventions included the following:

- Altering postural tone
- Increasing trunk extensor tone for postural control
- Increasing trunk flexor tone for stability and mobility
- Repeating newly acquired motor skills is necessary to develop function or motor learning

If the child requires immediate intervention and facilitation, the PT may choose not to delegate treatment to the PTA. Once the child begins to demonstrate some internal motor learning and control, the PTA could work on all of the above within that skill, working to the outer limits to allow the child the opportunity to practice, self-correct, and develop normal patterns of movement

QUESTIONS

1. What positions or postures could the PTA consider using with TC? Consider that his trunk tone is low, whereas his 3 extremities demonstrate high muscle tone.

2. Once postural tone is closer to normal and facilitated movement can be freer and easier, why would the PT ask the PTA to incorporate an activity where gravity is resisted?

3. Trunk extension must be balanced by trunk flexion. List 3 ways that you would develop trunk flexion strength.

4. Determine one functional posture in which you would place TC and explain what activity you would use to encourage repetition in order to get motor learning and eventually motor control.

5. When is it appropriate for the PTA to change or advance the child into new movement patterns?

Update on TC

TC is now 10 years old. He was receiving physical therapy twice weekly and then did not receive services for 9 months. When he returned, he had lost many of the skills he had previously achieved. Since that time, he has received therapy twice weekly focused on reducing his hypertonicity, maintaining and improving his ROM, and building strength to increase good functional alignment. His main modes of mobility are crawling and a motorized wheelchair that has been pursued and supported by his family. However, he has the ability to achieve ambulation with the use of a walker. He has progressed to being able to walk with moderate assistance for balance. TC has increased gross motor control of his left UE, allowing him to use it for assistance or support. There has been little to no follow-through of the therapist's suggested home programs, which has hampered his progress and motor learning. TC attends a regular classroom with an instruction aide but does not participate in extracurricular activities, limiting his social growth, self-confidence, and self-esteem. It is important to note that gains through therapy can still be made that will help him both medically and educationally.

Question

1. What has been the major reason for TC's slow or lack of progression?

CASE #2

JS and his twin sister were born 1 month prematurely, delivered by emergency cesarean section because his heart rate dropped during his mother's nonstress test. At birth, he weighed 3 pounds, 5 ounces, and he sustained an anoxic/ischemic event. He remained in the neonatal unit for 1 month, going home 1 week later than his twin, who had no complications. At 12 months of age, he was diagnosed with CP. He received some therapy initially after he was diagnosed. At 2.5 years, his family moved to another state, where he received physical and speech therapy for 2.5 years. At the time of evaluation in their new location, he presented with severe motor involvement as well as sensory dysfunction. All sensory systems were involved, which negatively influenced the motor system and caused a severe increase in muscle tone, irritability, and fear of movement. Increased muscle tone interfered with all movements of the extremities as well as the oral and facial muscles, affecting eating and sound production for speech. He did not have head or trunk control and could not be placed sitting or standing. He had no speech but communicated with crying.

He received intensive therapy consisting of physical therapy 3 times weekly and speech therapy one time weekly in a private clinic. Emphasis was placed on decreasing his extensor tone, increasing or maintaining his ROM, developing postural tone and control, increasing strength, and facilitating normal movement patterns. He had demonstrated potential for motor learning by showing significant improvement after 2.5 years of therapy. He was independent in sitting on the floor and in an appropriately fitting chair. He could pull himself to standing and maintain the upright posture to play. He could communicate verbally but lacked sufficient respiratory support for loud sound production. His left UE was used for playing, manipulating toys and objects, and feeding himself, while the right UE minimally assisted. He attended a regular kindergarten with the assistance of an aide. He rode in a therapeutic horseback-riding program once a week, where he gained further strength and postural control. JS's therapy has continued; his therapy will be ongoing until he is no longer making progress toward his goals both within the therapeutic setting and educationally. As children grow and mature, it is essential that they receive therapy to help them achieve their full potential.

QUESTIONS

1. Following the evaluation and during JS's initial therapy sessions, the PT delegated to the PTA sensory integration activities as part of intervention and functional skills such as swinging, spinning in a hammock, and bouncing on a ball in prone or sitting.

    What motor behaviors would a PTA be looking for during therapy that would indicate the child is improving?

2   How can the PTA work on increasing flexor and extensor postural tone to facilitate head and trunk strength and control? How would the PTA use therapeutic tools such as a ball, bolster, a swing, or one's knee to facilitate this control?

3. How would a PTA progress the child within an identified activity in order for the child to have greater internal control?

4. Between 2 and 6 months of initial treatment, JS's increased tolerance for processing sensory information permitted better organization of the motor system. He was less irritable, less fearful of movement, and he began to develop some head control in vertical. He was able to hold his head upright with neck elongation for 30 to 60 seconds. He began reaching for objects with his right UE that previously was held in flexion at the shoulder, elbow, and wrist. At this point in his therapy, the PTA was responsible through play for developing strength in the cervical and shoulder girdle musculature to promote good head control. This was done by placing the child in a mechanically aligned sitting posture both on hard and compliant surfaces. With support of his trunk, the PTA weight shifted him slowly, causing his COG to shift outside of his BOS (anterior and posterior and lateral). She then applied compression down through the shoulders, and then move to the hips. Then she used the hips as the pivotal point to cause perturbations. She was instructed to only perturb the BOS to the limit of the child's ability in order to allow him to practice successfully.

    How would the PTA know if the perturbations were too hard? What would the PTA look for in the child's behavior that would suggest the perturbations were creating appropriate learning?

5. During this same time period, the PTA was also responsible for developing head-righting reactions in sitting. She was taught how to support the trunk appropriately using control from the shoulders, mid-trunk, and hips. She learned to weight shift him in all planes. The LEs were inhibited from moving into flexion, adduction, and internal rotation during these activities by controlling the legs at the hips and thighs.

    What motor behavior by the child would the PTA use to know that the intervention was progressing in a positive direction? Why might noise or sudden movements by other individuals cause the child to lose control?

6. During this phase, the PTA was given responsibility for developing strength and stability of the child's UEs. She was instructed to place the child in prone in weight bearing, weight shift him initially on forearms, and then progress to extended arms as strength permitted. Initially, work on noncompliant surfaces on an angle off vertical, and work toward horizontal. As the child's strength and stability improve, the child was moved to compliant surfaces.

    Identify 2 motor behaviors exhibited by the child that would help the PTA know the goals of strength and stability of the UEs were being met.

7. During this phase, the PT increased the respiratory capacity through manual trunk mobilization, and the PTA was responsible for maintaining the mobility through side-lying and gentle rocking. Then, the PTA was instructed to follow with functional activities requiring blowing, sucking, and voicing.

What techniques might the PTA use to increase respiratory capacity?

8. Between 6 and 12 months of physical therapy, JS's head-righting had emerged and head control was developing. The PTA was given responsibility for developing trunk rotation. She was shown how to rotate the shoulder girdle and/or the pelvic girdle around the vertical axis in side-lying, prone, supine, and sitting postures. Use an activity that requires rotating first to one direction and then to the other. The body will follow the head in a righting reaction, which allows the child to move more freely. Creating an environment where the child is playing will motivate greater self-control and motor learning. For example, place a toy on one side of the child so that he has to reach to pick it up, and then rotate to the other side to complete the activity.

What motor behaviors by the child would clue the PTA that the PT needs to reassess and potentially change the program?

9. During this phase, the PTA was given the responsibility for developing transition skills from supine to prone to sitting as well as transition through various sitting postures available to him. Postural tone close to normal with proper alignment is necessary in order for movement to occur as fluidly and normally as possible. The PTA was instructed to guide him with as little or as much assistance as is necessary to help him achieve the movement successfully. As the child improved, the PTA was to slowly reduce the assistance while having the child still succeed at the activity.

Why is the previous sentence a clear indication that motor learning and control is in progress?

10. During this phase, the PTA was given the responsibility for developing strength and stability of the shoulder and pelvic girdle muscles by positioning in prone on forearms or in weight bearing on all fours or on hands and feet. Initially, the child was placed on elbows in prone and weight shifted from side to side. The child's head was stabilized (as if a turtle was poking his head out of a shell). The PTA must make sure the child was not only biomechanically resting on his joint structures instead of using his own muscle power. When a child only uses positioning to remain on-elbows, he will look as if his head was down in a shell and little postural control will be seen within the shoulder girdle. Once the child can hold with perturbations and begin to weight shift on his elbows, the PTA can use a toy to encourage reaching with one arm while supporting on the other. This activity can also be done on extended elbows or on all fours.

What would the PTA look for to make sure the child is gaining strength and greater stability?

Progression of Physical Therapist Assistant Intervention

Once most of these activities were developing and there was increased strength and mobility, the following activities were also delegated to the PTA:
- Increase cervical and upper thoracic muscle strength by placing him:

    a. In prone position, on forearms, while playing and weight shifting.

    b. On extended arms while reaching and playing.

    c. In prone position on a scooter board or platform swing or suspended in the PTA's arms while moving him through space.

- Develop trunk-righting responses by:

  a. Rolling in a horizontal position.

  b. Sitting on a lap, ball, or roll as a quiet sitting activity or during play.

  c. Swinging with trunk support. Use an appropriate swing that provides adequate support or, while the child is sitting on the lap of the therapist during the swinging activity, support the child at the pelvis and allow the child to respond to the imposed movements.

  d. Carry him facing away from the caregiver and with his hips on the caregiver's hip, thus encouraging the child to sit up using postural extension and socially interact with the environment for extended periods of time.

- Develop active trunk rotation around the vertical axis in sitting by having the child:

  a. Swing a bat or racket.

  b. Sit or straddle a roll while reaching and touching his feet or picking up objects off the floor with both hands (to one side and then to the other).

- Teach transitional movements (eg, supine to sit, rolling, all fours, knee standing to half-kneel, coming to standing from the floor or a chair, and facilitating gait by handling at the hips or shoulders):

  a. Supine to sit using diagonal movement patterns, which would be considered a partial rotation pattern from supine to sit.

  b. Moving the child from prone to all fours, handling from the hip. From prone, handling should guide the pelvic girdle back over the knees while encouraging the arms to weight bear.

  c. From side-sit, either have the child come up to or pull to knee standing, weight shift in kneeling. Then rotate the pelvis to encourage one leg to come into a half-kneeling position. Work or play in half-kneeling so the child weight shifts onto one leg and off the other. Then, have the child come to stand off the half-kneeling leg. Guidance can come from either the back at the hips or the front at the shoulder girdles, arms, or trunk.

- Increase standing balance while engaging the UEs in play by:

  a. Cruising on the furniture or wall.

  b. Standing while drawing.

  c. Catching and throwing a ball, Frisbee, etc.

  d. Riding a bike.

QUESTIONS

1. Are any of the previously mentioned interventions activities inappropriate to delegate to the PTA?

2. At what time if ever should the PTA go back to the PT to discuss the interventions?

Update on JS

JS is now almost 14 years old. He has continued to receive physical therapy several times per week. Therapy has continued to focus on decreasing tone, maintaining and improving ROM, and building strength to increase good functional alignment as he progresses in his motor learning. In 2008, a baclofen pump was surgically implanted that delivers a continuous low dose of baclofen, which has significantly decreased his hypertonicity and his ability to build strength and function. Unfortunately, JS has needed

2 subsequent surgeries to repair and then replace the pump. Prior to these surgeries, JS was not receiving the baclofen and thus tone increased, again limiting progress of his LEs. His mobility is limited to a motorized wheelchair that he can drive with either hand. He has consistently good head and trunk control in his chair. As his body has improved and he has developed better motor control, there has been good improvement in social interactions with his peers and others, allowing him to participate fully in scouting activities and hippotherapy. His family has been very involved and supportive of therapy and makes sure he is included in as many normal activities as possible. It is important to note that he has further potential, such as gaining sufficient LE control to be able to perform an independent transfer. It would be important for him to continue to have therapy to help him achieve both his medical and educational goals, particularly as he is still a child who will continue to grow and develop.

REFERENCES

1. Adams JH, Graham DI, Murray LS, Scott G. Diffuse axonal injury due to non-missile head injury in humans: an analysis of 45 cases. *Ann Neurol.* 1982;12(6):557-563.
2. Gaebler-Spira D. Overview of sensorimotor dysfunction in cerebral palsy. *Top Spinal Cord Inj Rehabil.* 2011;17(1):50-53.
3. Umphred DA, Lazaro R, Roller M, Burton G, eds. *Umphred's Neurological Rehabilitation.* 6th ed. St Louis, MO: Mosby; 2013.
4. Leahy BJ, Lam CS. Neuropsychological testing and functional outcome for individuals with traumatic brain injury. *Brain Inj.* 1998;12(12):1025-1035.
5. Van der Naalt J, Hew JM, van Zomeren AH, Sluiter WJ, Minderhoud JM. Computed tomography and magnetic resonance imaging in mild to moderate head injury: early and late imaging related to outcome. *Ann Neurol.* 1999;46(1):70-78.
6. Jennet B, Bond M. Assessment of outcome after severe brain damage: a practical scale. *Lancet.* 1975;1(7905): 480-484.
7. Kahn-D'Angelo L. The special care nursery. In: Campbell SK, ed. *Physical Therapy for Children.* Philadelphia, PA: WB Saunders; 1994.
8. Hoon AH, Stashinko EE, Nagae LM, et al. Sensory and motor deficits in children with cerebral palsy born preterm correlate with diffusion tensor imaging abnormalities in thalamocortical pathways. *Dev Med Child Neurol.* 2009;51(9):697-704.
9. Lee HM, Galloway JC. Early intensive postural and movement training advances head control in very young infants. *Phys Ther.* 2012;92(7):935-947.
10. Levine MS, Kliebhan L. Communication between physician and physical and occupational threats: a neurodevelopmentally base prescription. *Pediatrics.* 1981;68(2):208-214.
11. White-Trent RC, Nelson MN, Silvestri JM, Cunningham N, Patel M. Responses of preterm infants to unimodal and multimodal sensory intervention. *Pediatr Nurs.* 1997;23(2):169-175, 193.
12. Bly L. *Facilitation Techniques Based on NDT Principles.* San Antonio, TX: Therapy Skill Builders; 1997.
13. Bly L. *Motor Skills Acquisition in the First Year.* San Antonio, TX: Therapy Skill Builders; 1994.
14. Byl K, Byl N, Byl M, et al. Integrating technology into clinical practice in neurological rehabilitation. In: Umphred D, Lazaro R, Roller M, Burton G, eds. *Umphred's Neurological Rehabilitation.* 6th ed. St Louis, MO: Mosby; 2013:1113-1172.
15. Mobility Research. LiteGait. http://www.litegait.com/. Accessed December 28, 2012.
16. Kurz MJ, Wilson TW, Corr B, Volkman KG. Neuromagnetic activity of the somatosensory cortices associated with body weight-supported treadmill training in children with cerebral palsy. *J Neurol Phys Ther.* 2012;36(4):166-172.
17. Franki I, Desloovere K, De Cat J, et al. The evidence-base for conceptual approaches and additional therapies targeting lower limb function in children with cerebral palsy: a systematic review using the ICF as a framework. *J Rehabil Med.* 2012;44(5):396-405.
18. Franki I, Desloovere K, De Cat J, et al. The evidence-base for basic physical therapy techniques targeting lower limb function in children with cerebral palsy: a systematic review using the International Classification of Functioning, Disability and Health as a conceptual framework. *J Rehabil Med.* 2012;44(5):385-395.
19. Silva e Borges MB, Werneck MJ, da Silva Mde L, Gandolfi L, Pratesi R. Therapeutic effects of a horse riding simulator in children with cerebral palsy. *Arq Neuropsiquiatr.* 2011;69(5):799-804.

20. Snider L, Korner-Bitensky N, Kammann C, Warner S, Saleh M. Horseback riding as therapy for children with cerebral palsy: is there evidence of its effectiveness? *Phys Occup Ther Pediatr.* 2007;27(2):5-23.
21. Whalen CN, Case-Smith J. Therapeutic effects of horseback riding therapy on gross motor function in children with cerebral palsy: a systematic review. *Phys Occup Ther Pediatr.* 2012;32(3):229-242.
22. Zadnikar M, Kastrin A. Effects of hippotherapy and therapeutic horseback riding on postural control or balance in children with cerebral palsy: a meta-analysis. *Dev Med Child Neurol.* 2011;53(8):684-691.
23. Bongers BC, Takken T. Physiological demands of therapeutic horseback riding in children with moderate to severe motor impairments: an exploratory study. *Pediatr Phys Ther.* 2012;24(3):252-257.
24. Beinotti F, Correia N, Christofoletti G, Borges G. Use of hippotherapy in gait training for hemiparetic post-stroke. *Arq Neuropsiquiatr.* 2010;68(6):908-913.
25. Bronson C, Brewerton K, Ong J, Palanca C, Sullivan SJ. Does hippotherapy improve balance in persons with multiple sclerosis: a systematic review. *Eur J Phys Rehabil Med.* 2010;46(3):347-353.
26. Keren O, Reznik J, Groswasser Z. Combined motor disturbances following severe traumatic brain injury: an integrative long-term treatment approach. *Brain Inj.* 2001;15(7):633-638.
27. Silkwood-Sherer D, Warmbier H. Effects of hippotherapy on postural stability, in persons with multiple sclerosis: a pilot study. *J Neurol Phys Ther.* 2007;31(2):77-84.

SUGGESTED READINGS

Alberta Infant Motor Scale (AIMS)

Liao PM, Campbell SK. Examination of the Item Structure of the Alberta Infant Motor Scale. *Pediatr Phys Ther.* 2004;16(1),31-38.
Pagliarulo MA. *Introduction to Physical Therapy.* 4th ed. St Louis, MO: Mosby; 2012.
Yıldırım ZH, Aydınlı N, Ekici, B, Tatli B, Calişkan M. Can the Alberta Infant Motor Scale and the Milani Comparetti motor development screening test be rapid alternatives to Bayley Scales of Infant Development-II at high risk infants. *Ann Indian Acad Neurol.* 2012;15(3):196-199.

Assessment of Motor and Process Skills (AMPS)

Bonnier B, Eliasson A, Krumlinde-Sundholm L. Effects of constraint-induced movement therapy in adolescents with hemiplegic cerebral palsy: a day camp model. *Scand J Occup Ther.* 2006;13(1):13-22.
Center for Innovative OT Solutions. Assessment of Motor and Process Skills (AMPS). www.ampsintl.com/AMPS/. Accessed December 28, 2012.
Fisher AG, Bray JK. *Assessment of Motor and Process Skills. Vol. 1: Development, standardization, and administration manual.* 7th ed. Fort Collins, CO: Three Star Press; 2010.
Gol D, Jarus T. Effect of social skills training group on everyday activities of children with attention-deficit-hyperactivity disorder. *Dev Med Child Neurol.* 2005;47(8):539-545.
Payne S, Howell C. An evaluation of the clinical use of the assessment of motor and process skills with children. *Br J Occup Ther.* 2010;68(6):277-280.
Russo RN, Crotty M, Miller MD, Murchland S, Flett P, Haan E. Upper-limb botulinum toxin A injection and occupational therapy in children with hemiplegic cerebral palsy identified from a population register: a single-blind, randomized, controlled trial. *Pediatrics.* 2007;119(5):e1149-e1158.

Bayley Scale of Infant and Toddler Development (BSID-III)

Pearson. Assessment & Information. Bayley Scales of Infant and Toddler Development. 3rd ed. (Bayley-III). http://www.pearsonassessments.com/HAIWEB/Cultures/en-us/Productdetail.htm?Pid=015-8027-23X. Accessed December 5, 2012.

Brazelton—Neonatal Behavioral Assessment Scale (NBAS)

Boston Children's Hospital. The Brazelton Institute. Understanding the Baby's Language. www.brazelton-institute.com/intro.html. Accessed December 28, 2012.
Brazelton TB, Nugent JK. *Neonatal Behavioral Assessment Scale.* 3rd ed. London, England: Mac Keith Press; 1995.

Dubowitz—Neurological Assessment of Preterm and Full-Term Babies

Dubowitz L, Dubowitz V, Mercuri E. *The Neurological Assessment of the Preterm and Full-Term Newborn Infant.* 2nd ed. London, England: Mac Keith Press; 1999.

Dubowitz L, Ricciw D, Mercuri E. The Dubowitz neurological examination of the full-term newborn. *Ment Retard Dev Disabil Res Rev.* 2005;11(1):52-60.

Lissauer T. Physical examination of the newborn. In: Martin RJ, Fanaroff AA, Walsh MC, eds. *Neonatal-Perinatal Medicine: Diseases of the Fetus and Infant.* Vol 1. 9th ed. St Louis, MO: Elsevier Mosby; 2011:485.

Gross Motor Function Classification System (GMFCS)

Palisano RJ, Cameron D, Rosenbaum PL, Walter SD, Russell D. Stability of the gross motor function classification system. *Dev Med Child Neurol.* 2006;48(6):424-428.

Palisano RJ, Rosenbaum P, Bartlett D, Livingston MH. Content validity of the expanded and revised gross motor function classification system. *Dev Med Child Neurol.* 2009;50(10):744-750.

Piana AR, Viñals CL, Del Valle MC, et al. Neuromotor assessment of patients with spastic cerebral palsy treated with orthopedic surgery at the National Rehabilitation Institute [in Spanish]. *Acta Ortop Mex.* 2010;24(5): 331-337.

Gross Motor Function Measure (GMFM-66)

Russell D, Avery L, Walter SD, et al. Development and validation of item sets to improve efficiency of administration of the 66-item Gross Motor Function Measure in children with cerebral palsy. *Dev Med Child Neurol.* 2010;52(2):e48-e54.

Russell DJ, Rosenbaum PL, Avery L, Lane M. *Gross Motor Function Measure (GMFM-66 & GMFM-88) User's Manual.* London, England: Mac Keith Press; 2002.

Russell D, Rosenbaum PL, Cadman DT, Gowland C, Hardy S, Jarvis S. The gross motor function measure: a means to evaluate the effects of physical therapy. *Dev Med Child Neurol.* 1989;31(3):341-352.

Milani Comparetti Motor Development Screening Test (MCMDST)

Stuberg WA, White PJ, Miedaner JA, Dehne PR. *The Milani-Comparetti Motor Development Screening Test: Test Manual.* 3rd ed. Omaha, NE: University of Nebraska Medical Center, Meyer Children's Rehabilitation Institute; 1992.

Yildirim ZH, Aydinli N, Ekici B, Tatli B, Çaliskan M. Can the Alberta Infant Motor Scale and the Milani Comparetti motor development screening test be rapid alternatives to Bayley Scales of Infant Development-II at high risk infants. *Ann Indian Acad Neurol.* 2012;15(3):196-199.

Motor Assessment Scale (MAS)

Sabari JS, Lim AL, Velozo CA, Lehman L, Kieran O, Lai JS. Assessing arm and hand function after stroke: a validity test of the hierarchical scoring system used in the motor assessment scale for stroke. *Arch Phys Med Rehabil.* 2005;86(8):1609-1615.

Movement Assessment of Infants (MIA)

Chandler LC. Neuromotor assessment. In: Gibbs ED, Teti DM, eds. *Interdisciplinary Assessment of Infants: A Guide for Early Intervention Professional.* Baltimore, MD: Brookes; 1990.

Chandler L, Andrews M, Swanson M. *The Movement Assessment of Infants: A Manual.* Rolling Bay, WA: Infant Movement Research; 1980.

Pediatric Evaluation of Disability Inventory (PEDI)

de Brito BM, Gordon AM, Mancini MC. Functional impact of constraint therapy and bimanual training in children with cerebral palsy: a randomized controlled trial. *Am J Occup Ther.* 2012;66(6):672-681.

Haley SM, Coster WJ, Ludlow LH, et al. *Pediatric Evaluation of Disability Inventory (PEDI): Development, Standardization and Administration Manual.* Boston, MA: New England Medical Center Hospitals and PEDI Research Group; 1992.

Kao YC, Kramer JM, Liljenquist K, Tian F, Coster WJ. Comparing the functional performance of children and youths with autism, developmental disabilities, and no disability using the revised pediatric evaluation of disability inventory item banks. *Am J Occup Ther.* 2012;66(5):607-616.

Pearson. Clinical Assessment. Pediatric Evaluation of Disability Inventory (PEDI). www.pearsonassessments.com/HAIWEB/Cultures/en-us/Productdetail.htm?Pid=076-1617-647&Mode=summary. Accessed August 2, 2013.

Pediatric Functional Independence Measure (WeeFIM)

Davis MF. Measuring impairment and functional limitations in children with cerebral palsy. *Disabil Rehabil.* 2011;33(25-26):2416-2424.

Granger CR. *Guide for the Use of the Functional Independence Measure (Wee FIM) of the Uniform Data Set for Medical Rehabilitation.* Buffalo, NY: Research Foundation, State University of New York; 2000.

New South Wales Government. Lifetime Care & Support Authority. FIM and WeeFIM. www.lifetimecare.nsw.gov.au/fim_weefim.aspx. Accessed December 28, 2012.

Park EY, Kim WH, Choi YI. Factor analysis of the WeeFIM in children with spastic cerebral palsy [published online ahead of print December 3, 2012]. *Disabil Rehabil.*

Uniform Data System for Medical Rehabilitation. The WeeFIM II Advantage. www.udsmr.org/Documents/WeeFIM/WeeFIM_II_System.pdf. Accessed December 28, 2012.

Prechtl—Neurological Examination of the Full-Term Newborn Infant

Prechtl H. *The Neurological Examination of the Full-Term Newborn Infant.* 2nd ed. Philadelphia, PA: JB Lippincott; 1977.

Additional Suggested Readings

Goble DJ, Goble DJ, Hurvitz EA, Brown SH. Deficits in the ability to use proprioceptive feedback in children with hemiplegic cerebral palsy. *Int J Rehabil Res.* 2009;32(3):267-269.

Shamsoddini A. Comparison between the effect of neurodevelopmental treatment and sensory integration therapy on gross motor function in children with cerebral palsy. *Iran J Child Neurol.* 2010;4(1):31-38.

Yoshida S, Hayakawa K, Yamamoto A, et al. Quantitative diffusion tensor tractography of the motor and sensory tract in children with cerebral palsy. *Dev Med Child Neurol.* 2010;52(10):935-940.

Please see accompanying Web site at
www.healio.com/books/neuroptavideos

9

Clients With Genetic and Developmental Problems

Esmerita Roceles Rotor, PT, MAEd, PTRP
Darcy A. Umphred, PT, PhD, FAPTA
Eunice Shen, PT, PhD, DPT, PCS
Barbara H. Connolly, PT, DPT, EdD, C/NDT, FAPTA

KEY WORDS

- Chromosomal disorders
- Genetics
- Mitochondrial disorders
- Movement dysfunction
- Multifactorial disorders
- Neurodevelopmental condition
- Single-gene disorders

CHAPTER OBJECTIVES

- Describe genetic conditions with neurodevelopmental concerns that are commonly referred to physical therapy.
- Identify and discuss children with developmental problems that may or may not be related to genetics.
- Describe clinical features that affect motor development and movement.
- Identify tests and measures that are used in examination.
- Identify physical therapy strategies to address motor and movement issues.
- Discuss essential features when working with children with genetic conditions and/or developmental problems, including early intervention and working in collaboration with other professionals and programs that work with these children through childhood.

Umphred DA, Lazaro RT, eds.
Neurorehabilitation for the Physical Therapist Assistant,
Second Edition (pp 211-249).
© 2014 SLACK Incorporated.

INTRODUCTION

The World Confederation for Physical Therapy[1] states that part of the scope of physical therapy practice includes providing services to individuals and groups of individuals to develop, maintain, and restore maximum movement and functional ability throughout the lifespan. This includes infants and children with neurodevelopmental conditions brought about by genetic aberrations as well as other children who have developmental problems without specific genetic links. This chapter will present both areas of pediatric neurological conditions. No matter the cause, children with developmental delays have conditions that lead to long-term motor delays. These limit the child's ability to perform normal activities of daily living (ADL) and his or her ability to participate in many areas of life. Specific genetic links to developmental problems will be presented first, followed by a more general discussion of medical diagnoses leading to development delays.

GENETIC CONDITIONS LEADING TO NEUROLOGICAL AND MOTOR DEVELOPMENT CONCERNS

Although numerous genetic conditions have been reported, this chapter is limited to genetic conditions that are diagnosed immediately after birth and those that have neurological features that affect development. The discussion in this chapter will involve infants, children, and adolescents with genetic conditions.

The Human Genome Project, which started in 1990 and completed in 2003, aimed to identify all of the approximately 20,000 to 25,000 genes in human DNA.[2] This breakthrough has influenced health and medical practices. Currently, the importance of the role of genetics is being used in diagnosing, monitoring, and treating disease.[2]

Physical therapists (PTs) and other health care professionals may take on challenges brought about by strides made in genetics. Physical therapy professionals may find themselves in a position to suspect that a client may have a genetic condition,[3] and the professional should therefore have the knowledge and skills to recommend that appropriate clients seek further help.

There are 4 classifications of genetic disorders: single-gene disorders, mitochondrial disorders, chromosomal disorders, and multifactorial disorders.[4,5] Within these types, several conditions are diagnosed at birth or early childhood and will affect the neurological development of the child.

Chromosome disorders may be due to numerical abnormalities or structural abnormalities.[4] Conditions such as Down syndrome (DS) (trisomy 21), Edwards' syndrome (trisomy 18), and Patau syndrome (trisomy 13) are due to numerical abnormalities; there may be a missing or an extra chromosome. In the case of DS or trisomy 21, there is an extra chromosome on the 21st pair of chromosomes.

Structural abnormalities of the chromosome also lead to chromosome disorders. Cri du chat syndrome and Prader-Willi syndrome are examples of this. In cri du chat syndrome, there is a deletion of the short arm of chromosome 5, whereas in Prader-Willi syndrome, there is a structural defect on chromosome 15. Single-gene disorders or Mendelian disorders are caused by an error in a single unit of genetic information.[5] These disorders can be classified as autosomal dominant, autosomal recessive, and X-linked disorders. In an autosomal-dominant condition, one parent will have a defective gene than can be passed on to the child. Examples include achondroplasia and osteogenesis imperfecta. In autosomal recessive disorders, both parents are carriers of the defective gene. Parents are usually asymptomatic and may not know that they possess the defective gene until the child exhibits signs and symptoms. Examples of these are cystic fibrosis, sickle cell anemia, and Tay Sachs disease. In X-linked disorders, defective genes are on the X sex chromosome.

Females are carriers of these genes and pass it on to their male offspring. Examples of these are Duchenne muscular dystrophy (DMD) and hemophilia.

Multifactorial genetic conditions are brought about by a complex interaction of genetics with environmental factors,[4] resulting in birth defects, such as cleft lip, cleft palate, and spina bifida.

Lastly, mitochondrial disorders are due to defects in the genes within the cytoplasm of the mitochondria. These are usually rare conditions associated with aging. Mitochondrial disorders can be inherited only from the mother.

A list of disorders according to type, characteristics, clinical features, and examples can be found in Table 9-1.

The genetic conditions that result in neurological problems that affect development will be discussed in detail as these are the most common medical diagnoses a PT and physical therapist assistant (PTA) will encounter.

Down Syndrome (Trisomy 21)

DS, or trisomy 21, occurs in 1 in 800 live births, according to the Centers for Disease Control and Prevention.[6] This condition is the most frequent genetic cause of intellectual disability. DS is brought about by a chromosomal genetic condition in which there is an extra chromosome in the 21st pair of chromosomes. Persons with DS are easily identified by their stereotypical appearance. Their heads are of a smaller size, with a flattened neck area, excess skin at the nape, flattened nose, small and lower placed ears, and slanting eyes. A simian crease at the palm of each hand is also typical, although that is also found in children and adults without genetic abnormalities. The Committee on Genetics in 2001 provided data and information on the health supervision for children with DS. The Committee reports that children with DS exhibit mental impairment in varying degrees, from mild (intelligence quotient [IQ] 50 to 70) to moderate (IQ 35 to 50) and occasionally severe deficits (IQ 20 to 35).[7] Various medical conditions are associated with this condition, including congenital heart defects (50%), leukemia (< 1%), hearing loss (75%), otitis media (50% to 70%), Hirschsprung's disease (< 1%), gastrointestinal atresias (12%), eye diseases (60%), and thyroid disease (15%). It was found that children with DS had smaller cerebellar brain volume that could be responsible for motor coordination problems.[8]

Among the different developmental genetic conditions, PTs and PTAs get to work most frequently with children with DS. Physical therapy concerns for this population include hypotonia, joint laxity, muscle weakness, poor coordination, and sensory perceptual problems. For infants and toddlers, PTs and PTAs work toward attaining gross and fine motor skills, such as rolling, sitting, crawling, standing, and walking. As these basic skills are achieved, physical therapy could help young children master foundational movements and develop advanced motor abilities, such as running, throwing, catching, pedaling, and jumping, among others. As children with DS grow older, obesity may also be an issue. It is important that these children engage in activities that promote mobility, such as organized sports.

A study conducted by Shumway-Cook and Woollacott[9] on children with DS indicates that this group is functioning 18 to 24 months behind age level with a significant gradual decrease of performance in both static and dynamic balance tests. Functional balance issues normally seen in this group of children may be explained by problems in the postural control system.[9] This study found that DS children are able to respond to external perturbations in a manner similar to typically developing children except that they have a delayed activation of these responses. As a result of slow responses, these children have problems reestablishing and maintaining stability. Further, the children showed poor development of their ability to organize their responses to changing environmental contexts.

	Table 9-1

Overview of Genetic Disorders Affecting the Pediatric Age Group

Type of Disorder	Characteristic of Disorder	Name of Disorder	Clinical Features
Chromosome abnormalities	Deviation in number of chromosomes, 47, XY, +21*	Down syndrome (trisomy 21)	Characteristic facial features, including flat occiput, flat face; upward slanting eyes; hypotonicity; broad, short feet and hands; protruding abdomen; mental retardation; possible cardiac anomalies.
		Edwards' syndrome (trisomy 18)	Small stature; long, narrow skull; low-set ears; hypotonicity; rocker bottom feet; scoliosis; profound mental retardation.
		Patau syndrome (trisomy 13)	Microcephaly; cleft lip and palate; polydactyly of hands and feet; severe to profound mental retardation.
	Deviation in sex chromosomes	Turner syndrome (XO syndrome)	Congenitally webbed neck; growth retardation; ptosis of upper eyelids; lack of sexual development; congenital heart and kidney disease; scoliosis; low-normal intelligence.
		Klinefelter syndrome (XXY)	Long limbs; tall and slender build until adulthood when obesity becomes a problem (if no testosterone replacement therapy); small penis and testes; low-average to mild mental retardation; tremors; behavior problems.
	Partial deletion syndrome	Cri du chat syndrome (5p-)	High-pitched, catlike cry in infancy; microcephaly; low-set ears; hypotonicity; severe mental retardation; scoliosis; clubfeet; dislocated hips.
		Prader-Willi syndrome (15q–)	Low tone with feeding disorder in infancy; insatiable appetite develops in toddlerhood; moderate mental retardation; hyperflexibility; obesity; characteristic facial features, including almond-shaped eyes; and small stature, hands, feet, and penis.
		Williams syndrome (deletion near the elastin gene on chromosome 7)	Characteristic facial abnormalities, including prominent lips, medial eyebrow flare, and open mouth; mild microcephaly; mild growth retardation; short nails; mild to moderate mental retardation; cardiovascular anomalies.

(continued)

Table 9-1 (continued)
Overview of Genetic Disorders Affecting the Pediatric Age Group

Type of Disorder	Characteristic of Disorder	Name of Disorder	Clinical Features
Specific gene defects	Autosomal dominant	Neurofibromatosis	Areas of hyperpigmentation or hypopigmentation of skin inducing café au lait spots or axillary freckling; tumors along nerves, in connective tissue, eyes, or meninges; macrocephaly; short stature. May have skeletal abnormalities, including scoliosis, bowing of long bones, and dislocations.
		Tuberous sclerosis	Brain lesions causing seizures and mental retardation; skin lesions on cheeks around nose; café au lait spots; cyst-like areas in bones of fingers; kidney and teeth abnormalities.
		Osteogenesis imperfecta	Type I: Small stature; thin bones, bowing of the bones; fractures of long bones; hyperextensible joints; kyphoscoliosis; flat feet; thin skin; deafness in adult life; blue sclerae of eyes; blue or yellow teeth.
			Type II: Prenatal growth deficiency; short limbs; multiple fractures; hypotonia; hydrocephalus; frequent early death.
			Type III: Short stature; bowing and angulation of long bones; multiple fractures; kyphoscoliosis.
			Type IV: Osteoporosis leading to fractures; variable mild deformity of long bones; normal sclerae of eyes; may have poor teeth.
	Autosomal recessive	Spinal muscular atrophy	Progressive muscle atrophy and weakness; normal intelligence; normal sensation: weakness may begin before birth, in early childhood, or in later childhood.

(continued)

Table 9-1 (continued)			
Overview of Genetic Disorders Affecting the Pediatric Age Group			
Type of Disorder	**Characteristic of Disorder**	**Name of Disorder**	**Clinical Features**
		Sickle cell disease	A group of diseases characterized by blood disorders related to hemoglobin defects. Mostly seen in people of African or, infrequently, of Mediterranean descent. Sickle-shaped red blood cells cause anemia and crises of blockages in veins, causing a variety of conditions. These include leg ulcers, arthritis, acute pain, and problems in major organ systems, including the spleen, liver, kidney, bones, heart, and central nervous system. Children may exhibit weakness, pain, or fever and may have growth retardation.
		Hurler syndrome	Normal or rapid growth during the first year with deterioration during the second year; coarse facial features characterized by full lips, flared nostrils, thick eyebrows, low nasal bridge, and prominent forehead; still joints; small stature; small teeth, enlarged tongue; kyphosis, short neck; clawhand, hip dislocation, and other joint deformities; mental retardation.
		Phenylketonuria	Children cannot metabolize phenylalanine, causing mental retardation, growth retardation, hypertonicity, seizures, and pigment deficiency of hair or skin if left untreated. Can be successfully treated by limiting amount of phenylalanine in diet.
Sex-linked disorders (all affected are boys, X-linked)		Fragile X syndrome	One of the most common causes of mental retardation in boys. Characteristic facial features include elongated face, large ears and prominent jaw. Other characteristics include enlarged testicles in adulthood and prolapse of the mitral valve in the heart. Mental retardation is usually in the severe range, sometimes with aggressive behaviors. Some boys will have poor coordination and hypotonia.

(continued)

Table 9-1 (continued)
Overview of Genetic Disorders Affecting the Pediatric Age Group

Type of Disorder	Characteristic of Disorder	Name of Disorder	Clinical Features
	Abnormal gene on X chromosome	Duchenne muscular dystrophy	Onset at 1 to 5 years. Progressive, rapid weakness at onset stage; characteristic gait disturbances, including toe walking, abducted gait, lordosis, and waddling gait. Progressive weakness leads to w/c use, decreased independence in all areas, and finally death by respiratory or cardiac failure. Loss of ability to walk by age 9 or 10. Death by late teens.
		Lowe syndrome	Progressive mental deterioration leading to moderate to severe mental retardation; renal dysfunction; cortical cataracts with or without glaucoma leading to blindness later in life; hypotonicity; joint hyperextensibility; growth retardation; large, low-set ears; pale skin; blonde hair.
		Lesh-Nyhan syndrome	Moderate to severe mental retardation; hypertonicity leading to dislocated hips; clubfoot; growth retardation; movement disorders, including chorea, ballistic movements, and tremor. Self-mutilating behaviors including lip-biting and fingertip-biting characterize this disease.

*The normal number of chromosomes is 46; 47 indicates an extra chromosome present. XY refers to genetic male, +21 refers to the extra chromosome found on the #21 chromosome.
(This article was published in *Clinical Pediatric Physical Therapy*, Ratliffe KT, 219-274, Copyright Elsevier 1998.)

Prader-Willi Syndrome

Prader-Willi syndrome is brought about by a structural deformity of chromosome 15. It is relatively common, occurring in 1 of 15,000 to 1 of 30,000 births.[10] Like children with DS, these children also exhibit recognizable dysmorphic features such as a narrow bifrontal diameter, almond-shaped palpebral fissures, narrow nasal bridge, and thin upper lip. Hypopigmentation is notable with their fair hair, eyes, and skin color. Other clinical features include hypotonia and abnormal neurological functions, hypogonadism, developmental and cognitive delays, hyperphagia and obesity, short stature, and behavioral and psychiatric disturbances. Physical therapy is important in managing hypotonicity, motor delays, functional performance, and obesity.

Cri du Chat Syndrome

Cri du chat syndrome is a genetic disease that results from a deletion of the short arm of chromosome 5.[11] This rare disease occurs in 1 of 50,000 live-born infants.[11] Its distinct clinical feature is the infant's characteristic high-pitched cat-like cry from which the syndrome's name is taken. This is probably due to anomalies of the larynx, which is small, narrow, and diamond shaped. Infants have a distinct facial dysmorphism, microcephaly, and severe psychomotor and mental retardation (MR).[11] They initially present with hypotonia at birth, but this muscle tone is replaced by hypertonia as the child develops. A study on using the Denver Developmental Screening Test II established that half of the patients walk by themselves at 3 years old and all learn to walk by adulthood.[11] Twenty-five percent of children with cri du chat syndrome are able to use short sentences at 4.5 years old, 50% at 5.5 years, and all at 10 years. They are also able to achieve some skills for ADL such as feeding at 3.5 years and dressing at 5 years. Despite severe cognitive and psychomotor delays, these children are able to learn and achieve many skills in childhood.

For children with cri du chat, magnetic resonance imaging reveals atrophy of the brainstem, which includes the pons, cerebellum, median cerebellar peduncles, and cerebellar white matter.[11] This helps to explain the various motor dysfunctions that these children present.

PTs may be called on to help improve suction and swallowing in infants diagnosed with cri du chat. Early rehabilitation can help them develop motor skills and prevent some psychomotor delays. Because the children may have sensory-neural deafness and speech delays, PTs may find that it is critical to collaborate with speech pathologists.

Individuals with cri du chat syndrome have a good prognosis for survival once they overcome medical difficulties in the first years of life. The survival expectation is high.[11] Rehabilitative programs for children with cri du chat syndrome have led to improving psychomotor challenges that contribute to independent activities and social adaptation.

Rett Syndrome

Rett syndrome is a monogenic X-linked dominant disorder due to mutations in the methyl CpG binding protein 2 or MECP2 gene. This gene is responsible for making the protein MeCP2. The MeCP2 protein is found all over the body but is most numerous in the brain.[12] It seems that this protein plays an important role in the function of nerve cells and maintenance of synapses. In Rett syndrome, mutations of the MECP2 gene alter the structure or reduce the amount of the protein MeCP2.[13]

Rett syndrome occurs in 1 out of 10,000 births and is seen in females. The MECP2 gene is found in the X chromosome. Unlike females with 2 X chromosomes that allow them to survive on 1 normal X chromosome, the male child whose X chromosome is affected often does not survive in utero and results in miscarriage or stillbirth. If the males survive to birth, they usually have a very early death.[14]

A key characteristic of Rett syndrome is the neurological regression observed in patients that severely affects motor, cognitive, and communication skills.[12] Parents will often recount that their daughter was born "normal" and was developing normally before they noticed her losing certain skills or abilities. Around the first year of life, a slowing down of development will be observed, followed by regression in psychomotor abilities such as movement and speech.[15]

Children with Rett syndrome exhibit severe intellectual disability, seizures, dystonia, incoordination, orthopedic deformities, muscle wasting with contractures, dyspraxia, agitation, and sleep disturbances. They may experience abnormal breathing patterns and display with cold and blue extremities.[12] A classic clinical feature of Rett syndrome is loss of hand function and the appearance of stereotypical hand movements further limiting function.[12] Girls demonstrate continuous repetitive midline movements with hand wringing, hand washing, and clapping.

Physical therapy for Rett syndrome is aimed at maintaining physical fitness and function and decreasing secondary complications of immobility.[15] Secondary complications may include kyphoscoliosis and foot deformities such as equinus, equinovalgus, or equinovarus.

Edwards' Syndrome

Trisomy 18, or Edwards' syndrome, is less common than DS but is the second most common autosomal trisomy. This chromosomal abnormality occurs in 1 in 3000 births.[16,17] Females are affected more than males at a 3:1 ratio.[18] Although several abnormalities can manifest in this syndrome, 50% exhibit growth deficiency, psychomotor retardation, and hypertonicity.[17,18] Their physical features include having a prominent occiput, low-set rotated malformed ears, small palpebral fissures, micrognathism, and a short sternum. Congenital heart defect is also common.[17] Seventy-five percent of infants with Edwards' syndrome do not survive beyond 6 months.

Muscular Dystrophy

There are a variety of types of muscular dystrophies (MD), but all dystrophy medical diagnoses relate to muscle diseases that over time will weaken the musculoskeletal system. This weakness is caused by the death of muscle cells from defects in the proteins within the muscles themselves. The most common form is DMD, but other varieties include limb-girdle, Becker, facioscapulohumeral, myotonic, congenital, and distal dystrophy.[19] There are a few others types, but they are extremely rare. Males show a higher prevalence of these diseases, although females can also be diagnosed with MD. Although the predominant problem is seen in the peripheral musculoskeletal system, in time all muscle groups can be affected. Thus, the heart and respiratory systems experience critical system failures that ultimately lead to death. With MD, other organ systems, such as the vision, brain, gastrointestinal, and endocrine systems, can also be affected. Because these conditions are inherited and follow different courses, the diagnosis of MD is performed through muscle biopsies, electrocardiogram, electromyography, and DNA analysis. A common thread to these diseases is that the dystrophin gene within the muscles breaks down the muscle tissue itself, which leads to functional motor problems and in time diminishes the individual's ability to participate in normal childhood, adolescent, and adult activities.

As stated previously, the most common type of MD is DMD, and it is the type most frequently seen by PTs. A few decades ago, the diagnosis of DMD meant the child would not survive to adulthood. Today, many individuals with DMD survive into adulthood and middle age thanks to the use of corticosteroids and the prevention of other problems like pneumonia. The introduction of robotic assistive devices has already shown to help maintain the functional mobility in these children and allow them to continue to participate in life.[20,21] DMD will be the primary dystrophy discussed within the tests and measures as well as the intervention section.

DEVELOPMENTAL PROBLEMS WITHOUT SPECIFIC IDENTIFIED GENETIC CONDITIONS

Normal development is a lifelong process that is a result of the complex interplay of biological, psychological, cultural, and environmental factors (refer to Chapter 2). One approach to child development tracks this development within particular domains, such as gross motor, fine motor, social, emotional, language, and cognition skills or behaviors. Within each of these categories are sequences that reflect positive developmental changes and increase the child's ability to become independent in functional activities. These domains within normal development intertwine throughout life. A deficit in one area may cause secondary complications or impairments

Table 9-2
Developmental Milestones in the First 2 Years of Life

Milestone	Average Age of Attainment, mo	Developmental Implications
Gross Motor		
Head steady in sitting	2	Allows more visual interaction
Pull to sit, no head lag	3	Muscle tone
Hands together in midline	3	Self-discovery
Asymmetric tonic neck reflex gone	4	Child can inspect hands in midline
Sits without support	6	Increasing exploration
Rolls back to stomach	6.5	Truncal flexion, risk of falls
Walks alone	12	Exploration, control of proximity to parents
Runs	16	Supervision more difficult
Fine Motor		
Grasps rattle	3.5	Object use
Reaches for objects	4	Visuomotor coordination
Palmar grasp gone	4	Voluntary release
Transfers object hand to hand	5.5	Comparison of objects
Thumb-finger grasp	8	Able to explore small objects
Turns pages of book	12	Increasing autonomy during book time
Scribbles	13	Visuomotor coordination
Builds tower of 2 cubes	15	Uses objects in combination
Builds tower of 6 cubes	22	Requires visual, gross, and fine motor coordination
Communication and Language		
Smiles in response to face, voice	1.5	Child more active in social participation
Monosyllabic babble	6	Experimentation with sounds, tactile sense
Inhibits to "no"	7	Response to tone (nonverbal)
Follows one-step command	7	Nonverbal communication with gesture
Follows one-step command without gesture (eg, "Give it to me")	10	Verbal receptive language
Speaks first real word	12	Beginning of labeling
Speaks 4 to 6 words	15	Acquisition of object and personal names
Speaks 10 to 15 words	18	Acquisition of object and personal names

(continued)

Table 9-2 (continued)		
Developmental Milestones in the First 2 Years of Life		
Milestone	**Average Age of Attainment, mo**	**Developmental Implications**
Speaks 2-word sentences (eg, "Mommy shoe")	19	Beginning grammaticization, corresponds with 50+ word vocabulary
Cognitive		
Stares momentarily at spot where object disappeared (eg, ball dropped)	2	Lack of object permanence (out of sight, out of mind)
Stares at own hand	4	Self-discovery, cause and effect
Bangs 2 cubes	8	Active comparison of objects
Uncovers toy (after seeing it hidden)	8	Object permanence
Egocentric pretend play	12	Beginning symbolic thought (eg, pretends to drink from cup)
Uses stick to reach toy	17	Able to link actions and solve problems
Pretend play with doll (eg, gives doll bottle)	17	Symbolic thought

(This article was published in *Nelson Textbook of Pediatrics,* 17th ed; Behrman RE, Kliegman RM, Jenson HB, eds; Growth and development; Needlman RD; 44-50; Copyright Elsevier 2004.)

within another. Developmental delay is a common problem seen in pediatric physical therapy practice.[22] Refer to Table 9-2 for specific developmental milestones within the first 2 years of life.

Many children with abnormal genetic conditions show developmental problems within the first 2 years of life. Similarly, many children have developmental delays without identified genetic correlates. Children born prematurely are at risk of these developmental problems and are usually monitored by developmental specialists, physicians, and PTs or occupational therapists (OTs). Some of these children will be diagnosed with cerebral palsy; this specific topic is discussed in detail in Chapter 8 and will not be discussed further in this chapter. For other children without early markers such as MD to identify potential problems, parents are usually the ones to identify that something is wrong with the normal growth of their child and ask their pediatricians about these issues. It may be that some of these children have genetic problems and will be diagnosed through genetic tests, whereas others may in time fall into the category of "junk genetics" and have not yet been identified as a genetic problem. Some children may have had some sort of undiagnosed neurological insult in utero that has affected development. But there are many other children who do not reach acceptable developmental milestones who will later be diagnosed with learning disabilities (LD), MR, developmental coordination deficits (DCD), or autism, to mention just a few. Thus, developmental delays are considered delays in milestones that are typically expected of children within a specific age range. Refer to Table 9-3 for examples of typical delays seen within the first year. Table 9-4 lists signs of possible delays between the ages of 2 and 5.

Development of a child is so much more than physical size; it refers to the cognitive, social, fine motor, gross motor, and language skills of that individual and how those components interact with activities that are functional as well as societal. The PT or PTA may be asked to provide

Table 9-3
Signs of Possible Delay: First Year of Life

Age of Child	Problems Encountered
During week 2, 3, or 4	Sucks poorly and feeds slowly
	Does not blink when shown a bright light
	Does not focus on and follow a nearby object moving side to side
	Rarely moves arms and legs seem stiff
	Seems excessively loose in limbs or floppy
	Lower jaw trembles constantly, even when not crying or excited
	Does not respond to loud sounds
By the end of month 3	Still has no motor reflex after 4 months
	Does not seem to respond to loud sounds
	Does not notice her or his hands by 2 months
	Does not follow moving objects with her or his eyes by 2 to 3 months
	Does not grasp and hold objects by 3 months
	Does not reach for and grasp toys by 3 to 4 months
	Begins babbling but does not try to imitate any sounds by 4 months
	Does not babble by 3 to 4 months
	Does not bring objects to her or his mouth by 4 months
	Does not push down with her or his legs when feet are placed on a firm surface by 4 months
	Has trouble moving one eye or both eyes in all directions
	Crosses her or his eyes most of the time
	Does not pay attention to new faces, or seems very frightened by new faces or surroundings
	Still has the tonic neck reflex at 4 to 5 months
By the end of month 7	Seems very stiff with tight muscles
	Seems very floppy like a rag doll
	Head still flops back like a rag doll
	Reaches with one hand only
	Refuses to cuddle
	Shows no affection for the person who cares for her or him
	Does not seem to enjoy being around people
	One eye or both eyes consistently turn in or out
	Persistent tearing, eye drainage, or sensitivity to light
	Does not respond to sound around her or him

(continued)

	Table 9-3 (continued) **Signs of Possible Delay: First Year of Life**

Age of Child	Problems Encountered
	Has difficulty getting object to her or his mouth
	Does not turn head to locate sounds by 4 months
	Does not roll over in either direction (front to back or vice versa) by 5 months
	Seems inconsolable at night after 5 months
	Does not smile spontaneously by 5 months
	Cannot sit with help by 6 months
	Does not laugh or make squealing sounds by 6 months
	Does not actively reach for objects by 6 to 7 months
	Does not follow objects with both eyes at near ranges (1 to 6 feet) by 7 months
	Does not bear some weight on legs by 7 months
	Does not try to attract attention through actions by 7 months
	Does not babble by 8 months
	Shows no interest in games of peek-a-boo by 8 months
By the end of 12 months	Does not crawl
	Drags one side of body while crawling (for over 1 month)
	Cannot stand when supported
	Does not search for objects that are hidden while she or he watches
	Says no single word ("mama" or "dada")
	Does not learn to use gestures, such as waving or shaking head
	Does not point to objects or pictures

(Adapted from American Academy of Pediatrics, Shelov SP, Hanneman RE, Wray W, Gray A. *Caring for Your Baby and Young Child: Birth to Age Five.* New York, NY: Bantam Books; 1998.)

intervention for children with these delays, and it is important for the PT to differentiate whether these delays cross all categories of development or are identified only within specific categories. Children who have consistent delays in all categories usually have generalized retardation, whereas children who have inconsistent delays in developmental categories often fall into a larger group of children with LD that include motor coordination problems, general academic learning problems, and autism. All of these categories of developmental delays can be the reason why this child and his or her family are referred to physical therapy. Children with general LD are usually treated within the school system by PTs, OTs, and speech pathologists to try to facilitate academic learning.

There are also children with DCD. These children are usually diagnosed with DCD after the physician has eliminated various LD problems, autism, MR, and genetic abnormalities. DCD is primarily a problem of apraxia; the child demonstrates spatial organizational problems that cause the coordination difficulties. The problem affects gross and fine motor development and leads to academic challenges in school because of the demand to write a name, a sentence, or a math problem,

Table 9-4
Signs of Possible Delay: Second to Fifth Years of Life

Age of Child	Problems Encountered
By the end of 2 years	Cannot walk by 18 months
	Fails to develop a mature heel-toe walking pattern after several months of walking or walking on his or her toes
	Does not speak at least 15 words by 18 months
	Does not use 2-word sentences
	By 15 months, does not seem to know the function of common objects (eg, brush, telephone, bell, fork, spoon)
	Does not imitate actions or words
	Does not follow instructions
	Cannot push a wheeled toy
By the end of 3 years	Frequent falling and difficulty with stairs
	Persistent drooling or very unclear speech
	Cannot build a tower of more than 4 blocks
	Difficulty manipulating small objects
	Cannot copy a circle
	Cannot communicate in short phrases
	No involvement in "pretend" play
	Cannot understand simple instructions
	Little interest in other children
	Extreme difficulty separating from mother
By the end of 4 years	Cannot throw a ball overhand
	Cannot jump in place
	Cannot ride a tricycle
	Cannot grasp a crayon between thumb and fingers
	Has difficulty scribbling
	Cannot stack 4 blocks
	Still clings or cries whenever his or her parents leave him or her
	Shows no interest in interactive games
	Ignores other children
	Does not respond to people outside the family
	Does not engage in fantasy play
	Resists dressing, sleeping, and using the toilet
	Lashes out without self-control when angry or upset
	Cannot copy a circle
	Does not use sentences of more than 3 words
	Does not use "me" and "you" appropriately

(continued)

Table 9-4 (continued)
Signs of Possible Delay: Second to Fifth Years of Life

Age of Child	Problems Encountered
By the end of 5 years	Exhibits extremely fearful or timid behavior
	Exhibits extremely aggressive behavior
	Cannot separate from parents without major protest
	Is easily distracted and unable to concentrate on any single activity for more than 5 minutes
	Shows little interest in playing with other children
	Refuses to respond to people in general, or responds only superficially
	Rarely uses fantasy or imitation in play
	Seems unhappy or sad much of the time
	Does not engage in a variety of activities
	Avoids or seems aloof with other children and adults
	Does not express a wide range of emotions
	Has trouble eating, sleeping, or using the toilet
	Cannot differentiate between fantasy and reality
	Seems unusually passive
	Cannot understand 2-part commands using prepositions
	Cannot correctly give his or her first and last name
	Does not use plurals or past tense properly when speaking
	Does not talk about his or her daily activities and experiences
	Cannot build a tower of 6 to 8 blocks
	Seems uncomfortable holding a crayon
	Has trouble taking off clothing
	Cannot brush his or her teeth efficiently
	Cannot wash and dry his or her hands

(Adapted from American Academy of Pediatrics, Shelov SP, Hanneman RE, Wray W, Gray A. *Caring for Your Baby and Young Child: Birth to Age Five*. New York, NY: Bantam Books; 1998.)

as well as the fine motor expressive skills of speech. Prior to attending school, these children are seen as clumsy, and parents are often told they will just grow out of these problems. Whether they are treated by a PT or played with by the parents, the children need repetitive practice in gross and fine motor skill development to help them participate in normal motor activities and thus develop quality in their lives.[23–25] In terms of intervention that can be performed by the PTA, the handling techniques presented in the intervention chapter (Chapter 4) may assist in facilitating mobility in this population of patients. These children do not necessarily have cognitive deficits, but have great difficulty expressing their thoughts when using a hand to write or draw (holding a pencil, crayon, or pen) and when trying to express their thoughts verbally.[26] The specific causation of DCD is not known, but these children have problems with rhythmic coordination, catching and throwing, posture, balance, gait, and sensory perception[27] and thus are seen by PTs.

Task-oriented motor functions have been shown to be the best intervention strategies and fall directly under the scope of practice of PTs and OTs. Thus, a PTA may very likely see a child with DCD when working in a pediatric setting.[28]

Another population in whom developmental deficits are seen is children with autism. These children may have coordination problems but also have behavioral interaction problems. It is not within the scope of this chapter to cover the literature regarding autism. This specific developmental problem is pervasive and needs a multidisciplinary approach. Because of the complexity of these cases, intervention is not often delegated to a PTA.

Warning signs of developmental delays, whether caused by genetic factors, DCD, LD, or other possible diagnoses, require that the PTA identify and recognize these problems when working with children. Some of the most common signs are in Table 9-5.

Physical Therapy Management of Children With Genetic and Developmental Conditions: Common Examination Tools

The preceding sections discussed several clinical features of the selected genetic conditions and/or developmental delays that may be improved following physical therapy intervention. Problems with fine and gross motor skill development directly affect activities and participation. Impairments such as tone, muscle strength, and balance abnormalities obviously affect skill development and optimal function. Subsystem involvement, such as cognitive deficits, communication disorders, and oral motor delay, also confound not only the main problem, but also the potential for habilitation. As the child grows, additional problems, such as loss of range of motion (ROM), weakness, and decreased cardiovascular endurance, further complicate functional progress. Obesity either from dietary habits or immobility can lead to additional problems for these children.

The following section describes in detail some of the more important examination procedures to objectively assess the clinical problems of children with genetic conditions and developmental delays.

Motor Skill Development

Children with motor coordination problems or genetic conditions that affect neurological function will typically manifest with delays in acquisition of motor skills and abnormal movement patterns. Infants and children may have limitations in performing and participating in activities typically performed by age-equivalent individuals. This is true not only of children with genetic problems but also in a larger community of children with delays in development.

Past studies show that the rate of motor development of children with DS is slightly below that of non-DS children. Initially, the motor skills of infants with DS closely parallel those of children without the condition. By 12 months, the motor skills of infants with DS are approximately 5 months behind their peers without the syndrome, and by age 5, they are 2 years behind typically developing peers. At age 5, the child with DS performs activities at 50% to 70% below normal rate.[29]

The multisystemic issues present in children with Prader-Willi syndrome contribute to problems in movement and posture. Neurological issues include poor gross motor and fine motor coordination.[30] Their motor skills in sitting, kneeling, standing, and walking are delayed compared with typically developing children.[31] Hypotonia and severe obesity affects motor development in older children. Later on into adult life, these effects are observed in abnormal gait and postural instability. Poor motor coordination can result in delayed acquisition of motor skills.

Specific motor skills and stages of motor development can be measured, monitored, and compared to milestones of other children of comparable age. There are several motor skills assessment

Table 9-5			
Warning Signs of a Developmental Delay			
Behavioral	*Gross Motor*	*Vision*	*Hearing*
Does not pay attention or stay focused on an activity for as long a time as other children the same age.	Has stiff arms and/or legs.	Seems to have difficulty following objects or people with his or her eyes.	Talks in a very loud or very soft voice.
Focuses on unusual objects for long periods of time; enjoys this more than interacting with others.	Has a floppy or limp body posture compared with other children of the same age.	Rubs eyes frequently.	Seems to have difficulty responding when called from across the room, even when it is for something interesting.
Avoids or rarely makes eye contact with others.	Uses one side of body more than the other.	Turns, tilts, or holds head in a strained or unusual position when trying to look at an object.	Has difficulty understanding what has been said or following directions (after the age of 3 years).
Gets unusually frustrated when trying to do simple tasks that most children of the same age can do.	Has a very clumsy manner compared with other children of the same age.	Seems to have difficulty finding or picking up small objects dropped on the floor (after the age of 12 months).	Does not startle to loud noises.
Shows aggressive behaviors, acts out, and appears to be very stubborn compared with other children.		Has difficulty focusing or making eye contact.	Ears appear small or deformed.
Displays violent behaviors on a daily basis.		Closes one eye when trying to look at distant objects.	Fails to develop sounds or words that would be appropriate at her or his age.
Stares into space, rocks body, or talks to self more often than other children of the same age.		Eyes appear to be crossed or turned.	
Does not seek love and approval from a caregiver or parent.		Brings objects too close to eyes to see.	
		One eye or both eyes appear abnormal in size or coloring.	

(Adapted from Child and Adolescent Services Research Center. How Kids Develop. http://www.howkidsdevelop.com/developDevDelay.html. Accessed May 6, 2005.)

tests and measures available and used in physical therapy. These tools are discussed in Chapter 5 and include tests and measures that are appropriate for any child with a delay in development, whether or not that delay is due to a specific genetic deficit. Knowledge of the most frequently used tests can help guide the PTA to monitor the effectiveness of the plan of care for specific patients.

Gross Motor Function Measure

The Gross Motor Function Measure (GMFM) is a standardized observational criterion-referenced instrument to measure change in gross motor function over time. The GMFM has undergone revisions from its original form of 88 items to its current form of 66 items.[32] This test was originally developed to measure gross motor skills of children with cerebral palsy; however, it has been found to be a valid and reliable tool for children with DS and for children with various developmental delays.[32,33] This test can describe the child's current level of motor function and help determine treatment goals and allows clinicians to provide a more concrete way to explain to parents concerns regarding their child's progress. The GMFM measures how much of the activity the child can perform instead of how well the child will be able to perform it. The tool measures 5 dimensions of gross motor function: (1) lying and rolling, (2) sitting, (3) crawling and kneeling, (4) standing, and (5) walking, running, and jumping.

Bruininks-Oseretsky Test of Motor Proficiency, Second Edition

The Bruininks-Oseretsky Test of Motor Proficiency, Second Edition[34] (BOT-2), is a revision of the Bruininks-Oseretsky Test of Motor Proficiency.[35] This is a norm-referenced test that assesses the motor functioning of children from 4.5 to 21 years old. It measures gross and fine motor skills through 4 motor areas: (1) fine manual control, (2) manual coordination, (3) body coordination, and (4) strength and agility. The BOT-2 provides useful information that can help assess the motor skills of children, evaluate motor training programs, and assess serious motor dysfunctions and developmental disabilities in children. It has been found to be reliable in children with intellectual disabilities as well.[36]

Test of Gross Motor Development, Second Edition

The Test of Gross Motor Development, Second Edition[37,38] (TGMD-2), measures gross motor abilities that develop in the early years of life. The TGMD-2 measures 12 gross motor skills in 2 subtests among children from 3 to 10 years old. The test measure has a locomotor subtest that checks run, gallop, hop, leap, horizontal jump, and slide and an object control subtest that looks at striking a stationary ball, stationary dribble, catch, kick, overhand throw, and underhand roll. The TGMD-2 identifies children who are delayed in motor skills and can help plan and evaluate a gross motor program.

Peabody Developmental Motor Scales, Second Edition

Another measure of motor skills in very young children is the Peabody Developmental Motor Scales, Second Edition[39] (PDMS-2). This tool assesses motor skills in children from birth to 5 years of age. There are 6 subtests that can be scored under 2 composites: the gross motor quotient and the fine motor quotient. The subtests under the gross motor quotient are reflexes, stationary, locomotion, and object manipulation. The subtests under the fine motor quotient are grasping and visual motor integration. The results of the test can provide the examiner the age equivalents of the infants.[40]

Tone Abnormalities: Hypotonia and Hypertonia

Normal tone refers to that characteristic of muscle in its state of readiness. Tone should be high enough so that muscle activation can be initiated and maintained during a movement or postural contraction and yet low enough to allow normal range of movement against gravity.[41]

Hypotonia or hypotonicity is a common feature among children with genetic conditions such as DS and Prader-Willi syndrome. Low tone is also often found in children with developmental delays and/or cognitive retardation. Characteristics most frequently observed in children with hypotonia include decreased strength, hypermobile joints, and increased flexibility.[42] These characteristics are obtained mainly through observation of the child. At present, the French Angles Factor of the Infant Neurological International Battery (INFANIB) is meant to determine hypotonia but fails to discriminate findings from those of hypermobility. The French Angles include the scarf sign, heel to ear, popliteal angle, and abductor's angle.[43] The scoring sheet for the INFANIB can be retrieved from http://ptjournal.apta.org/content/66/4/548.full.pdf. This can guide the therapist on how to perform and score the test. Martin et al[42] proposed that there is a need to develop an operational definition of hypotonia to develop a valid test to determine the presence of this impairment and to assess effectiveness of intervention.

Hypertonicity and *spasticity* are often terms used interchangeably. However, the difference lies in how they are elicited. Clopton and colleagues[44] pointed out that spasticity is "velocity-dependent resistance of a muscle to stretch," whereas hypertonia is "increased resistance to externally-imposed movement." Both of these types of tone are often seen together. Stiffening of the limbs, tremors and/or clonus, weakness, and difficulty in movement are other symptoms that may be present along with spasticity and hypotonia. Children with neurogenetic conditions such as cri du chat exhibit hypertonia. Children with developmental delays, LD, or MR do not exhibit hypertonicity or spasticity. Their central nervous system problems are not identified as specific lesions or problems within the motor system that must be correlated with these specific tonal abnormalities. Children with cerebral palsy have specific lesions within the motor system and can simultaneously have delays in development, learning problems, or retardation, but their spasticity or hypertonicity is due to the motor system lesions or deficits.

One way to measure hypertonia is through the Modified Ashworth Scale, which is discussed in detail in Chapter 5 and also found in Table 5-3. The examiner passively moves a joint through its ROM at a standard speed and rates the resistance of the stretched muscles on a 6-point scale. Although prudence is suggested in using this test,[44,45] the grading system can guide therapists to develop realistic expectations when handling patients with hypertonicity. If a grade of 3 or 4 is given, then therapists should be more gentle and patient in moving an extremity. If a grade 1 or 1+ is given, then therapists can expect to move the extremity with ease.

Balance and Coordination Tools

The Pediatric Balance Scale is a revised version of the Berg Balance Scale (BBS). The original BBS was modified for use with children by rearranging the order of the test items, reducing time standards for maintenance of static postures, and clarifying directions to suit children.[46] The preliminary test was performed for children from 5 to 15 years with mild to moderate motor impairments, although a more recent study on typically developing children found that the test is more appropriate for children from 2 to 6 years old.[47] The test consists of 14 items arranged in functional sequence, with the most novel tasks placed in the end. Each item requires the tester to score the child from 0 to 4 depending on a set of criteria. The rater will sum up scores for each item; a total score of 56 is expected. To date, interpretation of scores has yet to be performed.

The gross motor measures discussed previously, such as the GMFM, BOT-2, and TGMD-2, also have the capability to provide insight on the balance and coordination of children with genetic and/or developmental problems.

PHYSICAL THERAPY INTERVENTION STRATEGIES

Genetic conditions with neurodevelopmental concerns often result in motor problems that result in movement dysfunctions. Similarly, children with various types of developmental delays also exhibit movement dysfunction that leads to motor delays. This requires the PT and PTA to be essential members of the health care team for these children. As mentioned previously, the

Figure 9-1. In supine, put rolled towels or pillow on lateral sides of the legs to prevent frog-like positioning of the legs. (Illustration by Anne Rivera.)

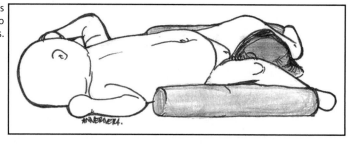

Figure 9-2. In prone, put a rolled towel or blanket to keep legs in midline and hips flexed. (Illustration by Anne Rivera.)

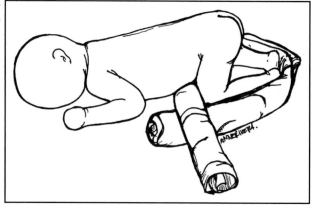

Figure 9-3. In side-lying, put a rolled towel to keep the spine straight and the hips flexed and slightly abducted. (Illustration by Anne Rivera.)

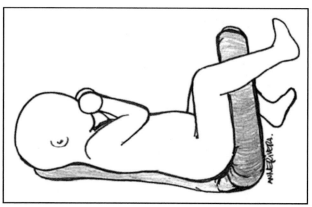

common impairments and activity limitations encountered in these conditions include tone abnormalities (hyper- and hypotonicity), weakness, delay in the development of fine- and gross-motor skills, and problems with balance and coordination. The following are interventions that can usually be delegated to the PTA.

Techniques for Managing Tone Problems

Proper positioning in infancy should be implemented at birth. Infants with low muscle tone tend to get into the frog-like posture in which the hips are flexed, abducted, and internally rotated and the knees are flexed.[48] A study conducted in 1991[49] among very premature infants showed significant positive motor development for those whose hips were supported with proper positioning. Upon reaching age equivalence to term, these same infants did not exhibit the typical hip/leg posturing commonly seen initially in hypotonic patients. These positioning techniques may be adapted for infants with hypotonia such as DS or Prader-Willi syndrome or for any child with developmental delays who exhibits this low tone. Figures 9-1 through 9-10 show examples of these positioning techniques.

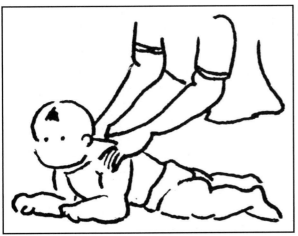

Figure 9-4. Prone on elbows. Support the child in the scapular area. (Illustration by Catherine M. Capio.)

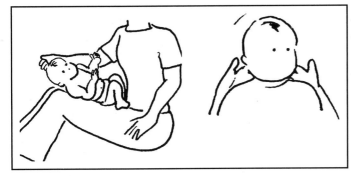

Figure 9-5. Position self in crook-lying facing the child. Give support to scapula and occiput. Lift the child while in this position and allow the child to contract his or her neck muscles. (Illustration by Catherine M. Capio.)

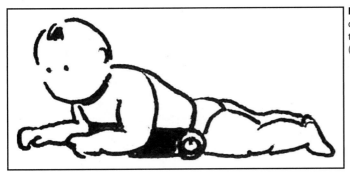

Figure 9-6. Put a rolled towel or blanket or a bolster under the chest to support the trunk in a prone-on-elbows position. (Illustration by Catherine M. Capio.)

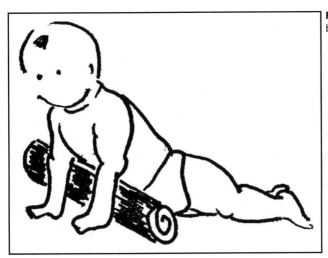

Figure 9-7. Prone-on-hands position with a bolster. (Illustration by Catherine M. Capio.)

Figure 9-8. From a prone on hands position, get the child into a quadruped or all-fours position by lifting the pelvis up and putting weight on the knees. (Illustration by Catherine M. Capio.)

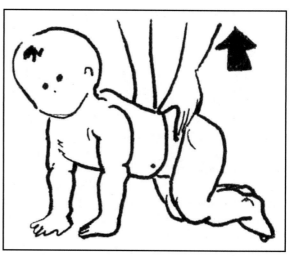

Figure 9-9. Sitting begins with bilateral arm support and progresses with the use of one hand for reaching or manipulating and eventually both hands. (Illustration by Catherine M. Capio.)

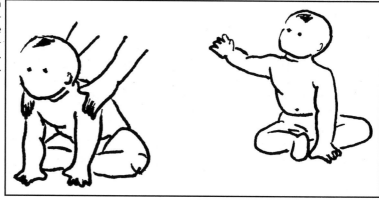

Figure 9-10. Kneeling can initiate standing by allowing the child to feel weight on the hips through the knees. (Illustration by Debbie Qua.)

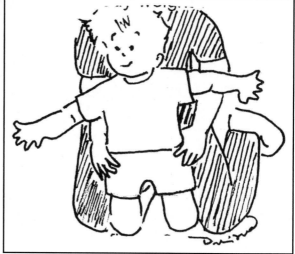

Handling Techniques to Guide the Child Into Normal Movement Patterns

As children mature and watch others move, they are highly motivated to move themselves. Thus, within the first year, a child will learn to roll, come to sit, sit independently, and come to stand. Some will even cruise independently and walk before their first birthday. These children continue to mature and gain motor control over more complex movement patterns, such as walking, running, climbing stairs, manipulating objects, throwing, independent feeding, and many additional movements that lead to independence and the ability to participate in age-related activities. Children with developmental delays, no matter the causation, do not experience these same learning opportunities. Thus, they do not develop normal postural control or functional control over moving from one position to another, and they do not gain the independence in motor control over their bodies, thus limiting their ability to participate normally in age-related activities. Handling techniques are designed to move these children through these developmental patterns to allow them the opportunities to gain motor learning experiences and control over their bodies. Handling a child to encourage rolling is usually performed by controlling one of the child's legs and flexing the knee and hip and guiding the child's pelvis and trunk into a rotation pattern in which the upper body will follow the lower body, followed next by the head. This pattern of rolling elicits a body-on-body-on-head righting reaction. The PTA must remember that for the child to learn a motor pattern, that pattern needs to be practiced over and over as the environment is changed by having various textures to roll on, external noises with a slow increase in volume and background sounds, and slight variations in the specific movements of hip and knee flexion with rotation. Through handling, a child can be moved from supine to prone, supine to side-lying to sit, various sitting positions, sit to 4-point, 4-point to kneeling, kneeling to half-kneeling, and half-kneeling to standing. The reader is referred to the video on handling techniques that accompanies this text.

One very effective way to learn handling techniques is to play with normal babies and feel their movements as you guided them from one position to another. Excellent resources on observing and development handling techniques can be found in a PowerPoint presentation by Lois Bly in April 2012 and in her books on the treatment of babies.[50,51] Also, spending time watching babies, children, adolescents, young adults, and aging adults is a wonderful way to learn to recognize normal movement and the transitions between one stable position to another. Another activity that can be used to help develop the background needed to develop handling techniques is to just move. Start by lying down on the floor and feeling what you experience as you roll over, come to sit, move into various sitting postures and move from sit to side-sit and then into 4-point. Then, rock back and sit on your knees and come up into hip extension or kneeling, then to half-kneeling and standing up. Then go through the same activities but with your eyes closed so you can truly feel what is normal and what a child should experience when begin handled. Then work with a colleague and have him or her go through those same patterns while you hold onto his or her head, then his or her arm, and then roll the leg. By going through these activities, the PTA can kinesthetically learn while visually identifying what those movements should look like. Then, as a clinician treating a child with developmental problems, the PTA can feel the effort or lack thereof when the child begins to assist with the movement and finally takes control over the patterns. Remember that the goal of treatment is to allow the child to feel normal transitions and experience success with minimal effort as movement is obtained from one position to another. The reader is also referred to Chapter 4 for additional ideas regarding handling under the Neuro-Developmental Treatment section.

Techniques for Facilitating the Development of Muscular Strength

Playing normally is the activity that a child uses to gain the muscular strength necessary to achieve motor control over postural positions and transitions between those postural patterns.

A child with developmental delays often lacks control over the necessary power of play and for that reason has difficulty moving from one position to another. Thus, developing the necessary strength needed to independently move may become part of the plan of care for children with these medical diagnoses. Again, strengthening needs to take place through play, and that play needs to be part of the plan of care. Using a ball in play begins with very young children and progresses to all ages. Using a balloon for children who have coordination problems allows them additional time to catch the ball. Medicine balls can have graded weights and can be used to assist in strength training of the upper extremities. If ball play is performed in standing, then having the child pick up the weighted ball can lead to lower limb and trunk strengthening as well. A question that therapists often ask is: "Should strength training be our goal versus using an assistive device?" According to a system review of the Cochrane Database regarding rehabilitation and strength training to prevent foot drop in neuromuscular disease, little long-term effect was found between control and experimental groups. These results may indicate that the use of an orthosis to assist with dorsiflexion of the foot may lead to the best long-term outcome.[52] Thus, identifying evidence that might guide the PT and PTA as to whether to begin or continue strength training can help in developing a plan of care for all children.

Many children will gain strength and then use that strength to participate and be functionally independent in movement activities valued by the child. But children diagnosed with some of these developmental and genetic delays need to be monitored more closely. Caution for specific medical diagnoses are identified in the following few paragraphs.

Progressive resistance training is found to be an effective program to improve strength among adolescents with DS.[53] Adolescents were placed in a twice-a-week program for 10 weeks that was designed according to the recommendations of the American College of Sports Medicine. They performed 6 exercises: latissimus pull-down, seated chest press, seated row, seated leg press, knee extension, and calf raise.

Gupta et al[54] suggested a more specific method for progressive resistance exercise for the lower limbs is to start at 50% of one repetition maximum. Exercises using sandbags were performed for hip flexors, abductors, extensors, knee flexors and extensors, and ankle plantarflexors. Two sets of 10 repetitions were performed for each muscle group, and the resistance was increased by half a kilogram when the child was able to complete the sets without difficulty.

Techniques for Improving Balance and Coordination

Shumway-Cook and Woollacott's research on postural control[9] suggests that treatment should focus on helping children develop and refine their postural responses by way of improving their spatiotemporal coupling between the different muscle groups that act together. These activities should engage children in activating specific muscle groups using appropriate body movements and proper timing. This lack of postural tone is consistent in children with LD, developmental coordination problems, developmental delays, genetic problems, and MR. Thus, balance and coordination problems are seen in many children with specific or general diagnoses that have led to delays in motor development.

A study conducted on young children with DS[54] concluded that balance improves when they are given a 6-week exercise training program that includes resistance exercises and balance training. For balance training, children ages 11 to 14 performed horizontal jumps, vertical jumps, one leg stance with eyes open, tandem stance, walking on a line, walking on a balance beam, and jumping on a trampoline. All these activities are within the scope of practice of the PTA.

Physical therapy interventions that facilitate the improvement of postural control are beneficial to this population of patients and clients. For PTAs, it is important to remember to optimize starting alignment and base of support (BOS) to provide a stable base for the trunk and lower extremity muscles. That allows the musculoskeletal system to be biomechanically optimized and will therefore facilitate more normal and functional movements.[55,56] This can be started with the patient sitting. Before starting an activity, it is important for the PTA to make sure that the patient's feet are on the floor to increase the stable BOS. Then the PTA can use verbal or tactile cues to improve alignment to ensure a stable proximal segment so that the child can move his or her distal segments (extremities) more efficiently. In terms of handling and facilitation, the PTA could use approximation techniques to facilitate co-contraction or coactivation of the postural muscles to optimize movement. As always, these could be incorporated into play activities. This way the child performs activities that are enjoyable and engaging while training to run motor programs that are not only automatic but also could facilitate cognitive loading or dual tasking. For example, the PTA could start with balloon-tossing activities with the child in sitting with proper support and alignment, with the necessary tactile cues and facilitation to optimize the position. The PTA could ask a helper to toss the balloon to the child, first just within a small base, and then progressing so the child moves his or her center of gravity outside the BOS. The same activity could be performed with the patient in kneeling, half-kneeling, standing, or standing on one foot. The PTA could provide tactile cues and approximation through the shoulders or pelvis while the child performs the specific activity.

The use of adaptive/orthotic or supportive devices could also be considered because they allow for better support and joint protection that could decrease pain and joint stress and facilitate movement.

Exercises that improve balance on compliant and noncompliant surfaces will improve the child's ability to optimize function and increase activity and participation. Going back to the previous example, the sitting and standing activities can be progressed by having the child sit or stand on foam, with appropriate guarding strategies by the PTA. A ball may be thrown to the child from different directions. Aside from throwing the ball, the PTA or child could also bounce it; this adds another component of complexity because the child will need both anticipatory and reactive control to be able to successfully catch and release the toy. Additionally, there are balls on the market that bounce unpredictably. Those types of balls would offer even more challenge to the child. There is no way to anticipate where the ball will go once it is bounced, and the child would have to respond automatically and quickly.

Another way to increase complexity and link to function is to change the environment to real-world situations. The PTA could configure activities outside of the clinic: playing on grass or asphalt or in an open environment where other people are moving, interacting, or playing with the child. This way, the child trains for his or her physical rehabilitation, along with social and emotional interaction.

Higher-level balancing activities disguised as play could also be effective in improving balance and coordination. An obstacle course with a series of starts and stops, perhaps played with Simon Says, allows the patient to run challenging motor programs while engaging in activities that improve attention and engagement. Playing hopscotch or jump rope allows single- and double-limb support while also moving the upper extremities. As important as these activities are to motor development, the exercises themselves help the cardiovascular and pulmonary systems, improve muscular and pulmonary endurance, increase oxygenation, and improve the child's ability to tolerate more strenuous activities.

Techniques to Improve Soft Tissue Mobility

Soft tissue mobilization has shown to improve muscle tone among toddlers with DS.[57] The tissue mobilization routine used in this study was conducted for 30 minutes twice a week. In supine, the legs and feet, stomach, chest, arms and hands, and finally the face were massaged. After this, the child was placed in a prone position and massage was given to the back. See Box 9-1 for a summary of the techniques.

Other techniques that involve mobilization of the soft tissues in pediatric populations include myofascial release and craniosacral techniques.[58] Both of these techniques require

---

Box 9-1
Soft Tissue Mobilization Techniques[57]

---

1. For the legs and arms, the therapist wraps the fingers around the child's leg/arm and then gives long milking and twisting strokes from the thigh to the ankles or from the upper arm to the wrist (Figure 9-11).

2. For the stomach, slow, circular, rubbing movements are administered to the stomach area using one hand and the palms; slide one palm at a time down the stomach in a hand-over-hand manner in a paddle-wheel fashion (Figures 9-12 and 9-13).

3. For the chest, the therapist places the palms of the hands on the child's sternum and strokes outward across the chest. Start at the sternum and stroke upward and over the top of the shoulders and down the sides of the ribs (Figures 9-14 and 9-15).

4. For the face, make circles to the entire scalp as if shampooing hair; with the flat aspect of the thumbs, while together on midline of forehead, stroke outward toward the temples. Stroke gently on eyes and brows. Progress the stroking from the bridge of the nose, across the cheekbones, to the ears. It is especially important to make circular movements under the chin, around the jaw line, around the ears, to the back of the neck, and to the rest of the scalp (see Figure 9-14).

5. For the back, one described technique starts at the top of the spine, alternating hand strokes across the back working down toward the tailbone but never pressing on the spine. Care must be taken by the PTA to make sure the hand strokes are not done vertically down along the spine because that creates an autonomic response and slows down all sympathetic motor responses, such as heart rate and breathing. Although this technique can be used to calm or relax an individual, it is not a mobilization technique and thus not used for that purpose.

---

additional training, and the PTA is encouraged to seek more information to incorporate these 2 important techniques in the PTA's intervention repertoire. Myofascial release comprises manual techniques that aim to remove fascial restrictions. It is postulated that the fascia is a 3-dimensional web of connective tissue that is intricately connected within the entire body. Any trauma, abnormal movements, or decreased mobility could affect the integrity of the fascia, including the formation of scar tissue that limits fascial mobility. Because it is postulated that the fascia is interconnected, it is possible that facial restrictions in one area could affect mobility in remote areas.

Craniosacral techniques also involve a series of specific manual, hands-on techniques that facilitate movements, decrease soft tissue restrictions, improve comfort, and decrease pain. Again, the techniques are highly specialized and require more training for the PTA.

Special-Focus Topics Specific to Selected Conditions

Fatigue in Children With Muscular Dystrophy

Fatigue in children with MD may be an indication of the severity of the myopathy.[59] Monitoring the child with MD during play and watching for development of incoordination or signs of fatigue is critical, and rest periods must be provided when those signs are observed. As in some types of MD, specifically DMD, the muscle loss can be pervasive and progressive, and heavy exercise may lead to further degeneration. Thus, play and strengthening should be of low intensity but regular to maintain the power potential of the child and to allow that child to participate in life.[60-62]

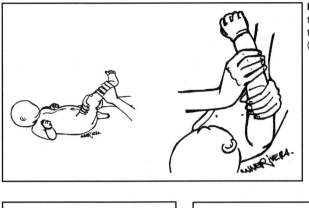

Figure 9-11. The PTA wraps the fingers around the child's leg and arm and gives long milking and twisting strokes in a proximal-to-distal direction. (Illustration by Anne Rivera.)

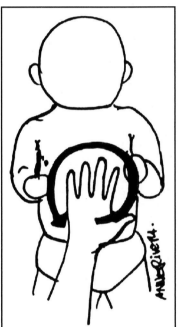

Figure 9-12. Rub the stomach in a slow, circular movement using one hand. (Illustration by Anne Rivera.)

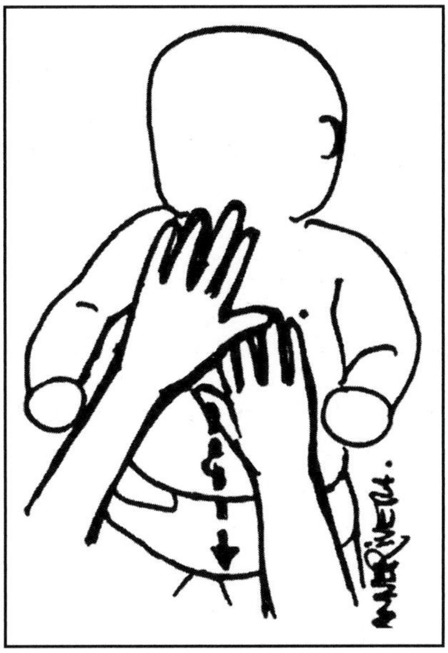

Figure 9-13. Using the palms, slide one palm at a time down the stomach in a hand-over-hand manner in a paddle wheel fashion. (Illustration by Anne Rivera.)

Cardiopulmonary Impairments in Children With Down Syndrome and Other Neuromuscular Diseases

Although not all children with DS have secondary complications, some of them are confronted with cardiopulmonary impairments that, if not identified, can lead to life-threatening problems.[63-65] The PTA, when playing with children to create strength training, needs to monitor heart rate and listen to the breathing. If the child begins to breathe heavily or take short but rapid breaths, then the activity may be too taxing for the cardiopulmonary system. If the PTA sees these behaviors, documenting and reporting them to the PT is very important. The PT can determine whether the child needs to be referred to the physician or whether the plan of care needs to be changed. Obviously, if the child seems to be in an acute life-threatening situation, the PTA needs to call 911 or medical staff immediately.

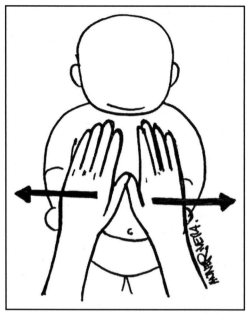

Figure 9-14. Place the palms of your hands on the child's sternum and stroke outward across the chest. (Illustration by Anne Rivera.)

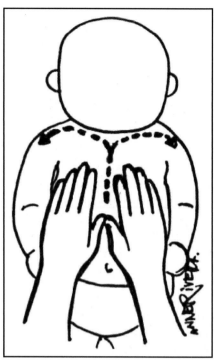

Figure 9-15. For the chest, starting at the sternum, stroke upward and over the top of the shoulders and down the sides of the ribs. (Illustration by Anne Rivera.)

Emerging Trends in Developing Motor Skills: The Use of Treadmills and Virtual-Reality Gaming Technology

The use of body weight–supported treadmill training has been shown to be an effective way to treat people with cardiovascular anomalies, spinal cord injury, and Parkinson's disease, among others (see Chapters 4, 8, 10, and 11). In recent years, the use of the treadmill for children with neurodevelopmental conditions has been reported in the literature with encouraging results.[25] For genetic conditions, the treadmill is used for infants and children with DS,[66-70] as well as for children with Rett syndrome.[58] The child can be placed in a body weight–supported harness to take away some of the body weight and need for power or strength. Then the treadmill can be used to trigger gait patterns. As the child improves in balance and strength, the amount of body support given by the harness can be reduced, thus encouraging strength development during movement and as a postural system. The difference in training these children is the slower rate needed for training and the use of a harness that fits the small child.

Children with developmental delays without a specific medical diagnosis of a disease or pathology might benefit from this high-tech equipment but would not qualify through the family's insurance for the cost of this type of intervention. When the child exhibits low tone without an abnormality such as spasticity, some parents might be able to adapt their home treadmills with a harness system so their child could get the repetitive practice of gait while having some body weight reduction.

Another modality that is being reported in the literature for children with developmental disabilities is the use of virtual reality–based activity, the most common of which is the Nintendo Wii. Studies have shown that computerized gaming can be used to work on visual-perceptual skills, postural control, and mobility in children with cerebral palsy[71,72]; to reduce hyperactive behavior in children with attention deficit hyperactivity disorder[73]; and to enhance sensory-motor functions in children with DS.[74] Although evidence is still limited as to its effectiveness and long-term outcomes, these studies indicate that gaming is a modality that can at the very least be an adjunct to regular therapy procedures. These gaming consoles are attractive to children and may help motivate these young individuals to perform physical activities. Refer to Chapter 4 for additional discussion of the use of technology as part of intervention strategies.

ESSENTIAL FEATURES IN THE MANAGEMENT OF NEURODEVELOPMENTAL CONDITIONS

Early Intervention

The strides gained in the field of genetics make it possible for physicians to identify and diagnose various genetic conditions at an early age. Identifying genetic conditions and syndromes as soon as possible allows parents to access medical and other health-related services for their child.

Early intervention is providing necessary and appropriate intervention at the soonest time possible. If patients with genetic conditions can be identified at birth, then referral to early intervention can begin immediately. Similarly, if a child does not progress in what is considered a normal developmental progression or rate considered within normal parameters, then that child may qualify for early intervention.

The basic tenet of providing early intervention is to minimize or reduce long-term costs and improve outcomes. For patients with acute or developmental lesions that affect the brain or spinal cord, the basic principles for enhancing neural outcomes include (1) growth of new cells, (2) regrowth of connections, and (3) retraining of existing growths.[69] The chance for each of these neural outcomes to happen depends on different factors, such as the area that is affected, the extent of damage, and the timing of injury. Regardless, research indicates that activity and specialty training are needed if the physical therapy interventions are to promote neuroplasticity and neuromotor control and to ensure functional outcomes.[69]

In the United States, the Individuals with Disabilities Education Act (IDEA) was amended in 1986 through Public Law (P.L.) 99-457 to include infants and toddlers with disabilities and their families as recipients of appropriate intervention. The amendments recognized the importance of addressing family concerns in the context of having to care for a child with special needs.[75] Bronfenbrenner,[76] in his depiction of the ecology of human development, emphasizes that a developing human being is influenced by and influences his or her immediate institutional structures, such as the family, school, or therapy center. Furthermore, the interactions between these institutions can have an effect on the developing child. The amendments of IDEA made through P.L. 99-457, therefore, takes this theory into consideration by addressing the family's needs and resources while providing appropriate care for the child with special needs.

Effectiveness of early intervention programs may be attributed to family characteristics, stressors, and resources for support.[77] This review of literature should help PTAs comprehend the benefits of early intervention. These insights may be applicable to all genetic conditions or developmental delays that affect neuromotor development, such as MR, DCD, and LD.

An environment that is generally stimulating through a moderately directive parenting style is found to be favorable in early intervention. To achieve such an environment, therapists must help parents gain confidence and increase their competence in the manner in which they interact with their infant or toddler with special needs. This indicates that instead of the therapist focusing an entire session working with the child and addressing therapy needs only, adequate time should also be spent in teaching parents how to hold, position, play with, and interact with the child. The parents will be the advocate for the child throughout most of the child's life and thus should be the ones who gain success from therapeutic intervention. It helps bond the parents to the child while enriching the child's environment. Teaching parents, by instructing, demonstrating, and giving feedback on how they can work with their children at home, can help empower them to care for and properly address their child's special needs. The PT and the PTA need to be sensitive to the needs of the parents, their frustrations, their expectations, and their fears. Incorporating the environmental and the personal factors of the parents/family will allow the PT and PTA to assess the problems the child will face in addition to those caused by body structure or function when interacting in activities. Refer to Chapter 1 and Figure 1-1 (the International Classification of Functioning, Disability and Health model from the World Health Organization) for additional discussion of impairments in body function, limitations in activities, and restrictions in participation.

Having adequate and timely information regarding the child's condition and possible resources that could help the family can help lessen the stress on the family. Therapists must always be ready to answer parents' questions correctly, provide sufficient and precise information, and lead or guide them to obtain the necessary support and resources that they need. At the time of diagnosis, parents are most interested to know more about whatever the condition might be, what caused the condition, what to expect from the condition, and how the condition will affect their child through life. As a PT or PTA, you may not be the first health care professional that the parents have encountered after receiving the medical diagnosis for their child. However, do not assume when you relay crucial data that the parents will immediately absorb all the information. Most parents will need to ask the same question over and over until they understand what either the doctor or the therapist is saying. Always be ready to address the information needs of the parents. It is important that you have accurate information. Apart from knowing about the condition, parents find it helpful if you can direct them to services that they need or for which they are eligible. In areas where a system is in place for early intervention services, knowing the process and reiterating that process to the family is often greatly appreciated.

Social networks can have a positive influence on the family's outlook on the care of the child with a genetic condition or delays in development. It is often valuable to direct families to organizations and groups that support and advocate for that specific condition. It may be a local support group that the family can easily access, or, if those groups are not available in the area, they might find technological advances and support through the Internet.

WORKING IN COLLABORATION WITH THE REHABILITATION TEAM

The developmental nature of conditions such as genetic abnormalities or developmental delays requires the involvement of several health care professionals in addressing pertinent problems and concerns. Human development is a complex process that requires attention to the different aspects of growth and development—physical, cognitive, and socioemotional. (Refer to Chapters 2 and 6 for additional information.) It is important that the PTA understands the different disciplines and the professionals that may be working with this population.

A child with MR may or may not have a genetic condition that is the causation of the retardation. One condition of retardation is that the developmental level across the spectrum of skills (cognitive, fine motor, gross motor, socialization) is constant, whereas a child with LD, motor coordination deficits, autism, DS, or another problem that causes developmental delays may exhibit areas of strength as well as areas of delay. Children with developmental delays often do not have a medical diagnosis to guide either the therapist or the parents toward available services. Yet, medical institutions have identified mechanisms to help children with developmental delays. Those mechanisms and the team responsible for services may be part of a larger state-run organization. Federal law requires that services be provided once a child's delay reaches certain criteria. Whether those services are part of a state-run children's services agency or are housed within a school-based program, they are often state specific. Parents will often identify these delays earlier than the medical system and may search for services that can help their child attain those developmental milestones and once again resume normal maturation. As the door to direct access opens more and more to physical therapy, parents may enter into physical services directly and the PT/PTA may engage in interventions that assist the child's central nervous system in learning cognitive and motor skills. Similarly, physical services may need to refer the parents and the child to other health care professionals to meet the complex nature of the developing child. A brief description of each profession has been included here for the PTA to become familiar with the entire health care team.

Physical Therapist and Physical Therapist Assistant

PTs and PTAs are concerned with movement and functional ability.[1] PTs are expected to perform a comprehensive examination of the patient, evaluate findings of the examination, and formulate a diagnosis, prognosis, and plan of care. In addition, PTs implement the treatment program, determine outcomes of interventions, and consult with and refer to other experts. PTs supervise and direct PTAs. The PTA may implement selected components of the treatment plan, obtain data related to the intervention provided, and make necessary modifications in the intervention at the direction of the PT.[78] Details on pertinent physical therapy management, including the role of the PTA, can be found in the next section.

Clinical Medical Geneticist

The American College of Medical Genetics (ACMG) defines the scope of practice of medical genetics as a broad and unique specialty of medicine that involves all organ systems, periods of life, and disease entities. The ACMG document on scope of practice[79] identifies members of the genetics health care team to include clinical and laboratory medical geneticists, genetic counselors, nurse geneticists, and metabolic disease dieticians.

Medical or clinical geneticists are physicians who are trained to diagnose and provide therapeutic procedures for patients with genetically linked diseases.[79] They are qualified to diagnose, treat, supervise, coordinate, and case manage individuals and families with known and suspected genetic disorders.

Genetic Counselor

Genetic counselors are involved in developing, documenting, and assessing family histories and facilitating genetic testing decision making and patient/family education. They are also able to address the psychosocial needs of patients and families.

Developmental-Behavioral Pediatrician

A developmental-behavioral pediatrician is a medical specialist who has gone through a residency or specialization in pediatrics and further trained for the subspecialty of developmental-behavioral pediatrics.[80] These medical specialists are equipped to evaluate, counsel, and provide treatment for children, adolescents, and families with a wide range of developmental and behavioral difficulties.

Occupational Therapist

Occupational therapy's primary goal is "to help patients and clients to participate in the things that they want and need to do through the therapeutic use of everyday activities."[81] The occupational therapy profession promotes health and well-being through occupation. An OT can provide a comprehensive and individualized evaluation and treatment plan to improve performance of ADL. For genetic conditions with neurodevelopmental concerns, OTs are helpful in addressing problems that interfere with feeding, attention, and movement. They are also able to provide comprehensive evaluation and recommend modification of the client's home and other significant environmental problems or barriers. OTs may also recommend and train in the use of assistive devices that will foster occupation.[81,82] A number of OTs work in school systems and focus specifically on the spectrum of problems considered LDs. Children with specific medical diagnoses such as DS, as well as those without medical diagnoses but with delays in motor development, often have various LDs or problems that will be treated by an OT.

Speech-Language Pathologist

Speech-language pathologists address typical and atypical communication and swallowing in the areas of speech production, resonance, voice, language comprehension and expression, cognition, feeding, and swallowing.[83] Speech-language pathologists are expected to screen, evaluate, diagnose, and provide treatment or intervention to patients with genetic conditions. Their role is more prominent and essential during the preschool and formal school years of children, when communication and socialization plays a vital role in children's social and cognitive development. These clinicians often work closely with other professionals addressing problems that stem from language, such as temporal sequencing and how it affects reading or language development.

Audiologists

Audiologists promote healthy hearing and communication competency.[84] These specialists identify, assess, and rehabilitate hearing, auditory function, balance, and other related systems while preventing additional problems within this area. Audiologists are important for children with hearing impairments and auditory problems. They closely work with speech-language pathologists.

THE PHYSICAL THERAPIST–PHYSICAL THERAPIST ASSISTANT TEAM: CONSIDERATIONS FOR EFFECTIVE COLLABORATION TO OPTIMIZE CARE

PTAs are indispensable members of the rehabilitation team. The PTA is tasked to implement activities, conduct exercises, and possibly apply modalities to patients under the PT's direction. A PTA may spend a considerable amount of time with the patient and his or her family and therefore have the opportunity to more closely follow the care of the child. When working with this population, the following considerations are important:

1. Always remember safety considerations. As discussed previously, while many conditions have similarities in presentation, other clinical aspects may be different. The PTA must be aware of those differences and must adjust the treatment protocol to accommodate these variations. For example, it may be harder to mobilize extremities of children with hypertonicity like Rett syndrome. Forcing an extremity to move through very high tone may result in injury of the child. In contrast, children with DS or Prader-Willi syndrome may be more mobile, but their balance is compromised. The PTA must always keep the environment safe to prevent falls and potential injuries to the child.

2. Ensure that the child is medically stable. Be sensitive to subtle changes in the child's behavior, participation in therapy, or level of alertness. These may indicate the presence of a medical issue. There may be times that the parents are the ones observing and reporting these changes. Immediately report these issues to the supervising therapist. Seizures are common among

children with Rett syndrome and cri du chat syndrome. A child with DS who has a significant decrease in mobility status may be experiencing cardiovascular compromise or other medical system disorders. In both these cases, physical therapy intervention may be altered or stopped completely until the child has been evaluated by an appropriate medical professional.

3. Listen to parents' stories and descriptions of their child and family life. Often they will disclose how their personal lives are being affected both positively and negatively by having a child with special needs. It is important that the child is given intervention, but it is just as important to keep the family system working for the child. You may need to report to the PT about these matters that affect therapy to update a plan of care or work out a more feasible and acceptable intervention for the child.

Working with children can be very fulfilling and satisfying. It is also not unusual to find yourself in challenging and frustrating situations. It is best to keep in mind that physical therapy primarily aims to improve mobility and enhance the patient's quality of life.

CASE STUDIES

CASE #1

The patient is a 4-year-old girl whose mother is concerned about her limited mobility skills. The child lives with her mother and father. She has 2 siblings, aged 21 and 16, who do not live with them anymore. Her father is a driver and her mother is a housewife. The child was born to a 33-year-old mother and had no remarkable events pre- and perinatally. When the child was 10 months of age, the mother noticed that she was not yet reaching or playing with toys. The child was brought to their local pediatrician, who diagnosed her with global developmental delay and referred her to physical therapy and occupational therapy services. The mother was not able to seek services immediately because of financial issues. The mother noticed that, at the age of 1 year, the child started losing her grip. At 1 year and 3 months, the mother was finally able to seek physical and occupational therapy services but was unable to go regularly—physical therapy once a week and occupational therapy once every 2 weeks. According to the mother's report, at 2 years old, the child was still able to W-sit independently (hips internally rotated and knees flexed) but eventually lost this skill by age 3.

After consultation with several specialists, the patient was diagnosed as having Rett syndrome. She usually ate finely chopped meat or vegetables and rice. On physical examination, the patient appeared well nourished. She was nonambulatory. She appeared lethargic. Tone assessment revealed 1+ spasticity on the Modified Ashworth Scale for both elbows and knees. The child had weak to fair control of head and neck in sitting; her head lagged when pulled to sit. She rolled from supine to prone and back using the log roll technique. She was able to assume and maintain prone on elbows. She was unable to assume quadruped, cross-sitting, or short-sitting. She was unable to creep or crawl. She was also not able to stand and walk. The child did not reach for any object independently. ROM testing revealed limitations in both hip flexion, both knee extension, and both ankle dorsiflexion and plantarflexion.

The plan of care included the following activities, which were delegated to the PTA. First, mobility exercises were performed to improve ROM of the trunk and extremities. Soft tissue mobilization techniques were performed to improve tissue mobility and release any restrictions due to scar tissue or tight muscles. Next, gentle, passive stretching activities were performed to improve ROM. The mother was also trained to perform these exercises as part of the home program. A referral to the orthotist for fitting of posterior ankle splints was also conducted.

The PTA was also responsible for administering the strengthening exercises for the trunk, postural muscles, and extremities. Examples of these exercises included pull-to-sit activities, prone extensions on a vestibular ball, and ROM activities in open- and closed-chain positions. Strengthening activities in short-sitting on a bench and cross-sitting on a mat were also performed. Play was incorporated with the child assuming these positions, with the PTA providing facilitation and tactile cues to maintain the positions and optimize alignment and BOS. Exercises were performed following a developmental sequence, beginning with the child prone on elbows, prone on hands, and then in the quadruped position. From these positions, the PTA trained the child to creep and crawl.

Next, sitting balance activities were performed. The child initially required moderate assistance to maintain the sitting position. The PTA optimized the position by correctly positioning the child's feet, keeping the child in proper biomechanical alignment before initiating any activities. In this position, the child performed bean bag toss, throwing the bean onto a board with targets, with assistance from the PTA. The activity was progressed to having the child sitting on foam, then a DynaDisc (Exertools). The patient also performed the activities in standing, first on a flat surface, then on foam. The PTA provided facilitation as appropriate to maintain good alignment and optimal engagement of the trunk muscles.

The child then started to perform sit-to-stand activities with the PTA. The PTA started this activity using a treatment table that could be raised and lowered. The PTA started with the table in a high position and then guided the child to stand up from the sitting position and then back down to sit. The PTA progressively lowered the table and then worked on the same movement, eventually training the child to stand up from sitting in a regular-height chair.

Next, the PTA worked on standing balance activities, first working on a hard, noncompliant surface, then progressing to foam. Again, play activities were incorporated, also to work on gross and fine motor movements of the upper extremities.

The child has now started to take a few steps with assistance from the PTA. She continues to be engaged in therapy and enjoys the interaction with the therapy staff.

All throughout this episode of care, the rehabilitation team has closely monitored the child's progress. The PTA regularly reported to the PT the child's progress and discussed how those changes might affect the plan of care. Once the PT identified the new plan of care, the PTA began to work toward those new goals. The PT and the PTA also involved the child's family in the rehabilitation process by optimizing adherence to the exercise program and participating in in-clinic activities.

QUESTIONS

1. Are there any inappropriate interventions that were delegated to the PTA during the intervention periods with this child?

2. If the PTA identifies that the child has reached an objective within the plan of care, is it okay to change the plan to progress the child?

CASE #2

Jonathan was born at 25 weeks' gestational age with a birth weight of 1 pound, 15 ounces. His mother reported that although Jonathan spent 2 months in the neonatal intensive care unit (NICU), he did not have any major medical problems. She stated that Jonathan sat at 9 months, crept on hands and knees at 12 months, cruised at 19 months, and walked at 24 months of age. He was started in an early intervention program (EIP) upon his discharge from the NICU and was seen on a twice-a-month basis until his discharge at 3 years of age. The PT who saw Jonathan in early intervention was concerned about his motor planning abilities because he had difficulty getting off the sofa, climbing in and out of large boxes, and changing direction when using a small riding toy at the time of discharge. Based on her recommendation, Jonathan was enrolled in a developmental preschool program after being in the EIP. At 8 years of age, he is currently enrolled in a regular second-grade class.

Jonathan was diagnosed as having developmental coordination disorder by an interdisciplinary evaluation team at age 7 years. He is currently receiving occupational and physical therapy services through the school system. Jonathan's teacher states he is distractible in the classroom and that he tends to give up if he is stressed by a task. Additionally, he rocks or fidgets frequently while sitting in his desk chair. She also notes that he chews on his pencil or other objects during the day. She further reports that he has difficulty keeping pace with his classmates when walking and that he bumps into other children frequently when walking in a line. On the playground, he prefers to be by himself and does not like to participate in age-related play.

On examination by the PT, Jonathan was found to exhibit these behaviors:

- Adequate attention span but distracted by extraneous visual or auditory stimuli
- Good understanding of requests
- Wants feedback often about his performance
- Decreased postural tone but normal deep tendon reflexes
- Postural assessment—flat feet, hyperextension of knees in stance, wide BOS during ambulation, increased lumbar lordosis, and protruding abdomen
- Inconsistent use of right and left hands during fine motor tasks; does not have a preferred hand for writing
- Unable to track with either eye; unable to separate eye and head movement; difficulty with convergence and divergence
- Difficulty with smooth control of movement; during game of Simon Says he performed movement faster than therapist; tends to plop when asked to sit down
- Diadochokinesia—unable to maintain rhythmical pattern with each arm or with both arms together
- Thumb to finger—unable to perform with either hand/both hands together; difficulty with sequencing
- Tongue to lip—good movement to lower lip, upper lip, and sides
- Co-contraction—decreased in arms, shoulders, and neck
- Asymmetric tonic neck reflex quadruped—positive when head turned to the left and right
- Equilibrium reactions—problems with response time when moved quickly in sitting and standing
- Supine flexion—could not assume
- Prone extension—could not assume
- Running—slightly uncoordinated
- Stands momentarily on either foot; unable to jump with both feet together or on one foot
- Skipping—refused

The following lists Jonathan's scores on the Sensory Integration and Praxis Test:

Scores Below Age Expectations

- Bilateral motor control
- Manual form perception
- Finger identification

- Motor accuracy
- Design copy
- Space visualization
- Standing and walking balance
- Postural praxis
- Sequencing praxis
- Figure ground
- Oral praxis
- Constructional praxis
- Postrotary nystagmus

Scores Within Age Expectation

- Graphesthesia
- Localization tactile stimuli
- Kinesthesia

The following is a list of physical therapy intervention activities:

- Increase attention to task using sensory input through use of weighted vest, slanted cushion
- Increase extensor and flexor tone
- Improve co-contraction of neck, shoulder, and pelvic musculature
- Facilitate use of both arms for bilateral motor coordination
- Improve motor planning using a cognitive approach
- Facilitate motor learning through the use of repetition and appropriate feedback scheduling

The PT is seeing Jonathan monthly at school, and the PTA is scheduled to work with Jonathan on a weekly basis. The PT is giving specific activities to the PTA that are to be practiced during the weekly sessions to achieve the stated objectives. When Jonathan has improved his motor function, responds automatically, and may be ready for new activities, the PTA should report to the PT and meet to discuss Jonathan's progress. The PT may decide that Jonathan needs more frequent visits or continue with the same intervention schedule. The PT will delegate treatment to the PTA once Jonathan's new needs are identified, and the PTA will be responsible for continuing practice and monitoring his progress.

QUESTIONS

1. What sensory input might be considered to use with Jonathan to increase his postural tone? How could these inputs be incorporated within the classroom setting?

2. Why do you think that Jonathan is rocking and fidgeting in the classroom?

3. What are some activities that might be suggested to encourage Jonathan to use both hands together?

4. Identify 3 activities that could be conducted with Jonathan to improve stability in the pelvic girdle. How would the PTA recognize that pelvis stability has been improved and that Jonathan is ready for new activities?

5. Identify 2 motor behaviors exhibited by Jonathan that would help the PTA know the goals of strength and stability of the UEs are being met.

6. When is it appropriate for the PTA to change or advance Jonathan into new movement patterns?

REFERENCES

1. World Confederation for Physical Therapy. Policy statement: Description of physical therapy. http://www.wcpt.org/policy/ps-descriptionPT. Accessed October 24, 2012.
2. US Department of Energy. Genome programs. http://www.genomics.energy.gov. Accessed June 18, 2012.
3. Long TM, Brady R, Lapham V. A survey of genetics knowledge of health professionals: implications for physical therapists. *Pediat Phys Ther.* 2001;13(4):156-163.
4. Sanger WG, Dave B, Stuberg W. Overview of genetics and role of the pediatric physical therapist in the diagnostic process. *Pediat Phys Ther.* 2001;13(4):164-168.
5. Smith M, Danoff JV, Jain M, Long TM. Genetic disorders: implications for allied health professionals: two case studies. *IJAHSP.* 2007;5(4).
6. Van Cleve SN, Cohen WI. Part I: clinical practice guidelines for children with Down syndrome from birth to 12 years. *J Pediatr Health Care.* 2006;20(1):47-54.
7. American Academy of Pediatrics. Committee on Genetics. American Academy of Pediatrics: health supervision for children with Down syndrome. *Pediatrics.* 2001;107(2):442-449.
8. Pinter JD, Eliez S, Schmitt JE, Capone GT, Reiss AL. Neuroanatomy of Down's syndrome: a high-resolution MRI study. *Am J Psychiatry.* 2001;158(10):1659-1665.
9. Shumway-Cook A, Woollacott MH. Dynamics of postural control in the child with Down syndrome. *Phys Ther.* 1985;65(9):1315-1322.
10. Cassidy SB, Driscoll DJ. Prader-Willi syndrome. *Eur J Hum Genet.* 2009;17(1):3-13.
11. Cerruti Mainardi P. Cri du Chat syndrome. *Orphanet J Rare Dis.* 2006;1:33.
12. Smeets EEJ, Pelc K, Dan B. Rett syndrome. *Mol Syndromol.* 2012;2(3-5):113-127.
13. Genetics Home Reference. MECP2. http://ghr.nlm.nih.gov/gene/MECP2. Accessed October 24, 2012.
14. US National Library of Medicine. PubMed Health. A.D.A.M. Medical Encyclopedia. Rett syndrome. http://www.ncbi.nlm.nih.gov/pubmedhealth/PMH0002503/. Accessed October 24, 2012.
15. Lotan M. Rett syndrome: guidelines for individual intervention. *Scientific World Journal.* 2006;6:1504-1516.
16. Seppo H, Markku R, Marko N, Pertti K. Detection of Trisomy 18 by double screening in a low-risk pregnant population. *Fetal Diagn Ther.* 1999;14(1):15-19.
17. Crandall BF. Genetic counseling and mental retardation. *Psychiatr Ann.* 1974;4(2):70-95.
18. Bharucha BA, Agarwal UM, Savliwala AS, Kolluri RR, Kumta NB. Trisomy 18: Edwards' syndrome (a case report of 3 cases). *J Postgrad Med.* 1983;29(2):129-132.
19. Understanding muscular dystrophy: the basics. WebMD. http://children.webmd.com/understanding-muscular-dystrophy-basics. Accessed August 24, 2013.
20. Esquenazi A, Packel A. Robotic-assisted gait training and restoration. *Am J Phys Med Rehabil.* 2012;91(11 Suppl 3):S217-S231.
21. Huang VS, Krakauer JW. Robotic neurorehabilitation: a computational motor learning perspective. *J Neuroeng Rehabil.* 2009;6:5.
22. Needleman H. Lead poisoning. *Annu Rev Med.* 2004;55:209-222.
23. Hielkelma T, Blauw-Hospers CH, Dirks T, Drijver-Messelink M, Bos AF, Hadders-Algra M. Does physiotherapeutic intervention affect motor outcome in high-risk infants? An approach combining a randomized controlled trial and process evaluation. *Dev Med Child Neurol.* 2011;53(3):e8-e15.
24. Magalhães LC, Cardoso AA, Missiuna C. Activities and participation in children with developmental coordination disorder: a systematic review. *Res Dev Disabil.* 2011;32(4):1309-1316.
25. Zwicker JG, Mayson TA. Effectiveness of treadmill training in children with motor impairments: an overview of systematic reviews. *Pediatr Phys Ther.* 2010;22(4):361-377.
26. Flapper BC, Schoemaker MM. Developmental coordination disorder in children with specific language impairment: co-morbidity and impact on quality of life. *Res Dev Disabil.* 2013;34(2):756-763.
27. Williams J, Omizzolo C, Galea MP, Vance A. Motor imagery skills of children with attention deficit hyperactivity disorder and developmental coordination disorder. *Hum Mov Sci.* 2013;32(1):121-135.
28. Wilson PH, Ruddock S, Smits-Engelsman B, Polatajko H, Blank R. Understanding performance deficits in developmental coordination disorder: a meta-analysis of recent research. *Dev Med Child Neurol.* 2013;55(3):217-228.
29. Connolly BH, Michael BT. Performance of retarded children, with and without Down syndrome, on the Bruininks Oseretsky Test of Motor Proficiency. *Phys Ther.* 1986;66(3):344-348.
30. McCandless SE, Committee on Genetics. Clinical report—health supervision for children with Prader-Willi syndrome. *Pediatrics.* 2011;127(1):195-204.
31. Cimolin V, Galli M, Vismara L, Grugni G, Priano L, Capodaglio P. The effect of vision on postural strategies in Prader-Will patients. *Res Dev Disabil.* 2011;32(5):1965-1969.
32. Russell DJ, Avery LM, Rosenbaum PL, Raina PS, Walter SD, Palisano RJ. Improved scaling of the Gross Motor Function Measure for children with cerebral palsy: evidence of reliability and validity. *Phys Ther.* 2000;80(9):873-885.

33. Russell D, Palisano R, Walter S, et al. Evaluating motor function in children with Down syndrome: validity of the GMFM. *Dev Med Child Neurol.* 1998;40(10):693-701.

34. Deitz JC, Kartin D, Kopp K. Review of Bruininks-Oseretsky Test of Motor Proficiency, Second Edition (BOT-2). *Phys Occup Ther Pediatr.* 2007;27(4):87-102.

35. Bruininks RH. *Bruininks-Oseretsky Test of Motor Proficiency Examiner's Manual.* Circle Pines, MN: American Guidance Service; 1978.

36. Wuang Y, Su C. Reliability and responsiveness of the Bruininks-Oseretsky Test of Motor Proficiency-Second Edition in children with intellectual disability. *Res Dev Disabil.* 2009;30(5):847-855.

37. Pearson. Gross Motor Development, Second Edition. www.pearsonassessments.com/HAIWEB/Cultures/en-us/Productdetail.htm?Pid=076-1618-201&Mode=summary. Accessed January 17, 2013.

38. Ulrich DA. *Test of Gross Motor Development Second Edition Examiner's Manual.* Austin, TX: Pro-Ed; 2000.

39. Folio MR, Fewell RR. *Peabody Developmental Motor Scales 2nd Edition Examiner's Manual.* Austin, TX: Pro-Ed; 2000.

40. Eldred K, Darrah J. Using cluster analysis to interpret the variability of gross motor scores of children with typical development. *Phys Ther.* 2010;90(10):1510-1518.

41. Boehme R. *Developing Mid-Range Control and Function in Children With Fluctuating Muscle Tone.* Tucson, AZ: Therapy Skill Builders; 1990.

42. Martin K, Kaltenmark T, Lewallen A, Smith C, Yoshida A. Clinical characteristics of hypotonia: a survey of pediatric physical and occupational therapists. *Pediatr Phys Ther.* 2007;19(3):217-226.

43. Ellison PH, Horn JL, Browning CA. Construction of an Infant Neurological International Battery (INFANIB) for the assessment of neurological integrity in infancy. *Phys Ther.* 1985;65(9):1326-1331.

44. Clopton N, Dutton J, Featherston T, Grigsby, A, Mobley J, Melvin J. Interrater and intrarater reliability of the Modified Ashworth Scale in children with hypertonia. *Pediatr Phys Ther.* 2005;17(4):268-274.

45. Mutlu A, Livanelioglu A, Gunel MK. Reliability of Ashworth and Modified Ashworth Scales in children with cerebral palsy. *BMC Musculoskelet Disord.* 2008;9:44.

46. Franjoine MR, Gunther JS, Taylor MJ. Pediatric balance scale: a modified version of the Berg Balance Scale for the school-aged child with mild to moderate motor impairment. *Pediatr Phys Ther.* 2003;15(2):114-128.

47. Franjoine MR, Darr N, Held SL, Kott K, Young BL. The performance of children developing typically on the Pediatric Balance Scale. *Pediatr Phys Ther.* 2010;22(4):350-359.

48. Martin K, Kaltenmark T, Lewallen A, Smith C, Yoshida A. Clinical characteristics of hypotonia: a survey of pediatric physical and occupational therapists. *Pediatr Phys Ther.* 2007;19(3):217-226.

49. Downs JA, Edwards AD, McCormick DC, Roth SC, Stewart AL. Effect of intervention on development of hip posture in very preterm babies. *Arch Dis Child.* 1991;66(7 Spec No):797-801.

50. Bly L. *Motor Skills Acquisition in the First Year: An Illustrated Guide to Normal Development.* San Antonio, TX: Therapy Skill Builders; 1998.

51. Bly L, Whiteside A, Medvescek R. *Baby Treatment Based on NDT Principles.* San Antonio, TX: Communication Skill Builders; 1999.

52. Sackley CM, van den Berg ME, Lett K. Effects of a physiotherapy and occupational therapy intervention on mobility and activity in care home residents: a cluster randomised controlled trial. *BMJ.* 2009;339:b3123.

53. Shields N, Taylor NF. A student-led progressive resistance training program increases lower limb muscle strength in adolescents with Down syndrome: a randomized controlled trial. *J Physiother.* 2010;56(3):187-193.

54. Gupta S, Rao BK, Kumaran SD. Effect of strength and balance training in children with Down's syndrome: a randomized controlled trial. *Clin Rehabil.* 2011;25(5):425-432.

55. Harris SR. Effects of neurodevelopmental therapy on motor performance of infants with Down's syndrome. *Dev Med Child Neurol.* 1981;23(4):477-483.

56. Harris SR, Roxborough L. Efficacy and effectiveness of physical therapy in enhancing postural control in children with cerebral palsy. *Neural Plast.* 2005;12(2-3):229-243, discussion 263-272.

57. Hernandez-Reif M, Field T, Largie S, Mora D, Bornstein J, Waldman R. Children with Down syndrome improved in motor functioning and muscle tone following massage therapy. *Early Child Dev Care.* 2006;176 (3-4):395-410.

58. Lotan M, Isakov E, Merrick J. Improving functional skills and physical fitness in children with Rett syndrome. *J Intellect Disabil Res.* 2004;48(Pt 8):730-735.

59. Angelini C, Tasca E. Fatigue in muscular dystrophies. *Neuromuscul Disord.* 2012;22(Suppl 3):S214-S220.

60. Sackley C, Disler PB, Turner-Stokes L, Wade DT, Brittle N, Hoppitt T. Rehabilitation interventions for foot drop in neuromuscular disease. *Cochrane Database Syst Rev.* 2009;(3):CD003908.

61. Grange RW, Call JA. Recommendations to define exercise prescription for Duchenne muscular dystrophy. *Exerc Sport Sci Rev.* 2007;35(1):12-17.

62. Jansen M, de Groot IJ, van Alfen N, Geurts ACh. Physical training in boys with Duchenne muscular dystrophy: the protocol of the No Use Is Disuse study. *BMC Pediatr.* 2010;10:55.

63. Chaoui R, Heling KS, Sarioglu N, Schwabe M, Dankof A, Bollmann R. Aberrant right subclavian artery as a new cardiac sign in second- and third-trimester fetuses with Down syndrome. *Am J Obstet Gynecol.* 2005;192(1):257-263.

64. Paladini D, Sglavo G, Pastore G, Masucci A, D'Armiento MR, Nappi C. Aberrant right subclavian artery: incidence and correlation with other markers of Down syndrome in second-trimester fetuses. *Ultrasound Obstet Gynecol.* 2012;39(2):191-195.

65. Zalel Y, Achiron R, Yagel S, Kivilevitch Z. Fetal aberrant right subclavian artery in normal and Down syndrome fetuses. *Ultrasound Obstet Gynecol.* 2008;31(1):25-29.

66. Angulo-Barroso R, Burghardt AR, Lloyd M, Ulrich DA. Physical activity in infants with Down syndrome receiving a treadmill intervention. *Infant Behav Dev.* 2008;31(2):255-269.

67. Angulo-Barroso RM, Wu J, Ulrich DA. Long-term effect of different treadmill interventions on gait development in new walkers with Down syndrome. *Gait Posture.* 2008;27(2):231-238.

68. Ulrich DA, Ulrich B, Angulo-Kinzler RM, Yun J. Treadmill training of infants with Down syndrome: evidence-based developmental outcomes. *Pediatrics.* 2001;108(5):E84.

69. Ulrich BD. Opportunities for early intervention based on theory, basic neuroscience, and clinical science. *Phys Ther.* 2010;90(12):1868-1880.

70. Ulrich DA, Lloyd MC, Tiernan CW, Looper JE, Angulo-Barroso RM. Effects of intensity of treadmill training on developmental outcomes and stepping in infants with Down syndrome: a randomized trial. *Phys Ther.* 2008;88(1):114-122.

71. Deutsch JE, Borbely M, Filler J, Huhn K, Guarrera-Bowlby P. Use of a low-cost, commercially available gaming console (Wii) for rehabilitation of an adolescent with cerebral palsy. *Phys Ther.* 2008;88(10):1196-1207.

72. Shih CH, Shih CT, Chu CL. Assisting people with multiple disabilities actively correct abnormal standing posture with a Nintendo Wii Balance Board through controlling environmental stimulation. *Res Dev Disabil.* 2010;31(4):936-942.

73. Shih CH, Yeh JC, Shih CT, Chang ML. Assisting children with attention deficit hyperactivity sisorder actively reduces limb hyperactive behavior with a Nintendo Wii remote controller through controlling environmental stimulation. *Res Dev Disabil.* 2011;32(5):1631-1637.

74. Wuang YP, Chiang CS, Su CY, Want CC. Effectiveness of virtual reality using Wii gaming technology in children with Down syndrome. *Res Dev Disabil.* 2011;32(1):312-321.

75. Bruder MB. Early childhood intervention: a promise to children and families for their future. *Excep Child.* 2010;76(3):339-355.

76. Bronfenbrenner U. *The Ecology of Human Development: Experiments by Nature and Design.* Boston, MA: Harvard University Press; 1979.

77. Van Hooste A, Maes B. Family factors in the early development of children with Down syndrome. *J Early Interv.* 2003;25(4):296-309.

78. American Physical Therapy Association. Role of a physical therapist assistant (PTA). http://www.apta.org/PTACareers/RoleofaPTA/. Accessed October 24, 2012.

79. American College of Medical Genetics. Medical Genetics Scope of Practice. http://www.acmg.net/StaticContent/SOP-for-WEB.pdf. Accessed October 24, 2012.

80. American Academy of Pediatrics. Division of Developmental Pediatrics and Preventive Services (DODPPS). http://www.aap.org/en-us/about-the-aap/departments-and-divisions/department-of-community-and-specialty-pediatrics/Pages/Division-of-Developmental-Pediatrics-and-Preventive-Services.aspx?nfstatus=401&nftoken=00000000-0000-0000-0000-000000000000&nfstatusdescription=ERROR%3a+No+local+token. Accessed February 15, 2013.

81. American Occupational Therapy Association. About occupational therapy. http://www.aota.org/Consumers.aspx. Accessed October 24, 2012.

82. World Federation of Occupational Therapists. Definition of occupational therapy. http://www.wfot.org/AboutUs/AboutOccupationalTherapy/DefinitionofOccupationalTherapy.aspx. Accessed October 24, 2012.

83. American Speech-Language-Hearing Association. Scope of practice in speech-language pathology [Scope of Practice]. http://www.asha.org/docs/html/SP2007-00283.html. Accessed October 24, 2012.

84. American Speech-Language-Hearing Association. Scope of practice in audiology [Scope of Practice]. http://www.asha.org/docs/html/SP2004-00192.html#sec1.3. Accessed October 24, 2012.

Please see accompanying Web site at

www.healio.com/books/neuroptavideos

Clients With
Spinal Cord Injury

Bret Kennedy, PT, DPT
Kelly Ryujin, PT, DPT
Claire E. Beekman, PT, MS, NCS

KEY WORDS

- Autonomic dysreflexia
- Crede
- Paraplegia
- Sacral sparing
- Tetraplegia

CHAPTER OBJECTIVES

- Explain the difference between a complete and incomplete traumatic spinal cord injury (SCI).
- Define sacral sparing.
- Define the motor level and sensory neurological levels of injury.
- Discuss the common characteristics of the clinical picture of a person with SCI.
- Define autonomic dysreflexia and discuss why it is a medical emergency and what the physical therapy assistant (PTA) should do when it occurs.
- Identify complications that may occur with SCI.
- Discuss why pressure sores occur in people with SCI and how they can be prevented.
- Identify and discuss the purposes of physical therapy for people with SCI.
- Discuss physical therapy interventions used by physical therapists and PTAs working with people with SCI.

INTRODUCTION

Traumatic spinal cord injury (SCI) is a devastating, life-changing injury that results in profound functional loss due to motor, sensory, and other impairments. The rate of occurrence in the

Umphred DA, Lazaro RT, eds.
Neurorehabilitation for the Physical Therapist Assistant,
Second Edition (pp 251-296).
© 2014 SLACK Incorporated.

United States is 40 cases per million. Teenagers and young adults are at greatest risk, and motor vehicle accidents (MVAs) are the most common etiology. Injuries are classified using the American Spinal Injury Association (ASIA) Impairment Scale to determine the spinal level and grading of the injury for prognostic value. Currently, with advances in technology, more treatment options are available to clinicians to assist their clients in achieving their highest functional capacity.

Treatment for a patient with SCI usually begins in the acute care setting, which may include the intensive care unit. When the patient is medically stable, he or she is often transferred to a rehabilitation unit to undergo intensive rehabilitative services. As medical stability improves and necessary functional gains are made, the patient may receive physical therapy services in the home and eventually the outpatient setting. Physical therapist assistants (PTAs) are an integral part of the rehabilitation team. PTAs will assist in improving or maintaining joint range of motion (ROM), increasing functional strength and endurance, optimizing safe functional mobility, and educating the patient, family, and caregivers.

EPIDEMIOLOGY OF SPINAL CORD INJURY

Incidence

According to the World Health Organization, 10% of civilian deaths globally are due to traumatic injuries in people aged 5 to 44 years.[1,2] For those suffering spinal trauma, mortality is 17%.[3] As recently as 2012, there were an estimated 40 new cases of SCI per million, or 12,000 per year, in the United States.[4] Young adults are primarily affected by SCIs, with the average age being 41 years since 2005.[5] It was reported that 80.6% of those with SCI are male.[4]

Etiology

MVAs account for almost 40% of reported cases of SCI. Falls and acts of violence, primarily gunshot wounds, are the next 2 most prevalent causes, respectively.[4] The proportion of injuries that are due to sports has decreased over the past 20 years, as has violence (14.6%). There has been a rise in SCIs due to falls (28.3%).[4] The number of injuries from acts of violence peaked in the 1990s and has decreased since then, as have SCIs due to MVAs.[4,5] MVAs, sports injuries, and falls were more likely to result in injuries of the cervical region of the spinal cord, whereas SCIs due to violence were more likely to result in injuries to the thoracic or lumbar and sacral regions of the spinal cord.[5]

Life Expectancy

Life expectancy for those with SCIs continues to increase but remains less than those without SCIs. Determinants of life expectancy are based on the level and extent of injury; those with a higher level of neurological injuries and/or ventilator-dependent individuals have the lowest life expectancy. Mortality rates are highest within the first year of injury. In the past, the leading cause of death was renal failure; today it is pneumonia and septicemia.[4,6]

Pathophysiology

Traumatic SCI often causes immediate and irreversible damage to the spinal cord. The initial injury involves primary and secondary injuries. The primary injury occurs from an external force or impact and causes immediate vascular hemorrhage and rapid cell death at the site of impact. This may result from compression, transection, distraction, and laceration of the spinal cord. The

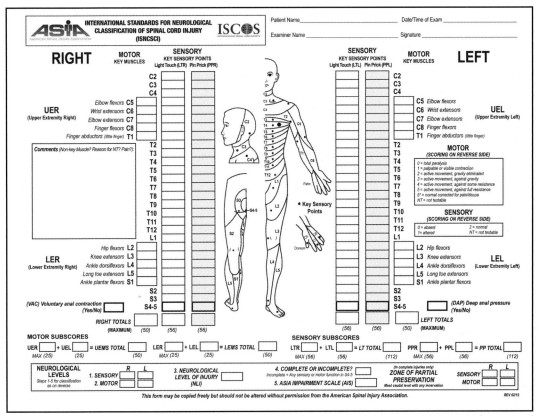

Figure 10-1. Worksheet to consistently document motor and sensory impairments, establish level of injury and determine ASIA impairment scale in persons with SCI. (Reprinted with permission from the American Spinal Injury Association. International Standards for Neurological Classification of Spinal Cord Injury, revised 2013; Atlanta, GA. Reprinted 2013.)

damage causes spinal shock and resultant flaccid paralysis below the level of the lesion. The initial insult or injury is followed by a cascade of secondary injuries that cause further tissue loss and mechanical damage. Edema around the spinal cord will be present and may spread to higher and lower spinal segments within the first 24 hours,[7] extending the neurological level of injury. The extent of the injury depends on the severity of the primary injury. SCIs are most common in the cervical region, C5 in particular.[8]

DESCRIBING THE NEUROLOGICAL INJURY

Neurological Level and Extent of Lesion

A lesion to the spinal cord can affect the transmission of sensory information to the brain and/or motor information to the periphery, depending on the location of the lesion within the spinal cord. Each spinal nerve root innervates a specific area of the skin called a *dermatome* (sensory) and a group of muscles called a *myotome* (motor). Although dermatomal patterns are similar in all people, the precise area of segmental innervation can vary. By accurately assessing a patient's sensation and muscle strength, a clinician can identify whether an injury is complete or incomplete and establish the neurological level of injury (Figure 10-1). Specific criteria described by the ASIA[9,10] are used to make these determinations. Using these criteria ensures that professionals

---

Table 10-1

American Spinal Cord Association Impairment Scale

A. Complete. No sensory or motor function is preserved in the sacral segments S4-S5.

B. Sensory Incomplete. Sensory but not motor function is preserved below the neurological level and includes the sacral segments S4-S5 (light touch, pinprick at S4-S5 or deep anal pressure), AND no motor function is preserved more than 3 levels below the motor level on either side of the body.

C. Motor Incomplete. Motor function is preserved below the neurological level*, and more than half of key muscle functions below the single neurological level of injury (NLI) have a muscle grade < 3 (grades 0 to 2).

D. Motor Incomplete. Motor function is preserved below the neurological level*, and at least half (half or more) of key muscle functions below the NLI have a muscle grade ≥ 3.

E. Normal. If sensation and motor function as tested with the ISNCSCI are graded as normal in all segments and the patient had prior deficits, then the AIS grade is E. Someone without an initial SCI does not receive an AIS grade.

---

*For an individual to receive a grade of C or D (ie, motor incomplete status), he or she must have either (1) voluntary anal sphincter contraction or (2) sacral sensory sparing with sparing of motor function more than 3 levels below the motor level for that side of the body. The standards at this time allow even non-key muscle function more than 3 levels below the motor level to be used in determining motor incomplete status (AIS B versus C).

Note: When assessing the extent of motor sparing below the level for distinguishing between AIS B and C, the motor level on each side is used; whereas to differentiate between AIS C and D (based on proportion of key muscle functions with strength grade 3 or greater) the neurological level of injury is used.

(Reprinted with permission from the American Spinal Injury Association. International Standards for Neurological Classification of Spinal Cord Injury, revised 2011; Atlanta, GA. Reprinted 2011.)

---

who work with people with SCIs will speak a common language, that outcomes of research will be comparable, and that functional predictors can be developed.[9,10]

Complete Versus Incomplete Injury

An incomplete SCI as defined by ASIA is the presence of sacral sparing, which is partial or complete preservation of motor function, sensory function, or both in the lowest sacral segments of the spinal cord (S4 and S5). Anal sensation and/or voluntary contraction of the external anal sphincter indicate sensory and motor incomplete injuries, respectively. Based on the sensory and motor evaluation, the ASIA Impairment Scale (AIS) classifies the patient's injury in 1 of 5 categories: A, B, C, D, or E[9,10] (Table 10-1). With an incomplete injury, motor and sensory function below the injury can vary, depending on the severity of the injury. Remember, a patient may exhibit partial sensory or motor function in segments below the designated neurological level; however, to be considered an incomplete injury, the lowest sacral segments (S4, S5) must have sensory or motor function (sacral sparing). In patients with a complete injury, a zone of partial preservation may exist.[10] This identifies the most caudal segment with some sensory or motor function.[9,10] For example, if a patient's injury is classified as C5, ASIA A, but has impaired sensation to T1, then T1 is said to be the sensory zone of partial preservation.

Level of Injury

The level of injury describes the neurological level of the spinal cord where normal function remains rather than the vertebral level affected. Specific segments of the cord innervate specific muscles. ASIA has deliberately chosen specific muscles for determining the motor level. Most of the chosen muscles are innervated by 2 spinal levels; they are easily accessible to test in supine, and they are significant in terms of functional mobility. For example, the radial nerve innervates the triceps brachii and is composed of nerves from spinal segments of C7 and C8; the C7 nerve innervates a sufficient number of motor units so that a person with a C7 lesion has at least Fair (F) strength (3/5) in the triceps brachii. The triceps brachii muscle is also active in many activities of daily living (ADL). Motor level of injury is determined by the last spinal segment that innervates key muscles at F strength, providing that the muscles innervated at the levels above are of Normal (N) strength.[9,10] Sensory level of injury is determined by the last spinal segment at which sensation is normal for both light touch and sharp/dull discrimination. People with SCIs may have different motor and sensory levels on the right and left sides of the body.

Tetraplegia Versus Paraplegia

Tetraplegia is the preferred term to describe a person with 4 extremities affected by an SCI, replacing the term *quadriplegia*. The extent of involvement in a person with tetraplegia can vary from complete loss of sensory and/or motor function of the upper extremities (UEs) and lower body to only partial loss of UE and lower-body function. Tetraplegia refers only to injuries that involve the spinal cord, not to injuries that affect only the peripheral nerves. T2 is the first level of injury at which the person is said to have *paraplegia*; in paraplegia, the UEs are not affected.

Upper Motor Neuron Lesions (Reflexic) Versus Lower Motor Neuron Lesions (Areflexic)

Most SCIs are considered to be upper motor neuron (UMN) lesions, or reflexic injuries, because the spinal cord is a part of the central nervous system. Symptoms of a UMN injury include spasticity, hypertonicity, and pathological reflexes. Lower motor neuron (LMN) lesions, or areflexic injuries, are seen when the damage is to peripheral nerves (eg, the cauda equina) or following an infarct to the cord. The clinical picture of an LMN injury includes flaccidity, atrophy, and absence of reflexes. It is possible for a patient to have both UMN and LMN involvement if there is spinal cord damage and the adjacent spinal root is involved. Areflexia also occurs during the period of spinal shock that follows anatomical or physiological transection or near transection of the cord.[11] During spinal shock, a transient suppression of reflex activity occurs below the injury. Proposed explanations for this phenomenon include decreased excitability of the spinal neurons, decreased descending facilitation, and increased spinal inhibition.[11,12]

Spinal Cord Injury Syndromes

Damage to specific areas of the spinal cord can result in unique sensory and motor clinical pictures. Based on their clinical presentation, these spinal cord injuries have been categorized into SCI syndromes including Brown-Séquard syndrome, central cord syndrome, anterior cord syndrome, conus medullaris syndrome, and cauda equina syndrome.[13]

Brown-Séquard Syndrome

Brown-Séquard syndrome results from a hemisection of the spinal cord. This type of injury can be caused by a spinal cord tumor, a spinal cord infection (eg, tuberculosis), inflammation of the

Figure 10-2. Brown-Séquard syndrome. Shading designates areas of injury in this schematic cross-section of the spinal cord. Complete hemisection results in the loss of ipsilateral motor function and proprioception and contralateral light touch and superficial pain sensations below the level of injury. (Reprinted with permission from Olson N. Brown-Séquard syndrome. http://en.wikipedia.org/wiki/File:Cord-en.png.)

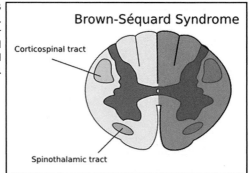

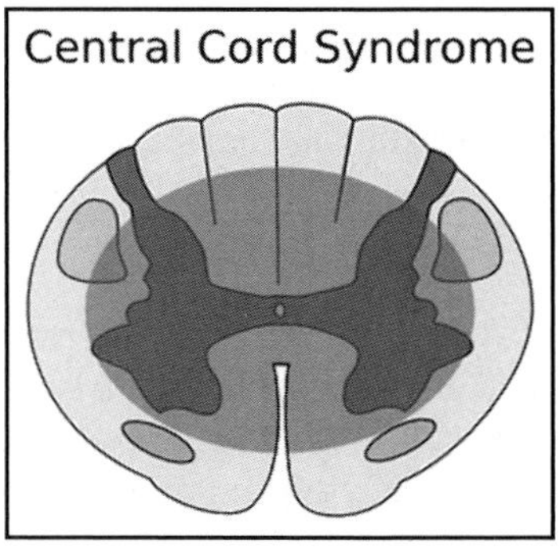

Figure 10-3. Central cord syndrome. Shading designates areas of injury in this schematic cross-section of the spinal cord. There is greater involvement of the upper extremities than the lower extremities because neurons within those tracks are organized by cervical, thoracic, and lumbar regions, with the cervical ones more central. (Reprinted with permission from Olson N. Central cord syndrome. http://en.wikipedia.org/wiki/File:Cord-en.png.)

spinal cord (eg, multiple sclerosis), or penetrating wounds to the spinal cord (eg, knife stabbing or gunshot wound). Because various sensory and motor tracts cross at different levels of the spinal cord, a distinctive clinical picture can be observed. Ipsilateral loss takes place below the level of the injury in the following sensory modalities: proprioception, vibration, 2-point discrimination, and fine touch. Ipsilateral loss may affect motor function below the level of the injury. Contralateral loss involves the following sensory modalities: pain sensation, temperature, and crude touch. A pure injury is rare, but a person can exhibit sensory and motor loss that approximates this distinctive pattern (Figure 10-2).

Central Cord Syndrome

Central cord syndrome usually occurs in the cervical spine, often in individuals with cervical spondylosis who have sustained a cervical hyperextension injury from a fall or MVA. This type of SCI is the most common of the SCI syndromes.[13] The person with central cord syndrome has greater involvement of the UEs than the lower extremities (LEs) because of the location of the spinal tracts and the UEs being more centrally located in the spinal cord than those innervating the LEs[14] (Figure 10-3). A person with central cord syndrome often exhibits bladder dysfunction and can present with varying degrees of sensory loss below the neurological level.

Anterior Cord Syndrome

Anterior cord syndrome is a type of SCI that primarily affects the anterior two-thirds of the spinal cord while sparing the posterior third (posterior columns). Anterior cord syndrome is usually associated with flexion injuries, direct bone fragments, or injuries causing vascular insufficiency. In anterior cord syndrome, the primary motor tract (corticospinal tract) and a sensory tract (spinothalamic tract) are damaged, causing variable motor paralysis with variable loss of pain, temperature, and indiscriminate touch sensation below the level of the lesion. However, because the posterior columns are spared, there is preservation of proprioception, kinesthesia, touch, 2-point discrimination, and vibration sense. Anterior cord syndrome has a poorer prognosis for functional improvement compared with other syndromes.[13]

Conus Medullaris Syndrome

The conus medullaris is the terminal end of the spinal cord, ending at approximately the first or second lumbar vertebrae. Conus medullaris syndrome occurs when there is a lesion in this region, most commonly caused by trauma and tumors. Conus medullaris syndrome presents clinically with a combination of UMN and LMN signs, including saddle anesthesia, areflexic bladder and bowel, and variable degrees of LE weakness.[13]

Cauda Equina Syndrome

Cauda equina syndrome occurs with injury to the lumbosacral nerve roots within the neural canal; therefore, it is not considered to be a true SCI.[13] Cauda equina syndrome is often caused by trauma, tumors, spinal stenosis, disk compression, infection, or postsurgical epidural hematoma.[13] As its etiology suggests, cauda equina syndrome can be caused by an acute process or a slowly progressive condition.

Cauda equina syndrome is considered a pure LMN lesion, without UMN signs. Clinically, cauda equina syndrome presents similarly to conus medullaris syndrome with saddle anesthesia, bladder and bowel dysfunction, and variable LE involvement that is often asymmetrical. It is suggested that cauda equina syndrome has a better prognosis than SCIs due to its being a LMN lesion, and nerve roots have the potential to regenerate. Early surgical decompression is one of the most important predictors for favorable recovery.[13]

CLINICAL PICTURE OF SPINAL CORD INJURY

Traumatic SCIs create various clinical pictures. These depend on many factors, including the neurological level of injury, the extent of injury, and medical complications that may accompany the initial injury. However, some common characteristics exist.

Motor Loss

Loss of motor function below the neurological level of injury is present in those with traumatic SCI. The motor loss may be complete or partial. Based on the segmental innervations of the muscles, ASIA has chosen key muscles to represent each of the neurological levels.[4,9,15,16] A list of the muscles representing each neurological level is provided in the Neurological Classification of Spinal Cord Injury worksheet (see Figure 10-1). These muscles are tested while keeping the patient in a supine position, which is the ASIA standard, and allows safe examination of patients who have an unstable spine. The physical therapist (PT) may ask the PTA to perform follow-up manual muscle tests of select muscles during the individual's rehabilitation. These procedures should follow the ASIA guidelines.

Involvement of Respiratory Muscles

Virtually all patients with SCI will have abnormal pulmonary function and increased risk of chronic respiratory symptoms, additional disability, and higher risk of early death from respiratory complications such as atelectasis and pneumonia.[17,18] Those with higher levels of injury may be ventilator dependent, which in turn is associated with lower functional status and a higher rate of skilled nursing home placement.[18] Those with lower-level injuries will also have compromised

Figure 10-4. Hand position for manual assisted cough. Note how fingers are below the xiphoid process and overlapped to localize force. The patient's head is to the left.

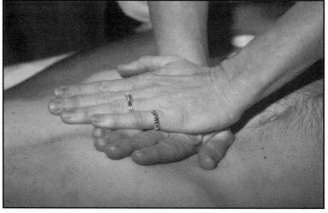

pulmonary function due to respiratory muscle involvement.[7] Forced vital capacity, a measure of restrictive dysfunction; peak expiratory flow rate, a measure of cough effectiveness; and forced expiratory volume in 1 second, a measure of obstructive dysfunction, increase with ascending SCI level, including pulmonary risk as low as L4.[17]

In people without SCI, inspiration is carried out by a combination of the diaphragm (innervated by C3 to C5) and intercostal muscles (innervated by T1 to T11). The intercostal muscles are also used in conjunction with the abdominal musculature (innervated by T8 to T12) for expiration, forced breathing, and coughing. The neck musculature (innervated by C2 to C4) are inactive in those without pathology but may show activity in those with cervical lesions.[19]

When adequate diaphragm function is lacking in those with SCI, patients must receive complete or partial mechanical ventilation. Those with injuries above T8 will be profoundly affected by the lack of expiratory effectiveness, limiting clearance of secretions and cough effectiveness, and will be more susceptible to lower respiratory tract infections.[20] Pneumonia is the leading cause of death among all patients with SCI over time. Patients may require manual assistance for coughing, a technique taught to patients and caregivers by the PT and PTA (Figure 10-4). Abdominal or quad coughing can increase stimulation for coughing and increase the cough flow up to 15% to 33%.[18]

Sensory Loss

After a traumatic SCI, a comprehensive physical examination is completed, including sensory testing that will give valuable information regarding injury level and classification and prognosis of neurological recovery.[21] Sensory loss is common in those suffering traumatic SCIs and presents as loss in a dermatomal pattern. Sensory testing according to ASIA standards includes light touch and pinprick in selected dermatomal areas. These areas are identified on an ASIA worksheet (see Figure 10-1). Sensation is graded as normal, impaired, or absent. When the patient is unable to discriminate between sharp and dull input at a given dermatome, sensation for pinprick is considered absent. Proprioception is also tested and graded. The results of proprioception tests help predict functional outcome because patients with impaired or absent proprioception will have difficulty controlling extremity movement, even with favorable motor function. With a complete injury, all sensation is lost below the level of injury. The PT may ask the PTA to repeat select sensory testing for individuals with an incomplete SCI to determine whether changes have occurred since the initial physical examination and the physical therapy examination. This may provide valuable prognostic information about recovery.

Spasticity

It has been reported that spasticity is seen in 25% of people with SCI. After the initial period of spinal shock, which lasts a variable amount of time after injury, spasticity may occur.[22] It affects skeletal muscles as well as muscles of the bowel, bladder, and sexual organs. The extent of spasticity and the muscles affected varies; it may be minimal or it may interfere with function and sitting position. Spasticity is measured using the Modified Ashworth Scale. Spasticity is often increased by noxious stimulants, such as a full bladder, pressure sores, or urologic infections. Treatment with medications (eg, baclofen, tizanidine) may be required to reduce interfering spasticity. New other measures to manage this problem include modalities and orthopedic surgical interventions such as tendon lengthening.[18] More recently, some patients with intractable spasticity are electing to receive an implantable intrathecal programmable pump that delivers spasticity medication (usually baclofen) into a very specific site near the spinal cord. Favorable results have been reported for spasticity and spasm reduction.[22]

Bowel, Bladder, and Sexual Dysfunction

The majority of people with SCI lose total or partial voluntary control of bowel and bladder function. The nature of the bowel and bladder dysfunction will be determined by whether the injury is reflexic or areflexic and whether it is complete or incomplete. People who lack volitional bladder control will require retraining or implementation of a compensatory voiding program. Methods of voiding urine include using an indwelling, condom, or suprapubic catheter; using intermittent catheterization; or performing a maneuver called *crede*, in which pressing on the bladder forces urine out. This is vital to long-term urinary and renal system integrity. People who lack volitional bowel function may experience incontinence and will require retraining of bowel function and elimination.[23,24] Constipation is very common post-SCI. Prescriptive medications may assist a bowel program. This population is 3 times as likely to have a cholecystitis (gallbladder inflammation).[7] Men with reflexive motor function are able to achieve a reflexive erection either spontaneously or by stimulation but are unable to ejaculate. Most men with areflexic injuries are unable to have erections or ejaculate. Women's menstrual periods may stop for up to a year following SCI,[25] but after that time, normal cycles usually return. Women are able to become pregnant following SCI. Premature infants are a known complication of childbearing in women with SCI.[7]

Autonomic Dysreflexia or Autonomic Hyperreflexia

Autonomic dysreflexia can be a life-threatening complication that can occur with an SCI at T6 or above, most commonly found in complete SCI. The splanchnic nerves, found in the mid-thoracic region, innervate the vessels in the viscera. The viscera are highly vascularized with a large blood supply. The increase in blood pressure (BP) is mostly due to shunting of blood away from the splanchnic vasculature, forcing it to enter the general circulation. Autonomic dysreflexia can vary in intensity, from mild discomfort to an emergency situation. It is caused by a noxious stimuli causing an uncontrolled generalized sympathetic response that causes widespread vasoconstriction and can result in a lethal rise in BP.[26] Normally, patients with an SCI at T6 or above have a relatively low systolic BP of 90 to 110 mm Hg in the sitting position. Therefore, a sudden increase of 20 to 40 mm Hg in systolic and diastolic BP over baseline can indicate an autonomic dysreflexia event is occurring. Paradoxically, bradycardia is often associated with autonomic dysreflexia due to the parasympathetic nervous system attempting to control the sudden increase in BP.

Bladder distention, bowel impaction, pressure sores, catheter irritation, LE hamstring stretching, tight clothing, a restrictive leg bag strap, or medical tests (eg, intravenous pyelogram or barium enema) are common noxious stimuli that can trigger this sympathetic response.[27,28] Signs and

---

Box 10-1

Signs and Symptoms of Autonomic Dysreflexia

- Elevated systolic and diastolic blood pressure (BP)
- Pounding headache
- Chills and goose bumps
- Nausea
- Sweating of the face and neck
- Flushing or blotchiness of the face, neck, and arms
- Restlessness or feelings of apprehension
- Bradycardia or tachycardia
- Blurred vision or spots in the visual field
- Nasal congestion
- Minimal or no symptoms other than elevated BP
- Cardiac arrhythmias

(Adapted from Acute management of autonomic dysreflexia: adults with spinal cord injury presenting to healthcare facilities. Consortium for spinal cord medicine. *J Spinal Cord Med.* 1997;20(3):284-307.)

symptoms of autonomic dysreflexia include increased BP; pounding headache; sweating, flushing, or blotchiness of the face; chills; and blurred vision (Box 10-1).

The following is an example of the normal sequence of events that occurs as the urinary bladder distends for individuals with an intact nervous system. As the bladder fills with urine, the stretch receptors in the bladder walls are activated and transmit impulses to the sacral portion of the spinal cord. As the bladder continues to fill and stretch, the impulses continue to ascend via sensory tracts and synapses in the sympathetic chain ganglia. The impulse continues to ascend to the brain, where the perception of a full bladder is sensed, and the person would likely urinate to inhibit further ascending impulses from the bladder. However, if the bladder is not emptied, there is a sympathetic nervous system response, which includes blood vessel constriction and increased BP. This increased BP is sensed by the baroreceptors in the carotid sinus, and a message is sent to the vasomotor center in the brainstem via the glossopharyngeal nerve. The vasomotor center in turn sends a message down the cord to the sympathetic chain ganglia, triggering a decrease in the sympathetic vasoconstrictive response and ultimately reducing BP.

In individuals with an SCI, as the bladder distends the sequence of events is similar as the ascending messages are sent from the bladder up the spinal cord to the sympathetic chain ganglion. However, the individual with an SCI will not experience a normal sensation of a full bladder and cannot react appropriately to relieve the pressure in the bladder. In people with an SCI at T6 or above, the descending impulse sent from the vasomotor center in the brainstem is unable to travel normally down the cord. The message does not reach the sympathetic chain ganglia, and the BP remains high.[27]

During an episode of autonomic dysreflexia, arterial BP may reach extremely high levels, be prolonged, and cause a cerebrovascular accident and death.[27,29] Because acute elevations of BP represent an immediate threat to the patient's life, autonomic dysreflexia is considered a medical emergency.[29] The source of the irritation that caused autonomic dysreflexia must be identified and eliminated.[27-29] Immediate treatment measures by the PTA would include monitoring the BP, loosening tight clothing or constrictive devices (eg, binder, stockings, or leg strap), getting the patient into the sitting position, making sure urine flow is unimpeded, and notifying the PT, nurse, and physician. All facilities that treat people with SCI should establish procedures for addressing this emergency and assign staff who can respond with the appropriate course of action.

The person with SCI must also recognize the importance of treating autonomic dysreflexia immediately and must be able to instruct others on how to help. In some facilities, patients receive written instructions for what to do should autonomic dysreflexia occur at home. Autonomic dysreflexia can sometimes be prevented by careful attention to bowel and bladder training, skin care, clothing, and catheters. If eliminating the precipitating cause is not sufficient to reduce BP, treatment with an antihypertensive drug will be required.[27-29]

Psychological Reaction to Loss

During the initial period following SCI, patients go through a series of adjustment phases of loss and grieving similar to those described by Kübler-Ross for people who are dying.[30] Patient responses to SCI can vary greatly and may include anger, depression, withdrawal, denial, and having unrealistic expectations about recovery. Those working with the patient can provide better support by understanding this process and helping him or her move through these phases by gaining independence and continuing to modify goals as progress is achieved.

Pain

Pain is a frequent complication to SCI. Pain has often been reported as an important factor in decreased quality of life and has been shown to adversely impact function and participation in a variety of activities (eg, sleep, ADL, community reintegration, recreation) in persons with SCI. Several studies have reported the prevalence to be 66%, with some estimates as high as 86%, with nearly 33% rated as severe pain.[31]

Research into pain following SCI has been limited by lack of consistent pain classifications and the inability to identify the mechanisms involved with the development of this pain. Two types of pain have been identified: (1) nociceptive pain, of which musculoskeletal pain is an example, and (2) neuropathic pain, which may be located above, at, or below the level of injury. Musculoskeletal pain is related to mechanical instability, inflammation, muscle spasm, and overuse of muscles and joints[32] and is described as dull, aching, and movement related.[33] It often involves the shoulder or wrist and may be from improper mobility techniques.[34-36] Transcutaneous electrical nerve stimulation (TENS) can be effective in reducing musculoskeletal pain.[32] Neuropathic pain has a different quality from nociceptive pain. It is described as sharp, stabbing, burning, or electrical pain and is associated with a painful, hypersensitive response to normally non-noxious stimuli.[32,33] The mechanism of neuropathic pain is not known but is thought to be related to damage to neurons within the spinal cord that transmit pain sensation.[33] Chronic neuropathic pain can be incapacitating, and conventional medical management is frequently not effective. Treatment with a combination of medications and modalities may be required.

Complications

Orthostatic hypotension is a drop in BP that often occurs as patients begin transitioning from the supine position (ie, assuming sitting or standing). The loss of the LE muscle pump and normal muscle tone below the level of the lesion can cause pooling of the blood in the legs and abdomen. Because of a decreased amount of blood and oxygen reaching the brain, a patient may become light-headed or even lose consciousness. An abdominal binder or corset and elastic stockings are used to substitute for lost muscle tone. Orthostatic hypotension usually resolves over time, although it may persist for 10 to 12 weeks or longer.[37] Use of a tilt table, recliner wheelchair (w/c), or medication may also be required to help the patient adapt to the upright position.

Deep vein thrombosis (DVT), a blood clot in a vein (usually of the leg), is associated with being inactive (physically, or lack of muscle contraction) or is due to prolonged bed rest. DVT is of medical concern because the clot could become dislodged, travel to the lungs, and cause a pulmonary embolus, which could be fatal. DVT is treated medically with anticoagulants or, if anticoagulants are contraindicated, with the surgical implantation of an inferior vena cava filter.

Common concomitant injuries are injuries that may occur at the same time as the SCI. Specific to SCI, they include fractures of the extremities, injuries to the brachial plexus or abdomen, and brain injuries. Brain injuries occur in more than 50% of people with SCI.[38] Brain injuries may affect the person's ability to participate in rehabilitation because of deficits in learning abilities or cognitive and emotional deficits.

Another complication is heterotopic ossification, an abnormal overgrowth of bone in the joint space and around the joint, which occurs with an incidence of 10% to 20%.[7] Common signs and symptoms are decreased ROM, localized swelling, and pain. It most commonly affects the hips, knees, shoulders, and elbows, in order of prevalence.[7] The PTA who works with the patient daily on functional activities and exercise may be the first person to note these changes. In people with SCI, heterotopic ossification occurs most commonly between the first and fourth month after injury. Risk factors include spasticity, age, pressure ulcers, and trauma to the joint.[7] It may not be visible on radiographs until the bone becomes mature. Treatment is ROM to the affected joint, use of medication (typically etidronate),[39] and, if necessary, surgical removal of the bone.[40]

Demineralization of bone, or decreased bone mineral density (BMD), occurs following complete SCI early after onset, and people with paraplegia and tetraplegia exhibit similar changes. BMD declines significantly during the first 3 months following SCI and reaches a loss of about 37% by 16 months.[40] Decreases in motor activity and marked decrease in weight-bearing activities are the main contributing factors. Once BMD has decreased 37%, the fracture index has been exceeded, and the person is at risk for fractures.[40] People with SCI should be aware of this late-occurring risk, and the PTA must exert caution when working with these people. Despite caution, fractures may occur during transfers or as the consequence of a fall, unusual movement, or LE passive ROM.

Another problem that occurs as a result of sympathetic nervous system dysfunction is impaired temperature regulation. The patient may complain about being cold and require warmer clothing. In the heat, however, the patient will be unable to sweat below the level of injury and can be at risk for heat stroke due to difficulty cooling the body. Problems associated with normal aging, such as musculoskeletal[41] and cardiovascular changes,[42] are magnified in people with SCI; therefore, it is important as a clinician to monitor such situations. Patients with injuries above the T6 level are at greater risk for cardiovascular compromise.[43]

Shoulder pathology is common for those with SCI that require use of manual w/cs for mobility. It is estimated that between 60% to 83% of those with paraplegia report pain since beginning use of a manual w/c.[44] Activities such as transferring to and from the w/c, performing pressure relief maneuvers, and w/c propulsion, as well as altered mechanics, put the patient at risk. Shoulder pathology is common in the extra-articular structures, including those under the subacromial arch, and intra-articular structures (bony surface, labrum). This pathology may be chronic, and patients can require dependent care if they require surgical intervention that immobilizes one arm.

Recovery Following Spinal Cord Injury

The most accurate method used to predict recovery from SCI is the standardized physical examination early after injury performed by the physician that uses the International Standards for Neurological Classification of Spinal Cord Injury. This examination makes it possible for clinicians to classify the degree of impairment and assist in creating a comprehensive plan of care for all disciplines. The information gathered by Model SCI centers using the international neurological standards is captured by the Model Spinal Cord Injury Systems database.[45]

Knowledge about the prognosis for neurological recovery following SCI allows the physician to counsel patients about the time during which recovery occurs and probable functional outcome. Studies have shown that neurological recovery is not related to sex, race, type of fracture, mechanism of injury, or timing or type of surgical procedures.[46] Rather, the most important prognostic variable is completeness of injury. Improved outcomes are seen in younger patients and those with a central cord or Brown-Séquard syndrome; both are incomplete injuries.[37,47] Research completed at the time of this publication has shown that high-dose steroids, usually methylprednisolone, significantly improved neurological outcomes for traumatic SCI when administered within 8 hours of injury and infused for a period of 23 to 48 hours.[48] Research for the efficacy of using high-dose steroid infusion for older children (8 to 16 years of age) is still under review.[49] Researchers have also shown that methylprednisolone may increase the prevalence of myopathy after high-dose infusion.[50] Motor recovery is the principal determinant of a patient's functional capabilities, and the primary determinant of motor recovery is completeness of injury at 1 month. Most motor recovery occurs within the first 6 months, and only a very few people (2%) experience a late conversion from a complete to an incomplete injury, although many may change ASIA classifications within 30 days of injury and have an improved functional prognosis.[45] Key muscles that are innervated at 1 month following injury usually recover to a grade of F or greater, while those that are graded at zero are unlikely to recover to a functional level of F.[51,52] Patients with complete injuries are unlikely to walk at a community level,[52] although they may walk with orthoses for exercise. A higher percentage of patients with incomplete injuries are likely to be community ambulators: 76% of patients with incomplete paraplegia and 46% of those with incomplete tetraplegia.[52]

MEDICAL TREATMENT: STABILIZING THE SPINE

Emergency personnel, paramedics, and emergency room staff must evaluate the extent of the person's injury while taking measures to save the person's life. This includes using medical treatments to stabilize the person's vital signs. If the spine is unstable because of a fracture or dislocation of the vertebrae or disruption of ligaments, stabilizing the spinal column is required. Stabilization of the bones ensures that loss of nerve function is minimized and that alignment and integrity of the spinal column is preserved. At the scene of an accident and before vertebral stabilization, care is taken to prevent movement of the neck or back, which could cause further damage to the spinal cord. Late symptoms of cervical instability include pain and tenderness at the site of the fracture or injury, increased radiating neck and arm pain, and increased loss of sensation or strength. When the patient reports symptoms of this nature, treatment must be stopped and the PT and physician notified immediately.

There is strong evidence that early surgical stabilization of patients with unstable spinal columns has favorable outcomes. A systematic review by Dimar et al[53] showed shorter hospital and intensive care unit stays, fewer days on mechanical ventilation, and a lower rate of pulmonary complications. This effect was found in those with more severe injuries.[53]

Nonsurgical stabilization (if not surgically stabilized, and/or in addition to) may allow earlier mobilization. This is achieved by the application of orthotics. Depending on the nature of the injury, the appropriate orthosis is applied (usually custom made by an orthotist).

A halo vest (Figure 10-5) or collar (Figure 10-6) for neck injuries or a thoracolumbosacral orthosis (TLSO), also called a *body jacket* (Figure 10-7), for thoracic and lumbar injuries may be applied. The length of time the patient wears the device and restrictions on movement and activities during the time of healing depend on the type of fracture and stabilization, how well the fracture heals, and the protocol of the physician and facility. The PTA must look for and pay close attention to any restrictions listed in the medical record. It is important to check the patient's skin for redness or breakdown when the brace is being applied or removed and discuss with nursing and the physician if these problems arise.

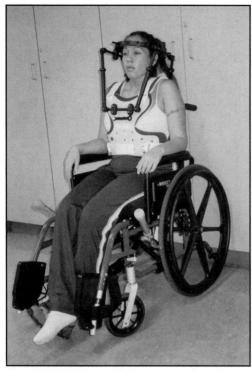

Figure 10-5. Patient with cervical vertebral fracture immobilized in a halo vest.

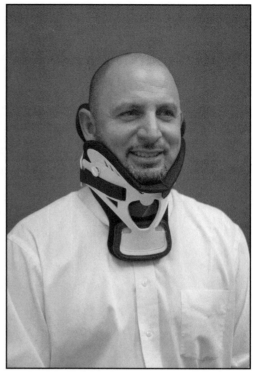

Figure 10-6. Miami collar.

Figure 10-7. Thoracolumbosacral orthosis.

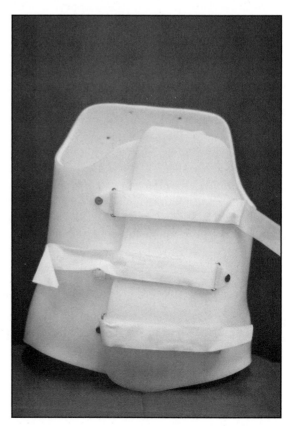

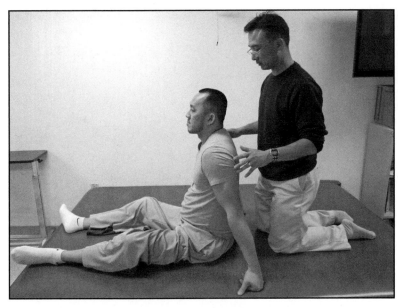

Figure 10-8. Clinicians need to avoid inadvertently overstretching the back extensor muscles, which can occur when the person with tight hamstring muscles leans forward to perform functional activities in long sitting.

PHYSICAL THERAPY INTERVENTIONS

Prevent Deformity and Maintain and Protect Joint Range of Motion

Positioning, passive ROM exercises, and the use of orthoses or splints can prevent loss of joint motion. This is especially important when the person is unable to move his or her extremities or when an imbalance between agonist and antagonistic muscles occurs because of the level of injury or hypertonic muscles. For example, an individual with C5 tetraplegia will often rest his or her elbows in a flexed position because the elbow flexors are innervated but the elbow extensors are not. Splints can help hold elbows in extension when the person is not using the arms for functional activities, helping to avoid elbow flexion contractures. Elbow flexion contractures for individuals with SCI can be extremely limiting for mobility and ADL, especially for individuals without triceps strength. In people with cervical injuries, the shoulders are particularly vulnerable to developing limited ROM and associated pain. Close attention to maintaining ROM, especially abduction and external rotation of the shoulder, and interventions to reduce pain, such as heat, cold, or TENS, are important to prevent a disabling pain cycle.

All joints should be kept mobile; however, some joints need to be protected from overstretching. Clinicians need to avoid inadvertently overstretching the back extensor muscles, which can occur when the person with tight hamstring muscles leans forward with the knees straight in the long sitting position (Figure 10-8). If the trunk muscles and ligaments are overstretched, the trunk will tend to elongate during transfers, making it more difficult to clear the buttocks. For patients with high cervical injuries, rolling will also be more difficult with an overstretched trunk because the upper trunk will roll without the lower trunk following.

Even individuals with complete tetraplegia who are not expected to ambulate must maintain adequate ROM of hips, knees, and ankles. For example, if the hip and knee flexors are tight, there is an increased chance of skin breakdown in the heels and the sacral/coccygeal region when the patient is lying supine. The hip and/or knee flexion contractures will not allow the weight to be distributed through the surface area of the thighs and legs, thereby increasing the pressure on

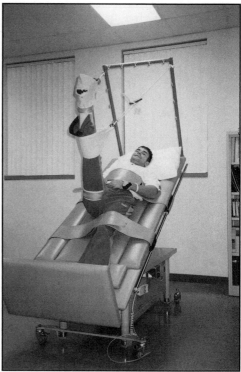

Figure 10-9. Using a tilt table also allows for stretching the weight-bearing plantarflexors and assists with acclimating to the vertical position.

the bony prominences of the pelvis and feet. Patients are encouraged to lie prone to lengthen hip flexors and knee flexors and improve trunk extension. Lying prone for extended periods will also allow improved blood flow to the buttocks and areas that are frequently compromised because of prolonged periods of sitting. Also, ankle plantarflexion contractures can make it difficult for the feet to stay on the w/c foot rests and also decrease the stability of the foot/ankle (base of support) during transfers.

People with complete SCI who will be performing ADL in long sitting (eg, dressing, scooting, recreating, exercising) need 100 to 110 degrees of hamstring range, as determined by flexing the hip with the knee straight (straight leg raise [SLR]). By maintaining approximately 110 degrees of SLR, an individual can rely on the passive insufficiency of the muscles to provide stability in long sitting for ADL. Stretching the hamstrings is most effective when performed for long durations one LE at a time with the pelvis stabilized as much as possible in the supine position. A device such as the one in Figure 10-9 may be used. Initially, physical therapy personnel will need to provide passive LE ROM. People with adequate UE function can learn to perform their own passive LE ROM, typically with the assistance of a strap.

People with tetraplegia who lack triceps function need full elbow extension and wrist extension to lock the elbows for functional activities (eg, transfers and sitting balance). Because of the shape of the ulna and distal humerus, passive stretching of the elbow may cause soft tissue damage. Using a resting splint can help maintain full ROM.

For patients who have wrist extension (C6 innervation) but do not have innervation to the finger flexors (SCI above C8 level), the long finger flexors and the flexor pollicis longus are allowed to become functionally shortened. This allows the patient to flex the fingers and oppose the thumb to the index finger when the wrist is extended. This is called *functional wrist tenodesis*. PTAs play an active role in providing interventions to prevent deformity and increase or maintain ROM and in performing goniometric measurements to demonstrate progress. They may also be involved in teaching the individual and family members how to perform stretching and ROM.

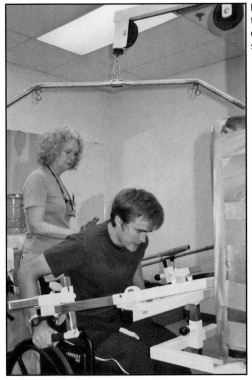

Figure 10-10. The PTA assists the patient to maintain a forward trunk position while performing upper extremity–strengthening exercises. The patient is performing reverse dips to strengthen the elbow and shoulder extensor muscles.

Strengthen Weak Muscles

Muscles that are innervated below the level of injury will lose function or demonstrate weakness. Bed rest is common after SCI and is associated with diminished muscle function and endurance. Muscles with remaining function must be strengthened by progressive resistive exercise to provide the maximum strength possible for performing functional activities (Figures 10-10 and 10-11). In people with complete SCI, the UE muscles must substitute for those lost in the LEs for transfers and w/c propulsion. Specific muscles most vulnerable to fatigue during w/c propulsion are the pectoralis major, supraspinatus, middle and posterior deltoid, subscapularis, and middle trapezius.[54] People with tetraplegia are at greater risk of shoulder pathology because their UE muscles are weaker than those of able-bodied people and people with paraplegia,[55] and activities such as grooming will require different patterns of muscular activity than those used by able-bodied people.[56] People with incomplete injuries also require strengthening of LE muscles (Figure 10-12). The PTA will need to perform periodic manual muscle tests of specific muscles to modify the patient's exercise program and determine when advancing the functional program is warranted. The American College of Sports Medicine (ACSM) recommends performing 2 to 4 sets of 8 to 12 repetitions (failure occurs between the 8th and 12th repetition) and performing 8 to 10 exercises that train the major muscle groups. It is recommended that exercise for each muscle group occur on 2 or 3 nonconsecutive days each week with moderate intensity level (6 on a 10-point ordinal scale).[57] Specificity of training should be used. Nonstandard positions may be preferred, as patients with SCI will likely use altered mechanics and positions for functional mobility and need to be strong in these alternative positions. Progressive resistive training can be performed using weights, pulleys, machines such as a Rickshaw machine (Figure 10-13), or the patient's own body weight (Figure 10-14).

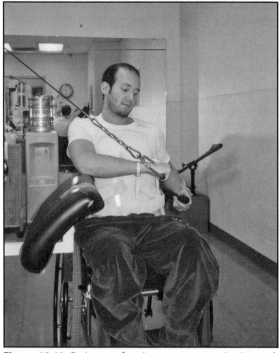

Figure 10-11. Patient performing upper extremity internal rotation exercise with weights. The patient lacks lower trunk musculature and uses his left arm to help stabilize his body while performing the exercise.

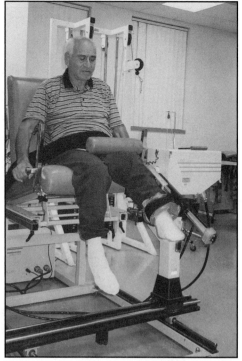

Figure 10-12. Patient with incomplete tetraplegia performing quadriceps strengthening exercises using an isokinetic machine.

Figure 10-13. The Rickshaw machine.

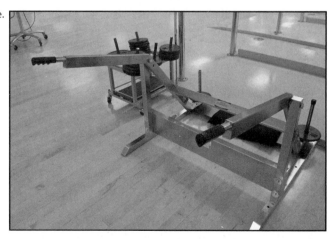

Develop Endurance

Endurance training is aimed at improving muscular performance and aerobic capacity to improve the efficiency of mobility and improve overall health. Disproportionately high rates of cardiovascular disease and hypertension occur in people with SCI compared with able-bodied individuals.[42] Some people have difficulty maintaining an ideal body weight because of limited ability to exercise, which may cause functional decline. Endurance can be achieved by weight training with low weights and a high number of repetitions, use of an UE ergometer or similar device, and w/c propulsion, all of which are interventions appropriate for the role of the PTA.

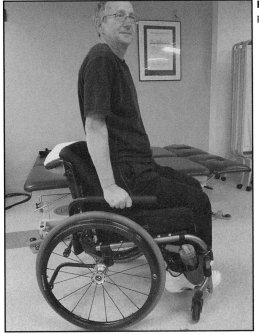

Figure 10-14. Strengthening the upper extremities using the patient's own body weight.

The ACSM guidelines for muscular endurance include moderate intensity exercise (6 of 10), 15 to 20 repetitions to failure, 2 to 4 sets.[57] ACSM guidelines for cardiovascular endurance include moderate-intensity cardiorespiratory exercise training for 30 or more minutes a day on 5 or more days per week. Vigorous intensity cardiorespiratory exercise is recommended 20 or more minutes for 3 or more days a week. These can be combined to achieve an energy expenditure of more than 500 to 1000 metabolic equivalents per week.[57]

Respiratory Program

People with thoracic-level injuries initially demonstrate lower respiratory measurements than able-bodied people. Respiratory function returns to able-bodied levels when they undergo UE muscle training.[58] The respiratory program for people with cervical-level injuries focuses on interventions for developing strength and endurance in the respiratory muscles; maintaining rib cage mobility; and learning assisted cough, bronchial hygiene, and postural drainage for home use. People who are ventilator dependent can learn specialized voluntary breathing techniques, such as neck breathing[59] or glossopharyngeal breathing.[60]

High compliance with a structured inspiratory training program using diaphragm weights (Figures 10-15A and B) or an inspiratory muscle trainer 15 to 30 minutes per day, 5 to 7 days a week for 6 to 8 weeks, has been shown to result in increased vital capacity (VC), inspiratory capacity, and maximal expiratory pressure.[61,62] Lerman and Weiss describe a variety of respiratory exercises that can be incorporated into a respiratory program, including breath holding, taking triple breaths for rib cage expansion, and neck exercises.[62] Exercises can be made more difficult by increasing resistance, increasing the time that the exercise is performed, and changing the patient's position. Weekly monitoring of VC is used to assess patients' progress and modify the respiratory program, as needed. VC is greater in people with cervical injuries in supine[14] and in people with lower injuries in sitting. Using a consistent position allows for more accurate assessment of respiratory function. A corset or abdominal binder can assist with respiration when the patient is sitting, as it helps substitute for the abdominal muscles and improve the lung volume. People with C6 injuries may have a VC of 20% to 30% of normal initially but typically have a VC of 65% of normal at more

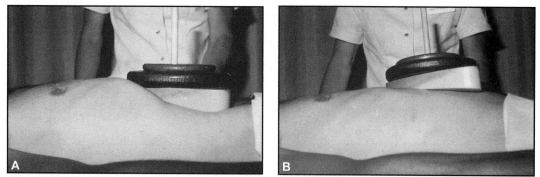

Figure 10-15. Inspiratory training using diaphragm weights. The triangular weight part is designed to fit in the area below the xiphoid process. Note position of the diaphragm (A) before the patient takes a breath, and (B) after. The patient's head is on the left.

long-term follow-up.[63] PTAs working in rehabilitation settings serving patients with SCI may be actively involved in providing all of the interventions discussed above, including testing VC.

Learn Functional Skills

The person with a complete SCI or residual impairments from an incomplete SCI will need to perform functional activities in a modified manner. The extent of independence achieved and the way in which these activities are performed will depend on the level and completeness of injury. Functional activities include bed mobility and transfers; sitting pressure relief; eating; grooming; dressing; bathing; hygiene; ensuring adequate bowel and bladder function; driving, walking, and moving around in the community; and meal and home management activities. See Table 10-2 for a summary of select activities for given levels of SCI, and refer to the Consortium for Spinal Cord Medicine publication *Outcomes Following Traumatic Spinal Cord Injury: Clinical Practice Guidelines for Health-Care Professionals* for more detail on expected outcomes.[64] As mentioned above, patients with injuries above C8 can use a tenodesis grip to manipulate objects. Tenodesis is the passive closing of the fingers and opposition of the thumb to the index finger when the wrist is actively extended. When practicing mat activities, like propped sitting, care must be taken to maintain finger flexion needed for a tenodesis grip; overstretching of the long finger flexors can severely impair hand function for these patients. Patients who have manual muscle grade of 3 of 5 (fair) in their biceps but lack shoulder strength may be fitted with mobile arm supports (Figure 10-16). This device attaches to the w/c to help support the shoulder while the patient bends his or her elbow for activities such as eating and combing hair.

PTAs play a key role in providing functional training interventions and assessing the current level of assistance required by the patient with an SCI.

Head-Hips Relationship

When teaching new functional mobility skills, it is important to teach the patient the concepts of head-hips relationship, levers, unweighting extremities, and the use of momentum.

The concept of head-hips relationship becomes very important in bed mobility and functional transfers. As the patient moves his or her head in one direction, the hips move in the opposite direction. For example, if the patient is in short sitting with arms on the mat in elbow extension and moves his or her head down toward the feet, the hips will lift up; if while lifting the buttocks off the mat with the UEs the head is turned to the left, the hips will then move to the right.

			Table 10-2		
			Select Functional Outcomes for Persons With		
			Complete Spinal Cord Injury		

SCI Level	Muscles Present*	Transfer Type	Functional Capabilities	Wheelchair Type
C1 to C3	Scalenes, partial SCM, trapezius	Mechanical lift; dependent	Mouthstick activities. Sip and puff, possibly chin control or mouth joystick for ECU. Power-assisted pressure relief, mechanical vent (bedside and portable). Total assist for eating and all ADL.	Power w/c with recliner or tilt-in-space with sip and puff, mouth or possibly head control joystick
C4	Diaphragm (partial), SCM, upper trapezius	Mechanical lift; dependent	Mouthstick activities. Sip and puff, possibly chin control or mouth joystick for ECU. May use MAS. May be able to breathe without a vent. Total assist for eating and all ADL.	Power w/c with recliner or tilt-in-space with sip and puff, mouth, or possibly head control joystick; may need tray
C5	Diaphragm, deltoids, <u>biceps</u>, brachialis, brachioradialis, possibly rhomboids, serratus anterior (possibly)	Mechanical lift; dependent, possibly assisted sliding board	Self-feeding, light grooming, light functional activities, computer use with wrist and hand orthoses. Forward pressure relief, possibly with loops.	Power w/c with recliner or tilt-in-space with hand control, possibly in midline
C6	<u>Radial wrist extensors</u>, pectoralis major (clavicular portion), serratus anterior, latissimus dorsi (partially)	Sliding board with assistance or independently; possibly depression lift	Rolling, coming to sit, dressing, grooming, short and long sitting balance. Forward pressure relief. Drive car with assistive devices.	Power upright with hand control, possibly ultralight manual with friction rims
C7	<u>Triceps</u>, wrist flexors, finger extensors, pectoralis major, sternal portion, latissimus dorsi	Depression lift; may require a sliding board	Rolling, coming to sit, dressing, grooming, short and long sitting balance, w/c into car. Depression or forward pressure relief.	Ultralight manual w/c, possibly with friction rims; possibly power w/c
C8	<u>Flexor digitorum profundus</u>, finger flexors, thumb movements	Depression lift	Depression pressure relief. Independent functional activities except floor and stairs.	Ultralight manual w/c

(continued)

Table 10-2 (continued)

Select Functional Outcomes for Persons With Complete Spinal Cord Injury

SCI Level	Muscles Present*	Transfer Type	Functional Capabilities	Wheelchair Type
T1	Intrinsic muscles of the hand, <u>abductor digiti minimi</u>	Depression lift	Same as C8.	Ultralight manual w/c
T2 to L1	Increasing innervation of the intercostals, trunk flexors and extensors	Depression lift	Ambulation with RGOs and UE assistive devices, for exercise only. Modified independent for all functional activities.	Ultralight manual w/c
L2	<u>Iliopsoas</u>, quadratus lumborum, hip flexors	Depression lift	Ambulation with KAFO or RGOs and UE assistive devices, for exercise only. Modified independent for all functional activities.	Ultralight manual w/c
L3	<u>Quadriceps</u>	Stand or squat pivot	Ambulation with AFO and UE assistive devices. Modified independent for all functional activities.	Typically still requires lightweight or ultralight manual w/c
L4-L5	<u>Tibialis anterior (L4)</u>, <u>extensor hallucis longus (L5)</u>, ankle dorsiflexors, knee flexors, hip abductors	Stand pivot	Ambulation with AFOs. May not require UE assistive devices. Modified independent for all functional activities.	May require a w/c for long distances
S1	<u>Gastrocnemius/ soleus</u>, plantarflexors, hip extensors	As able bodied	Ambulation with no orthoses or UE assistive devices. Independent functional activities.	May be modified independent for bowel and bladder care; no w/c

*New muscles at each level are in addition to previously innervated muscles. Underlined muscles are ASIA key muscles for that level (ISNCSCI, 2002).

AFO=ankle-foot orthosis; ECU=environmental control unit; KAFO=knee ankle foot orthosis; MAS=mobile arm support; RGO=reciprocating gait orthosis; SCM=sternocleidomastoid muscle.

Modified independent: independent with adaptive equipment.

Guidelines may require modification for cardiovascular, musculoskeletal, neurological, or other problems.

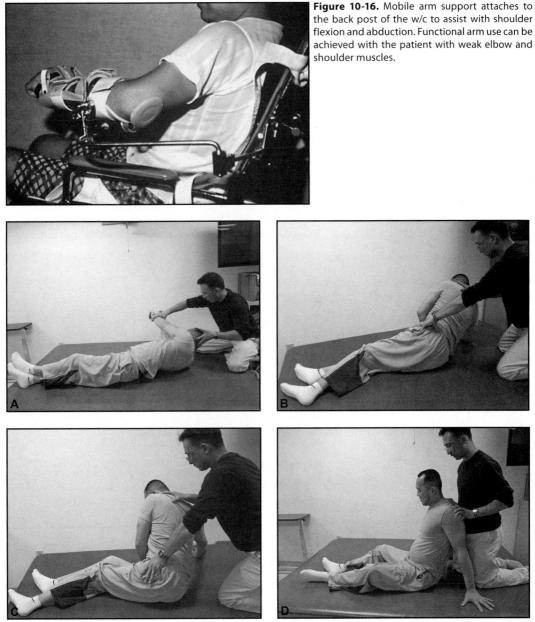

Figure 10-16. Mobile arm support attaches to the back post of the w/c to assist with shoulder flexion and abduction. Functional arm use can be achieved with the patient with weak elbow and shoulder muscles.

Figure 10-17. Bed-mobility activities with a patient with T7 ASIA A SCI. (A) Coming to sit on the mat. The patient rolls to his side and the PTA assists him to initiate the sitting movement. (B) The patient moves his arm up on the mat in preparation for pushing to sitting. (C) The patient continues to move his arms around in front of him until he is sitting upright. (D) The patient continues to move his arms around until he is in the long sitting position. He will be able to do this independently, with practice.

Bed Mobility

Bed mobility consists of rolling, scooting, moving up and down in bed, balance activities, coming to sitting (Figures 10-17A through D), long and short sitting (Figure 10-18) balance, LE management, and self-ROM. Speed of movement and momentum are especially important for patients with tetraplegia.

Figure 10-18. Patient with T7 ASIA A SCI in short sitting, practicing balance activities with the PTA.

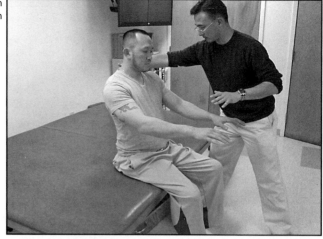

Figure 10-19. The PTA assists a patient with T7 ASIA A SCI in practicing a depression lift on the mat. Practicing this skill will make transfers easier to perform.

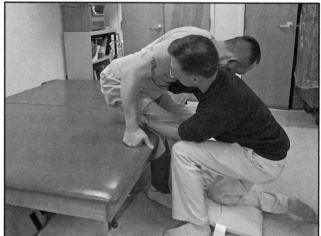

Transfers

Transfers allow the person to move from place to place, including to or from a lower or higher surface. For the person with high tetraplegia, a dependent transfer or use of a mechanical lift will be required. A sliding board can assist people who have UE weakness or are unstable during movement. A depression transfer, or a lift-pivot transfer, can be used by people with greater UE strength and better body awareness. A depression transfer is accomplished when the person straightens his or her elbows, depresses the shoulders, lifts the buttocks off the supporting surface, uses head-hips relationship, turns, and moves onto a nearby surface (Figures 10-19 and 10-20). A stand- or squat-pivot transfer is used by people with sufficient motor function to take weight on their LE. Transfers to all surfaces are practiced, including to a mat or the floor (Figures 10-21A through C), a bed, a toilet, a w/c, a bathtub, a car, the ground, and other sitting surfaces. The PT or PTA must be skillful in assisting the patient during the transfer, and the patient must have confidence in the person assisting. Initially, the patient may fail to lean far enough forward or move his or her shoulders and head enough to transfer efficiently. Details on how to perform functional activities for people at varying levels of injury can be found in the book *Spinal Cord Injury: Functional Rehabilitation*, by Somers.[65]

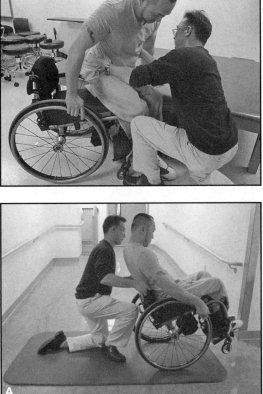

Figure 10-20. The PTA assists a patient with T7 ASIA A SCI with depression transfer to the w/c. Note how the patient turns his head to the right as he lifts his body to facilitate movement of his buttocks to the left onto the w/c (head-hips relationship).

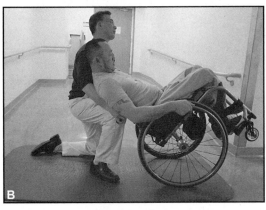

Figure 10-21A. Transfer activities. The PTA assists a patient with T7 ASIA A SCI in practicing w/c to floor transfers. PTA lowering the patient to the floor. Brakes are locked to help control the descent.

Figure 10-21B. Patient controls his knees with his arm for protection as he is further lowered to the ground.

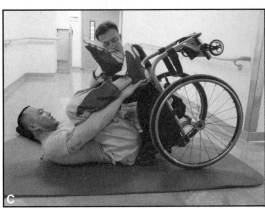

Figure 10-21C. After the patient is lowered to the floor, the PTA unlocks the brakes. The patient controls his lower extremities with his hands as the PTA pulls the w/c out from under the patient.

Figure 10-22. The PTA walking with a patient with C6 tetraplegia, ASIA D. Bilateral arm troughs on the walker are needed because of weakness in the triceps and finger flexors. Under his trousers, the patient is wearing bilateral polypropylene AFOs with a dorsiflexion assist and dorsiflexion stop. Cosmesis with this type of AFO is excellent.

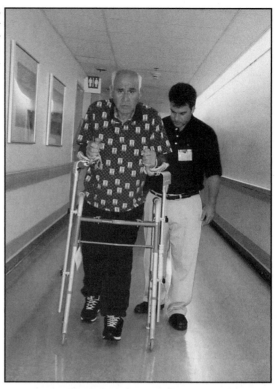

Wheelchair Mobility Training

W/C mobility training involves learning to maneuver in tight spaces: over uneven terrain, like gravel or grass; over a threshold; up and down ramps; through doors; and backward, forward, and to the sides. A person using a manual w/c who has sufficient UE motor control may learn more advanced w/c skills, such as how to navigate curbs and go up and down stairs. The position of the wheel axle in relation to the patient's hips, the angle of the seat (anterior to posterior), the amount the wheels flare out (camber), and the patient's position in the w/c are important in maximizing the efficiency of w/c propulsion.

A person in a manual w/c learns to perform a wheelie, balancing on the large wheels while tilted backward. Patients can practice this while attached to an overhead safety cord or being spotted by the clinician, usually using a gait belt attached to a sturdy part of the w/c frame. Helping the patient find the balance point while in a wheelie is critical in mastering this skill.

The surface the person pushes on affects velocity, with tile being easier than carpet. In a manual w/c, a person with a higher injury level may push at a slower speed and will likely travel shorter distances than a person with a lower level injury. People with C6 tetraplegia are so limited by UE weakness that they are unable to navigate a 4% grade and no method of manual propulsion is efficient.[66]

Gait training is an important part of functional training for people who have sufficient motor recovery in their LEs, particularly those with incomplete injuries. People with SCIs who ambulate may require LE orthoses to substitute for weak muscles.[67] An ankle-foot orthosis (AFO) can substitute for weak dorsiflexor muscles to prevent foot drop in swing and loading response. An AFO can also substitute for weak plantarflexor muscles by preventing unrestrained dorsiflexion in stance (Figure 10-22). A knee-ankle-foot orthosis (KAFO) is used to substitute for weak quadriceps muscles (Figure 10-23). An erroneous, yet commonly held, belief of many clinicians is that use of an LE orthosis will prevent a muscle from contracting and, therefore, impede return of strength.

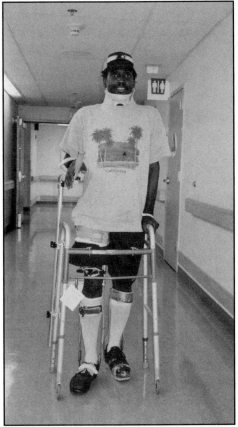

Figure 10-23. Patient with tetraplegia walking with trial orthoses. Using these temporary orthoses—right KAFO and left AFO—allows ambulation before the patient's permanent orthoses are ordered and fabricated. The arm trough helps support the patient's right arm, which has weakness of the triceps muscle.

This concept has not been supported in research of calf muscle function in people with SCI,[68] so an AFO should be used when it improves patient function during gait or transfers. More extensive orthoses, such as a hip-knee-ankle-foot orthosis (HKAFO), are usually too cumbersome, although a reciprocating gait orthosis (RGO), which controls the hip, may be used to provide assistance in advancing the leg and, therefore, may be used by people with low cervical or thoracic injuries.

Body weight–support devices, provided by an overhead unweighting system, combined with treadmill walking or over ground can facilitate ambulation in people with incomplete SCI (Figure 10-24). Trainers or mechanical devices assist the patient in moving his or her legs in a normal gait pattern, and speeds approaching those of normal walking are attained. No evidence currently exists that this intervention has carryover to walking over ground in people with complete injuries.

Although people with complete lesions are usually unable to rely on walking as their primary mode of mobility, they may use it as a form of exercise. The high energy cost of lifting the body with the arms, the slow velocity at which people in KAFOs or RGOs travel, and the demand on the shoulder musculature make this type of walking impractical. Another method of exercise ambulation uses electrical stimulation to activate the LE muscles. The energy cost per meter traveled is similar for walking with KAFOs, RGOs, and electrical stimulation aides.[69]

At the time of this publication, robotic technology for ambulation specific for patients with SCI is being researched. Researchers have been developing various robotics, some of which are programmable for use with body weight–supported treadmill gait training, and some of which are programmable, mobile, battery-operated, wearable exoskeletons.[70,71] ROM limitations, such as hip flexion, knee flexion, or ankle plantarflexion contractures, will interfere with the person's ability

Figure 10-24. Body weight–supported treadmill training. Staff are positioned to assist in moving the legs and to control trunk rotation and weight shift.

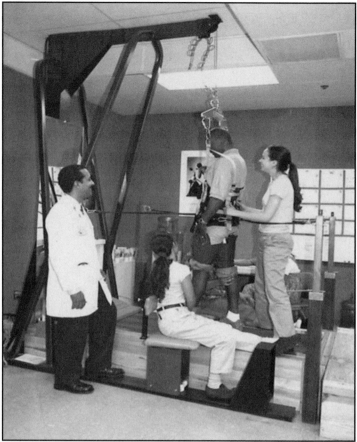

to walk. Plantarflexion contractures can usually be decreased by stretching in standing or using serial casts whereby sequential casts are applied to the ankle as the contracture is lessened. To stretch hip-flexion contractures, the opposite hip must be flexed sufficiently to stabilize the pelvis. In supine, the hip being stretched hangs off the table in neutral abduction, with weights to help pull the leg down. Patients are also encouraged to lie prone to lengthen hip flexors and improve trunk extension. Abnormal tone may also interfere with general mobility. Antispasticity medications taken orally or delivered through an implanted pump may assist in managing abnormal muscle tone that can interfere with normal movement patterns.

Provide Community Reentry Activities

Visits into the community, with trips to movies, restaurants, or amusement parks; introduction to w/c sports; and similar activities are coordinated by a multidisciplinary team. In some communities, outreach programs provide an opportunity for individuals to participate in competitive sports and outdoor recreation.

Obtain Adaptive Equipment

The PT and occupational therapist (OT) are 2 team members responsible for selecting and prescribing most of the appropriate adaptive equipment. The PT may ask the PTA for input and suggestions, especially if the PTA has been practicing these functional activities with the patient and is more aware of the patient's status. Depending on an individual facility's policies, the PTA

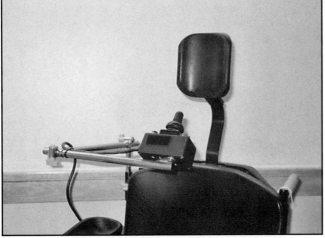

Figure 10-25. Power w/c with head and chin control.

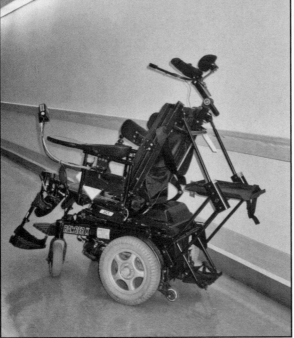

Figure 10-26. Power w/c with ventilator tray. The cheek switch to operate the power recliner is attached to the headrest. Accessories include trunk supports and arm troughs.

may be responsible for ordering and obtaining some of the equipment once it has been selected by the team.

Wheelchair

Many people with an SCI rely on a w/c for mobility. The most appropriate w/c for a given person depends on many factors, including the person's level of injury, age, UE strength, vocational or school plans, living situation, resources, or whether he or she has other medical problems. People who are older or weaker or have medical problems may require a power w/c, even with paraplegia or an incomplete injury. Patients with C1 to C4 injuries will require a power w/c with head, chin (Figure 10-25), or sip and puff control to drive the chair. People who lack the ability to perform pressure relief will need a w/c with power recline or tilt (Figure 10-26). Even people who walk

Figure 10-27. Ultralight manual w/c.

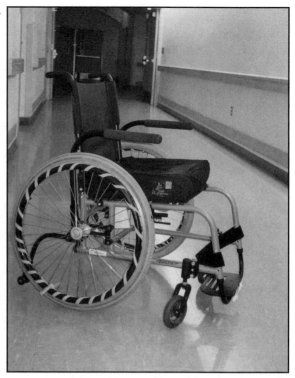

limited distances may require a w/c for community mobility. A rigid-frame ultralight manual w/c (Figure 10-27) is often recommended over a folding w/c for people who are more active or those who require a lighter, more efficient w/c due to UE weakness. The energy cost for pushing a rigid, ultralight w/c is less than for the heavier, collapsible w/cs because the majority of the propulsive energy goes into the wheels rather than into the joints of the collapsible chair.[72] Many w/c components, such as the back height and type, seat to floor height, wheel and caster size, tire type, armrests, "bucket" (the amount the seat back is lowered compared with the front), wheel camber (the amount the wheels flare away from the chair at the floor), and foot plates, can be customized for each patient's needs. Specialized hand rims, such as plastic covered or with projections, allow better contact with the push surface when hand function is limited, such as in the person with C6 to C8 tetraplegia (Figure 10-28). People who will rely on a w/c for mobility must learn enough about w/c maintenance and upkeep to prolong the life of the chair and ensure that it will remain in good working condition.

Adaptive Equipment

Adaptive equipment includes a cushion, bathtub bench, raised toilet seat, and equipment that facilitates function, such as a reacher, a UE orthosis (Figure 10-29), or gloves. A cushion, which helps to better redistribute pressure and provide sitting support, may be foam, gel, air-filled, or a combination. Anecdotal reports indicate that standing devices are helpful in reducing bladder problems, but clinical trials do not exist, and third-party payers may not consider this piece of equipment medically necessary.

Preventing Pressure Sores

Pressure sores, also called *bedsores* or *pressure ulcers*, are damage to the skin and or underlying tissues caused by excessive pressure or shear over bony prominences. Pressure on blood vessels

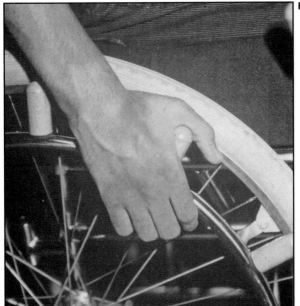

Figure 10-28. Specialized handrims.

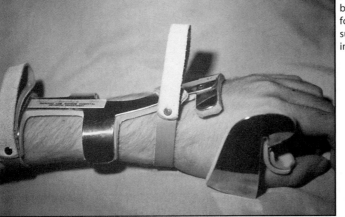

Figure 10-29. A wrist-hand orthosis stabilizes the wrist while the patient performs functional activities. Implements, such as utensils and pens, can be inserted into the palm.

limits the flow of blood and its oxygen supply to the tissues, just as the water supply is diminished when a garden hose is twisted or stepped on. Subsequently, the tissues supplied by these blood vessels die, and ulceration occurs. Pressure sores are common over any bony prominence, with some locations being more vulnerable than others, depending on the position the person assumes. For example, the sacrum is at most risk when the person is in supine or in a sitting position in bed, the heels are most vulnerable in supine, and the ischial tuberosities are vulnerable in sitting.[73] When pressure is relieved, the blood supply returns to the area and tissues are spared. Typically, people with SCI are at risk for pressure sores because they lack protective sensation and have a limited ability to move. Other factors that may cause pressure sores are thick, rough clothing (eg, decorative seams or rivets on jeans), lumpy or folded sheets, cushion covers, or clothing; moisture, especially due to bladder accidents; heat; burns (Figure 10-30); ill-fitting clothing; poor nutrition; injuries due to carelessness with insensate skin; and orthopedic deformities (eg, scoliosis and pelvic obliquity).[73]

The 2 most important methods for preventing pressure sores are use of special pressure-relieving cushions (Figures 10-31A through C) and mattresses and periodic relief of pressure over

Figure 10-30. Patients with sensory impairments are at risk for being burned. The PTA could educate the patient to be cautious because the water may be too hot.

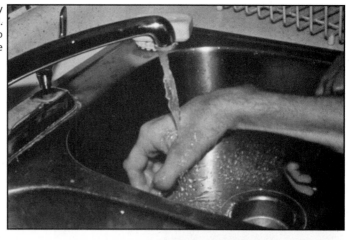

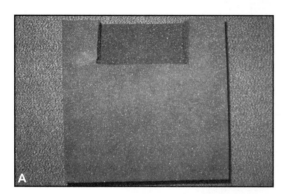

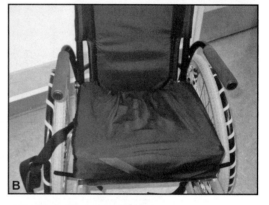

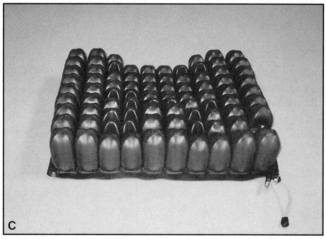

Figures 10-31. Pressure-relieving cushions. (A) Four-inch laminated foam w/c cushion (high density over extra high density) with ischial cutout. The cutout goes three-quarters of the way through the height of the cushion, thereby maintaining integrity of the cushion while eliminating pressure under the ischial tuberosities. (B) Gel cushion over a contoured foam base. Redistribution of sitting pressure is achieved with this cushion. The gel is primarily in the area of the ischial tuberosities. (C) Air w/c cushion. This provides excellent pressure redistribution for persons who have bony deformities of the pelvis. Cushion must be checked daily to ensure that it is inflated adequately to prevent pressure sores.

Figure 10-32. This easy-to-remember acronym, "RAISED," describes lifting the body weight off the ischial tuberosities for pressure relief. (Reprinted with permission from Rancho Los Amigos National Rehabilitation Center, Downey, CA).

RAISED

Reposition to

Alleviate

Ischial

Skin

Embarrassment and

Destruction

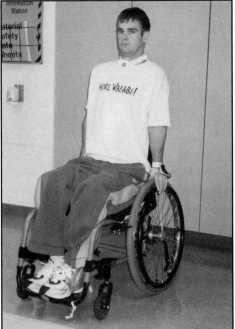

Figure 10-33. Patient with tetraplegia performing depression pressure relief.

the bony prominences. To help people remember to perform pressure relief, the acronym RAISED was coined[74] (Figure 10-32). This term conveys the process of lifting pressure off the ischii when sitting, which may be easier for the patient to remember than "pressure relief."

Studies of the optimum frequency of pressure relief are limited. In general, people with paraplegia or those who can use their arms for pressure relief are instructed to perform their pressure relief for 15 seconds every 15 minutes. Other recommended time frames are 30 seconds of pressure relief every 30 minutes or 1 minute of pressure relief every hour. Further research is required to determine whether these time frames are sufficient to allow recovery of blood oxygen to resting levels.[75] While in the sitting position, pressure can be relieved by lifting the buttocks from the seat (Figure 10-33), leaning forward enough to raise the ischial tuberosities off the seat (Figure 10-34)

Figure 10-34. Patient with tetraplegia performing forward pressure relief.

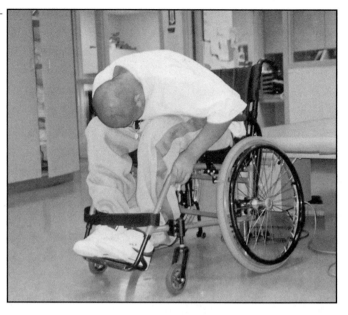

or leaning side to side. In people with a power w/c equipped with a recliner or tilt system, pressure relief is accomplished by lying down or tilting backward at least 65 degrees.[75]

Special equipment, such as a mattress, can help relieve pressure over bony prominences or redistribute pressures over larger and less bony areas. Just as in sitting, pressure relief is required in addition to any pressure redistribution provided by the mattress. Pressure relief is provided by turning the person in bed every 2 hours, using an air pressure–changing mattress, or having the person lie prone or semi-prone. In the prone or semi-prone position, pillows are used to bridge bony areas, including the pelvis and knees. People who are able to lie in one of these positions can sleep for longer periods without turning, because pressure on prominent bony areas is minimized. The person is able to rest better, and the amount of nursing or attendant care required is decreased.

Pressure mapping with computerized pressure-sensing devices is a form of assessment the PT performs to provide additional information about sitting pressures. Pressure can be measured on various pieces of adaptive equipment, such as mattresses or cushions, and the effectiveness of modified equipment or positions that relieve pressure can be compared. The PT and PTA can use the resulting pressure map as an education tool. The best screening for areas of excess pressure in sitting is by palpation of the bony prominences with the PT's or PTA's hands. When areas of excess pressure are identified, the cushion or sitting position can be altered to minimize pressures.

Pressure sores take a toll on the person with SCI and on society—physically, socially, and monetarily. To prevent sores or to identify them before they become severe, people with SCI are taught to inspect their skin morning and evening using a long-handled mirror and assistance, if needed.

Pressure sores may occur very quickly (eg, within 30 minutes) and may take up to a week for even a stage I sore to heal. If a pressure sore does occur (Table 10-3), complete relief of pressure by staying off the sore is optimal to allow healing. The person who has a pressure sore may need to avoid or severely limit sitting.[53] If pressure sores progress to stage III or IV, surgery may be required.[76]

Patient and Family Education

Family members and hired attendant personnel must learn how to assist the person with SCI at home. People with SCIs who are unable to care for themselves must learn how to direct others to provide their care. Many rehabilitation programs have classes for patients with SCIs covering a

Table 10-3
Classification of Pressure Sores

Stage I	Nonblanchable erythema of intact skin (USPHS). In persons with dark skin, discoloration of the skin, warmth, edema, induration, or hardness may also be indicators.
Stage II	Partial-thickness skin loss involving the dermis, epidermis, or both.
Stage III	Full-thickness skin loss involving damage to or necrosis of subcutaneous tissue that may extend down to, but not through, underlying fascia. The ulcer is a deep crater, with or without undermining adjacent tissue.
Stage IV	Full thickness skin loss with extensive destruction, tissue necrosis, or damage to muscle, bone, or supporting structures such as tendon or joint capsule.
*Nonstagable	Sore is covered with eschar so that one is unable to determine the condition of the tissue below.

*Used at Rancho Los Amigos National Rehabilitation Center, Downey, CA. (Adapted from Treatment of Pressure Ulcers. Clinical Practice Guideline #15 [AHCPR Publication #95-0652]. Rockville, MD: US Department of Health and Human Services; 1994.)
Note: It is not appropriate to reverse-stage a healing ulcer (eg, stage III will NOT become a stage II). The damaged tissue is not replaced by the same type; it is replaced by granulation tissue. Document the wound improvements by its characteristics (eg, size, depth, amount of necrotic tissue, amount of exudate).

variety of subjects. These may include the nature of SCI and how it affects the body, research on spinal cord regeneration, sexual function, adaptive vehicles, w/c maintenance, dealing with w/c vendors, hiring an attendant, and other topics that will assist the patient once he or she leaves the hospital.

Evaluate the Home for Accessibility

A visit to the individual's home may be recommended to ensure architectural barriers are minimized. The therapists will assess the outside and the interior layouts of the patient's home and make recommendations to maximize functional independence. Possible recommendations may include ramping entryways, moving/removal of furniture, changing flooring, lowering commonly used items, altering doorways, removing shower doors, hand-held shower head, placement of medical equipment, and kitchen and bathroom alterations. The PTA will assist in contributing to the problem-solving process during and/or after the home visit.

Discharge From the Rehabilitation Program and Reintegration Into the Community

Most people with SCI are discharged home, although people with more severe injuries or fewer resources may require discharge to an assisted living situation, such as a board-and-care, skilled nursing, or subacute facility. People with tetraplegia, and some with paraplegia, will require assistance from family members, friends, or a paid caregiver. Some communities have support groups to help people with SCI and their families continue to cope with the changes in their lives. A period of time is required for the person with SCI to adapt physically and emotionally to his or her new lifestyle, but successful social and vocational reintegration is an achievable goal. During the time following discharge from rehabilitation, the person may take advantage of vocational training to determine how the work environment and tasks can be modified for physical limitations that are present and how adaptive equipment can be used. People who have a valid driver's license may learn to drive with hand controls. Some medical centers have gyms that people with SCI can access, or they may be able to modify exercise methods to use a commercial gym. Medical follow-up is required to monitor bladder function and overall health and to ensure that late complications are minimized. Each individual with SCI deserves to have a fulfilling and meaningful life and can achieve one with support and assistance.

CASE STUDY

The following case study illustrates an episode of care in the physical rehabilitation of a person with SCI.

Background

The patient, Matt, is a 35-year-old man who is married with 2 boys, ages 9 and 12. Prior to his injury, he was employed by an energy company as a senior chemical engineer, managing 16 employees in his department. He enjoys traveling abroad, playing tennis, and watching his children play soccer and baseball. The patient was involved in a MVA, sustaining a T4 complete SCI (ASIA A). He lives in a 2-story home, with the bedrooms on the second floor. There are 2 steps to enter the home.

Matt underwent surgery for stabilization with placement of Harrington rods from T2 to T8, and he was given intravenous steroids to reduce inflammation and secondary damage to the spinal cord. He was then admitted to the acute neurological unit for 10 days until he was medically stable. The physician has prescribed a TLSO brace (clamshell type) for the patient to wear for 8 to 10 weeks. Acute therapists worked together to decrease his pain, improve his sitting tolerance, and increase his UE strength and endurance. During treatment, Matt experienced a severe headache; the PTA treating him assessed his BP as 180/100, immediately contacted the nurse, and began examining Matt for possible reasons for the rise in BP. The PTA found that Matt's urinary catheter was twisted and kinked at the proximal end. After straightening the catheter, Matt remained sitting up in his w/c; after 20 minutes, his BP came down to his baseline of 92/60. The nurse was prepared to administer nitroglycerin gel if his BP did not return to baseline. This was Matt's first experience of autonomic dysreflexia. Matt presented with pitting edema in bilateral feet and legs, and prior to Matt's transfer to rehab, his LEs were assessed for DVT using a Doppler ultrasound. He wore compressive thigh-high stockings to help reduce the dependent edema.

Inpatient Rehabilitation

Matt was transferred to the inpatient rehab center after he was medically stable and could tolerate an intensive rehabilitation program. The inpatient rehab team evaluating Matt consisted of a physician, registered nurse, PT, OT, neuropsychologist, dietician, and social worker. During his first week, the clinicians presented their findings to one another at the initial team conference to establish the plan of care. The individualized care plan and his length of stay were based on Matt's medical problems, neurological level and projected functional outcome levels (T4 ASIA A), cognitive and emotional status, physical impairments, functional deficits, SCI educational needs, and discharge disposition, as well as patient and family goals. Some inpatient rehab centers invite the patient and family members to participate in the team conference. Oftentimes, family members offer information that will help the team better understand different qualities of the patient and create a more complete treatment plan. In this setting, the patient stated the following goals: take care of himself, return to work, participate in his children's life, and help care for his family.

The following goals were set during inpatient rehabilitation:

1. Be independent with his specific home exercise program for ROM and strengthening UEs, passive ROM, etc.

2. Maintain/increase hip, knee, and ankle ROM.

3. Independently assume the sitting position from supine with the TLSO on without using the bedrails (he will continue to require moderate assistance from caregivers to don and doff TLSO because of spinal precautions).

4. Maintain the short sitting position independently at the edge of bed, with UE support.

5. Independently transfer from his w/c to a bed, toilet, couch, and tub transfer bench; car transfers with transfer board and minimal assistance.

6. Demonstrate 3 different types of w/c pressure reliefs every 30 minutes.

7. Independently propel w/c through doorways and up and down American With Disabilities Act (ADA)—compliant ramps.

8. Independently propel w/c over a 2-inch curb, curb cutouts, and uneven terrain.

The following goals were set for the family:

1. The family will demonstrate independence with assisting Matt with standard height curbs and stairs.

2. The family will also demonstrate an understanding of how to perform a dependent transfer from floor to w/c for fall recovery.

Tests and Measures

Cardiovascular/pulmonary:

Vitals at rest: BP, 110/70 mm Hg (supine), 96/60 mm Hg (sitting); heart rate, 80 beats per minute; respiratory rate, 20 respirations per minute in sitting; oxygen (O_2) saturations, 98% in supine, 94% in sitting (using pulse oximeter).

Strength: Bilateral UEs = normal (5/5); bilateral LEs = absent (0/5); trunk = intercostal muscles intact to T4 level, abdominal muscles are not innervated.

Sensation (sharp/dull discrimination, light touch): Bilateral UEs = normal/intact; bilateral LEs = absent; trunk = intact for both sharp/dull and light touch modalities to T4 dermatome, absent below T4.

ROM: UE active ROM, within normal limits for all UE joints; LE passive ROM, within normal limits, except hip flexion (SLR) = 0 to 60 degrees bilaterally and ankle dorsiflexion to neutral.

Deep tendon reflexes (0 to 4): Biceps (C5 to 6), 2; brachioradialis (C5 to 6), 2; triceps (C7), 2; quadriceps (L3 to4), 3; plantarflexors (S1), 4.

Functional Abilities

Matt was active and independent for all functional skills prior to his injury. At the time of the evaluation, his functional mobility was as follows:

Donning/doffing TLSO: Matt needed total assistance to don and doff the TLSO brace (clamshell) before getting out of bed. The TLSO brace interfered with all functional mobility skills.

Bed mobility: He needed moderate assistance for rolling, maximal assistance for supine to long sitting position, and maximal assistance from supine to short sitting at the edge of bed. Initially, he needed time to acclimate to the upright position because of orthostatic hypotension.

Sitting balance: He needed minimal to moderate assistance to maintain a sitting position at the edge of the bed with bilateral hands either in front or behind his hips (propping). He was not able to change hand position without moderate to maximal assistance to maintain his balance.

Transfers: He needed maximal assistance from one person for all basic transfers, and total assistance for advanced transfers (eg, floor to w/c transfer, car transfers). He was not yet able to apply the head-hips relationship.

W/C mobility: He was independent for propulsion on level terrain for short distances (< 50 feet). He required total assistance for all high-level w/c skills (eg, steep ramps, wheelies, curbs, stairs). He was able to demonstrate 3 w/c pressure-relieving techniques with minimal assistance (ie, leaning forward onto thighs to relieve pressure on coccyx and sacrum, lateral lean to relieve pressure on the ischial tuberosities, and lifting his entire buttock off the seat using a depression-lift technique).

Physical Therapy Program

Team communication: As Matt continues to improve in his functional mobility, it is important that all members of the team understand his level of assistance needed for activities, as well as movement strategies. A team conference will be held at least weekly, and at some rehab facilities, a team "huddle" will occur daily or as needed to ensure all team members have current information. An information board is updated daily in Matt's room to keep the staff current and inform Matt and his family about his progress.

Teaching problem-solving strategies: It is important to allow Matt to problem solve as he is learning new movement strategies. Because of Matt's educational background, he is able to understand the physics and mechanics behind the new skills. However, applying the skills is very challenging without normal sensation or motor control below the level of the lesion. New situations will arise during treatment sessions and throughout his day in rehab; it is important to allow him time to problem solve on his own to help him become self-sufficient. On a regular basis, the clinicians will ask Matt what his goals are to ensure he is involved in his plan of care.

UE strengthening exercises: With manual muscle testing, Matt demonstrated having normal strength and ROM throughout his UEs; however, because he will be using his UEs for all functional mobility tasks, the muscle strength of the scapulothoracic and glenohumeral joints is critical to decrease the risk of shoulder pain and injury. Posterior musculature (rhomboids, trapezius, rotator cuff, posterior deltoids) must be strengthened to avoid a muscle imbalance because the majority of functional movements use primarily the anterior shoulder musculature. The latissimus dorsi, serratus anterior, triceps, deltoids, and pectoralis major muscles are also very important for functional transfers. It is critical for Matt to strengthen his UEs in positions that **do not** decrease the integrity of the spine surgery or create more kyphosis. The PT and PTA will work together to provide an exercise program that he will perform independently using exercise machines, as well as mat exercises using weights or his own body as resistance, or with the PTA providing manual resistance through important ROMs specific for functional mobility.

Bed mobility skills: Bed mobility activities require proper technique, speed, momentum, and timing; adequate ROM; and an understanding of how to unweight extremities. Overstretching the back muscles and ligaments will often make rolling more difficult, causing the lower trunk to not move with the upper trunk as it is rotating. The rehab staff will need to help Matt don his TLSO brace prior to teaching bed mobility skills. To roll, Matt needs to use momentum from swinging his UEs while simultaneously rotating and flexing the head/neck. Rolling to the prone position will be useful in reducing pressure on bony prominences on his back, sacrum, coccyx, and heels. Proning is initiated by the therapists for 1 to 2 hours per day, carried over by nursing, and eventually Matt will be fully responsible for his proning schedule. When Matt is independent, assuming the prone or semi-prone position with pillows protecting bony prominences, he can reduce the amount of turning he must do at night, reducing the amount of assistance required. From the side-lying position, Matt will be able to assume the long sitting position by crawling around toward his feet and then pushing up into long sit. Remember, it is important that his hamstring length is adequate (SLR of 100 to 110 degrees) to prevent excessive posterior pelvic tilt, and overstretching his back when in the long sitting position. Initially, Matt's SLR was inadequate and he needed to assume the frog-leg position in long sitting (hips abducted and externally rotated, with knees flexed), or the therapist allowed his legs to drape over the edge of the mat. Matt's abdominal musculature is not innervated, but because his ROM and strength in his UEs are within functional limits throughout, he can assume the long sitting position directly from supine using momentum, speed, and power without rolling to the side-lying position. This direct method is more efficient; however, many times the rolling from supine to side-lying to long sit progression will be taught before the supine to long sit progression because it is easier to master. From side-lying or the long sitting position, he will learn how to manage his LEs and trunk to assume short sitting at the edge of the mat/bed.

Transfer training and functional activities: The PT and PTA will work together to improve basic transfers and begin advanced transfer training. The natural progression of transfers is usually mastered in the following order: w/c to/from mat, bed, toilet, tub transfer bench, car, and floor. Sitting balance is a critical component in mastering transfers. Although Matt does not have sensation below the nipple level (T4), he will learn to balance himself using his upper trunk, head/neck, and arms. He must learn to maintain balance with his hands in front of his hips and behind his hips, one arm support, and without UE support. Counterbalancing is an important mobility skill as he becomes more dynamic in sitting. For example, positioning his LEs in preparation for a transfer requires balancing on one arm, then counterbalancing to lift and reposition the LE with the other arm. As his long sitting and short sitting balance improves, depression lifts are taught, implementing the head-hips relationship. The PTA needs to allow Matt to find his balance point during the lift. It is important to provide Matt with enough space to lean forward, drop his head down, and lift his hips off the mat. While finding his balance point during a depression lift, Matt will often fall quickly backward onto the mat or forward into the clinician; remaining vigilant and in the correct position to catch him is critical. Matt will initially use a transfer board to bridge the distance from surface to surface, until his depression lift-pivot transfer technique is safe to travel over the necessary distance without risk of falling. Because of Matt's need to wear his TLSO brace when out of bed, his ability to master many skills may be difficult. When his TLSO brace is finally discontinued (8 to 10 weeks), he may have difficulty finding his balance once again and will need to learn how to manage his body during functional activities, and more advanced skills will be taught without the brace interfering (eg, floor transfers). As his mobility and balance improves, he will be taught how to load his w/c independently into a car; he most likely will not be able to master this skill prior to discharge from rehab.

W/C mobility exercises: W/C mobility training involves learning to maneuver in tight spaces, over uneven terrain (eg, gravel or grass), over a threshold, up and down ramps, and through doorways. A person using a manual w/c who has sufficient UE motor control may learn more advanced w/c skills, such as how to navigate curbs and go up and down stairs. Matt must be taught how to propel his w/c efficiently on level and uneven surfaces. On a flat, smooth surface, patients will often excessively push their w/c instead of allowing it to coast and resting the UEs. Pushing his w/c on uneven surfaces (eg, grass, stepping stones, sand) will challenge Matt's balance and his ability to shift weight to maintain traction on the rear wheels. The PTA must be sure to secure Matt by using the w/c seat belt because he may fall forward while practicing high-level skills. Matt has difficulty negotiating doorways, especially those with automatic door closers; he will be taught methods to open and close doors by using the door and the doorframe to get through doorways efficiently. There are many ramps that are not ADA compliant in Matt's community. When propelling up ramps, he will be taught to keep his trunk flexed forward to decrease the risk of tipping backward. He will also be taught to descend steep ramps (not ADA compliant) rolling backward, with his trunk flexed forward on his thighs, and slowly allowing the w/c rims to glide through his hands to manage his speed. Ascending and descending curbs are also an occasional necessity. In preparation for curbs, wheelies will be taught by using a gait belt around the rear of the w/c frame or rear axle to enable the PTA to catch Matt when falling backward. The clinician will assist him to find his balance point in the w/c and learn how to keep his hands on the top-most part of the rims, allowing equal movement to push the rims forward and backward when finding his balance. Once Matt has gained some proficiency in performing wheelies, he will practice maintaining a wheelie while propelling the w/c down the hallway (wheelie glide). He will then learn how to ascend and descend a 2-inch curb popping up the front casters onto the curb, transferring his weight forward, and quickly and forcefully pushing the w/c onto the curb. He will also learn how to descend a curb backward with his trunk flexed forward onto his thighs and also forward in a wheelie glide. Most patients are not proficient or safe with ascending/descending curbs or stairs at discharge from rehab. It is necessary to teach caregivers how to help negotiate curbs and stairs.

W/C and cushion prescription: Because of Matt's neurological level and ASIA classification (T4 ASIA A), it is very unlikely for him to be a functional ambulator; therefore, an ultralight rigid w/c will be prescribed. Factors to consider will be discussed with the patient, such as needing to independently transfer his w/c into a car, accessibility in his home and work environment, and insurance issues. Matt will be able to try a few different w/c models with different specifications and will be educated on their specific features (ie, weight, size, frame dimensions, seat-to-back angle, axle position, camber angle, tires, spokes, caster size). Matt's body type puts him at high risk for pressure ulcers; therefore, a seating evaluation using a computerized pressure mapping system will be performed to determine the most appropriate w/c cushion. The PTA will also work with Matt to teach basic w/c maintenance (eg, fixing a flat tire and adjusting wheel camber, casters, and brakes).

Home evaluation: The PT or PTA and an OT will complete a home evaluation with Matt and his family present. Recommendations for equipment and home modifications will be documented and discussed with the family and the rehab team members. Equipment such as a raised toilet seat, drop-arm commode, bath bench, and grab bars may be recommended. Other home modifications may include installing a ramp in the entrance, removing or installing double-hinged doors to widen entrances, removing sliding bath/shower doors, clearing floors of clutter for w/c accessibility, relocating common items to his level, and removing or securing area rugs. Near the end of his rehab stay, Matt will be scheduled for a day pass with his family to examine some of the potential problems and logistics to returning home.

Patient and family education: Many rehab centers provide educational reading materials and classes taught by various disciplines on topics specific to SCIs. Matt and his wife will attend classes on bowel and bladder management, preventing pressure ulcers, community resources, and sexuality. SCIs can greatly affect the caregivers physically, mentally, and emotionally. Neuropsychologists and social workers are trained to help caregivers with understanding SCIs, potential issues, and emotional assistance. Matt and his caregivers will be informed regarding support groups in the area and recreational outreach programs. The Internet has become an excellent resource for patients, caregivers, and family members. There are many Web sites and videos that provide information on everything from potential movement strategies to the newest technological advancements in mobility.

Final Results

Matt underwent a 5-week rehabilitation program with only a few setbacks, including a small stage II decubitus ulcer on his coccyx and the beginnings of heterotopic ossification in his right hip that was controlled with medication, and passive ROM exercises. During the first week, the physician discussed with him the importance of his rehabilitation program, his current status, and his prognosis. Matt reported that this information was disheartening and at the same time somewhat motivational. During the first 2 weeks, the PT and PTA began working with Matt to improve his hamstring ROM, UE strength, bed mobility, sitting balance, performing w/c pressure relief, basic transfer skills, and basic w/c mobility skills. By the end of the third week, Matt was dressing himself with minimal assistance, performing his self-care with supervision/minimal assistance, performing bed mobility skills with supervision assistance and minimal verbal cues for technique, achieving tub and toilet transfers with moderate assistance, and performing depression transfers to and from the mat and bed with contact guard/minimal assistance. He was able to pop up into a wheelie and hold for 3 to 5 seconds. During this week, his PTA found his right hip passive ROM was becoming less flexible and reported it to the PT and the physician. He was diagnosed with heterotopic ossification of the right hip and began a course of medication along with continued passive ROM exercises. He was also able to perform self-catheterization independently and check his skin with a flexible mirror independently. Matt was also on a bowel program with nursing. By the end of the fourth week, he was able to perform bed mobility skills with modified independence (after receiving assistance to don/doff TLSO), transfer from his w/c to the bed with supervision/ modified independence, transfer to the toilet and bath bench (managing LEs) with minimal assistance, and transfer to the car with minimal assistance using a sliding board. He was able to perform a wheelie in a w/c and maintain a wheelie while gliding 20 feet with supervision, ascend and descend a 2-inch curb with minimal assistance and verbal cues, propel w/c up and down a non-ADA—compliant ramp independently, and propel his w/c through grass and gravel with modified independence. The home evaluation was performed during this week by the PT and OT, who documented and discussed recommendations with the patient and family. A w/c and seating evaluation was performed this week with a vendor; an ultralight w/c with a foam and air combination cushion was ordered because of Matt's history of pressure ulcers and postural concerns. By the end of the fifth week, he was modified-independent with bed mobility skills (except for donning and doffing TLSO) and w/c transfers to bed, toilet, and tub transfer bench. He required supervision for car transfers with a sliding board. He and his family were educated on how to assist him in the areas of concern and demonstrated the skills proficiently.

When Matthew was discharged from the hospital, the family rented a ramp until a permanent ramp could be built. He then began a course of home health care (PT, OT, registered nurse, social worker) to make the adjustment to home and to become independent in the home and community. The home health therapists continued making recommendations on home modifications as issues arose. He lived on the first floor of his home for the first 2 months, while a stair glide was installed. The second floor is now accessible to him; however, he needed to purchase another w/c for use on the second floor. After he became independent at home, he was discharged from home health care and then began a course of outpatient therapies to continue working on improving UE strength, maintaining ROM in LEs, advanced w/c skills, advanced transfer techniques, and updating his home exercise program. Matt returned to work at the energy company, continuing his previous level of employment. The company is making efforts to accommodate his disability.

CASE STUDIES

CASE #1

John, age 22, sustained a C6 level SCI, ASIA A, in a MVA 2 months ago. He was a student at a local community college studying computer science.

1. What muscles remain innervated?
2. Will he be able to continue using his computer?
3. What kind of adaptive equipment will be required to use the computer?
4. The PT has identified sliding board transfers as a goal for the patient. What activities or interventions might the PTA be asked to do prior to initiating or attempting transfers?
5. What kind of w/c will he probably need, given his vocational goals?

CASE #2

A patient is on the tilt table having his hamstrings stretched to gain ROM for an SLR. His injury level is T2. He starts sweating and complaining of a headache.

1. What do you suspect has occurred?

2. What should you do first?

3. If his BP is elevated, what should you do?

CASE #3

You are working with a patient with an SCI at L1 level, ASIA C, which he sustained 2 months ago. You know that the doctor has talked to the patient about recovery and the level of his injury. The patient now has Poor minus (P– or 2/5) to Poor (P or 2/5) strength in the hip flexor and quadriceps muscles and Trace (Tr or 1/5) in his dorsiflexor, hamstring, and hip abductor muscles.

1. Is it important to continue to strengthen the muscles in his LEs?

2. Can he get stronger?

3. Would he still benefit from exercise if it were 13 months post-injury? Why?

CASE #4

A PTA was asked to work with a patient who has T6 paraplegia and is sitting on a gel cushion. Yesterday was his first day sitting, and he had no problems with dizziness. The PT asks the PTA to implement an education program on pressure relief and prevention of pressure sores.

1. What points would the PTA want to cover with this patient?

2. What does the patient need to know about his cushion?

CASE #5

The PTA is running a class on power w/c mobility for patients with C2 to C5 tetraplegia.

1. What activities would be important for these people to learn to be able to function in the community?

2. What additional activities would be important if it were a class for patients using manual w/cs and at a higher level of function?

CASE #6

A PTA is working with a patient with T7 paraplegia.

1. What functional activities would the PTA work on in preparation for a car transfer?

2. What are some precautions to tell the patient when performing this skill?

RESOURCES

American Spinal Injury Association

An organization for physicians and other health care professionals specializing in care of patients with SCI.

2020 Peachtree Road NW
Atlanta, GA 30309
Phone: (404) 355-9772
www.asia-spinalinjury.org
Email: ASIA_Office@shepherd.org

Christopher & Dana Reeve Foundation
A foundation committed to funding research to develop cures and treatment for paralysis due to SCI. Also provides grants for quality of life for people living with disabilities.
636 Morris Turnpike, Suite 3A
Short Hills, NJ 07078
Phone: (800) 225-0292
www.christopherreeve.org

National Spinal Cord Injury Association
Provides information on a variety of topics related to SCI and an online newsletter.
75-20 Astoria Blvd
Jackson Heights, NY 11370
Phone: (718) 803-3782
www.spinalcord.org

Spinal Cord Injury Model System Information Network
Provides information about research projects and statistics about SCI provided by the University of Alabama—Birmingham.
529 Spain Rehabilitation Center
1717 6th Ave S
Birmingham, AL 35249-7330
Phone: (205) 934-3283
www.spinalcord.uab.edu

Other Web Sites and Social Media

www.ninds.nih.gov/disorders/sci/sci.htm
A site of the National Institute of Neurological Disorders and Stroke, National Institutes of Health, which supports biomedical research on disorders of the brain and nervous system.

www.makoa.org/sci.htm
The Spinal Cord Injury and Disease Resources' site has multiple resources, including general resources, facts, statistics, rehabilitation, email groups and listserves, message boards, newsletters, magazines, articles, and books.

Facebook pages:
Life After Spinal Cord Injury
Spinal Cord Injury Health/Wellness Web site
Spinal Cord Injury Model Systems
Spinal Cord Injury Non-Profit Organization

Twitter:
@faceDisability
https://twitter.com/FaceDisability
Peer support for families.

@SCI_MS
http://www.msktc.org/sci/
The Model Systems Knowledge Translation Center summarizes research, identifies health information needs, and develops information resources to support the Model Systems programs in meeting the needs of individuals with traumatic brain injury, SCI, and burn injury. Funded by the National Institute on Disability and Rehabilitation Research.

@spinalinjuries
https://twitter.com/spinalinjuries
A user-led organization that works to support and promote the well-being of the 40,000 people with SCI in the United Kingdom.

REFERENCES

1. World Health Organization. World Health Statistics 2009. Cause-specific mortality and morbidity, Table 2. http://www.who.int/whosis/whostat/EN_WHS09_Table2.pdf. Accessed August 12, 2012.
2. Hasler RM, Exadaktylos AK, Bouamra O, et al. Epidemiology and predictors of spinal injury in adult major trauma patients: European cohort study. *Eur Spine J.* 2011;20(12):2174-2180.
3. Pirouzmand F. Epidemiological trends of spine and spinal cord injuries in the largest Canadian adult trauma center from 1986 to 2006. *J Neurosurg Spine.* 2010;12(2):131-140.
4. National Spinal Cord Injury Center Statistical Center. Spinal cord injury: facts and figures at a glance. Birmingham, AL. https://www.nscisc.uab.edu/PublicDocuments/fact_figures_docs/Facts%202012%20Feb%20 Final.pdf. Accessed January 19, 2012.
5. Jackson AB, Dijkers M, Devivo MJ, Poczatek RB. A demographic profile of new traumatic spinal cord injuries: change and stability over 30 years. *Arch Phys Med Rehabil.* 2004;85(11):1740-1748.
6. Krause JS, Saunders LL. Health, secondary conditions, and life expectancy after spinal cord injury. *Arch Phys Med Rehabil.* 2011;92(11):1770-1775.
7. Livecchi MA. Spinal cord injury. *Continuum (Minneap Minn).* 2011;17(3 Neurorehabilitation):568-583.
8. Oyinbo CA. Secondary injury mechanisms in traumatic spinal cord injury: a nugget of this multiply cascade. *Acta Neurobiol Exp (Wars).* 2011;71(2):281-299.
9. Marino RJ, Barros T, Biering-Sorenson F, et al. International standards for neurological classification of spinal cord injury. *J Spinal Cord Med.* 2003;26(Suppl 1):550-556.
10. American Spinal Injury Association. *International Standards for Neurological Classification of Spinal Cord Injury.* Chicago, IL: Author; 2002.
11. Atkinson PP, Atkinson JLD. Spinal shock. *Mayo Clin Pro.* 1996;71:384-389.
12. Dittunno JF, Little JW, Tessler A, et al. Spinal shock revisited: a four-phase model. *Spinal Cord.* 2004;42:383-395.
13. McKinley W, Santos K, Meade M, Booke M. Incidence of outcomes of spinal cord injury clinical syndromes. *J Spinal Cord Med.* 2007;30(3):215-224.
14. Merriam WF, Taylor TK, Ruff J, McPhail MJ. A reappraisal of acute traumatic central cord syndrome. *J Bone Joint Surg Br.* 1986;68(5):708-713.
15. Kirshblum SC, Waring W, Biering-Sorensen F, et al. Reference for the 2011 revision of the international standards for neurological classification of spinal cord injury. *J Spinal Cord Med.* 2011;34(6):547-554.
16. American Spinal Injury Association. *American Spinal Injury Association Reference Manual for the International Standards for Neurological Classification of Spinal Cord Injury.* Chicago, IL: Author; 2003.
17. Linn W, Adkins R, Gong H, Waters R. Pulmonary function in chronic spinal cord injury: a cross-sectional survey of 222 Southern California adult outpatients. *Arch Phys Med Rehabil.* 2000;81(6):757-763.
18. McKinley WO, Gittler MS, Kirshblum SC, Stiens SA, Groah SL. Medical complications after spinal cord injury: identification and management. *Arch Phys Med Rehabil.* 2002;83(Suppl 1):S58-S64.

19. Short DJ, Silver JR, Lehr RP. Electromyographic study of sternocleidomastoid and scalene muscles in tetraplegic subjects during respiration. *Int Disabil Stud.* 1991;13(2):46-49.

20. Jain NB, Sullivan M, Kazis LE, Tun CG, Garshick E. Factors associated with health-related quality of life in chronic spinal cord injury. *Am J Phys Med Rehabil.* 2007;86(5):387-396.

21. Kirshblum S, Millis S, McKinley W, Tulsky D. Late neurologic recovery after traumatic spinal cord injury. *Arch Phys Med Rehabil.* 2004;85(11)1811-1817.

22. Guillaume D, Van Havengergh A, Vloeberghs M, Vidal J, Roeste G. A clinical study of intrathecal Baclofen using a programmable pump for intractable spasticity. *Arch Phys Med Rehabil.* 2005;86(11):2165-2171.

23. Consortium for Spinal Cord Medicine. *Neurogenic Bowel Management in Adults with Spinal Cord Injury.* Washington, DC: Paralyzed Veterans of America; 1998:11.

24. Benevento BT, Sipski ML. Neurogenic bladder, neurogenic bowel, and sexual dysfunction in people with spinal cord injury. *Phys Ther.* 2002;82(6):601-612.

25. Rehabilitation Institute of Chicago. Spinal cord injury: sexuality. http://lifecenter.ric.org/index.php?tray=content&tid=top3&cid=2560. Accessed January 19, 2013.

26. Gundu H, Binak DF. Autonomic dysreflexia: an important cardiovascular complication in spinal cord injury patients. *Cardiology J.* 2012;19(2):215-219.

27. Comarr AE. Autonomic dysreflexia (hyperreflexia). *J Am Paraplegia Soc.* 1984;7(3):53-57.

28. Acute management of autonomic dysreflexia: adults with spinal cord injury presenting to health-care facilities. Consortium for spinal cord medicine. *J Spinal Cord Med.* 1997;20(3):284-307.

29. Naftchi NE, Richardson JS. Autonomic dysreflexia: pharmacological management of hypertensive crises in spinal cord injured patients. *J Spin Cord Med.* 1997;20(3):355-360.

30. Kübler-Ross E. *On Death and Dying.* New York, NY: Macmillan Publishing; 1969.

31. Teasell RW, Mehta S, Aubut JL, et al. A systematic review of pharmacologic treatments of pain after spinal cord injury. *Arch Phys Med Rehabil.* 2010;91(5):816-831.

32. Burchiel KJ, Hsu FP. Pain and spasticity after spinal cord injury: mechanisms and treatment. *Spine (Phila Pa 1976).* 2001;26(245 Suppl):S146-S160.

33. Siddall PJ, Loeser JD. Pain following spinal cord injury. *Spinal Cord.* 2001;39(2):63-73.

34. Gellman H, Sie I, Waters RL. Late complications of the weight-bearing upper extremity in the paraplegia patient. *Clin Orthop Relat Res.* 1998;233:132-135.

35. Subbarao JV, Klopfstein J, Turpin R. Prevalence and impact of wrist and shoulder pain in patients with spinal cord injury. *J Spinal Cord Med.* 1995;18(1):9-13.

36. Curtis KA, Drysdale GA, Lanza RD, Kolber M, Vitolo RS, West R. Shoulder pain in wheelchair users with tetraplegia and paraplegia. *Arch Phys Med Rehabil.* 1999;80(4):453-457.

37. Dittunno JF, Little JW, Tessler A, Burns AS. Spinal shock revisited: a four-phase model. *Spinal Cord.* 2004;42(7):383-395.

38. Davidoff G, Morris J, Roth E, Bleiberg J. Closed head injury in spinal cord injured patients: retrospective study of loss of consciousness and post-traumatic amnesia. *Arch Phys Med Rehabil.* 1985;66(1):41-43.

39. Banovac K. The effect of etidronate on late development of heterotopic ossification after spinal cord injury. *J Spinal Cord Med.* 2000;23(1):40-44.

40. Garland DE. A clinical perspective on common forms of acquired heterotopic ossification. *Clin Orthop Relat Res.* 1991;263:13-29.

41. Thompson L, Yakura J. Aging related functional changes in people with spinal cord injury. *Top Spinal Cord Rehabil.* 2001;6:69-82.

42. Bauman WA, Adkins RH, Spungen AM, Kemp BJ, Waters RL. The effect of residual neurological deficit on serum lipoproteins in individuals with chronic spinal cord injury. *Spinal Cord.* 1998;36(1):13-17.

43. Sisto SA, Lorenz DJ, Hutchinson K, Wenzel L, Harkema S, Krassioukav A. Cardiovascular status of individuals with incomplete spinal cord injury from 7 NeuroRecovery Network rehabilitation centers. *Arch Phys Med Rehabil.* 2102;93(9):1578-1587.

44. Nawoczenski D, Riek LM, Greco L, Staiti K, Ludewig PM. Effect of shoulder pain on shoulder kinematics during weight-bearing tasks in person with spinal cord injury. *Arch Phys Med Rehabil.* 2102;93(8):1421-1430.

45. Kirshblum S, Millis S, McKinley W, Tulsky D. Late neurologic recovery after traumatic spinal cord injury. *Arch Phys Med Rehabil.* 2004;85(11):1811-1817.

46. Pollard ME, Apple DF. Factors associated with improved neurologic outcomes in patients with incomplete tetraplegia. *Spine (Phila Pa 1976).* 2003;28(1):33-39.

47. Roth EJ, Lawler MH, Yarkony GM. Traumatic central cord syndrome: clinical features and functional outcomes. *Arch Phys Med Rehabil.* 1990;71(1):18-23.

48. Bracken MB. Steroids for acute spinal cord injury. *Cochrane Database Syst Rev.* 2012;18(1):CD001046.

49. Arora B, Suresh S. Spinal cord injuries in older children: is there a role for high-dose methylprednisolone? *Pediatr Emerg Care.* 2011;27(12):1192-1194.

50. Qian T, Guo X, Levi AD, Vanni S, Shebert RT, Sipski ML. High-dose methylprednisolone may cause myopathy in acute spinal cord injury patients. *Spinal Cord.* 2005;43(4):199-203.

51. Waters RL, Adkins R, Yakura J, Sie I. Functional and neurologic recovery following acute SCI. *J Spinal Cord Med*. 1998;21(3):195-199.

52. Waters RL, Adkins RH, Yakura JS, Sie I. Motor and sensory recovery following incomplete tetraplegia. *Arch Phys Med Rehabil*. 1994;75(3):311.

53. Dimar J, Carreon J, Riina J, Schwartz D, Harris M. Early versus late stabilization of the spine in the polytrauma patient. *Spine (Phila Pa 1976)*. 2010;35(21 Suppl):S187-S192.

54. Mulroy SJ, Gronley JK, Newsam CJ, Perry J. Electromyographic activity of shoulder muscles during wheelchair propulsion by paraplegic people. *Arch Phys Med Rehabil*. 1996;77(2):187-193.

55. Powers CM, Newsam CJ, Gronley JK, Fontaine CA, Perry J. Isometric shoulder torque in subjects with spinal cord injury. *Arch Phys Med Rehabil*. 1994;75(7):761-765.

56. Gronley JK, Newsam CJ, Mulroy SJ, Rao SS, Perry J, Helm M. Electromyographic and kinematic analysis of the shoulder during four activities of daily living in men with C6 tetraplegia. *J Rehab Res Dev*. 2000;37(4):423-432.

57. Garber CE, Blissmer B, Deschenes MR, et al. Position stand. Quantity and quality for developing and maintaining cardiorespiratory, musculoskeletal, and neuromotor fitness in apparently healthy adults: guidance for prescribing exercise. *Med Sci Sports Exerc*. 2011;43(7):1134-1359.

58. Silva AC, Neder JA, Chiurciu MV, et al. Effect of aerobic training on ventilatory muscle endurance of spinal cord injured men. *Spinal Cord*. 1998;36(4):240-245.

59. Gilgoff IS, Barras DN, Jones MS, Adkins HV. Neck breathing: a form of voluntary respiration for the spine-injured ventilator-dependent quadriplegic child. *Pediatrics*. 1988;82(5);741-745.

60. Warren VC. Glossopharyngeal and neck accessory muscle breathing in a young adult with C2 complete tetraplegia resulting in ventilator dependency. *Phys Ther*. 2002;82(6):590-600.

61. Liaw MY, Lin MC, Cheng PT, Wong MK, Tang FT. Resistive inspiratory muscle training: its effectiveness in patients with acute complete cervical cord injury. *Arch Phys Med Rehabil*. 2000;81(6):752-762.

62. Lerman RM, Weiss MS. Progressive resistive exercise in weaning high quadriplegics from the ventilator. *Paraplegia*. 1987;25(2):130-135.

63. Linn WS, Spungen AM, Gong H Jr, Adkins RH, Bauman WA, Waters RL. Forced vital capacity in two large outpatient populations with chronic spinal cord injury. *Spinal Cord*. 2001;39(5):263-268.

64. Consortium for Spinal Cord Medicine. *Outcomes Following Traumatic Spinal Cord Injury: Clinical Practice Guidelines for Health-Care Professionals*. Washington, DC: Paralyzed Veterans of America; 1999:9,10-20.

65. Somers MF. *Spinal Cord Injury: Functional Rehabilitation*. Norwalk, CT: Appleton and Lange; 1992.

66. Newsam CJ, Mulroy SJ, Gronley JK, Bontrager EL, Perry J. Temporal-spatial characteristics of wheelchair propulsion. *Am J Phys Med*. 1996;75(4):292-299.

67. Waters RL, Miller L. A physiologic rationale for orthotic prescription in paraplegia. *Clin Prosth Orthot*. 1987;11(2):66-73.

68. Beekman CE, Miller-Porter L, Schoneberger M. Energy cost of propulsion in standard and ultralight wheelchairs in people with spinal cord injuries. *Phys Ther*. 1999;79(2):146-158.

69. Waters RL, Mulroy S. The energy expenditure of normal and pathologic gait. *Gait Posture*. 1999;9(3):207-231.

70. Wu M, Landry JM, Schmit BD, Hornby TG, Yen SC. Robotic resistance treadmill training improves locomotor function in human spinal cord injury: a pilot study. *Arch Phys Med Rehabil*. 2012;93(5):782-789.

71. Koopman B, van Asseldonk EH, van der Kooij H, van Kijk W, Ronsse R. Rendering potential wearable robot designs with the LOPES gait trainer. *IEEE Int Conf Rehabil Robot*. 2011;2011:5975448.

72. Beekman C, Perry J, Boyd LA, Newsam CJ, Mulroy SJ. The effects of a dorsiflexion-stopped ankle-foot orthosis on walking in individuals with incomplete spinal cord injury. *Top Spinal Cord Inj Rehabil*. 2000;4(4):54-62.

73. Treatment of Pressure Ulcers. Clinical Practice Guideline #15 (AHCPR Publication #95-0652). Rockville, MD: US Department of Health and Human Services; 1994.

74. *Methods of Ischial Pressure Relief for Patients With Spinal Injury*. Downey, CA: Rancho Los Amigos Medical Center; 1980.

75. Coggrave MJ, Rose LS. A specialist seating assessment clinic: changing pressure relief practice. *Spinal Cord*. 2003;41(12):692-695.

76. Rubayi S, Pompan D, Garland D. Proximal femoral resection and musculocutaneous flap for the treatment of pressure ulcers in spinal cord injury patients. *Ann Plast Surg*. 1991;27(2):132-138.

Please see accompanying Web site at
www.healio.com/books/neuroptavideos

11

Clients With
Traumatic Brain Injury

Dennis Klima, PT, MS, PhD, GCS, NCS

KEY WORDS

- Coma
- Coup/contrecoup injury
- Diffuse axonal shearing
- Glasgow Coma Scale
- Persistent vegetative state
- Rancho Los Amigos Levels of Cognitive Function
- Traumatic brain injury

CHAPTER OBJECTIVES

- Describe major causes of traumatic brain injury (TBI).

- Discuss mechanisms of injury and medical complications associated with TBI.

- Describe the major categories of the Glasgow Coma Scale.

- Outline the major levels and associated cognitive behavior included in the Rancho Los Amigos Levels of Cognitive Function.

- Describe key components of the physical therapist's (PT's) examination for patients recovering from a TBI.

- Identify common cognitive, musculoskeletal, and neuromuscular body structure/function deficits seen in this special patient population.

- List physical therapy management precautions for individuals with TBI.

- Describe major interventions performed for those musculoskeletal and neuromuscular deficits noted in the PT's examination.

- Discuss techniques for integrating both cognitive and functional training strategies to advance the patient toward those established goals.

Umphred DA, Lazaro RT, eds.
Neurorehabilitation for the Physical Therapist Assistant,
Second Edition (pp 297-324).
© 2014 SLACK Incorporated.

- Describe key activities associated with patient discharge planning, home programs, equipment procurement, and community integration.

- Describe an exercise progression used to prepare athletes for safe return to play in a designated sport.

- Describe primary, secondary, and tertiary blast injuries associated with high-order explosion.

TRAUMATIC BRAIN INJURY: OVERVIEW

Managing clients with traumatic brain injury (TBI) presents a major challenge for all health care professionals working with this special patient population. More than 1 million people sustain a TBI each year in the United States; moreover, 80,000 to 90,000 individuals will have a lifelong disability secondary to the injury.[1,2]

A TBI may be defined as an "alteration in brain function, or other evidence of brain pathology, caused by an external force."[2] TBI accounts for one-third of all injury-related deaths in the United States, although the majority of all treated injuries are classified as mild.[1,3]

Major causes of head injury include motor vehicle and recreational vehicle accidents, as well as firearm-related injuries. TBI rates are higher for males in all age brackets, and individuals between the ages of 0 to 4 years and 15 to 19 years and adults over 65 years of age demonstrate the greatest risk for a TBI.[4] Motor vehicle accidents are a leading cause of head injury in minorities, and violence and pedestrian vehicle trauma account for greater incidences of injury than in nonminority populations.[5] No significant differences exist, however, in functional recovery patterns between minority and nonminority groups.[5] For individuals 65 years or older, the leading cause of TBI is a fall-related episode; moreover, TBI-related hospitalization and death rates are highest among adults aged 75 and older.[4,6]

Head injury sequelae can be devastating and affect virtually every component of the quality of life: self-care, home management, work responsibilities, and leisure activities.[7] Poor recovery outcomes can eventually lead to long-term institutional placement if caregiving demands exceed available resources in the home environment. Public awareness has increasingly focused on injury prevention through vigilance, with fall prevention strategies for older individuals and increased helmet use during recreational sports and cycling activities. Local and national brain injury associations serve as strong advocacy catalysts for children and adults recovering from a TBI.

THEORETICAL FRAMEWORK: ROLE OF THE PHYSICAL THERAPIST ASSISTANT

Physical therapist assistants (PTAs) perform interventions associated with deficits at all levels of the International Classification of Functioning, Disability and Health (ICF) model: body structure/function, activity, and participation components.[8] This framework is outlined in Figure 11-1. In addition, these domains may be affected by environmental as well as personal factors. Neurological interventions with this special patient population require a level of expertise beyond entry-level practice. PTAs working with these clients have gained experience through mentoring, continuing education, and shadowing activities in the clinical arena. Clinical expertise and additional responsibilities may have also developed through a career ladder progression in the rehabilitation setting. Physical therapists (PTs) and PTAs with expertise in neurological patient management serve as powerful expert mentors in facilitating clinical expertise among novice clinicians and students.[9]

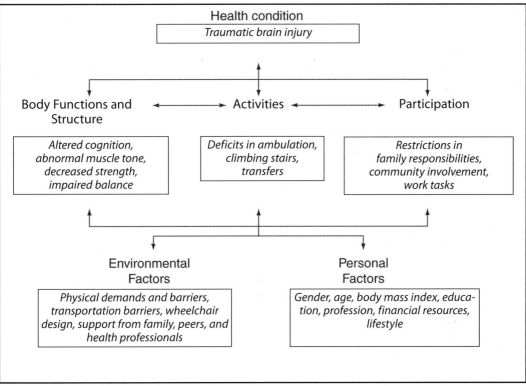

Figure 11-1. Integration of the International Classification of Functioning, Disability and Health framework with physical therapy management of clients with traumatic brain injury.

It should be noted that PTs and PTAs may initially elect to approach patient management through a team effort to enhance the PTA's intervention skills with patients with TBI. The seasoned PTA may then be delegated select interventions for more complicated patients for whom patient and situational considerations are less stable and predictable.[10] For example, functional activities with the agitated patient dictate immediate modification of intervention strategies given potential outbursts of hostility or inappropriate behavior. Effective delegation strategies are enhanced by ongoing communication with the supervising PT to optimize interventions performed by the PTA in the trajectory of care.

MEDICAL AND RECOVERY ISSUES

Mechanisms of Injury

Following a traumatic insult, the initial site of impact to the brain is known as the *coup* injury. Because of the rebound effect that occurs in the cranium following the initial impact, a *contrecoup* injury will often occur (Figure 11-2). The term *diffuse axonal shearing or injury* refers to neuronal damage associated with traumatic rotational acceleration and deceleration of the brain during unrestricted movement.[11] Extensive brain tissue deformation occurs through shearing forces and inertial loading incurred during the injury. Head injuries generally fall into 2 categories: open and closed. The skull and meninges remain intact following a closed-head injury, whereas open injuries cause fracture and rupture of these protective structures. *Contusions* refer to more localized hemorrhages that occur at the site of injury and are commonly seen in the frontal and temporal regions of the brain.

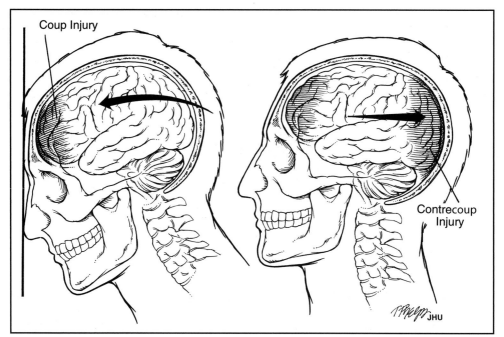

Figure 11-2. Mechanisms of injury: coup and contrecoup injuries. (Illustrations by Tim Phelps.)

Injuries sustained within the cranial vault may also be accompanied by concomitant edema, which adversely increases intracranial pressure (ICP). Normal ICP levels of between 0 and 15 mm Hg can substantially escalate to near-fatal levels. In addition, cerebral perfusion pressure may be impaired following a sustained head injury and neural oxygen supply becomes inadequate.[12] Additional secondary damage results from tissue hypoxemia or infection, with infection more commonly arising when open penetration to the skull occurs during the injury.

Complications

Unfortunately, TBI rarely occurs in isolation without other orthopedic or internal organ trauma. Skull fractures may be present and are classified by the specific type of fracture line or location. Common fractures include linear, depressed, and basilar skull fractures; additionally, each type of fracture is associated with unique characteristics. For example, depressed skull fractures often occur following a blow to the skull, whereas basilar skull fractures are associated with a high incidence of cranial nerve damage and meningitis.[13] In addition to these complications, patients can also experience multiple facial fractures and scalp lacerations. Facial fracture severity is outlined in the LeFort classification system.[14] Extremity fractures and internal organ damage further create potential life-threatening complications, which lengthen recovery periods. Common areas of injury include pelvic, femoral, and humeral fractures. The presence of heterotopic ossification, a condition characterized by the formation of ectopic bone in patients following spinal cord injury and TBI, may cause further joint motion restrictions.[15]

Another complicating factor to recovery is the presence of a hematoma after the head injury (Figure 11-3). Subdural hematomas refer to rupture of the cerebral bridging vein complex with resultant bleeding into the subdural space. Fluctuating periods of lucency characterize this type of bleeding episode.[16] An epidural, or extradural, hematoma, is usually caused by a tear in the middle meningeal artery. Patients sustaining these types of hematomas can experience varying degrees of altered consciousness, headaches, or other signs and symptoms specific to the areas of the lesion.[16] Intracerebral hematomas are located deeper within the brain and accompany more

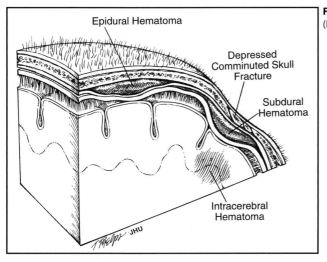

Figure 11-3. Complications from TBI. (Illustration by Tim Phelps.)

Epidural Hematoma

Depressed Comminuted Skull Fracture

Subdural Hematoma

Intracerebral Hematoma

severe traumatic injuries and basilar skull fractures. Extensive hematoma formation may require surgical evacuation though a craniotomy procedure. These massive hematomas can potentially cause a hemispheric midline shift because of the size of the space-occupying lesion. Patients sustaining severe injuries undergo radical craniotomy procedures with burr hole drilling and resultant removal of portions of the skull. Subsequent cranioplasty procedures with bone grafting are later performed to ensure neural tissue protection.

Seizures present further medical complications following TBI and may vary from mild in nature to those of the tonic-clonic variety. Seizures can occur immediately following the injury or can develop later in the course of recovery. Recent evidence suggests that the development of late post-traumatic seizures is linked to more extensive brain damage.[17] Patients are placed on prophylactic anticonvulsant medications, such as Dilantin (phenytoin), following a head injury to manage the recurrent seizure activity. Health care professionals who work with patients recovering from TBI should be versed in emergency procedures for those patients having post-traumatic seizure episodes to ensure patient safety during a seizure event. Patients should be protected during the episode and the type and duration of behavior should be well documented.

Recurrent, spontaneous seizure activity necessitates medication management. Common medications used for seizure management include Dilantin, Tegretol (carbamazepine), and phenobarbital. Pertinent adverse effects of seizure medications should also be recognized in the rehabilitation setting. Specifically targeting the motor cortex, Dilantin inhibits abnormal electrical discharge activity in the brain.[18] Major side effects include ataxia, nervousness, and confusion. Phenobarbital and Tegretol may both induce drowsiness as a potential side effect, and patients should be monitored for problematic oversedation while in therapy.[18] Zonegran (zonisamide), a more recent medication introduced in the United States, demonstrates fewer adverse cognitive side effects, although may induce distal upper-extremity dyskinesias.[19]

Intensive Care Unit Management

Following TBI, appropriate medical intervention must immediately address direct injuries as well as secondary complications. Multitrauma patients are often transported to local or regional trauma centers. Severe injuries necessitate intubation and the need for multiple intravenous lines. An ICP monitor may be placed to record ongoing pressure changes and gradients. Osmotic diuretics, such as mannitol, are used to decrease adverse ICP.

Damage to the abdominal or thoracic cavities can warrant chest tube placement, and those patients requiring extensive ventricular or fluid monitoring may have a specialized pulmonary artery monitor, the Swan-Ganz catheter, inserted.

Table 11-1
Glasgow Coma Scale

Eyes	Open	Spontaneously	4
		To verbal command	3
		To pain	2
	No response		1
Best motor response	To verbal stimulus	Obeys command	6
	To painful stimulus	Localizes pain	5
		Flexion-withdrawal	4
		Flexion-abnormal (decorticate rigidity)	3
		Extension (decerebrate rigidity)	2
		No response	1
Best verbal response	Oriented and converses		5
	Disoriented and converses		4
	Inappropriate words		3
	Incomprehensible sounds		2
	No response		1
Total range			**3-15**

(Adapted from Teasdale G, Jennett B. Assessment of coma and impaired consciousness: a practical scale. *Lancet.* 1974;2[7872]:81-84.)

In the very acute stage of medical intervention, patients will be evaluated using the Glasgow Coma Scale, and resultant scores will categorize the severity of the injury. The instrument assesses 3 domains of function in individuals following head injury: motor performance, eye opening, and verbal response (Table 11-1).[20] The scale is composed of 15 points, and injury severity is depicted through summation of the points from each of the 3 sections. Glasgow Coma Scale scores between 13 to 15 designate mild injury, 9 to 12 moderate injury, and 3 to 8 severe TBI.[11,21] Patients with mild brain injury generally demonstrate less severe loss of consciousness (< 20 to 30 minutes) and post-traumatic amnesia (< 24 hours).[22] Manifestations of moderate and severe brain injury are more pronounced and linked to brainstem injury. Factors associated with poorer outcomes include associated secondary injuries, persistent coma, and lingering post-traumatic amnesia.[23] The rehabilitation team members should be aware of the initial Glasgow score and ensuing complications at the time of injury to modify any examination or intervention activities.

Classification of Levels of Recovery

Recovery from TBI depends on a multitude of factors related to the extent of the injury, associated medical complications, and the patient's premorbid status. The Rancho Los Amigos Levels of Cognitive Function are often used to categorize patients following TBI and to describe behavioral patterns in the sequence of recovery (Table 11-2).[24] Composed of 8 levels, this scale illustrates a recovery continuum that begins with the patient's initial unresponsive status and then tracks

Table 11-2
Rancho Los Amigos Levels of Cognitive Function

I. No Response

The patient appears to be in a deep sleep and is completely unresponsive to any stimuli.

II. Generalized Response

The patient reacts inconsistently and nonpurposefully to stimuli in a nonspecific manner. Responses are limited and often the same regardless of the stimulus presented. Responses may be physiologic changes, gross body movements, and/or vocalization.

III. Localized Response

The patient reacts specifically but inconsistently to stimuli. Responses are directly related to the type of stimulus presented. The patient may follow simple commands in an inconsistent, delayed manner, such as with closing of the eyes or squeezing the hand.

IV. Confused/Agitated

Behavior is bizarre and nonpurposeful, relative to the immediate environment. The patient does not discriminate among persons or objects and is unable to cooperate with treatment efforts. Verbalizations are frequently incoherent and/or inappropriate to the environment. Confabulation may be present. Gross attention to the environment is very short and selective attention is often nonexistent. The patient lacks short-term recall.

V. Confused/Inappropriate

The patient is able to respond to simple commands fairly consistently. However, with increased complexity of commands or lack of any external structure, responses are non-purposeful, random, or fragmented. The patient has gross attention to the environment, but is highly distractible and lacks ability to focus attention to a specific task. With structure, the patient may be able to converse on a social-automatic level for short periods of time. Verbalization is often inappropriate and confabulatory; moreover, memory is severely impaired. The patient often shows inappropriate use of objects. He/she may perform previously learned tasks with structure but is unable to learn new information.

VI. Confused/Appropriate

The patient shows goal-directed behavior but is dependent on external input for direction. He/she follows simple directions consistently and shows carry-over for relearned tasks with little or no carry-over for new tasks. Responses may be incorrect due to memory problems but appropriate to the situation. Past memories show more depth and detail than recent memory.

VII. Automatic/Appropriate

The patient appears appropriate and oriented within the hospital and home settings. He/she goes through daily routines automatically and frequently in a robot-like fashion. The patient has minimal-to-absent confusion but has shallow recall of activities. There is carry-over for new learning, but at a decreased rate. With structure, the patient is able to initiate social or recreational activities. Judgment remains impaired.

VIII. Purposeful/Appropriate

The patient is able to recall and integrate past and recent events and is aware of and responds to the environment. He/she shows carry-over for new learning and needs no supervision once activities are learned. The patient may continue to show deficiencies, relative to premorbid abilities, in quality and rate of processing, abstract reasoning, tolerance for stress, and judgment in emergencies or unusual circumstances.

(Reprinted with permission from Hagen C, Malkmus D, Durham P. Levels of cognitive functioning. In: *Rehabilitation of the Head Injured Adult: Comprehensive Physical Management*. Downey, CA: Professional Staff Association of Rancho Los Amigos Hospital; 1979.)

cognitive improvement to the final behavioral category.[25] The initial 3 levels reflect the patient's minimally responsive phase. Level I denotes no response, whereas Level II reflects an observed generalized response to a designated stimulus.[24,25] Such generalized responses often are characterized by gross body movements or an increase in vital signs. Patients in the third level begin demonstrating more specific elicited response patterns, such as a hand squeeze or visual tracking in response to a verbal stimulus. It should be noted that patients with massive injuries and severe brain damage can permanently remain within these initial classification levels. The fourth level of the Rancho scale describes behavior related to the agitated patient. At this level, the patient is unable to integrate the multitude of sensory experiences in the immediate environment. The patient's gross attention to the environment is very limited. Aggression may arise when periods of overstimulation occur, and the patient becomes distracted very easily.[24,25] Young nonverbal pediatric patients may exhibit continual crying at this phase. The physician or PT needs to differentiate agitation from anger. Patients who are angry will often bite, use inappropriate verbal sayings, or strike at the clinician. Those people are beyond a level of agitation and confusion and are reacting to an environment they do not like with intent and awareness of that environment.

Levels V through VIII demonstrate gradual resolution of cognitive deficits toward behavior that is both purposeful and appropriate. In Level V, agitated behavior wanes, although the patient continues to demonstrate substantial deficits in language, memory, and praxis. The patient remains highly distractible and shows difficulty focusing on a specific task and demonstrates inappropriate behavior. Confused appropriate behavior is designated in the sixth level, and the patient begins demonstrating increased goal-directed behavior with the ability to follow simple commands.[24,25] In the remaining 2 Rancho levels (VII-Automatic/Appropriate and VIII-Purposeful/Appropriate), the patient becomes increasingly oriented and demonstrates improved learning capacity. In addition, responses become more automatic in nature. Judgment may continue to remain impaired in the final levels. The patient, for example, may have difficulty performing appropriate activities during emergency situations at home.

Following the acute rehabilitation phase, patients will be discharged to receive further rehabilitation at a rehabilitation center, subacute facility, or nursing home. Patients may even return home provided that sufficient care and monitoring can be provided by the caregiver. Inpatient settings may initially be preferred to offer more intense therapy on a daily basis. Rehabilitation centers, however, often have specific policies that dictate minimum Rancho levels for admission, and placement may be difficult for patients at lower functional levels.[26]

PHYSICAL THERAPY MANAGEMENT

Examination

The PT will perform an examination prior to the initiation of select intervention activities by the PTA. Given the patient's potential altered mental status, pertinent social history and home environment information may have to be obtained through family members or other caregivers. In performing a detailed systems review and examination, the PT will ascertain the degree to which the patient's injury has affected the overall baseline cognitive and functional status. Target tests and measures will further assess the extent of impairments and functional limitations.

The PTA should be clearly aware of those alterations in arousal, mentation, and cognitive status that may be encountered when dealing with patients with TBI. Examination findings may indicate varied levels of arousal impairment consistent with coma or persistent vegetative state. The term *coma* refers to a lack of responsiveness to verbal stimuli, variable responses to other forms of stimuli, and an absent sleep-wake cycle.[16] *Persistent vegetative state* denotes similar patterns of unresponsive behavior and tends to reflect a condition that will be of longer duration. Severe disturbances in cognition, arousal, and communication may impede standard testing procedures. For instance, patients are often able to follow only simple one-word commands, and examination strategies must be augmented. Key components of the cognitive examination area include orientation, level of consciousness, and memory. Confusion and disorientation may be considerable, and residual lethargy and sluggishness are often associated with delirium following head injury.[27] Furthermore, the patient may exhibit a concomitant period of post-traumatic amnesia (the time duration between the injury and subsequent ability to recall persons and events) and display persistent memory deficits during the recovery period.

Additional neurological testing will include assessment of select cranial nerves, sensation, and coordination. Patients with cerebellar deficits should be screened for extremity deficits, such as dysmetria and dysdiadochokinesia; moreover, trunk and axial ataxia patterns may be noted in sitting posture or gait activities. Neurological tests may uncover important findings that have implications for interventions by the PTA. For example, sensory disturbances may call for therapeutic handling adaptations, and cranial nerve deficits require intervention adjustments because of such conditions as hemianopsia.

A detailed musculoskeletal examination will yield findings related to muscle tone, strength, and joint range of motion (ROM). Abnormalities in tone may be found in any one or all extremities. Patients with more severe injuries may demonstrate postural patterns consistent with decorticate or decerebrate rigidity. Patients with decerebrate rigidity display strong extension posturing in all 4 extremities. Patients with decorticate rigidity demonstrate grossly flexed upper extremities with a similar lower extremity extension positioning. The PT may elect to quantify tonal disturbances through the Modified Ashworth Scale. In this scale, muscle tone is described through varying resistance felt throughout the available ROM.[28] Given the potential for joint contractures and limitations due to abnormal posturing or heterotopic ossification, joint integrity must be thoroughly assessed. Detailed goniometric measurements will underscore pertinent ROM limitations. When cognitive deficits impede formal testing procedures, examination of muscle performance may be completed through motor pattern analysis demonstrated in gravity-eliminated and antigravity planes. Patients at higher functional levels may be candidates for more traditional strength testing techniques.

Examination of the integument involves a systematic skin inspection to detect any possible skin irritation, rashes, or pressure ulcer areas. Patients who have begun posturing extremities are particularly at risk. The therapist must examine those areas that are particularly vulnerable for pressure sore development. These include the ischial tuberosities, greater trochanters, and sacrum. Patients who are bed-confined should be inspected for less common areas of skin compromise, such as the spine of the scapula or olecranon process. Protection devices may be indicated when the patient is unable to volitionally change positions in bed.

For patients at a higher level of function, examination activities will continue with assessment of all areas of functional mobility. Bed-mobility activities, including bridging, rolling, and supine-to-sit transitions, will be observed for level of assistance required and qualitative performance strategies. Static and dynamic balance will be assessed to investigate postural control in sitting and standing. Common balance instruments used to identify fall risk in the elderly have been extrapolated to quantify balance performance in individuals with head injury and include the Performance Oriented Mobility Assessment[29] and the Berg Balance Test.[30] (Refer to Chapter 4 for additional information.) These tools have not been thoroughly validated in the population of patients with TBI, although the PT may elect to use these instruments with geriatric patients who have sustained a head injury because of a fall.

Careful examination of the patient's gait and locomotion status will identify such important findings as pertinent gait deviations, required level of assistance, and muscle substitution patterns. Lastly, aerobic capacity and functional endurance will be measured through vital sign response to activity, perceived exertion, or other standardized measures of aerobic capacity. These baseline measures are particularly important for patients recovering from severe brain injuries because of reported diminished exercise capacity and fitness levels.[31]

Table 11-3
Practice Patterns Associated With Adult Head Injury[7]

Pattern 5D: Impaired motor function and sensory integrity associated with nonprogressive disorders of the central nervous system acquired in adolescence or adulthood

Pattern 5I: Impaired arousal, range of motion, and motor control associated with coma, near coma, or vegetative state

---

Evaluation, Diagnosis, and Prognosis

Following the examination, the PT will formulate a summation of findings in the evaluation and establish a diagnosis and prognosis. Diagnoses may be related to impaired mobility, motor function, or sensory integrity secondary to the TBI. Parameters of management for patients with TBI are delineated in the *Guide to Physical Therapist Practice, Second Edition*.[7] Two key practice patterns address management of the adult patient with head injury and include related practice content, such as the expected range of number of visits, factors affecting the duration of care, and applicable tests, measures, and interventions (Table 11-3). Prognostication for patients with TBI is based on characteristics of the injury, comorbidity conditions, and previous level of function. The PT's clinical decision-making process regarding the patient's prognosis will also be based on current evidence to support those short- and long-term goals established. For example, the PT must consider that patients with decreased awareness of their limitations following head injury tend to set less realistic goals.[32] In addition, brain injury severity, lower-extremity hypertonicity, and concomitant lower-extremity injuries are factors that have been shown to predict ambulation potential in children and adolescents following TBI.[33] Complications such as heterotopic ossification have been associated with poorer functional outcomes following TBI.[15]

Interventions

Initiating interventions within the PT's plan of care requires careful analysis of those mitigating impairments and functional limitations identified in the initial examination. Moreover, the PTA must carefully review the results of the PT's tests and measures to effectively target effective interventions aligned with those established goals within the plan of care. ROM goniometric measurements and muscle test grades will corroborate specific areas to be addressed. Furthermore, attention to upper motor neuron deficits will effectively allow the PTA to incorporate therapeutic exercise strategies to improve the patient's motor control. Patients recovering from TBI may demonstrate varying levels of hemiplegia in accordance with the severity of the insult. Motor performance may progress through Brunnstrom's recovery sequence, and active dissociation should be recognized to track and facilitate recovery patterns.[34] For example, the PTA must note progress through increased complexity of extremity movement combinations as compared with abnormal synergy patterns. Finally, functional mobility activities will be implemented to address major deficits in bed and wheelchair (w/c) mobility, transfers, balance, and gait performance. Along with the PT evaluation, the PTA should look at the occupational therapy and speech/language pathology evaluations and progress notes for additional information pertinent to the patient's plan of care. These evaluations will provide information related to perceptual, communication, and cognitive impairments that may be present that impact performance of essential activities of daily living.

SPECIFIC INTERVENTIONS FOR IMPAIRMENTS AND FUNCTIONAL LIMITATIONS

Seating Considerations

Careful consideration of all aspects of the patient's condition should be weighed when creating an initial seating system for the patient. The PTA may work in conjunction with the supervising PT in making adaptive changes to the w/c for optimum positioning and seating alignment. Patients lacking postural control may benefit from a tilt-in-space w/c with attached head positioning.[35] A recliner w/c may be used for patients with orthopedic fixation devices and associated fractures. Patients with residual hemiparesis deficits may find hemi-height w/cs effective for propulsion maneuvers given the reduced seat-to-floor height. When adapting any seating system for the patient's needs, it becomes important to recognize the advantages and disadvantages of any change that is proposed. For example, the addition of desk-style armrests to a w/c may be beneficial for approaching any table surface, although they may impede a patient's ability to perform a sit-to-stand maneuver if upper-extremity assistance is required.

For patients first using w/cs, appropriate time should be allotted for instruction in propulsion maneuvers and parts management. Patients should be taught brake-locking maneuvers, leg-rest management, and general propulsion strategies for level surface and turn negotiation. Important points of safety should be reinforced when cognitive deficits exist and judgment is impaired. Frequently an initial short-term goal for the patient will be to independently propel between the physical therapy department and the rehab gym for scheduled sessions (Figure 11-4).

Therapeutic Exercise

The PTA may be delegated selected activities involving the application of various therapeutic exercise programs for impaired joint integrity or muscle performance.[7] Given the prevailing weakness that develops from either the injury itself or the adverse effects of bed rest, patients may exhibit considerable deficits in muscle performance. The PTA should be cautious in scrutinizing examination findings to discern specific muscle grades of tested muscles or the ratings of muscle tone to effectively position and stabilize affected areas. Appropriate therapeutic exercise programs and mobility activities should be implemented based on these test findings. For example, in an analysis of patients with TBI, Duong et al[36] found that those patients having less than 3/5 lower-extremity strength on admission required greater assistance with transfers and locomotion. Passive ROM and active-assisted strategies may be indicated for flaccid limbs, and the PTA may be required to don and doff various splints, braces, or other orthoses to effectively position an extremity.[37] Splints should not be used in place of comprehensive stretching programs but rather as an adjunct to treatment.[38] Aggressive-passive ROM regimens are necessary to maintain joint integrity when hypertonicity results in prolonged flexed or extended posturing of extremities. In a study of 105 patients diagnosed with moderate or severe brain injury, it was noted that a major predisposing factor to ankle contracture development included dystonia in the inversion and plantarflexion musculature.[39]

Depending on the resultant impairments from TBI, neurofacilitation techniques may be required to enhance optimum motor performance with upper motor neuron deficits (Figure 11-5). Active dissociation patterns can be used in conjunction with functional activities to promote active use of hemiparetic extremities.[40] In addition, strategies employing techniques such as weight bearing can facilitate stabilization in flaccid extremities. (Refer to Chapter 5 for additional suggestions.) PTAs may elect to have patients perform bilateral extremity patterns for activation of weakened muscle groups.[41] Using air splints may be beneficial to position an extremity during

Figure 11-4. Initial short-term goals for the patient include performing w/c parts management independently and propelling to and from therapy sessions.

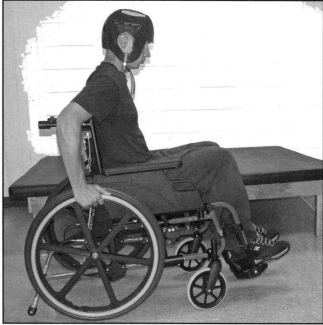

Figure 11-5. Neurofacilitation techniques are performed to enhance optimum motor performance when upper motor neuron deficits are present.

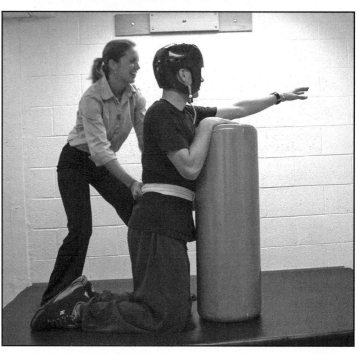

an activity. Current interventions involving constraint-induced movement therapy in stroke rehabilitation have also proven to be beneficial in individuals recovering from TBI.[42] This procedure involves restraining the patient's unaffected upper extremity in an effort to promote increased functional use of the hemiparetic extremity.

The effective clinician should be innovative in adapting therapeutic regimens around prevailing cognitive deficits. Patients may benefit more from exercise activities within the context of a

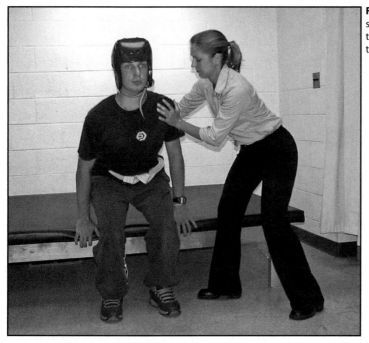

Figure 11-6. Activities, such as the sit-to-stand transition allow patients to perform exercise programs within the context of a task.

task rather than conventional cardinal plane performance (Figure 11-6). Patients sustaining additional extremity or spinal fractures may require additional adjustment of therapeutic exercise programs based on the location and severity of the fracture. Caution should be used when handling any extremity with a cast or external fixator apparatus.

Functional Mobility Training

Functional training interventions are germane to the patient's rehabilitative success. It is within this domain that PTAs can effectively and strategically progress the patient toward the short- and long-term mobility goals established by the supervising PT. In accordance with both cognitive and mentation recovery, appropriate mobility maneuvers will guide patients in achieving optimum functional independence. Patients at lower functional or cognitive levels require extensive practical training in transfer techniques and bed mobility sequences.[43] Patients with severely impaired coordination, dense hemiparesis, or orthopedic trauma may initially require a dependent transfer strategy in an effort to maneuver from surface to surface. Patients sustaining TBI with associated fractures or other complications present a challenge. Extensive fractures and orthopedic complications necessitate modified transfer strategies secondary to weight-bearing restrictions on multiple extremities. Furthermore, fixation devices, such as halo vests, alter balance responses[44] and normal postural transitions, such as supine to sit. Sliding boards and upper-extremity fracture platform devices are beneficial to perform transfers and bed mobility tasks.

The PTA should guide the patient toward independence in all bed mobility skills, including bridging, rolling, and supine to sit. Sit-to-stand transitions may be especially difficult during recovery.[45] Patients having hemiparetic extremities should be taught strategies to use and facilitate use of these limbs. Activities such as bridging merge functional tasks with active dissociation patterns. Adjuncts to treatment, such as physio balls and bolsters, may prove helpful in securing patient positioning.

Figure 11-7. The PTA can manipulate the sensory systems that modulate balance through the use of foam for higher-level patients.

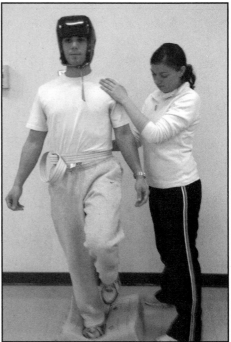

Interventions for Balance Impairments

Patients recovering from TBI may demonstrate balance impairments related to their injury. Balance interventions are aimed at maintaining the body's center of mass within the limits of stability given environmental factors and the individual's own biomechanics.[46] The regulation of balance reflects contributions by the vestibular, somatosensory, and visual systems to effectively maintain postural control. The PTA may elect to challenge or manipulate these sensory systems by having the patient stand on foam or reduce the patient base of support in tandem stance (Figure 11-7). The interaction of these systems illustrates a systems approach to motor control and represents an integrated, multisystem network among various structures within the central nervous system to modulate balance responses. (Refer to Chapters 4 and 5 for additional ideas on intervention and examination.) This more current model better displays the dynamic nature of the central nervous system compared with previous hierarchical paradigms.

The initial examination by the PT should clarify the extent of the balance impairment and the degree to which functional sitting and standing require attention. The PTA should recognize key components, as well as score interpretation, of common balance instruments. The Performance-Oriented Mobility Assessment,[29] also known as the Tinetti instrument, was formulated to assess balance and gait disturbances in the geriatric population. The instrument contains 28 available points, and a simple ordinal scale is used. The Berg Balance Scale is a simple battery used to assess an individual's balance control during a series of tasks, which are graded on a 4-point scale. Fifty-six available points are possible from performance on the 14 skill categories.[30] Subjects must perform a variety of tasks that include a transfer, picking up an object from the floor, and alternately touching a step stool with each foot. For patients at a higher functional level, the therapist may elect to use the functional High-Level Mobility Assessment Tool (HiMAT) to assess the ability to perform advanced activities, such as running, hopping, and walking backward.[47] Scores from the PT's initial examination may point to those target interventions that are needed in the rehabilitation program. For example, patients having difficulty with the sit-to-stand maneuver on a standardized balance instrument may require preliminary activities such as strengthening activities or arising from varied surfaces to successfully master the activity.

It should be noted that patients demonstrating balance improvements from rehabilitation programs may not necessarily have concomitant gait progress.[48] Moreover, medical complications from the patient's acute care hospitalization affect balance performance. In a recent multicenter analysis of factors associated with balance deficits among patients recovering from TBI, it was found that the incidence of medical complications (eg, respiratory complications and urinary tract infections) was strongly related to sitting balance impairment.[49]

Balance impairments can be caused or further exacerbated by existing muscle weakness. The presence of abductor weakness may result in a compensated abnormal trunk lean in unilateral stance toward the more affected side.[50] This compensation strategy becomes especially treacherous if the patient has a decreased upper-extremity protective response because of hemiplegia or processing latency. Simple light touch contact with a cane or other assistive device may prove beneficial in improving postural control by enhancing hip abductor activation.[51]

Balance training should also reflect activities with attention to designated strategies used to maintain postural control. The sequential ankle, hip, and stepping strategies may be interrupted because of motor control problems or abnormal coactivation. (Refer to Chapter 5, Figures 5-11 and 5-12, for examples of these strategies.) Also, flexibility limitations at the hip and ankle may further impede strategy activation. Recent evidence in the application of tai chi techniques suggests that this intervention approach has demonstrated efficacy in improving standing balance with individuals who sustained a severe head injury.[52] (Refer to Chapter 15 for additional information on complementary therapies.) Patients with severe balance impairments or vestibular dysfunction require more advanced interventions by the PT.

Unfortunately, persistent dizziness following TBI has been shown to be a major barrier to reemployment among patients desiring to return to work following their injury.[53]

Gait and Locomotion Training

Gait interventions are major constituents in the functional mobility program of the patient. It is essential that qualitative and quantitative parameters of gait performance be addressed. Patients should not be advanced with gait-training activities without the appropriate muscle activity or assistive device to support a limb or advance the lower extremities in gait. Patients often achieving independent functional ambulation within 3 months of their TBI include those who are younger, less severely injured, and have a better functional ambulation profile prior to the onset of rehabilitation.[54]

Gait quality for the patient with TBI becomes a major priority in rehabilitation training. PTAs should link gait deviation causality to those concomitant impairments. For example, tightness in the gastrocnemius muscle may be linked to a genu recurvatum tendency in stance phase. Likewise, residual weakness in the ankle dorsiflexors may induce a steppage or circumducted swing pattern.[50] Because of the duality in roles of the dorsiflexor muscles in stance and swing phases, an abrupt slap may be observed during the loading response. Persistence of gait deviations should be communicated to the supervising PT to assess the patient for possible orthotic candidacy.

Patients with resultant spastic hemiplegia in the lower extremities may have additional gait deviations. Particular problematic gait issues include the adductor/scissoring gait, the stiff knee, and the equinovarus foot.[55] Specific interventions should be employed to address gait quality. Stretching techniques can be performed to elongate spastic muscle groups. Aggressive stretching is indicated following select chemodenervation procedures, such as Botox injections or phenol nerve blocks, to improve gait quality.[55] In addition, the PTA may assist with advanced tone management procedures. The PT frequently elects to perform serial casting with a patient who has moderate to severe plantarflexion tone to achieve improved ankle ROM for gait or w/c footplate positioning for

Figure 11-8. The PT may apply a serial cast to gain ankle ROM for patients who have moderate to severe hypertonicity.

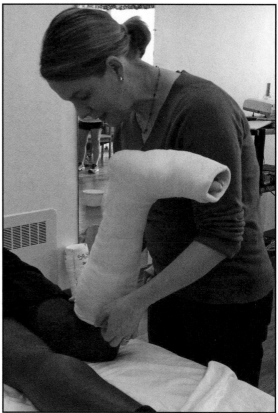

nonambulators. The procedure involves the application of a plaster or fiberglass cast for a series of days to achieve the desired ROM gain (Figure 11-8).[56]

Correction strategies during gait and locomotion training are implemented to normalize gait quality and to improve quantitative parameters, such as speed, distance, and base of support. Independence in ambulation for short distances may take 6 months or longer for those individuals recovering from severe injuries.[43] Selection of the appropriate gait device may be problematic when extensive cognitive deficits persist. Patients often exhibit difficulty with sequencing and placement of the cane, crutches, or walker. Patients at higher functional levels should be trained on all surfaces and should perform activities on inclines, curbs, and uneven surfaces. Instruction in floor transfers is also an integral part of the management plan for the patient who is at risk for falls (Figure 11-9). Often slight gait deviations are persistent following TBI, and patients attempt to maximize safety through a slower walking pattern and increased guardedness.[57] Body weight–support treadmill training interventions have been used to improve gait performance as well as aerobic capacity in the rehabilitation plan of care (Figure 11-10).[58]

The PTA should be aware that walking speed is an integral part of community navigation and the return to participation. A gait speed of 1.2 meters per second is required to effectively navigate the community and cross streets.[59] The PT may initially measure this velocity by timing ambulation across a 4-meter path, with appropriate acceleration and deceleration distances allotted prior to and following the designated path. Gait velocity is determined by dividing 4 meters by this measured time. The PTA should incorporate speed drills and dual-task activities to prepare patients functioning at a higher level of motor performance for traffic light changes and changing task demands on the gait cycle.

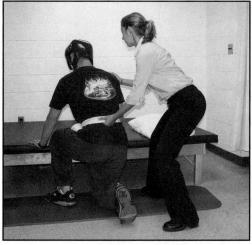

Figure 11-9. Instruction in floor transfers is an integral part of interventions for higher-level patients.

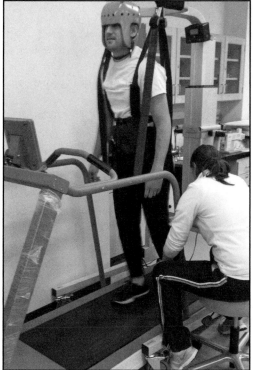

Figure 11-10. The PT may use body weight–support treadmill training to improve gait performance and aerobic capacity.

SPECIAL CONSIDERATIONS FOR THE PATIENT WITH BRAIN INJURY

Coma Emergence

Patients with severe TBI may require extensive medical management on the intensive care unit. Following medical stabilization, patients will be discharged to facilities where coma-emergence programs may be implemented. The PT may track progress through a standardized coma-emergence rating form. Three commonly used instruments include the JFK-Revised instrument, the Coma/Near Coma Scale, and the Western Neuro Sensory Stimulation Profile.[60] These tools assist in quantifying designated responses to standardized sensory stimuli. Patients reaching maximum scores on these instruments may then have more advanced goals and intervention plans established. Patients emerging from minimally responsive states may be progressively mobilized through the use of tilt table or standing-frame activities. Patients are begun on a sitting schedule to gradually increase sitting time. Vital signs should be carefully monitored for orthostatic changes and adverse physiological responses to positional changes. Patients can demonstrate abnormal fluctuations in blood pressure and diaphoresis. PTAs often work in tandem with supervising therapists in coma-emergence programs given the complexity of the multiple medical issues and ongoing need for reexamination. In addition, patients often require 2 people for lifts, positioning, serial casting, and standing activities.

The Agitated Patient

Perhaps one of the most challenging issues for all rehabilitation team members is management of the agitated patient. Significant agitation can contribute to the patient's length of stay, hinder functional independence, and ultimately hinder impending discharge to home.[61] PTs and PTAs must be attentive to the multitude of sensory experiences that are communicated to the patient during this stage because of potential adverse responses from the patient. Patients often become anxious and aggressive when they cannot process the immediate sensory information within their environment. Moreover, patients may overreact in the presence of relatively minor requests or tasks.

The PTA must effectively strategize interventions to deliver appropriate sensory experiences. Sessions should be structured properly to prevent sensory overload.[24] Often, quiet areas are helpful in reducing distractions, and reducing voice volume may be more calming. Treatment sessions may have to be modified to multiple shorter sessions. Time-out periods can be implemented when undesired behavior is unable to be redirected. Caution must be taken with verbal and manual cues during mobility maneuvers, as agitated patients may demonstrate periods of tactile defensive behavior. Before assuming that the agitated or negative behavior presented by the patient is due to the TBI, the therapist should first assess the environment and behavior of the clinicians to determine if a change in the therapist's techniques or voice or the surrounding environment may eliminate the patient's unwanted behavior.

Integration of Cognitive and Neuromuscular Interventions

The ultimate challenge in head trauma rehabilitation is to integrate cognitive and functional training strategies to effectively guide the patient toward established target goals and to maximize independence. The added cognitive dimension within therapeutic interventions adds a level of complexity that necessitates the skills of the experienced PTA. Cognitive impairments following TBI may be substantial. Sleep disorders arising after the injury can also interfere with treatment sessions.[62] Patients may demonstrate slower processing and require increased time to optimize task performance.[63] Diminished attention span is also apparent, and patients require ongoing redirection to the designated task. Simple strategies, such as reducing background distraction noise can be helpful. The PTA must consider that learning often occurs at a considerably diminished rate in the rehabilitation activity. Appropriate time allotment and cue sequence must be constructed within a treatment session to facilitate skill attainment. The effective PTA will recognize processing latencies when teaching motor tasks and allow appropriate time for problem solving. Finally, physical therapy clinicians must be reminded that the issue of impaired judgment is still evident, even in the latter stages of the Rancho scale. Cognitive and motor recovery rates do not necessarily occur in synchrony, and while independent in mobility skills, the patient with poor judgment creates a potentially dangerous situation if left unsupervised in the clinic or home environment or out in the community.

Cognitive and functional interventions are frequently fused in a variety of ways. The PTA can perform gait interventions while requiring that the patient perform the necessary speed changes needed during an emergency situation, such as exiting a building during a fire drill. Reinforcing safety strategies taught during previous sessions will assist the patient in identifying critical components of a desired task. PTAs should employ critical problem-solving strategies to maximize patients' ability to prepare for home or community situations. Such activities might include performing safety maneuvers with rail support in dim lighting during stairs negotiation or practicing dialing 911. A patient's cognitive recovery can be monitored through a cognitive log.[64] This is a simple bedside tool that tracks progress in measures, such as memory, language, attention, and reasoning. Progress achieved and patient outcomes may also be monitored through such assessment measures, such as the Functional Independence Measure tool. This outcomes measure has demonstrated validity with patients recovering from TBI.[65]

Precautions

Functional mobility programs and interventions for patients with TBI require attention to several key issues. Patients who are agitated should be monitored closely and should never be left alone if 24-hour direct supervision is required. Furthermore, rehabilitation professionals should make sure assistance is immediately available within the treatment area if a sudden occurrence of agitation should occur. Functional activities in enclosed areas, such as stairwells, dictate additional personnel nearby. Policies should be in place for a silent "show of force" pending significant outbursts of aggressive behavior. For example, multiple staff may be required to rush to a patient's room to diffuse a hostile behavioral event. PTAs must be cognizant of policies implemented to protect patients who have been victims of family abuse or assault; moreover, alias names are used as part of the facility's procedures to maintain patient protection and confidentiality.

Managing patients at lower levels of function also mandates precautionary measures. Patients who have undergone craniotomy procedures may require helmet use. Patients are regularly required to wear a helmet when out of bed. When patients are mobilized without the helmet, care should be taken not to put excess pressure over the affected area. Rehabilitation team members must also demonstrate competency with management of catheters, oxygen canisters, and tube-feeding lines during treatment sessions.

DISCHARGE PLANNING AND COMMUNITY REENTRY

Equipment Procurement and Family Training

The PTA will be involved in all aspects of discharge planning following the designated course of rehabilitation. Appropriate ordering of durable medical equipment will be required at the time of discharge, and the PTA will participate in the ordering of required assistive device and ambulation needs. If a w/c is required, appropriate features should be ordered to sufficiently address the patient's needs. For example, appropriate seat width and depth should accommodate the patient's size, and front-rigging features should provide for necessary lower-extremity support and orthopedic considerations.[35] Elevating leg rests may also be required for individuals with lower-extremity fractures or circulatory impairments.

An important component of the discharge disposition will include family training activities for those patients being discharged who require care and assistance at home. The PTA will effectively train the caregiver in mobility strategies that are linked to those functional needs of the patient.

Table 11-4
Key Questions Addressed During the Home Visit

---

1. Will the patient be able to enter and exit the living environment safely?
2. What environmental barriers are present?
3. Are any grab bars or additional devices needed in the bathroom?
4. If a wheelchair is to be used, will it be able to clear the doorways?
5. Where are steps encountered in the home?
6. Are rails available in stairways? If so, right or left?
7. Are safety devices present, such as smoke alarms or telephone access?
8. Will the patient be able to navigate around furniture in all rooms?

These activities may include transfer techniques, ambulation guarding, w/c management skills, and supervision of home exercise programs. Family training programs should also address car transfers and both stairs and curb negotiation.

In conjunction with recommendations by the supervising PT, the PTA may suggest the need for continued therapy interventions. Patients may require a course of outpatient or home therapy in an effort to continue work toward the long-term goals established for the patient in the plan of care. Patients who are at higher functional levels may benefit from a community reentry program to transition into previous employment and societal roles.

Home Assessment

Prior to discharge, the PTA or supervising PT may elect to conduct a home visit to assess the patient's home environment and identify potential environment barriers. The setting should be thoroughly inspected for possible safety issues that may arise when the patient returns home. Scrutiny of doorway widths, inclines, and floor surfaces is especially important for the patient who will be returning home in a w/c. In addition, the PTA should analyze major entrance and exit passageways to the home. In some rehabilitation settings, patients may be allowed to return home for a scheduled visit prior to discharge for a trial run of mobility skills acquired. Often rehabilitation team members perform a joint home assessment to address multiple areas of potential patient needs (Table 11-4). The PTA serves as an important conduit to the supervising PT for identifying issues related to the discharge disposition and recommendations.

Home Programs

Creating an individualized home program following discharge from an inpatient rehabilitation stay requires careful attention to all components of the patient's functional status. Exercise interventions should target weakened muscle groups and incorporate functional activities; moreover, the exercises should be sufficient in quantity to address pertinent needs yet not overwhelming in number. Home programs should provide for ambulation activity with the caregiver where possible.

It is crucial that the program extend beyond a simple instructional sheet. Performance logs will help ensure adherence, especially when caregiver supervision is not optimum. Written instructions should be clearly written with large print and should contain key terms familiar to the patient and caregiver.[66] Using medical jargon or unknown terms becomes detrimental to the teaching process. Diagrams are often useful, especially when the PTA wants to accentuate important performance strategies or points of emphasis in the program. Effective home programs take into account those residual cognitive deficits that may still be pervasive at the time of discharge. Caregivers supervising home programs should receive appropriate instructions regarding strategies to facilitate optimum performance in lieu of any attention or processing deficits.

Community Integration

Patients who are recovering from TBI often begin community reentry activities during the inpatient rehabilitation stay. The rehabilitation team members may accompany patients, for example, on a community outing to the mall or a recreation activity. Patients who display behavior consistent with the final Rancho stages, Levels VII and VIII, are particularly appropriate for such activities, and the PTA will be able to observe such phenomena as abstract reasoning processes and social interactions. Gait and locomotion progress within the environmental context can also be analyzed during community outings to gauge the patient's readiness for participation.

Patients may also continue community reentry activities with adult day programs designed for this special patient population. These programs assist patients in transitioning to employment initiatives and also provide important psychosocial support. Important activities aimed at optimizing problem-solving skills are addressed because of those residual cognitive deficits that still exist.[67] Factors associated with a good quality of life following TBI include inveterate community and social support.[68] Key factors impeding patients' successful return to employment include significant cognitive impairment and low education levels.[69] Day programs can also provide resource assistance for those patients who experience depression, which is one of the most common secondary conditions associated with TBI.[70]

SPECIAL POPULATIONS OF PATIENTS WITH TRAUMATIC BRAIN INJURY

Concussion

Recent attention on local, national, and international levels has focused on managing the athlete following a sustained concussion. Operationally, a concussion is a clinically diagnosed brain injury caused by traumatic biomechanical forces with or without a loss of consciousness.[71] It is important to underscore that a concussion, while often mild, is a TBI. Concussions may occur through organized and unorganized sports, including bicycling and playground activities. PTAs may work with patients following concussion to improve deficits in balance and coordination, and participate in the multidisciplinary effort to safely return an athlete to contact or noncontact play. In their published consensus statement of sports-related concussion (Table 11-5), McCrory and colleagues established guidelines to progress athletes through a continuum of activities and maximize neural preparedness for safe return to play.[71]

Blast Injuries

Soldiers returning from service duty in active military zones have sustained unique injuries associated with warfare: blast injury. Blast injuries occur when, following detonation, high-order explosives propel expanding gases and create a blast wind. Three types of injuries have commonly been described.[72] Primary injuries occur from the impact of the blast wave. Structures with an air-solid interface, such as the lungs and tympanic membrane, are especially susceptible. Secondary injuries can occur when soldiers are hit by shrapnel (ie, rocks and pellets) from detonated improvised explosive devices. Tertiary injuries occur when soldiers are thrown off their feet and propelled into objects, sustaining various traumatic injuries and fractures.[72]

Table 11-5

Therapeutic Interventions Aligned for Phases of Return to Play in the Management of Athletes With Concussion

Rehabilitation Stage	Functional Intervention Example	Objective
No activity	Complete cognitive and physical rest	Brain recovery
Light aerobic conditioning	Walking, swimming	Add movement
Sport-specific exercise	Running sprint in soccer or lacrosse	Add movement
Noncontact training drills	Passing in football or lacrosse	Multitask Intensity
Full-contact practice	Normal training activities (with medical clearance)	Return to sport-specific intensity

(Adapted from McCrory P, Meeuwisse W, Johnston K, et al. Consensus statement on concussion in sport: the 3rd International Conference on Concussion in Sport held in Zurich, November 2008. *Amer Acad Phys Med Rehabilit*. 2009;1[5]:401-418.)

Soldiers returning from active duty with injuries may be managed through the veterans' network continuum of care, including polytrauma rehabilitation centers. PTAs working with soldiers in these settings will perform interventions aligned with the severity of injuries, including body weight–supported treadmill training to increase gait endurance and distance.[73] Vestibular and ocular exercises may be performed to alleviate symptoms of dizziness occurring at rest or during activities requiring exertion.[74]

CONCLUSION

Rehabilitating individuals with TBI offers the PTA the unique opportunity to interlock principles of functional training with key cognitive strategies to improve the overall quality of life for their clients. Carefully planned intervention programs, molded from clinical expertise and best-practice evidence, range from bed mobility to locomotion activities to community reentry activities.[75] Interventions by the PTA are pivotal components of the ICF and Patient/Client Management Model as they relate to managing patients with TBI.[76] The approach to individuals with complex deficits in body structure/functions and activities should be one of partnership between the PTA and the supervising PT to effectively facilitate the patient's return to community participation. The effective PT/PTA team will successfully assemble appropriate intervention and reexamination activities, in conjunction with ongoing communication, to optimize functional and neurobehavioral outcomes for the patient.

CASE STUDY

The patient, Leszek, is a 19-year-old Polish student who was an unrestrained passenger in a motor vehicle accident. He suffered a right frontal cerebral contusion with diffuse axonal shearing. He also sustained a mild subdural hematoma in the right frontal lobe pole. The initial Glasgow Coma Scale score was 12 in the emergency room. His acute care admission was significant for episodes of post-traumatic seizures, which lengthened his stay considerably. Following medical stabilization, he was transferred to a rehabilitation setting where an initial examination was performed by the PT. The patient's cognitive status was consistent with Rancho Level VI.

On admission, the PT performed the examination. Findings include:

History and systems review: Information was obtained from the patient's family because of the patient's memory deficits. Leszek's parents are Polish immigrants who moved to this country 16 years ago. He is a student at the university and is majoring in accounting. Leszek works as a waiter at a local restaurant on weekends. His medical history is significant for asthma, and he has had no major surgeries. He enjoys dancing and playing soccer. They characterize Leszek as a "quick learner." He lives with his family in a 2-story home. There are 8 steps between floors. The family has a pet dog, Borek, who is in good health. The patient has one sister, who will be getting married in 1 month. The patient's current medications include Dilantin and albuterol.

Tests and Measures

Orientation: Oriented to name only.

Arousal/mentation: Lethargic; slow in initiating activity.

Short-term memory: Poor/unable to remember 3 objects.

Cranial nerves: Intact I-XII.

Sensation: Intact to light touch and proprioception in all extremities.

ROM/joint integrity: No upper extremity limitations noted passively. Lower extremity passive ROM is significant for a lack of full hip extension on the right by 5 degrees and a lack of 10 degrees on the left. Knee and ankle joints demonstrate no limitations. No significant muscle tone abnormalities detected.

Strength: Upper extremity: 4/5 in major shoulder and elbow muscle groups.

5/5 wrist and hand musculature.

Lower extremity: Proximal weakness: 3+/5 hip abductors and extensors.

4/5 hip rotators, flexors.

4/5 quadriceps/hamstrings.

5/5 ankle/foot musculature.

Reflexes: 2+ biceps, triceps, brachioradialis, 1+ quadriceps, 2+ gastrocnemius.

Coordination: Mild right upper extremity dysmetria noted in the finger-to-nose test.

Balance: Maintains static unsupported sitting > 3 min. Patient loses balances when reaching outside base of support. Standing: Unable to stand unsupported; demonstrates a (+) Romberg.

Bed mobility: Moderate assistance/supine to sit.

Minimal assistance/bridging.

Minimal assistance/rolling.

Moderate assistance/sit to stand.

Gait and locomotion: Patient ambulates 10 feet with a rolling walker with moderate assistance; he demonstrates decreased step and stride lengths and displays strong tendency to shuffle feet in gait. (+) Trendelenburg noted bilaterally.

W/C mobility: Supervision required for parts management. Propels 20 feet with minimal assistance and extensive cues for turns and direction changes.

Aerobic capacity: Resting heart rate of 64 beats/min. Following ambulation: 88 beats per minute. No shortness of breath observed following ambulation. Oxygen saturation: Resting: 95%, post-ambulation: 92%.

Lungs: Clear to auscultation other than mild congestion heard in upper airways.

Goals: *Long-term goals (3 weeks)*

1. Supervision with household ambulation with assistive device (distances: 100 feet) with verbalized safety precautions.

2. Independent transfers and bed mobility.

3. Supervision with stairs negotiation with right rail and correct step sequencing.

4. Supervision with home exercise program.

5. Hip strength: 4/5 bilaterally and ROM: 15 degrees passive hip extension for stairs negotiation.

6. Durable medical equipment procurement.

7. Completion of family training activities.

8. Dancing with supervision with family members in preparation for upcoming wedding.

Short-term goals (1 week)

1. Ambulation 40 feet with minimal assistance with rolling walker.

2. Transfers with minimal assistance and minimal cues for safety.

3. Rolling and bridging with supervision and minimal cues; sit to stand with minimal assistance.

4. W/C propulsion to and from physical therapy sessions with supervision.

5. Independent w/c parts management.

6. W/C pressure relief with supervision.

Evaluation, prognosis, and diagnosis: The PT noted that Leszek demonstrates excellent rehabilitation potential because of his current functional profile, age, and minimal restrictions by comorbidity conditions. The prognosis for improving his overall functional mobility status is good, although impaired cognition may impede immediate involvement with previous community and work-related activities. The PT's diagnosis conveys impaired motor function associated with the TBI, along with related balance impairments and functional limitations in transfers, bed mobility, and gait.

Plan of care: The patient will receive physical therapy for 1 hour daily for gait training, therapeutic exercise, balance activities, and transfers. Appropriate durable medical equipment procurement and family training activities will be included. The patient's estimated length of stay is 3 weeks.

INTERVENTIONS

Following the initial examination, the PTA began seeing the patient daily. Leszek was also followed by occupational therapy and speech therapy. A w/c and temporary seating system was prepared. Leszek performed a daily regimen of functional training involving those activities included in the plan. Therapeutic exercises included extremity exercise band activities, w/c push-ups, sit to stand repetitions, and pelvic lifts. Passive stretching of the hip joint was also included. Gait training focused on increasing distance while decreasing the overall level of assistance required. Consistent with Rancho Level IV, he followed simple directions well, although he displayed difficulty learning new tasks. The PTA used repetition and visual cues to enhance the learning process (eg, the w/c brakes were covered with colored tape to serve as a reminder to lock the brakes prior to a transfer). In addition, the PTA learned some key Polish terms to emphasize particular skill components. Signs were also placed in the patient's room to indicate times for scheduled activities, and the patient maintained a daily log of activities performed in physical therapy. In each physical therapy session, the patient would verbalize those key safety strategies involved in the performance of the particular skill. Leszek began transporting himself independently to therapy sessions.

The patient steadily progressed through his therapy regimen and incrementally achieved designated goals. Leszek's cognition also improved, along with his speed of processing in mobility maneuvers. The PTA was soon able to introduce a straight cane with contact guarding in ambulation activities. As Leszek's balance progressed, the PTA had the family bring in his soccer ball to perform more challenging dynamic activities. Moreover, the ball represented a past activity that he enjoyed and could now revisit in therapy. The PTA progressed the patient with more advanced activities, such as floor transfers and uneven surface ambulation. He scored a 48 on the Berg Balance Test during the PT's reexamination, and he began working on tasks involved with the instrument's most demanding categories. The PTA challenged his judgment with various emergency maneuvers, such as running to dial 911. In the final week of therapy, he was able to perform a quick polka step in preparation for his sister's upcoming wedding. Discharge planning activities included a family training session and ordering of required equipment. Leszek still required a temporary w/c for longer community ambulation distances. A foam cushion and straight cane were also ordered. His parents demonstrated safe and effective guarding in gait, stairs negotiation, and car transfer techniques. A full home exercise program was formulated and reviewed with Leszek and his parents. A course of outpatient therapy was recommended. Two weeks following discharge, the PTA received a photo in the mail of Leszek dancing at the wedding.

PHYSICAL THERAPIST–PHYSICAL THERAPIST ASSISTANT COLLABORATION

Throughout the intervention regimen, the supervising PT and PTA discussed the patient's progress toward the established goals. On one occasion, the PT was asked to examine a developing skin rash on the patient's distal upper extremities. In addition, the PTA communicated to the therapist that Leszek's gait had been noticeably more unsteady over the past few days. Following the assessment, the physician was notified and it was determined that the rash was due to an adverse side effect of the patient's Dilantin.

QUESTIONS

1. What are some of the red flags seen in the initial evaluation that the PTA needs to consider when carrying out the plan of care?

2. Given the long-term goals set by the PT and the plan of care identified, was there anything that was outside the potential scope of practice of the PTA?

3. When would it be appropriate for the PTA to contact the PT outside of their normal discussion periods regarding this patient?

REFERENCES

1. Thurman DJ, Alverson C, Dunn KA, Guerrero J, Sniezek JE. Traumatic brain injury in the United States: a public health perspective. *J Head Trauma Rehabil.* 1999;14(6):602-615.
2. Brain Injury Association of America. BIAA adopts new TBI definition. http://www.biausa.org/announcements/biaa-adopts-new-tbi-definition. Accessed January 10, 2013.
3. Cassidy JD, Carroll LJ, Peloso PM, et al. Incidence, risk factors, and prevention of mild traumatic brain injury: result of the WHO collaborating center task force on mild traumatic brain injury. *J Rehab Med.* 2004;(43 Suppl):28-60.
4. Centers for Disease Control and Prevention. Traumatic brain injury. http://www.cdc.gov/TraumaticBrainInjury/index.html. Accessed January 10, 2013.

5. Burnett DM, Kolakowsky-Hayner SA, Slater D, et al. Ethnographic analysis of traumatic brain injury patients in the National Model Systems Database. *Arch Phys Med Rehabil.* 2003;84(2):263-267.

6. Brain Injury Association of America. 2013. http://www.biaa.org. Accessed January 10, 2013.

7. *Guide to Physical Therapist Practice.* 2nd ed. Alexandria, VA: American Physical Therapy Association; 2001.

8. Svestkova O, Angerova Y, Sladkova P, Bickenbach JE, Raggi A. Functioning and disability in traumatic brain injury. *Disabil Rehabil.* 2010;32(1):S68-S77.

9. Jenson GM, Gwyer J, Shepard KF, Hack LM. Expert practice in physical therapy. *Phys Ther.* 2000;80(1):28-43.

10. Watts NT. Task analysis and division of responsibility in physical therapy. *Phys Ther.* 1971;51(1):23-30.

11. Smith DH, Meaney DF, Shull WH. Diffuse axonal injury in head trauma. *J Head Trauma Rehabil.* 2003;18(4):307-316.

12. Murdock KR. Physical therapy in the neurologic intensive care unit. *J Neurol Phys Ther.* 1992;16(3):17-21.

13. Murdock KR, Klein P. Physical therapy intervention for acute head injury. *Phys Ther Prac.* 1994;3:19-36.

14. LeFort classification system. http://emedicine.medscape.com/article/1283568-overview#showall. Accessed August 27, 2013.

15. Johns JS, Cifu DX, Keyser-Marcus L, Jolles PR, Fratkin MJ. Impact of clinically significant heterotopic ossificans on functional outcome after traumatic brain injury. *J Head Trauma Rehabil.* 1999;14(3):269-276.

16. Paz JC, West MP, eds. *Acute Care Handbook for Physical Therapists.* 2nd ed. Boston, MA: Butterworth-Heinemann; 2002.

17. Englander J, Bushnik T, Duong TT, et al. Analyzing risk factors for late posttraumatic seizures: a prospective, multicenter investigation. *Arch Phys Med Rehabil.* 2003;84(3):365-373.

18. Keltner NL, Folks DG. *Psychotropic Drugs.* Philadelphia, PA: Mosby; 2002.

19. Glenn MB, Hoch MB, Daly L. Anticonvulsants. *J Head Trauma Rehabil.* 2003;18(4):383-386.

20. Teasdale G, Jennett B. Assessment of coma and impaired consciousness: a practical scale. *Lancet.*1974;2(7872):81-84.

21. Graham DI. Pathophysiological aspects of injury and mechanisms of recovery. In: Rosenthal M, Griffith ER, Kreutzer JS, Pentland B, eds. *Rehabilitation of the Adult and Child With Head Injury.* 3rd ed. Philadelphia, PA: FA Davis; 1999:42-52.

22. Kay T, Harrington DE, Adams R, et al. Definition of mild traumatic brain injury. *J Head Trauma Rehabil.* 1993;8(3):86-87.

23. Evans RW. Predicting outcome following traumatic brain injury. *Neurol Rep.* 1998;22:144-148.

24. Malkmus D. Integrating cognitive strategies into the physical therapy setting. *Phys Ther.* 1983;63(12):1952-1959.

25. Hagen C, Malkmus D, Durham P. Levels of cognitive functioning. In: *Rehabilitation of the Head Injured Adult: Comprehensive Physical Management.* Downey, CA: Professional Staff Association of Rancho Los Amigos Hospital; 1979.

26. Gray DS, Burnham RS. Preliminary outcome analysis of a long-term rehabilitation program for severe acquired brain injury. *Arch Phys Med Rehabil.* 2000;81(11):1447-1456.

27. Nakase-Thompson R, Sherer M, Yablon SA, Nick TG, Trzepacz PT. Acute confusion following traumatic brain injury. *Brain Inj.* 2004;18(2):131-142.

28. Bohannon RW, Smith MB. Interrater reliability of a modified Ashworth scale of muscle spasticity. *Phys Ther.* 1987;67(2):53-54.

29. Tinetti M. Performance-oriented assessment of mobility programs in elderly patients. *J Am Ger Soc.* 1986:34(2):119-126.

30. Berg KO, Wood-Dauphinee SL, Williams JI, Maki B. Measuring balance in the elderly: validation of an instrument. *Can J Public Health.* 1992;83(Suppl 2):S7-S11.

31. Bhambhani Y, Rowland G, Farag M. Reliability of peak cardiorespiratory responses in patients with moderate to severe traumatic brain injury. *Arch Phys Med Rehabil.* 2003;84(11):1629-1636.

32. Fischer S, Gauggel S, Trexler LE. Awareness of activity limitations, goal setting and rehabilitation outcomes in patients with brain injuries. *Brain Inj.* 2004;18(6):547-562.

33. Dumas HM, Haley SM, Ludlow LH, Carey TM. Recovery of ambulation during inpatient rehabilitation: physical therapist prognosis for children and adolescents with traumatic brain injury. *Phys Ther.* 2004;84(3):232-242.

34. Sawner K, LaVigne J. *Brunnstrom's Movement Therapy in Hemiplegia.* 2nd ed. Philadelphia, PA: JB Lippincott; 1992.

35. Falk Bergen A. The prescriptive wheelchair: an orthotic device. In: O'Sullivan SB, Schmitz TJ, eds. *Physical Rehabilitation: Assessment and Treatment.* 4th ed. Philadelphia, PA: FA Davis; 2001:1061-1091.

36. Duong TT, Englander J, Wright J, Cifu DX, Greenwald BD, Brown AW. Relationship between strength, balance, and outcome after traumatic brain injury: a multicenter analysis. *Arch Phys Med Rehabil.* 2004;85(8):1291-1297.

37. Blanton S, Grissom SP, Riolo L. Use of a static adjustable orthosis following tibial nerve block to a residual plantar-flexion contracture in an individual with brain injury. *Phys Ther.* 2002;82(11):1087-1097.

38. Lannin NA, Horsley SA, Herbert R, McCluskey A, Cusick A. Splinting the hand in the functional position after brain impairment: a randomized, controlled trial. *Arch Phys Med Rehabil.* 2003;84(2):297-302.

39. Singer BJ, Jegasothy GM, Singer KP, Allison GT, Dunne JW. Incidence of ankle contracture after moderate to severe acquired brain injury. *Arch Phys Med Rehabil.* 2004;85(9):1465-1469.

40. Platz T, Winter T, Müller N, Pinkowski C, Eickhof C, Mauritz KH. Arm ability training for stroke and traumatic brain injury patients with mild arm paresis: a single-blind, randomized, controlled trial. *Arch Phys Med Rehabil.* 2002;82(7):961-968.

41. Mudie MH, Matyas TA. Can simultaneous bilateral movement involve the undamaged hemisphere in reconstruction of neural networks damaged by stroke? *Disabil Rehabil.* 2000;22(1-2):23-37.

42. Karman N, Maryles J, Baker RW, Simpser E, Berger-Gross P. Constraint-induced movement therapy for hemiplegic children with acquired brain injuries. *J Head Trauma Rehabil.* 2003;18(3):259-267.

43. Watson MJ, Hitchcock R. Recovery of walking late after a severe traumatic brain injury. *Physiotherapy.* 2004;90(2):103-107.

44. Richardson JK, Marr Ross AD, Riley B, Rhodes RL. Halo vest effect on balance. *Arch Phys Med Rehabil.* 2000;81(3):255-257.

45. Zablotny CM, Nawoczenski DA, Yu B. Comparison between successful and failed sit-to-stand trials of a patient after traumatic brain injury. *Arch Phys Med Rehabil.* 2003;84(11):1721-1725.

46. Shumway-Cook A, Woolacott MA. Normal postural control. In: Shumway-Cook A, Woolacott MA, eds. *Motor Control: Theory and Applications.* 2nd ed. Philadelphia, PA: Lippincott Williams & Williams; 2001:163-191.

47. Williams GP, Robertson V, Greenwood KM, Goldie PA, Morris ME. The high-level mobility assessment tool (HiMAT) for traumatic brain injury. Part 2: content validity and discriminability. *Brain Inj.* 2005;19(10):833-843.

48. Wade LD, Canning CG, Fowler V, Felmingham L, Baguley IJ. Changes in postural sway and performance of functional tasks after traumatic brain injury. *Arch Phys Med Rehabil.* 1997;78(10):1107-1111.

49. Greenwald BD, Cifu DX, Marwitz JH, et al. Factors associated with balance deficits on admission to rehabilitation after traumatic brain injury: a multicenter analysis. *J Head Trauma Rehabil.* 2001;16(3):238-252.

50. Lippert LL. *Clinical Kinesiology for the Physical Therapist Assistant.* Philadelphia, PA: FA Davis; 2000.

51. Jeka JJ. Light touch contact as a balance aid. *Phys Ther.* 1997;77(5):476-487.

52. Shapira MY, Chelouche M, Yanai R, Kaner R, Szold A. Tai Chi Chuan practice as a tool for rehabilitation of severe head trauma: 3 case reports. *Arch Phys Med Rehabil.* 2001;82(9):1283-1285.

53. Chamelian L, Feinstein A. Outcome after mild to moderate traumatic brain injury: the role of dizziness. *Arch Phys Med Rehabil.* 2004;85(10):1662-1666.

54. Katz DI, White DK, Alexander MP, Klein RB. Recovery of ambulation after traumatic brain injury. *Arch Phys Med Rehabil.* 2004;85(6):865-869.

55. Esquenazi A. Evaluation and management of spastic gait in patients with traumatic brain injury. *J Head Trauma Rehabil.* 2004;19(2):109-118.

56. Singer BJ, Jegasothy GM, Singer KP, Allison GT. Evaluation of serial casting to correct equinovarus deformity of the ankle after acquired brain injury in adults. *Arch Phys Med Rehabil.* 2003;84(4):483-491.

57. McFadyen BJ, Swaine B, Dumas D, Durand A. Residual effects of a traumatic brain injury on locomotor capacity: a first study of spatiotemporal patterns during unobstructed and obstructed walking. *J Head Trauma Rehabil.* 2003;18(6):512-525.

58. Mossberg, KA, Orlander EE, Norcross JL. Cardiorespiratory capacity after weight-supported treadmill training in patients with traumatic brain injury. *Phys Ther.* 2007;88(1):77-87.

59. Fritz S, Lusardi M. Walking speed: the sixth vital sign. *J Geriatr Phys Ther.* 2009;32(2):2-5.

60. Duff D. Review article: altered states of consciousness, theories of recovery, and assessment following a severe traumatic brain injury. *Axone.* 2001;23(1):18-23.

61. Bogner JA, Corrigan JD, Fugate L, Mysiw WJ, Clinchot D. Role of agitation in prediction of outcomes after traumatic brain injury. *Am J Phys Med Rehabil.* 2001;80(9):636-644.

62. Castriotta RJ, Lai JL. Sleep disorders associated with traumatic brain injury. *Arch Phys Med Rehabil.* 2001;82(10):1403-1406.

63. Ríos M, Periáñez J, Muñoz-Céspedes JM. Attentional control and slowness of information processing after severe traumatic brain injury. *Brain Inj.* 2004;18(3):257-272.

64. Alderson AL, Novack TA. Reliable serial measurement of cognitive processes in rehabilitation: the cognitive log. *Arch Phys Med Rehabil.* 2003;84(5):668-672.

65. Corrigan, JD, Smith-Knapp K, Granger CV. Validity of the Functional Independence Measure for persons with traumatic brain injury. *Arch Phys Med Rehabil.* 1997;78(8):828-834.

66. Mostrum E, Shepard KF. Teaching and learning about patient education. In: Shepard KF, Jenson GM, eds. *Handbook of Teaching for Physical Therapists.* 2nd ed. Boston, MA: Butterworth Heinemann; 2002:287-319.

67. Rath JF, Hennesy JJ, Diller L. Social problem solving and community integration in postacute rehabilitation outpatients with traumatic brain injury. *Rehabil Psychol.* 2004;48(3):137-144.

68. Kalpakjian CZ, Lam CS, Toussaint LL, Merbitz NK. Describing quality of life and psychosocial outcomes after traumatic brain injury. *Arch Phys Med Rehabil.* 2004;83(4):255-265.

69. Franulic A, Carbonell GC, Pinto P, Sepulveda I. Psychosocial adjustment and employment outcome two, five, and ten years after TBI. *Brain Inj.* 2004;18:119-129.

70. Gordon WA. Community integration of people with traumatic brain injury: introduction. *Arch Phys Med Rehabil.* 2004;85(4 Suppl 2):S1-S2.

71. McCrory P, Meeuwisse W, Johnston K, et al. Consensus statement on concussion in sport: the 3rd International Conference on Concussion in Sport held in Zurich, November 2008. *Amer Acad Phys Med Rehabil.* 2009;1(5):401-418.

72. Taber KH, Warden DL, Hurley RA. Blast-related traumatic brain injury: what is known? *J Neuropsychiatry.* 2006;18(2):141-145.

73. Scherer M. Gait rehabilitation with body weight-supported treadmill training for blast injury survivor with traumatic brain injury. *Brain Inj.* 2007;21(1):93-100.

74. Scherer MR, Shelhamer MJ, Schubert MC. Characterizing high-velocity angular vestibulo-ocular reflex function in service members post-blast exposure. *Exp Brain Res.* 2011;208(3):399-410.

75. Bland DC, Zampieri-Gallagher C, Damiano DL. Effectiveness of physical therapy for improving gait and balance in ambulatory individuals with traumatic brain injury: a systematic review of the literature. *Brain Inj.* 2011;25(7-8):664-679.

76. Ptyushkin P, Vidmar G, Burger H, Marincek C. Use of the International Classification of Functioning, Disability and Health in patients with traumatic brain injury. *Brain Inj.* 2010;24:1519-1527.

Please see accompanying Web site at
www.healio.com/books/neuroptavideos

Clients With Stroke

Becky S. McKnight, PT, MS
James M. Smith, PT, DPT, MA

KEY WORDS

- Affective disorder
- Anosognosia
- Aphasia
- Apraxia
- Body-weight support during gait training
- Cerebrovascular accident
- Constraint-induced movement therapy
- Dysphagia
- Dysphasia
- Hemiparesis
- Hemorrhagic stroke
- Homonymous hemianopia
- Ischemic stroke
- Lacunar infarction
- Learned nonuse
- Pusher syndrome
- Shoulder pain after stroke
- Stroke
- Transient ischemic attack
- Unilateral neglect

CHAPTER OBJECTIVES

- Describe the types of cerebrovascular accidents.
- Read and appropriately process the physical therapist's (PT's) initial evaluation to guide decisions related to the implementation of selected interventions.

Umphred DA, Lazaro RT, eds.
Neurorehabilitation for the Physical Therapist Assistant,
Second Edition (pp 325-373).
© 2014 SLACK Incorporated.

- Identify when the directed interventions are beyond the scope of work of the physical therapist assistant (PTA).

- Identify when it is necessary to communicate with the PT regarding the patient's status and response to interventions.

- Explain the rationale for selected interventions to achieve patient goals as identified in the PT's plan of care.

- Identify common safety issues and precautions that should be monitored when working with patients who have had a stroke.

- Describe strategies for effective physical therapy interventions, including patient- or client-related communication and instruction and procedural interventions that may be included within a PT's plan of care for a patient who has had a stroke.

- Describe the impairments in body functions and limitations in activities and participation that typically accompany stroke and identify strategies that a PTA may use to accommodate for these during the provision of physical therapy interventions.

- Describe strategies and identify tests a PTA may use to monitor the patient's response to selected interventions and to determine a patient's progress within the PT's plan of care.

- Describe strategies a PTA may use to progress interventions based upon the patient's responses.

- Discuss confounding factors that can affect the patient's ability to participate in physical therapy and describe methods to accommodate the patient's unique needs.

INTRODUCTION

Cerebrovascular disease refers to any disorder involving the blood supply to the brain. When cerebrovascular disease results in the death of brain tissue, a stroke, also called a *cerebrovascular accident* (CVA), occurs. Diverse symptoms can develop depending on the location and size of the brain injury. Stroke is, unfortunately, common; in the United States, about 750,000 strokes occur each year, making it the most common neurological disorder and the leading cause of disability among adults.[1,2] Physical therapy interventions are usually indicated for the impairments in body functions and limitations in activities and participation that follow a stroke. Appropriately applied physical therapy interventions can diminish the limitations related to stroke symptoms.

Types of Stroke

There are 2 broad categories for stroke: ischemic and hemorrhagic. Ischemic stroke, which is more common, involves loss of the blood supply to part of the brain. This develops because of a blockage of one or more arteries that supply blood to the brain. The obstruction can occur from pathological changes that gradually occlude the blood vessel, such as atherosclerosis, or from an embolus that blocks a blood vessel. There are 2 additional categories of ischemic stroke: lacunar infarction and transient ischemic attack (TIA). A hemorrhagic stroke, also referred to as an *intracranial hemorrhage*, occurs when a blood vessel in the brain ruptures, resulting in blood flooding into the surrounding tissues (Figure 12-1).

Ischemic Stroke

Ischemia involving the brain is of great concern because of the high-energy demands of brain tissue. There is no mechanism to store metabolic reserves in the brain, so adequate blood supply is required to provide all of the glucose, oxygen, and nutrients used by these tissues. When a

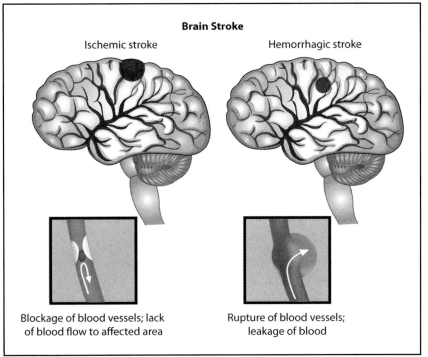

Figure 12-1. Image of ischemic and hemorrhagic stroke.

blood vessel becomes blocked, the blood supply is interrupted distal to the blockage. In the area of complete or near-complete interruption of blood supply, ischemic necrosis, or death of the tissue, occurs within a couple of minutes. This cell damage is irreversible. Surrounding the area of necrosis is an area where the blood supply is diminished but not completely interrupted. The tissues in this area will have diminished functioning during the time of ischemia but can return to normal function if blood supply is restored quickly. If, however, blood supply is not restored within a short period of time, the necrotic area will expand, resulting in greater tissue death and greater disability. Because of this, immediate medical attention is imperative.[1] The patient's presentation (impairments in body structures and functions and limitations in activities and participation) will depend on the size and location of the lesion as well as the nature and function of the structures involved, the availability of collateral blood flow, and early acute management (Table 12-1).

Lacunar Infarction

Lacunar infarcts are small strokes deep inside the brain that are named for their crescent-shaped appearance. They are common in the putamen, basal ganglia, thalamus, and internal capsule. As with all strokes, the symptoms associated with lacunar infarctions vary depending on the exact structures that are involved (internal capsule, thalamus, etc). Although these involve a small area, the effects can be quite dramatic because the areas involved can serve a variety of functions (weakness of the face, dysarthria, ataxia, weakness, etc).[1]

Transient Ischemic Attack

TIAs are caused by a temporary interruption in blood supply to the brain and result in sudden onset of impairments in body functions or limitations in activity, such as extremity weakness, sensory deficits, and difficulties with functional mobility. TIA symptoms vary in duration, but most are resolved within 1 hour. Within 24 hours there is a full recovery from all symptoms. TIAs often precede a stroke and require medical attention although the symptoms do resolve.[1]

Table 12-1

Body Function Impairments Commonly Associated With Cerebrovascular Accident

Primary Impairments	Secondary Impairments
• Impaired muscle strength	• Changes in alignment and mobility
• Changes in muscle tone	• Changes in muscle and soft tissues
• Impaired motor control	• Pain
• Impaired somatosensation	• Edema
• Impaired perception	• Diminished cardiovascular endurance
• Aphasia	• Skin breakdown
• Cognitive impairments	
• Urinary incontinence	

Hemorrhagic Stroke

The major effects of a hemorrhagic stroke are damage from the lost circulation and damage from the leaked blood itself. The blood that leaks into the brain tissue has volume (ie, it takes up space), but the skull cannot accommodate the increase in volume. This results in compression of brain tissue, which results in direct injury to neurons. It may also cause compression of adjacent blood vessels, resulting in those vessels narrowing or closing down. While this effect is greatest in the area of the bleeding, the enclosed nature of the skull may result in an elevated intracranial pressure throughout the brain, requiring special medical management. Another effect of the leaked blood is irritation of the adjacent tissues. The chemical composition of the blood is noxious to brain tissue, causing further damage.[1]

PATIENT ENTRY INTO PHYSICAL THERAPY CARE

A patient who is in the process of having a stroke is admitted to an acute hospital for medical intervention. The patient will initially receive medical care to identify the type of stroke and to implement the appropriate medical intervention to minimize the stroke and its sequelae. Of prime importance is to determine whether the stroke is ischemic or hemorrhagic. This is typically accomplished through radiologic imaging (computed tomography). For ischemic strokes, if tissue plasminogen activator can be administered within the first 3 hours of initial stroke, the person is 30% more likely to recover from the stroke.[1] Medical treatment of hemorrhagic stroke depends greatly on the extent of the stroke as well as the underlying cause (eg, arterial malformation). Frequently, medical management consists of administration of antihypertensive medication. Various procedures can also be used to evacuate the hematoma or to repair an arterial malformation or damage.

Physical therapy in the acute care setting is initiated early via a referral from a physician or through a critical pathway established at the institution. In the contemporary health care system, a patient typically has a short stay in the acute care environment. Once the patient has become medically stable, the care team will consider which setting the patient should be moved to, where the focus will be on rehabilitation efforts to facilitate patient recovery. Frequently, patients are moved into an inpatient rehabilitation facility where they will receive a minimum of 3 hours of rehabilitation services a day from the physical therapy, occupational therapy, and speech therapy

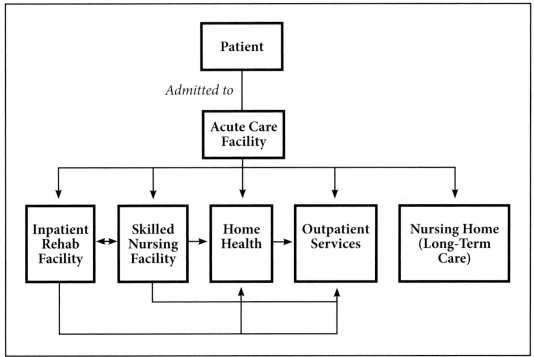

Figure 12-2. Patient pathway through the health care system.

departments. Alternatively, patients who are not able to participate at that level of intensive therapy can receive therapy services in a skilled nursing facility (SNF). Some patients who have mild disorders and a good support system at home can be discharged to home to receive therapy through home health services or on an outpatient basis. Finally, patients with limited capacity to improve functioning may be discharged to a nursing home or long-term care setting where physical therapy can be provided. Occasionally patients who have transferred to an SNF or nursing home make improvements and demonstrate potential for significant improvements and then are transferred into an inpatient rehabilitation setting for intensive therapy at a later date (Figure 12-2).

ROLE OF THE PHYSICAL THERAPIST ASSISTANT

Although symptoms from a stroke can vary widely depending on the size and location of the brain injury, recovery from a stroke often follows a predictable pattern. When a patient is medically stable and the stroke symptoms appear to be following the predictable prognosis, the physical therapist (PT) may choose to direct the physical therapist assistant (PTA) to provide selected physical therapy interventions. The PTA functions as a member of the entire team working to assist the patient to meet various medical, functional, and social goals. Team members can include medical personnel, other rehabilitation personnel, and other health care professionals (Table 12-2).

Within this team, the PTA provides interventions, as directed by the PT, to address impairments in body functions or limitations in activities and participation. These interventions are designed to help the patient progress from his or her current status to meet therapy goals (set by the PT) focused on helping the patient regain the ability to participate in normal activities. To help structure the intervention session, the PTA must take into consideration a variety of factors and pieces of information. The model depicted in Figure 12-3 will function as a framework to discuss these factors.

Table 12-2

Team Members Involved in the Care of a Patient Who Has Had a Stroke

- Physician
  - Physiatrist
  - Neurologist
  - Others as appropriate (eg, cardiologist)
- Nursing staff
- Pharmacist
- Neuropsychologist
- Physical therapist and physical therapist assistant
- Occupational therapist and occupational therapy assistant
- Speech therapist
- Recreational therapist
- Orthotist
- Social worker

Since the PTA's primary role is in the implementation of interventions, the PTA should order his or her clinical decision making around interventions directed by the PT. Once the PTA has established the interventions that will be provided, he or she should consider the impairment(s) and activity limitation(s) the PT expects to address with those interventions. For example, balance activities can be used to address trunk muscle strength deficits or motor control deficits. It is important that the PTA recognizes which impairments are being addressed to choose the specific balance activities and intervention strategies that will be most effective in addressing the problem. To further refine the intervention choices, the PTA next needs to consider the patient's current status as related to the impairment(s) or activity limitation(s) being addressed. These should be addressed in light of the goals the PT has set for these specific deficits. This will allow the PTA to plan effective intervention strategies to use. Strategy considerations include assistive or adaptive devices, amount and type of feedback, and specific activities to incorporate in the intervention session. Considering the current status in light of the goals will also help the PTA be prepared to progress the patient appropriately. All of these clinical decisions are made within the context of the medical diagnosis and expected prognosis, which is frequently influenced by confounding factors such as comorbidities or other impairments of body factors (eg, communication deficits). Other factors that can influence patient participation and progress include personal and environmental factors.

To ensure patient safety, the PTA must be familiar with common contraindications and precautions associated with working with patients with CVA as well as those associated with conditions that are frequent comorbidities for these individuals. The PTA must take all of these various factors into consideration when planning the specific parameters of the interventions prescribed by the PT.

Prior to implementing each session, the PTA should determine the patient's readiness for participation. When tests and measures and patient responses indicate readiness, the PTA then is able to implement the tailor-made intervention activities. The PTA uses formal and informal assessment processes during a session, at the end of a session, and at intervals as required by the plan of care to make decisions related to modification, progression, or discontinuation of any or all intervention activities and communicates this to the PT in a timely fashion.

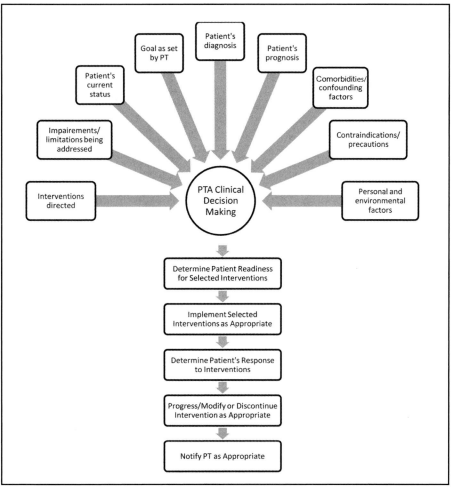

Figure 12-3. PTA clinical decision-making model.

The remainder of this chapter will use this framework to discuss details that the PTA needs to consider when working with patients recovering from stroke.

SELECTED INTERVENTIONS

By definition in the *Guide to Physical Therapist Practice* (the *Guide*),[3] physical therapy interventions include 3 components: (1) coordination, communication, and documentation; (2) patient- or client-related instruction; and (3) procedural interventions. Each of these components of providing an intervention must be included in the PT's plan of care for an individual recovering from a stroke. The PTA will participate in each of these areas as directed by the PT (Table 12-3). Intervention categories commonly used with patients who have had a stroke focus on a combination of compensatory strategies to compensate for lost functioning and remediation strategies to recover motor and functional abilities.

Table 12-3

Interventions

- **Coordination, communication, documentation**
- **Patient-/client-related instruction**
- **Procedural interventions**
- Therapeutic exercise
  - **Aerobic capacity/endurance conditioning or reconditioning**
  - **Balance, coordination, and agility training**
  - Body mechanics and postural stabilization
  - **Flexibility exercises**
  - **Gait and locomotion training**
  - **Neuromotor development training**
  - Relaxation
  - **Strength, power, and endurance training for head, neck, limb, and trunk**
  - Aquatic programs
- **Functional training in self-care and home management, including activities of daily living (ADL) and instrumental activities of daily living (IADL)**
- **Functional training in work (job/school/play), community, and leisure integration or reintegration, including IADL, work hardening, and work conditioning**
- Manual therapy techniques, including mobilization/manipulation
- **Prescription, application, and, as appropriate, fabrication of devices and equipment (assistive, adaptive, orthotic, protective, supportive, or prosthetic)**
- Airway clearance techniques
- Integumentary repair and protective techniques
- **Electrotherapeutic modalities**
- Physical agents and mechanical modalities

Bold interventions are those most commonly used when working with patients who have had a stroke and are those addressed in this chapter.

Coordination, Communication, Documentation

Because of the diverse symptoms that may be present, the coordination of services is very important when working with individuals who have had a stroke. Most patients recovering from a stroke will be receiving care from other health care providers, including a physiatrist, occupational therapist, speech-language pathologist, nurse, neuropsychologist, and others. It is important that all disciplines coordinate the care provided to ensure the patient will have the time and the energy necessary to participate in all of the treatment sessions and rehabilitation activities. In some settings, multidisciplinary meetings will allow for coordination and communication between the different health care providers working with the patient. This will provide the PT and PTA with invaluable information regarding: (1) the patient's impairments of body structures and functions that are not directly addressed by the physical therapy procedural interventions, (2) the patient's abilities, and (3) strategies to manage these issues. Skilled communication includes the verbal interactions between the PTA and the PT (and other health care providers) as well as appropriate documentation by the PTA that clearly delineates the interventions provided and the patient's response(s) to those interventions. (Refer to Chapter 7 on documentation for additional information.)

Patient-/Client-Related Instruction

Providing patient- or client-related instruction should be a part of every physical therapy session. The PTA should document the patient's response to this instruction. Documentation typically includes a description of the individual's ability to follow directions or comprehend instruction as evidenced by the presence or absence of behavioral changes. As patients learn more about their condition, including unique impairments and functional limitations, they will be better prepared to take control over their own care even if independent physical functioning is an unlikely outcome. Additionally, when caring for a patient recovering from a stroke, it is common that the patient's family and caregivers will require education related to providing care and support for the patient. In summary, education should be a priority within the interventions provided to the patient who has had a stroke.

Procedural Interventions

The plan of care designed by the PT will be unique to each patient receiving physical therapy following a stroke. Therefore, the PTA must be able to interpret that plan of care and apply it to the individual needs of each patient. This can be a daunting challenge because diverse therapeutic strategies and techniques have been advocated for promoting improvements in body functions and the patient's ability to perform functional activities and participate in a variety of social roles following a stroke. To guide the PTA in this process, the authors recommend the conceptual framework for therapeutic interventions for neuromuscular disorders described by Fell.[4] Fell categorized interventions as those related to motor learning and practice, those related to characteristics of a movement or task, and as other parameters for interventions (which will be described shortly). This framework is summarized in Table 12-4 and will be useful for streamlining the clinical decision making when providing physical therapy interventions to persons who have had a stroke.

Further discussion related to procedural interventions will focus on intervention categories as delineated in the *Guide*. The discussion will begin with the area of neuromotor development training that includes motor training and neuromotor reeducation. Principles related to neuromotor reeducation are foundational to working with patients with motor deficits associated with neurological conditions. These basic principles are applied to other types of therapeutic interventions, such as strength training and functional training.

Therapeutic Exercise Interventions for Neuromotor Development/Neuromotor Reeducation

One component of the therapeutic exercise interventions for a patient who has had a stroke is the fostering of a change in abilities through motor learning. The need for learning will vary with each individual and with the types of tasks the individual must perform. Examples include learning how to obtain movement from weakened limbs, learning how to use something new (eg, an assistive device), or learning new strategies for ambulating in crowded areas. To promote learning, the PTA must apply strategies that have proven effective for motor learning. The essential strategies for this are variability in practice, practicing components of movement, task attention, feedback, and environmental progression.[4] Each of these strategies is discussed in Chapter 3 and will be built on here; in the clinic, the PTA should consider these individually and collectively when providing interventions.

Table 12-4

Progressing Therapeutic Intervention in Patients With Neuromuscular Disorders

---

Parameters Related to Motor Learning and Practice

- Variability in practice (eg, blocked practice → random practice)
- Practicing components of movement (eg, part-task training → whole-task training)
- Task attention (eg, minimal distractions → cognitive/attentional demands)
- Feedback (eg, extrinsic feedback (knowledge of performance, knowledge of results) → intrinsic feedback)
- Environmental progression (eg, simple → complex)

Parameters Related to Characteristics of a Movement or Task

- Amplitude or magnitude of movement (eg, small range → large range of movement, mass synergy → isolated movement)
- Velocity (eg, slow gait → fast gait)
- Amount of work (eg, increase the frequency, intensity or duration of activity/exercise)
- Endurance (eg, increase the capacity to persevere at a task)
- Regional (eg, isolated movement → multi-joint movement, proximal movements → distal movements)

Other Parameters

- Developmental sequence (eg, low → high center of gravity, large → small base of support
- Supportive device (eg, ankle-foot orthotic or cane)
- Assistance given (eg, verbal cues for guidance → minimal cues, moderate assistance → minimal assistance)

(Adapted from Fell DW. Progressing therapeutic intervention in patients with neuromuscular disorders: a framework to assist clinical decision making. *J Neurol Phys Ther.* 2004;28[1]:35-46.)

Practice Strategies

Practice is a well-recognized technique for improving performance. This applies whether the learner is a canoer learning a paddle stroke, a child just learning how to walk, or a person rehabilitating from a stroke who needs to learn how to move a limb. The PTA should recognize that each session of providing physical therapy interventions is the patient's opportunity for practice and that the practice is an essential component of improving the ability to move and to function. Therefore, each session should be designed for motor learning and should include those strategies that will make the act of practicing most successful for the patient. Skilled applications of motor learning and practice strategies should be applied to **all** therapeutic exercise interventions so that the patient can gain the optimal benefit from physical therapy.

When designing practice of a new movement or task, a common strategy is to have the patient repeat a single component of the action. For example, the PTA may choose to have the patient who has had a stroke repeatedly practice transferring from sitting to standing to sitting, or the PTA may have the patient practice walking on a flat, smooth surface. This type of practice, which relies on repeating the same component of a task under the same conditions, is called *blocked practice.* Blocked practice assists with the preliminary learning of the movements or components of the task; therefore, it should be used in the early stages of learning. However, "it has been found that recall and transfer of motor skills, as well as learning, retention, and refinement of a skill, are best facilitated by random repetition over blocked repetition."[4] This means that varying the activities being practiced (ie, random practice) has the potential to improve the learning. For example, the PTA may have the patient practice transferring from sitting to and from standing from chairs of different heights, or the PTA may have the patient practice walking on irregular surfaces or on an obstacle course. An appropriate progression of the intervention would be to advance exercises from the consistency of blocked practice to the variability of random practice of a task.[4]

Another strategy to advance learning in the early stages of the acquisition of motor learning is part practice (or part-task training), in which the components or the movements that constitute a task are practiced. Once these components have been practiced, the intervention should be progressed to whole practice (whole-task training) to foster motor learning. For example, a patient who has had a stroke may practice standing weight shifting, then progress to stepping forward and backward with the right leg, and then stepping with the left leg for part practice. This may later be progressed to ambulating, which represents the strategy of whole practice.[4]

Attention

The patient's initial motor learning will be greatest if he or she is able to pay close attention to the task or exercise that is being learned. Stroke is a brain injury, and as described earlier, there is a risk for symptoms of altered cognition or attention. Therefore, a PTA should use an environment with minimal distractions, and that may mean planning interventions in a quiet room or during quieter periods in the therapy area (Figure 12-4). As learning advances, the PTA must also consider the anticipated outcome for the patient. If the patient is preparing for discharge to an environment with multiple distractions (eg, social gatherings, restaurants, or religious services), the individual will require the ability to manage complex demands on attention. Therefore, the interventions applied should prepare for those demands by progressing practice sessions toward complex environments (eg, walking in a busy hallway [Figure 12-5] or by increasing cognitive demands (eg, holding a conversation while ambulating).[4]

Research has shown that patients post-stroke who are provided with explicit information regarding task goals before beginning practice have improved motor learning. Evidence on individuals without neurological impairments suggests that instruction with an external focus (the results of the movement) rather than those with an internal focus (the movement itself) were associated with better outcomes. For example, during gait training to increase step length, the PTA can provide instruction for the patient to "put the cane out farther" instead of to "take a larger step."[5]

Feedback

Feedback is any of the sensory information that a person uses for learning and improving his or her performance. Intrinsic feedback is the information that an individual gathers on his or her own, such as the kinesthetic sensations of movement from the limbs. This type of feedback can be augmented by techniques such as using a mirror to allow a patient to observe his or her posture and how the posture changes as a result of movements. Extrinsic feedback is when the physical therapy provider gives information to the patient to improve performance. Extrinsic feedback is characterized as knowledge of performance, which is information about the components or quality of movement(s), or knowledge of results, which is information about the outcome achieved from the movement(s). A PTA must use feedback as a tool to shape and improve his or her patient's motor performance and learning. To achieve this, Fell has advised that, as interventions are advanced with a patient, "regardless of the type and source of feedback, there should always be a progressive decrease in extrinsic feedback provided" to promote learning.[4] The PTA should also be considerate of the amount of feedback provided because excessive feedback will distract from the patient's ability to attend to the task at hand. The timing of feedback should also be considered. In many situations, the optimal time for feedback is delayed for a few seconds following the completion of the task, when feedback can be used to augment the patient's reflection and assessment of his or her performance of the task.[4]

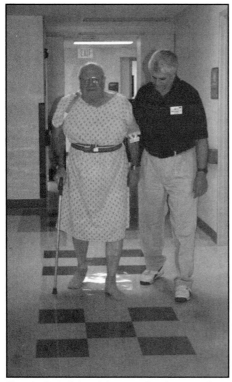

Figure 12-4. Gait training a patient in an environment with minimal distractions.

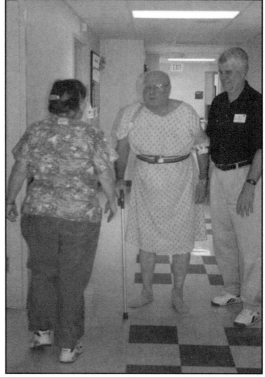

Figure 12-5. As the patient's attention to task improves, the environment should become more complex during the functional activity.

Environmental Progression

The context in which physical therapy interventions are provided will influence the motor learning based on the demands placed on the patient during the learning process. To better understand this, it is helpful to look at the taxonomy of tasks developed by Gentile (Table 12-5).[6] She has identified the following incremental demands, which depend on the type of task (described here as progressing from less to more complex):

- The person is stationary—the person is moving or being moved while performing the task (eg, riding in a wheelchair [w/c]).

- The task remains consistent each time—the task varies with each performance.

- The person's posture is stable—the person is moving him- or herself during the task (eg, walking).

- The task does not require manipulation—the task requires manipulation (eg, buttoning a shirt).

As described by Gentile, these parameters can be combined (see Table 12-5) to identify the level of complexity of a task and, therefore, to categorize the types of demands that are imposed by different types of tasks or by different therapeutic exercise interventions.[6] The PTA should be able to apply these general concepts for progression of the interventions provided to a patient receiving physical therapy interventions for stroke symptoms. This is best achieved by identifying, through the goals established by the PT, the types of environments and demands that the patient is likely to encounter. The exercise interventions must begin in the less demanding components described here and advance according to the patient's response and success of performance. Advancement should follow these concepts to foster the patient's achievement of the physical therapy goals.

Table 12-5
Gentile's Taxonomy of Tasks

	Body Stability No Manipulation	*Body Stability Manipulation*	*Body Transport No Manipulation*	*Body Transport Manipulation*
Stationary No intertrial variability	Closed Consistent Motionless Body stability	Closed Consistent Motionless Body stability Manipulation	Closed Consistent Motionless Body transport	Closed Consistent Motionless Body transport Manipulation
Stationary Intertrial variability	Variable Motionless Body stability	Variable Motionless Body stability Manipulation	Variable Motionless Body transport	Variable Motionless Body transport Manipulation
Motion No intertrial variability	Consistent Motion Body stability	Consistent Motion Body stability Manipulation	Consistent Motion Body transport	Consistent Motion Body transport Manipulation
Motion Intertrial variability	Open Variable Motion Body stability	Open Variable Motion Body stability Manipulation	Open Variable Motion Body transport	Open Variable Motion Body transport Manipulation

(Adapted from Gentile AM. Skill acquisition: action, movement and neuromotor processes. In: Carr J, Shepherd R, Gordon J, et al, eds. *Movement Science: Foundations for Physical Therapy in Rehabilitation*. Rockville, MD: Aspen Publishers; 1987:93-154.)

For example, a patient whose goal or anticipated outcome includes the expectation of ambulation in public areas (eg, restaurant or place of worship) will need to achieve the ability for body transport **and** be able to perform this when intertrial variability (eg, obstacles and other people also walking by) is occurring. If the earlier interventions are performed in a quiet physical therapy gym to foster attention for successful learning, it is expected that the patient will develop the ability to walk in a consistent (nonvariable) environment. However, the addition of variables, such as walking in a hallway in which other people are also walking so that the patient now has to respond to and avoid those people, results in a more complex task that places greater demands on the patient. If this is not practiced, it cannot be expected that the patient will develop the necessary abilities to succeed with the task. Therefore, the therapeutic exercise interventions should be intentionally designed to advance the exercises to include this type of practice and, therefore, prepare the patient for the task and make the patient more likely to succeed when outside of the physical therapy environment.[4]

Factors Relating to the Movement or Task

The exercises used should also be directed at advancing the ability to move a region of the body, including advancing the strength of the movement and the quality (skill) of the movement. For example, if a patient who has had a stroke has an impairment of weakness of the knee extensor muscles, which contribute to a functional limitation of requiring assistance to stand up from a chair, there are many exercise options that will promote strengthening of the knee extensor muscles. However, for the exercise to be therapeutic, the interventions should be designed so that the patient is exercising and practicing at the level that challenges that individual to improve

Figure 12-6. Characteristics of a task and how to progress it.

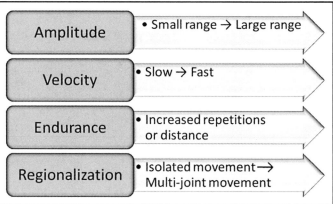

performance for that movement or task. The following are examples of characteristics of a task or movement that should be advanced or progressed as the patient's improving performance allows:

- The amplitude (or amount) of movement that occurs (eg, progress from moving through a small range to large range of movement or progress from moving large regions of the body to isolated or fine movements).

- The velocity of the movement (eg, progress from training at a slow gait speed to a fast gait).

- The amount of work being performed (eg, increase the frequency, intensity, or duration of the exercise or the task that is being practiced).

- The patient's capacity for work (endurance) should be advanced (eg, increase the repetitions performed or the distance walked during gait training).

- Progression can be based on the region(s) of the body being addressed (eg, the challenge may be increased by training for proximal movements before distal movements or for the performance of isolated movement before multijoint movements) (Figure 12-6).[4]

Other Parameters

The ability to perform a task may be improved through the use of a supportive or adaptive device, allowing for practice and improved capability with that task. For example, a patient may use an ankle-foot orthosis (AFO) to improve the ability to walk or a grab bar to provide additional support while rolling. Progression may be achieved by reducing the amount of support or the amount of reliance placed on the device, or by adjusting or adapting the device. For example, a patient may initially walk while supporting him- or herself with parallel bars, followed by progression to a quad cane and then a straight cane.[4] Discussion of the use of assistive, adaptive, and supportive devices and orthotics will occur later in this chapter.

Another consideration during the provision of therapeutic exercise interventions is the amount or type of assistance provided by the PTA. This progression is commonly recognized for physical assistance, in which the PTA gradually and intentionally decreases the amount of support provided while the patient increases the amount of work she or he is able to perform. Progression can also be achieved by reducing other supports, such as the amount of verbal cues provided for guidance during task performance, with the progression being achieved by intentionally reducing the amount of cues provided to the patient.[4]

Therapeutic Exercise Interventions for Aerobic Capacity/Endurance

An overarching concern when implementing therapeutic exercise interventions is impaired exercise capacity. The American Heart Association has recommended that the major rehabilitation goals following a stroke are preventing inactivity and disuse, decreasing the risk of a recurrent

Table 12-6

Summary of Exercise Programming Recommendations for Stroke Survivors from the American Heart Association

Mode of Exercise	Major Goals	Intensity/Frequency/Duration
Aerobic		
• Large-muscle activities (eg, walking, treadmill, stationary cycle, combined arm-leg ergometry, seated stepper)	• Increase independence in ADL • Increase walking speed/efficiency • Improve tolerance for prolonged physical activity • Reduce risk of cardiovascular disease	• 40% to 70% peak oxygen uptake; 40% to 70% heart rate reserve; 50% to 80% maximal heart rate; RPE 11 to 14 (6 to 20 scale) • 3 to 7 days/week • 20 to 60 min/session (or multiple 10-min sessions)
Strength		
• Circuit training • Weight machines • Free weights • Isometric exercise	• Increase independence in ADL	• 1 to 3 sets of 10 to 15 repetitions of 8 to 10 exercises involving the major muscle groups
Flexibility		
• Stretching	• Increase ROM of involved extremities • Prevent contractures	• 2 to 3 days/week (before or after aerobic or strength training) • Hold each stretch for 10 to 30 seconds
Neuromuscular		
• Coordination and balance activities	• Improve level of safety during ADL	• 2 to 3 days/week (consider performing on the same day as strength activities)

(Reprinted with permission from Gordon NF, Gulanick M, Costa F, et al. Physical activity and exercise recommendations for stroke survivors: an American Heart Association scientific statement from the Council on Clinical Cardiology, Subcommittee on Exercise, Cardiac Rehabilitation, and Prevention; the Council on Cardiovascular Nursing; the Council on Nutrition, Physical Activity, and Metabolism; and the Stroke Council. *Circulation*. 2004;109[16]:2031-2041.)

stroke or cardiovascular disorder, and increasing aerobic fitness.[2] To achieve this, each patient should engage in physical exercise as soon as possible to enhance his or her general activity level. When the PTA is providing therapeutic exercise interventions, he or she must be very considerate of providing sufficient aerobic challenges, preferably through upright activities (eg, training for gait or stair climbing) while monitoring the patient's response to those exercises.[2] Sample activities are described in Table 12-6. The PT will be a resource for determining precautions and thresholds for aerobic training (eg, target and maximum heart rates and acceptable blood pressure [BP]). However, the PTA should also be aware of general guidelines for cardiovascular conditions for patients who demonstrate those comorbidities. Some patients may have inadequate capacity for planned exercise interventions, and in those situations, the PTA should modify the intervention appropriately, such as decreasing the exercise intensity or duration while increasing the frequency of exercise sessions. (Refer to Chapter 14, Cardiopulmonary Issues Associated With Patients Undergoing Neurorehabilitation.)

Therapeutic Exercise Interventions for Balance and Coordination

Individuals who have had a stroke frequently demonstrate deficits in balance and coordination. These impairments can also be referred to as deficits in postural control and motor control. The deficits are a result of a combination of impairments common for individuals who have had a stroke (see discussion of impairments later in this chapter). Postural control or balance should be addressed in the sitting and standing positions (as the patient is able). The primary focus of postural control is trunk control. Trunk control is imperative for functional movement, including weight shifting and reaching. Initially activities should focus on helping the patient to obtain and maintain symmetrical upright control, in which the patient weight bears equally on both ischial tuberosities in sitting or both feet in standing. Once midline control has been achieved, weight-shifting activities can be initiated. These activities help the patient reestablish the appropriate synergistic relationship between the agonist and antagonist muscle groups. Simple weight-shifting activities are followed by more challenging dynamic activities, such as reaching and manipulating objects or taking steps forward/backward. At each step, the PTA should monitor for appropriate postural control and modify the activity based on the patient's abilities.[5] The importance of initiating sitting activities is emphasized by Carr and Shepherd when they state, "In the acute state post-stroke, major goals are to prevent medical complications associated with the supine position and bed rest and to retrain balance in sitting. Reestablishing sitting balance early is critical since it impacts positively on many functions. It provides greater stimulus for gaseous interchange and facilitates coughing, enables more effective swallowing, encourages eye contact and focusing attention, communication and more positive attitudes, stimulates arousal mechanisms, and discourages learned 'sick role' behavior."[7]

Therapeutic Exercise Interventions for Flexibility

Following a stroke, there is a high risk for losing flexibility in the involved limbs, and traditionally stretching is applied. For example, a patient with involvement of the hand often develops greater activity in the finger flexor muscles over time, with accompanying spasticity and posturing into finger flexion. Stretching is typically provided to prevent or correct for stiffness or contracture involving flexion of the fingers. However, evidence has indicated that stretching interventions have no appreciable benefit on joint mobility, spasticity, or pain.[8] Therefore, routine stretching may not benefit a patient following a stroke, although the PT's plan of care may include a specific stretching intervention based on the unique needs of a patient.

Therapeutic Exercise Interventions for Gait and Locomotion Training

Like balance and coordination, much of what is discussed regarding gait and locomotion training falls under motor control and motor learning strategies. In addition, gait training often uses various types of assistive or adaptive equipment. Specifics related to using assistive devices will be discussed below. Within this section, the PTA will find descriptions of gait deviations that are commonly seen with individuals who have had a stroke and discussion of general strategies not described in other areas.

Discussion of interventions for gait often starts with a description of pre-gait activities. Pre-gait activities include mat activities, such as bridging to improve hip extension in a weight-bearing position, tall kneeling, or half-kneeling. Research has not shown these activities to be effective in facilitating improvements in gait outcomes.[5] However, these activities may be appropriate for patients who are not safe to work with in the standing position. Other pre-gait activities include interventions to focus on range of motion (ROM) or strength deficits that lead to identified gait deviations.

During gait training activities it is important for the PTA to monitor and be aware of gait deviations as listed in Table 12-7. Determining the most likely cause of a gait deviation is the responsibility of the PT, as multiple factors can be the cause. Knowledge of common gait deviations displayed

---

Table 12-7

Common Gait Deviations Seen in Individuals With Hemiparesis

- Heel strike to midstance
  - Excessive forward trunk flexion
  - Limited ankle dorsiflexion
  - Lack of knee flexion
- Midstance
  - Inability to control knee
    - Lack of knee extension
    - Knee hyperextension
  - Limited hip extension
  - Limited ankle dorsiflexion
  - Excessive lateral weight shift
  - Inability to transfer weight appropriately
- Late stance/pre-swing
  - Lack of knee flexion
  - Lack of ankle plantarflexion
- Early and mid-swing
  - Limited knee flexion
  - Limited hip flexion
  - Limited ankle dorsiflexion
- Late swing
  - Limited knee extension
- Parameters of gait
  - Decreased walking speed
  - Short and/or uneven step and stride lengths
  - Increased stride width
  - Increased double support phase
  - Dependence on support through upper extremities

---

by individuals who have had a stroke, however, will allow the PTA to be better prepared to provide gait training interventions and make modifications.

There has been interest in using partial body-weight support during gait training. This technique involves gait training on a treadmill or over land while the patient is suspended in a harness that supports the lower trunk and proximal lower extremities (LEs) (Figure 12-7). This harness supports a portion of the person's body weight so that he or she may practice the task of walking with a low risk for falling and with a reduction of gait deviation(s). This technique has achieved restoration of greater walking ability, as demonstrated by significantly less reliance on assistance, greater walking speed, and greater walking endurance.[9,10]

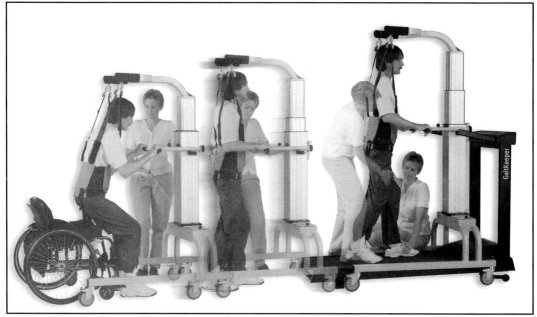

Figure 12-7. Gait training with a body weight–support system on a treadmill. (Reprinted with permission from Mobility Research, Inc, Tempe, AZ. www.litegait.com.)

This intervention typically involves walking on a treadmill while supported in the harness while 2 or 3 PTs and/or PTAs assist the patient to achieve the desired movement. Their manual assistance involves guidance with weight shifting, stance, and the swing and stance movements of the more involved LE. Progression of this intervention may be achieved by (1) decreasing the amount of assistance as the patient's skill improves, (2) providing less support through the harness (ie, increasing the weight-bearing demands on the patient's LEs), and/or (3) increasing the speed of walking on the treadmill.[9,10] Another option with body-weight support gait training that shows promise is the use of a robotic device to provide movement and/or support of the LEs during the practice of walking.[9]

Locomotor training includes w/c mobility training. This will be part of the plan of care for patients who will be using a w/c either exclusively or for community integration. W/C mobility includes instructing the patient on how to maneuver the w/c with the stronger extremities. This is frequently accomplished through the patient using the stronger leg to maneuver and propel the w/c with assistance of the stronger arm. An alternative is the use of a one-arm drive w/c. Patients should be instructed in maneuvering around obstacles to mimic the environments in which they will be functioning. Instruction should include w/c use up and down ramps, through doors, and on and off elevators.

Therapeutic Exercise Interventions for Strength and Endurance

Interventions that address strength deficits in individuals who have had a stroke are frequently referred to as *muscle or movement reeducation activities*. The strength deficits associated with a stroke, as with other neurological deficits, are due to a unique combination of upper neuron involvement, motor control deficits, and muscular deconditioning (Figure 12-8). As such, several exercise principles come into play when addressing these deficits. Exercise principles that govern all strength programs include the Reversibility Principle, the Overload Principle, and the Specific Adaptation to Imposed Demands Principle[11] (Table 12-8). In addition, aspects of motor control and motor learning discussed earlier in this chapter should guide the PTA when making decisions related to strengthening programs for patients who have had a stroke.

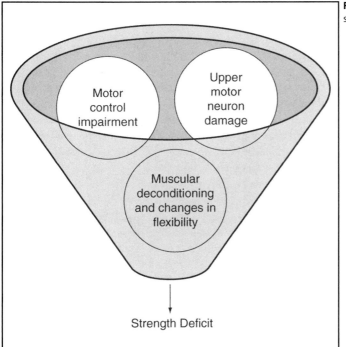

Figure 12-8. Components that lead to strength deficit.

Table 12-8

Principles of Exercise as Applied to Patients Who Have Had a Stroke

Principle of Exercise	Description	Application to Patients With Cerebrovascular Accident
Overload Principle	For training adaptation to take place, a greater-than-normal stress (or load) must be place on the body system being targeted.	Use interventions that work the patient near the limit of her or his abilities functionally, aerobically, motorically.
SAID Principle (Specific Adaptation to Imposed Demands)	Certain exercise or type of training produces adaptations specific to the activity performed and only in the body systems stressed by the activity.	Use interventions to train for activities that are relevant to the patient's needs for functioning and participation.
Reversibility Principle	Training-induced changes (such as increased strength) are transient unless regularly used for functional activities.	Engage the patient in behavioral changes that emphasize activity and use involved body segments (ie, overcome learned nonuse).

Many individuals who have a neurological condition such as a stroke also demonstrate movement patterns that are dominated in a synergistic pattern (common synergistic patterns). To address these abnormal movement patterns, principles of movement reeducation should be implemented. Movement reeducation is designed to increase strength and movement control on 4 levels. The first level is the ability to recruit individual muscles. At this level, the PTA focuses on helping the patient learn to activate muscles to work selectively with concentric, eccentric, and isometric contractions without being dominated by synergistic movement patterns. For example, a therapy session may focus on the patient being able perform elbow flexion without the synergistic movement of shoulder flexion occurring. The second level is the movement component level. At this level, groups of muscles in an extremity or the trunk are training to work together synergistically to produce a desired functional movement. For example, the patient will work on bringing a hand to the top of the head. The third level is the movement sequence level. At this level, multiple muscles from various body parts are trained to work together. Movement sequences are primarily used for transitional movements, such as rolling. The fourth and final level is the functional movement level. At this level, muscles are trained to work together to accomplish complex movements required for function, such as reaching for a glass.[12] An important consideration of movement reeducation is ensuring appropriate biomechanical alignment during movement. It has been recognized that poor muscle alignment can be a factor in strength deficits and can facilitate inappropriate (even synergistic) muscle activation.

Multiple studies have indicated that strength gains can occur even in patients who are in the chronic stage after traditional therapies are typically discontinued. Therefore, it is important to incorporate strengthening activities at all stages of recovery from a stroke. Strengthening activities can include traditional resistive exercises; however, to facilitate strength gains that are associated with functional activities, task-specific training is preferred.[13–16]

Functional Training

One challenge when working with patients following a CVA is determining the types of postures or activities that will be used as the foundation for the practice that is necessary to foster the reattainment of functional abilities. A frequently used framework for determining therapeutic exercise interventions is a developmental progression. According to Fell, this is typically biomechanically based and progressed by elevating the center of gravity and/or narrowing the base of support (BOS).[4] Examples of activities include exercises in prone or prone on elbows, rolling or crawling activities, exercises in quadruped or during creeping, exercises in kneeling or half-kneeling, and standing and ultimately walking activities (Figure 12-9).[4] For example, a patient who is limited in the ability to transition from a supine to a sitting posture should receive exercise interventions addressing that task with activities of a similar nature. Exercises lower on the developmental progression (eg, prone on elbows) will provide insufficient challenge to facilitate improvement, and exercises higher on the developmental progression (eg, standing) will reduce the likelihood of success during practice.

Another framework for determining therapeutic exercise interventions is to choose tasks necessary to the patient and design exercise interventions to advance ability for that task. This is an important consideration given the wide scope of activities that may be relevant to an individual within his or her discharge environment (Figure 12-10). These tasks may range from self-care (eg, getting up from the floor or putting on a coat) to recreation (eg, handling a fishing rod or walking on a beach); therefore, potential tasks to be considered are too numerous to list. Instead, the PTA must be considerate of this and keep in mind the following when choosing postures or activities for exercise interventions: (1) the types of tasks and demands unique to each patient's needs upon discharge from physical therapy, (2) the patient's current functional ability, and (3) those postures or activities that represent a developmental progression that the patient should practice.

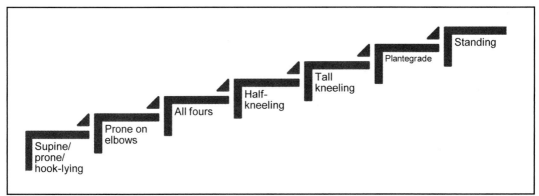

Figure 12-9. Developmental progression framework for functional training.

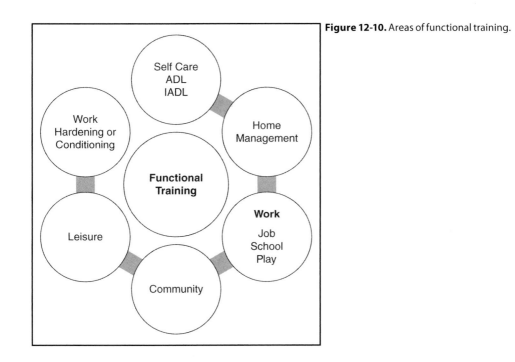

Figure 12-10. Areas of functional training.

The authors recommend that the choice of activities for therapeutic exercise interventions be guided by the following considerations:

- The activity is, or is similar to, a task that is necessary (relevant) to the patient.

- Learning and improved function will be fostered when:

  ○ The patient is capable of some successful performance of the activity.

  ○ The activity is sufficiently challenging (difficult) for the patient during the practice sessions.

Note that the developmental progression is not a sequential progression or an advancement of activities that should be followed. Also, a patient may be able to skip some activities and should increase his or her practice with those activities that have the greatest relevance to physical therapy goals.[4]

Devices and Equipment

A variety of assistive and adaptive devices are used as part of the therapeutic intervention strategy in physical therapy. Some devices are used only during an intervention session to provide additional support or feedback for the patient during task-oriented activities; other devices are used on a temporary basis (days, weeks, or months) to help the patient be more independent and safe while working toward established goals. Some devices, however, are used on a long-term basis as part of a compensatory approach to deal with long-term deficits. Selecting and using assistive, adaptive, supportive, or orthotic devices should be considered carefully regardless of the time frame for use. Each device used should be used in a prescriptive fashion with a clear understanding of the goals and intentions for their use. The PTA may decide to use some devices, such as an air-sleeve or a knee splint, during an individual treatment session to provide feedback to the patient and to act as a second pair of hands allowing the PTA the opportunity to focus the patient's attention and efforts on other areas. For example, a knee splint may be used to stabilize the weaker lower limb during standing balance activities while the PTA facilitates appropriate trunk control. Devices used on a temporary (not limited to an individual therapy session) or long-term basis will be the decision of the PT. The PTA will be made aware of the PT's expectations through the plan of care. Devices such as a w/c, a hemi cane or an AFO may be used either on a temporary or a long-term basis. In the event of temporary use, the PT's plan of care will specify the expected time frame when the patient should be advanced to a different device or to independent activity without an assistive device. As with all interventions, the PTA will monitor the patient's abilities as related to use of the device. This should include monitoring for appropriate fit and alignment, as well as safe and appropriate use of the device during use. If the patient's progression is faster or slower than anticipated, the PTA should bring this to the PT's attention and make suggestions based on the patient's presentation and response to therapeutic intervention. The following are examples of devices and equipment commonly used with patients who have had a stroke.[17]

Bedside Equipment

Pillows, wedges, towels, and other positioning devices can be used when the patient is in bed, especially in the early stages of recovery after a stroke. These are used to position the patient in bed or when sitting in a chair to decrease the development of secondary impairments such as ROM deficits or pressure sores. Once the patient is able to move around in bed, these devices are no longer necessary.

Wheelchairs

W/Cs should have a solid seat instead of a sling seat, which facilitates poor posture and trunk control. An appropriate seat cushion is necessary. The type of cushion will depend on the patient's mobility status and prognosis. A lower seat height is preferred to allow patients to propel the chair with the less affected LE. A supportive device for the affected upper extremity (UE) is also recommended (Figures 12-11 and 12-12).

Canes

Although wheeled walkers (with or without forearm attachment) are on occasion used with patients who demonstrate adequate upper limb strength and movement control, the majority of patients requiring an assistive device for ambulation after a stroke use some type of cane. A variety of canes are available, but they all fall into the basic categories of hemi cane, quad cane, and straight cane. A hemi cane is typically used only early in the recovery process as it provides a very large BOS for initial standing and gait activities and provides a sense of security for the patient. Few patients use a hemi cane on a long-term basis, as it is cumbersome because of the large BOS. When a patient demonstrates adequate trunk control, typically a quad cane is used. Quad canes can have larger or smaller bases to accommodate the stability needs of the patient; the larger the base, the more it will slow the patient's walking speed. The least amount of stability is provided by

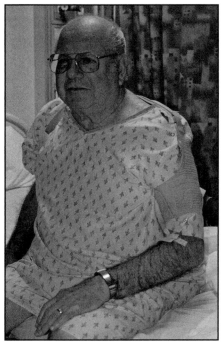 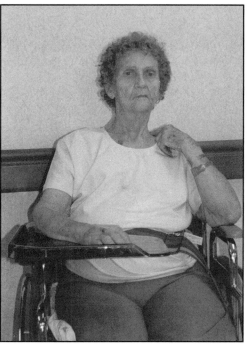

Figure 12-11. Patient with cuff supporting the shoulder of the hemiplegic upper limb.

Figure 12-12. Patient using arm support on w/c to support the weakened upper extremity.

a straight cane. Straight canes can, however, be adapted by adding a large tip. Straight canes are typically used with patients who demonstrate mild balance or LE strength and control deficits.

The PTA will instruct the patient on the use of the assistive device during gait on a variety of surfaces congruent with the patient's discharge needs. This may include gait training with an assistive device on stairs, up and down a curb, on uneven terrain (gravel, grass, etc), or on carpet. The PTA should monitor for appropriate fit of the assistive device and determine patient safety during use of the device. The patient and/or the patient's caregiver should be instructed on how to clean and adjust the cane and how to monitor for wear.

Orthotics

The most common orthotic device used with patients who have had a stroke is an AFO. AFOs help to ensure foot clearance during the swing phase of gait and help the patient heel strike. AFOs can be set at neutral or into slight dorsiflexion or plantarflexion to produce effects at the knee joint. When a patient demonstrates a tendency toward hyperextension because of poor knee control, the AFO can be set to a mild amount of dorsiflexion to produce a flexion moment at the knee. The PTA will need to monitor the patient's skin to ensure proper fit of the AFO, especially because patients who have had a CVA frequently have altered or absent sensation in their involved limb. The PTA should instruct the patient and/or the patient's caregiver on how to assess skin integrity and monitor for skin breakdown. In addition, the patient should be taught how to don and doff the device and how to clean and maintain it.

On occasion, other orthotic devices, such as a knee-ankle-foot orthosis (KAFO) or a hyperextension knee brace, may also be prescribed by the PT for the patient. Basic principles of use and patient training/instruction are the same.

Hand Splints and Slings

Hand splints and slings have traditionally been used to provide support and protection for the more involved UE. Controversy over the use of hand splints has primarily revolved around the evolving understanding of the cause of tonal issues observed in patients with UE involvement from a stroke. A contemporary understanding focuses on providing a neutral functional splint that promotes functional training and hand use. The splint is designed to hold the wrist and hand in a position of orthopedic neutral as opposed to the traditional resting position, which placed the wrist in some extension and the hand in mild flexion. This functional splint is primarily used during the day only.[17]

UE slings are used to support the glenohumeral joint in an effort to prevent subluxation. Various slings are available; however, no research has been conducted that assesses the sling's effect on the trunk or scapular position. No available shoulder sling is able to provide the scapula with support to maintain the upward rotation required for appropriate scapulohumeral mechanics. As such, use of an UE sling must accompany strengthening and muscle reeducation of the trunk and scapular musculature.

The ideal shoulder sling will help maintain the normal alignment of the glenoid fossa and decrease the tendency for the humerus to internally rotate. Shoulder immobilizer slings should be avoided. Shoulder sling options include shoulder saddle slings, humeral cuff slings, and clavicle supports.[17]

Electrotherapeutic Modalities

Neuromuscular electrical stimulation (NMES) can be effective at increasing movement strength, making it an appropriate physical therapy intervention for some people who have had a stroke. Intervention strategies with NMES vary depending on the impairment or functional limitation being targeted. This intervention should only be a component of, or adjunct to, a therapeutic exercise program. NMES can be applied to the shoulder to reduce glenohumeral joint subluxation and the accompanying pain by stimulating the supraspinatus and posterior deltoid muscles.[18,19] Another NMES application has been directed at improving UE performance with functional tasks. This strategy requires stimulation to the weakened muscle groups that is performed concurrently with a task that requires those muscles. This application may improve patterns of movement that are weak following a stroke, such as impaired strength for wrist and finger extension.[20,21] There have been few reports on the role of NMES interventions to the LEs following stroke. It appears to improve the recruitment of muscles[22] and gait (during the stimulation),[23] but the persistence of functional benefits has not been established.

Additional Intervention Strategies in Stroke Rehabilitation

Another strategy for rehabilitation of motor (movement) abilities following stroke is constraint-induced movement therapy (CIMT). This intervention evolved from a fascinating series of investigations into learned nonuse, in which it was discovered in the laboratory of psychologist Edward Taub that a monkey relieved of sensation in a UE will cease to use that limb. The monkey has the potential to use the limb, but doing so is laborious. That level of effort is negative reinforcement, while use of the limb in which sensation is intact is easy and provides positive reinforcement. The combination reinforces the avoidance of using that limb, which Taub has identified as learned nonuse. Taub applied this understanding to the development of an intervention in which the limb that is not impaired is constrained by strapping it to the trunk, and the monkey is then required to use the impaired limb to feed itself and perform other essential functions. This results in constraint-induced movement of the limb and a restoration of the ability to use it functionally.[24]

This technique has proven effective in the rehabilitation of movement ability of either the UE or the LE when the ability to move and use the limb is impaired following stroke. The intervention involves constraint of the less-involved extremity for 14 days, and during that period, the patient participates in training activities and tasks using the involved limb for 6 hours each weekday and for additional exercise periods on the weekends. This intervention is effective in increasing the amount and quality of movement in the involved limb and the use of the limb for functional tasks. The benefits from the intervention are sustained over time. The research on this protocol has been impressive in that it confirmed the efficacy of this intervention when massed practice (constraint of the less-involved limb paired with approximately 70 hours of training activities) is provided to the patient.[24–26] For additional information on CIMT, refer to www.usc.edu/uscnews/stories/9548. html.

It appears that CIMT interventions are rarely used outside of those clinics that specialize in this intervention.[27] The barriers to widespread use of this intervention may be related to the need for massed practice sessions, which encompass a full day of activities over 2 weeks.[25,26] This presents a problem for scheduling treatment sessions as well as achieving reimbursement by insurers. Fortunately, there is recent evidence that modifying the schedule also achieves benefits because improved movement control and functional use of the limb has also been demonstrated following training sessions for 1 hour, 3 times a week over a 10-week period.[28]

In the past decade, there has been growing interest in using virtual-reality gaming devices to enhance therapeutic exercise interventions. Anecdotal evidence suggests more and more clinical environments are beginning to use gaming devices; many of them are skilled nursing and long-term settings. Recent research has demonstrated that including virtual-reality gaming technology does provide some benefit for motor improvements in individuals who have had a stroke.[29,30] Because this is a new strategy, more research is needed to determine parameters to ensure effective use with this patient population.

Typical Impairments and Functional Limitations Being Addressed

Once the PTA knows which interventions will be implemented, he or she must confirm which impairments of body function or activity limitation are to be addressed by each intervention. This is necessary because each intervention can be used to address one or more deficits depending on the patient's problems and the PT's plan to address those problems. For example, using electrotherapeutic modalities can be to address pain issues or can be used to facilitate motor recovery. Parameters will need to be adjusted based on the specific impairment or deficit being addressed (Table 12-9).

It is therefore important that the PTA has a basic understanding of common impairments in body functions and limitations in activities seen in patients who have had a stroke. In addition, the PTA should be familiar with contemporary intervention strategies that can be used to address them.

Impairments in Motor Planning and Apraxia

Praxis is the performance of intentional action(s) or skills. Apraxia, therefore, is an acquired impairment in the performance of purposeful movements. As defined by Shumway-Cook and Woollacott, apraxia "is a disorder of the execution of movement that cannot be attributed to weakness, to incoordination or sensory loss, or to poor language comprehension or inattention to commands."[31] It can develop after a stroke and appears to result from an inability to mentally formulate a plan of action for a motor task. The disruption in the formation or implementation of a plan may result in surprising functional limitations: the inability to comply with a request to lie down on a bed or comb one's hair, consistently putting clothes on inside out, drinking from an empty cup, or attempting to cut one's food with a spoon.[31]

Symptoms among persons with apraxia vary greatly. The following list includes some of the types of apraxia that may be encountered in the clinic[32,33]:

- Ideational apraxia: Failure to conceive or formulate an action, either spontaneously or to command.

Table 12-9

Impairments and Their Corollary Procedural Interventions and Tests and Measures

Impairments	Procedural Interventions								Tests and Measures to Objectify Progress
	Motor Control	Aerobic Capacity	Balance & Coordination	Flexibility	Gait/locomotion	Strength & Endurance	Functional Training	Devices & Equipment	
Motor planning/ apraxia	X		X		X	X	X		• Observation of functional tasks • Nose-finger-nose • Rapid alternating movement • Heel to shin
↓ Aerobic capacity/ endurance		X					X		• Observation of patient level of exertion • Heart rate and rhythm • Respiratory rate • Blood pressue • O_2 saturation • 6-minute walk test
↓ Strength	X					X	X	X	• Observation of functional movements • Manual muscle testing • Hand-held dynamometry
Shoulder pain	X			X		X		X	• Pain scale
Balance deficits	X		X			X	X	X	• Observation of sitting, standing and functional tasks • Timed Up and Go • Berg Balance Test • Timed unipedal standing
Functional limitations	X	X	X	X	X	X	X	X	• Barthel Index • Fugl-Meyer Assessment • Rivermead ADL • National Institutes of Health Stroke Scale

- Ideomotor apraxia: The patient may know and remember the planned action, but he or she cannot execute it with either hand.

- Kinetic limb apraxia: Clumsiness and maladroitness of a limb in the performance of a skilled act that cannot be accounted for by paresis, ataxia, or sensory loss.

- Facial-oral apraxia: Patient is unable to carry out facial movements to command (lick the lips, blow out a match, etc).

- Motor impersistence: An inability to sustain a physical action; is usually identified when a patient cannot close the eyes, protrude the tongue, or raise the nonparetic arm on request and persist in the action for 20 seconds.

One-third of patients with a first stroke will have symptoms of apraxia, and it is more common among those who have had a left hemisphere lesion.[34] Apraxia present at the time of hospital admission for a stroke indicates there will be a higher dependency on others to support the patient upon discharge. When providing interventions to a person with apraxia, the PTA should recognize the tasks that are impaired by apraxia and focus on the patient's learning of strategies for those tasks. For example, if a patient is impaired in the initiation of an activity, the emphasis should be placed on instruction, and if the problem is one of performance errors, the emphasis should be placed on feedback to enhance error detection.[35]

Diminished Aerobic Capacity

People who have had a stroke have impaired fitness (ie, capacity to perform physical activity and work). The following list includes reasons for this acquired activity intolerance:

- Decreased cardiorespiratory fitness

- Energy demands that accompany hemiparesis, sensory loss, and incoordination

- Deficient motor planning and deconditioning from bed rest and inactivity[2,36,37]

In addition, current clinical practices for inpatient rehabilitation appear to contribute to deconditioning because activity levels among individuals receiving rehabilitation services during the 14 days following a stroke are very low. Bernhardt et al found that among patients receiving inpatient rehabilitation, only 13% of an individual's day included participation in therapeutic activities that contribute to the recovery of mobility.[38] The cumulative effect is that the leading cause of mortality among individuals who survive a stroke is vascular disease affecting either the heart (eg, cardiovascular disease) or the brain (eg, stroke).[2]

This has implications for the physical therapy interventions applied following stroke. Gordon et al[2] recommend that exercise programs should be directed at the following goals:

- Regaining the endurance to participate in activities as soon as possible

- Aerobic training for the benefits of decreasing body fat and improving glucose regulation

- Improving aerobic fitness to minimize the functional limitations and mortality that accompany stroke[2]

To achieve these goals, the exercise program, as designed by the PT, may contain elements similar to a cardiac rehabilitation program. That is, the exercise will need to be of sufficient frequency and duration and of a type that the patient can perform to achieve training benefits. To individualize and safely implement the exercises, the PTA must collect data about the patient's response during exercise interventions. The data collection should include data on cardiovascular (ie, heart rate, BP, and arrhythmia monitoring) and cardiopulmonary (ie, respiratory rate and oxygen saturation) responses and the patient's perceived exertion.

Impaired Strength or Motor Control

Eighty-nine percent of patients admitted to the hospital following a stroke have weakness.[39] The severity of the weakness or paralysis that develops following stroke varies according to the location of the damaged brain tissue. The weakness is more a representation of the locale (ie, structures) damaged than it is the size (ie, volume of brain area) of the stroke.

Hemiparesis is the term that describes weakness of either the right or left half of the body, and *hemiplegia* describes a similar unilateral weakness combined with loss of sensation(s). Historically, the weakness that develops following a stroke has been described as hemiparesis or hemiplegia that involves the contralateral side (ie, the extremities and trunk of the half of the body opposite the side of the brain injured from the stroke). However, the loss of strength also involves the extremities and trunk ipsilateral (same side) to the stroke, although to a lesser extent. Therefore, the terms *weaker side* and *stronger side* are recommended for accuracy when describing the pattern of weakness that follows a stroke. This pattern of weakness is important when performing physical therapy interventions because exercise to improve strength should be directed at both sides of the body and not just to the weaker side.[40]

Less than 15% of people who have a stroke will fully recover motor function, and the more severe the weakness, the poorer the prognosis. That is, individuals who have the greatest weakness following a stroke are expected to have a slower recovery and will remain weaker than those with lesser strength deficits. In addition, the severity of post-stroke weakness is related to the severity of functional limitations for transfers, standing, ambulating, and stair climbing.[39]

Shoulder Pain After Stroke

Developing shoulder pain following a stroke can cause psychoemotional distress and limit function. This is a frequent complication, with the literature indicating that it affects 34% to 84% of persons who have had a stroke.[41] Several theories have been proposed to explain the pathology responsible for this disorder, including this summary by Turner-Stokes and Jackson[42]:

- Development of muscle imbalance from the competing symptoms of spasticity and flaccidity, resulting in malalignment of the glenohumeral joint

- Development of adhesive capsulitis (ie, frozen shoulder) with inflammation of the joint capsule restricting flexibility

- Joint subluxation with incongruity of the glenohumeral joint developing due to inadequate muscular support to compensate for the tractioning effect of gravity

- Inflammation of extracapsular structures, such as irritation or tears of the rotator cuff muscles or tendons

- Nerve damage from traction or entrapment of peripheral nerves

- Development of complex regional pain syndrome (eg, reflex sympathetic dystrophy)

These theories propose that the pain develops because of irritation or repetitive trauma to the tissues about the shoulder joint, indicating that a proactive approach designed to prevent the development of shoulder pain is the preferred intervention strategy. Unfortunately, strong evidence supporting a specific method does not exist. Protective strategies have included adhering to a static positioning program and using a sling or other supportive device for the involved UE. The support devices are used to combat gravity's tractioning pull on the glenohumeral joint. An arm sling will effectively support the limb; unfortunately, it also limits and discourages active use of that UE. Another option is a cuff support that encircles the proximal humerus and is suspended from the upper trunk and opposite shoulder (see Figure 12-11). Placing an axillary roll or pad suspended under the involved limb has fallen out of favor because it does not adequately support the glenohumeral joint. Individuals in a chair can also support the arm in an arm trough attached to a lap tray or directly on the lap tray[42] (see Figure 12-12).

Another protective strategy is preserving flexibility about the shoulder joint. This can be achieved through passive ROM. However, care should be taken to inhibit (relax) the shoulder muscles, which may resist the movement because of spasticity or spasm.[42]

NMES is an electrotherapy intervention appropriate for a patient with hemiparesis and can be applied as a component of physical therapy interventions to achieve contraction of the supraspinatus or posterior deltoid muscles. The goal of NMES intervention is to preserve muscle strength in the flaccid or weakened shoulder through peripheral stimulation. By doing so, the subluxation of the glenohumeral joint is reduced or prevented, with benefits of decreased pain or increased mobility.[42]

Balance Deficits

The risk of falling is greater after stroke because of impaired balance. This is expected, because normal balance requires effective performance of the systems for sensation (visual, vestibular, and somatosensation) and motor control (including the strength, coordination, and rate of the person's response), and these abilities are often impaired following stroke. Therefore, a person who has had a stroke may require interventions to remediate impaired balance when sitting, standing, or walking.[43]

In addition to these balance disturbances, there is a subset of about 5% of patients who have had a stroke who demonstrate "pusher" behavior. As described by Roller, "*pusher syndrome* in patients post-stroke is characterized by leaning and active pushing toward the hemiplegic side with no compensation for instability"[44] while maintaining the head in a mostly upright position. The person with this disorder will resist correction, and when a caregiver attempts to assist the person toward a neutral (upright) posture, the patient will complain that they are falling, and the pushing behavior will persist.

This "pusher" behavior develops because the brain injury from the stroke leaves the individual unable to sense and correctly interpret an upright posture (either in sitting or standing). This misinterpretation leads the individual to think he or she is upright when, in fact, he or she is leaning to the side. The individual may also have the sense of falling while being supported in the upright position by the PT or PTA. Therefore, the individual's response is to continue to lean, or push, away from the correct upright position.[45] Interventions performed by the PTA should include focusing the patient's attention on the available sensations—which may include vision, vestibular sensation, or proprioception—and awareness of the support surface. Interventions should augment this sensory feedback, such as using a mirror or training sitting balance on a firm (rather than soft) surface. Practice is a necessary strategy for improving the patient's ability to detect errors and then to develop corrective strategies.[44]

Functional Limitations

The severity of the functional limitations that follow a stroke varies according to the location of the damaged brain tissue and the presence of the previously described impairments. Functional limitations may affect the patient's ability to move alone, change positions, or complete activities of daily living (ADL). The *Guide*[3] outlines the following functional limitations:

- Difficulty planning movements
- Difficulty with manipulation skills
- Frequent falls
- Loss of balance during ADL
- Difficulty negotiating terrains

PATIENT'S CURRENT STATUS

As noted previously, the clinical presentation of individuals following a stroke will be diverse and range from the individual requiring total assistance for all ADL to those with no obvious impairments or limitations in functioning. In addition, the stroke may influence any of the brain's functions so that cognitive skills, such as communication, praxis, or even the ability to stay awake, may be impaired. It is also important to note that the symptoms will vary over time for each patient. For the PTA to be able to form a clear picture of the patient's current status to inform intervention-related decisions, the PTA will review the PT's initial evaluation. In addition to indicating deficits that will be addressed by physical therapy interventions, the PT's evaluation will provide information about other impairments in body functions that can influence the patient's ability to participate in therapy and affect the patient's progress. The following section will discuss various evaluation tools and measurements used by the PT that can provide useful information to help the PTA develop appropriate expectations and make good clinical decisions related to provision of selected interventions. Following this discussion, impairments will be identified that are common to individuals who have had a stroke but not directly addressed by physical therapy interventions and can affect the treatment choices and patient progress.

EXAMINATION TOOLS, TESTS, AND MEASURES

The PT's examination will identify baseline measures of the patient's impairments in body functions and limitations in abilities and participation. These data are evaluated by the PT and inform the prognosis and the development of the PT's plan of care. As physical therapy has moved into evidence-based practice, it is more common to see PTs incorporate standardized tests and measures during the initial examination and evaluation and subsequent evaluations. Some of these standardized tests and measures are referred to as outcome measurements or scales. Two excellent resources for these types of scales are Lewis and McNerney's *The Functional Toolbox*[46] and *The Functional Toolbox II*.[47] Upon review of the PT's evaluative note for a patient, the PTA will have expectations for how the patient will present and behave. The PTA will want to take note of the data collected and the tests and measures used by the PT in the evaluation to choose the appropriate techniques for data collection to monitor the patient's response to the interventions provided, as delegated by the PT.

Motor Control: Strength and Coordination

Strength is measured as a component of the PT's examination, although the method of collecting these data varies depending on the patient's capabilities (eg, ability to follow instructions and severity of weakness). Strength measures may be taken through manual muscle testing or hand-held dynamometry or through a record of functional capabilities (eg, the ability to transfer from sitting to standing). Historically, there has been debate about the role of measuring the strength of patients who have had a stroke or related upper motor neuron lesion (ie, damage to the brain accompanied by symptoms that include spasticity); however, the evidence has indicated that measuring strength following stroke will provide reliable and valid data and that this is valuable information in determining prognosis.[48]

As identified in the section on impaired strength following a stroke, it is common to have weakness that is greater in the extremities opposite from the side of the stroke (eg, following a right middle cerebral artery CVA, the left arm and leg will exhibit more pronounced weakness than the right arm and leg). In a majority of individuals, the strength will improve over time, although impairment of strength will persist.[39]

However, as the strength improves, another impairment that often becomes evident is the inability to isolate extremity movements. That is, when attempting to move a single joint, the other joints in that limb also move in a pattern identified as a synergy (refer to Table 5-4). One of the goals of physical therapy interventions will be to reduce the tendency for movement in these patterns and improve the ability to isolate movements.

Symptoms of coordination impairment that may be affected following stroke include the following:

- Dysdiadochokinesia, which is a deficiency in the ability to perform rapidly alternating movements
- Dysmetria, in which the ability to control the distance, power, and speed of movement is impaired
- Action tremor, which indicates that a tremor or shaking occurs during the performance of voluntary (intentional) movements
- A general slowing of movements, with additional delays in the ability to initiate a movement and to terminate a movement

Refer to Chapter 5 for testing procedures for coordination.

Flexibility

Passive ROM is usually measured to identify any preexisting impairments that need to be addressed (eg, arthritis). In addition, these baseline data are collected because of the risk for the development of stiffness in the muscles affected by stroke. That is, in addition to the resistance to stretch that accompanies spasticity, the muscles often develop a gradual loss of flexibility because of a reduction of elasticity.

Functional Limitations

Following a stroke, a patient may have limited capabilities with the functions of bed mobility, transferring from sitting to standing or standing to sitting, ambulating, stair climbing, and many other ADL. Documenting functional abilities may be performed by describing the patient's ability to perform the function, by timing the patient's performance of the function, or by physical therapy outcome measurement scales.

The description of the patient's functional abilities should be based on efficiently and accurately describing the patient's (not the caregiver's) ability or contribution to performing the function. The descriptors from the Functional Independence Measure are effective for this and were described in Chapter 5.

Timed measurement of a patient's performance of tasks also provides valuable clinical data. Examples include using a stopwatch to time the functions of transferring from sitting to standing and ambulation speed. Transfers can be timed for the time needed to stand up from a chair once, the time needed to stand up 3 consecutive repetitions, or the number of repeated transfers (from sitting to standing to sitting) that can be completed within 10 seconds. Measures such as the 6-minute walk test are designed to measure exercise capacity and may be used for some patients following stroke.[24] However, patients with much lower ambulation or exercise capacity will be better described through measures such as rate of ambulation. One technique is to determine the time it takes an ambulating patient to traverse 10 feet. This should be measured during a period of walking because starting and stopping will alter the results. Gait speed can then be easily calculated as the distance divided by the duration. A patient who ambulates across 10 feet in 5 seconds has a gait speed of 2 feet per second, while the speed of a patient who requires 15 seconds is 0.67 feet per second.

Another important distinction in the ability to ambulate is the patient's ability to accommodate to different environments. The surface that is being walked on can alter performance because of the appearance (eg, visual contrast), texture (eg, tile versus carpeting), or presence of obstacles. Environmental complexity will alter performance because the presence of obstacles, local activity (eg, other people walking nearby), or other distractions in the area may impair performance. For example, a patient may be able to walk effectively in a quiet physical therapy department, but his performance may deteriorate when he walks in a busy hospital hallway. When this occurs, the difference should be recorded and reported to the PT.

Common standardized examination tools used by the PT during the examination include the Barthel Index, the Fugl-Meyer Assessment of Sensorimotor Recovery After Stroke, the Rivermead ADL Scale, and the National Institutes of Health Stroke Scale. It is helpful for the PTA to become familiar with these tools to understand the PT's findings. In addition, some of these tools may be used to determine the patient's response to the intervention(s) provided and objectify the patient's progress. For the PTA to be able to do this accurately, the PTA should review the tool with the PT to identify the data collection technique(s) to be used within the plan of care and the methods to use to correctly perform each technique for collecting necessary data.

Balance Measures

PTs use standardized tests to measure balance in the initial evaluation to provide a baseline and to assist the PT in determining the prognosis and plan of care. All of these tools can also be used to demonstrate the patient's progress; therefore, the PTA should be able to implement all of them appropriately. As described above, the PTA should communicate with the PT to ensure the correct performance of the technique. The following are examples of balance measures:

- Timed Up & Go
- Berg Balance Scale
- Functional Reach Test
- Unipedal standing (timed for duration)

In general, the PTA will want to note the patient's balance reactions based on position (sitting versus standing) and in relation to a functional activity. Often, the patient will have increasing difficulty with balance as the demands of the task increase. This information should be noted, documented, and relayed to the PT. Chapter 5 provides more in-depth information on assessing balance.

Cardiovascular Endurance

Exercise capacity is impaired following stroke. Some of this impairment may result from the hemiparesis because the patient must accommodate for weakness. However, cardiorespiratory fitness is also affected. Mackay-Lyons and Makrides reported that within 1 month after the stroke, the capacity to exercise was reduced to 60% of the typical capacity of a healthy, sedentary person, a response that is equivalent to that for a person recovering from a myocardial infarction.[37] The PT's examination will contain measures of the patient's response to exercise to determine the baseline and because the reduced capacity raises the potential for an adverse response during exercise.

The data collected will usually contain information about the amount of exercise and the patient's response to that level of activity. The PTA should note the amount of activity, such as whether the patient was able to transfer repeatedly, ambulate a specific distance, or ascend a flight of stairs. This information will aid the PTA when determining the exercises and activity expectations for the first intervention session with the patient. The PT's examination should also contain information about the patient's response to exercise. This is usually identified through measuring (at rest and with activity) the patient's heart rate, respiratory rate, BP, and/or oxygen saturation (pulse oximetry). The PTA should continue to collect these data during exercise interventions to make sure the exercises are within the patient's cardiopulmonary capacity.

COMMON IMPAIRMENTS NOT DIRECTLY ADDRESSED BY PHYSICAL THERAPY

Impaired Vestibular Sensation

The vestibular system senses head movement and head position relative to gravity. This information is used to inform the movement system for the extremities and trunk and to improve visual acuity. When a stroke interrupts the transmission or interpretation of vestibular information, it may cause symptoms of vertigo (an illusion of motion), nystagmus (involuntary back-and-forth movements of the eye), disequilibrium (a sense of imbalance), ataxia (incoordination of movement that is not a result of weakness), or a combination of these symptoms. The symptoms of vertigo or disequilibrium may cause nausea, and medications may reduce the nausea sufficiently to allow the patient to participate in physical therapy interventions.

Cognitive Impairments

Cognitive abilities include the mental processes of comprehension, reasoning, and decision making that guide our behaviors and actions. When a portion of the brain has been injured, there will be a disruption in the way that the brain receives, processes, interprets, or responds to information; the behaviors we observe following a stroke are a result of the disruption of these processes.[31] The cognitive impairments most frequently encountered while working with people who have had a stroke are neglect, apraxia (discussed above), anosognosia, and communication disorders. These impairments are confusing to recognize and can present barriers to the patients' participation in physical therapy interventions, to their improvement, and to their attainment of goals. Therefore, when providing selected physical therapy interventions, a PTA should be able to recognize and respond appropriately to the behavioral expressions of these cognitive impairments.

Another contributor to cognitive performance in some individuals is an alteration in perception, which is the process of converting sensations into meaningful and understandable information. Because of the amount and types of sensory disturbances that may occur following a stroke, it is not surprising that these individuals have impaired cognition. When this type of impairment contributes to deterioration in cognitive performance, the PTA should work to augment sensory inputs (examples are provided below) and to educate the patient, family, and other caregivers about strategies to compensate for the sensory or perceptual deficit.

Unilateral Neglect

Unilateral neglect is a disorder that is important to recognize because of its frequency and its influence on the rehabilitation process. The symptoms of unilateral neglect are an inability to report, attend to, or recognize sight, sound, and/or touch opposite to the side of the brain affected by stroke.[49] It is also referred to as *neglect, visuospatial neglect, hemispatial neglect,* or *left neglect.*

Neglect is a frequently encountered impairment, with a reported incidence following stroke between 10% and 82%.[43] Neglect is classically associated with stroke involving the right half of the brain, causing neglect (inattention or unawareness) of the left environment or body; however, it may also be observed when a left hemisphere lesion causes a right neglect, although that form is more likely to resolve 4 to 8 weeks following the stroke.[50,51]

The PTA must be concerned with the functional impact from the symptoms that accompany the inability to attend to the left or right components of the patient's environment. The symptoms will present as deficiencies in the domains of memory (mental representation and recall), action-intention (motor performance), or attention (response to sensations).[50] Neglect involving memory is quite striking because the patients may be impaired in their ability to describe aspects of their home based on the mental perspective from which they are recalling it. For example, a patient with a left unilateral neglect may not be able to recall the railing on his stairs if he is picturing the stairs from the perspective of the bottom of the stairs with the railing on the left, but he will be able to recall the same railing if he changes his perspective to the top of the stairs with the railing on his right. When neglect involves motor intention, the patient will be impaired in his ability to act or plan movements involving the right or left half of the body. This will adversely affect function as seen by behaviors, such as not recognizing that food is on the left side of a plate and, subsequently, not eating that half of a meal; not dressing or applying makeup to half of the body; or not accounting for objects (eg, door frames) to one side and then walking into them, causing injury or falls. When the neglect involves attention, there may not be a response to stimuli that occurs within a portion of the individual's environment. For example, a person with a neglect involving the left side of his or her environment may not respond to sounds, sights, and/or touch that originates from the left regardless of his or her integrity to those sensations. Another example is when an individual may not be able to identify when a car is approaching from the left side while the individual is crossing the street.

Neglect is associated with a poorer outcome following stroke because people with neglect require longer programs of inpatient rehabilitation, achieve less recovery of functional abilities, and require greater assistance with ADL.[43] Pierce and Buxbaum[49] comprehensively reviewed the interventions for unilateral neglect, which, briefly summarized, are categorized as interventional techniques directed at the following to alleviate neglect:

- Achieving arousal through the following:
  - Medications that stimulate excitatory neurotransmitters (such as dopamine)
  - Feedback, either auditory or auditory and visual, that alerts the patient to his or her area of neglect
- Improving visual attention through interventions to increase visual tracking into the neglected visual field or through visuoperceptual training.
- Improving hemispatial representation (eg, awareness) through interventions directed at the impaired side that include the following:
  - Activation or movement of the hemiparetic limb(s)
  - CIMT
  - Mental imagery training
  - Optical training with prism lenses to reorient the visual fields
  - Patching of one eye, or the modification of eyeglasses to block a hemifield of vision for both eyes, to reorient visual attention
  - Caloric stimulation (placing cold water in the outer ear canal)
  - Optokinetic stimulation via visual stimuli moving horizontally across the visual field
  - Vibratory stimulation to the posterior neck muscles
  - Trunk rotation (passive)

All of these interventions have demonstrated some benefit in reducing the effects of unilateral neglect. However, when reviewed in total, the evidence on these interventions remains limited.[49]

Recognizing the conflicting evidence on the response to interventions for unilateral neglect is important for the PTA because this will result in the PT using different strategies for interventions based on the patient's symptoms and the evolving evidence for this problem. Given the diverse intervention strategies, it is unlikely for a PTA to become trained in applying all of them, and when the PTA encounters an unfamiliar technique, she or he must request guidance from the PT. Also, the PTA needs to identify when a patient is or is not responding to an intervention for unilateral neglect and communicate that information to the PT.

Anosognosia

Anosognosia is the denial of one's own neurological symptoms, such as weakness, functional limitation, and other deficits. Examples that have been observed following stroke include the denial of hemiparesis, visual loss, aphasia, movement disorder, and apraxia. This is typically observed by the PTA through the persistent denial of post-stroke impairments, the minimizing of weakness, and the indifference to the effects of the weakness (eg, blaming it on arthritis, fatigue, or trauma to a limb). Common concurrent stroke symptoms are hemisensory disturbances, unilateral neglect, dressing or constructional apraxia, reduced intellectual functions, motor impersistence, and prosopagnosia (impaired recognition of familiar faces), although memory is usually spared. The incidence of anosognosia is greater than is recognized by most clinicians; the literature indicates an occurrence of 28% to 85% among people who have had a right hemisphere stroke and 0% to 17% among patients who have had a left hemisphere stroke. Although this symptom usually resolves 12 to 22 weeks after the onset of a stroke, the presence of anosognosia is generally considered a poor prognostic indicator for functional recovery.[52,53] The authors are not aware of intervention strategies for those cases in which anosognosia persist. Fortunately, that occurs among less than 10% of persons with this symptom.

Communication Disorders

Dysphasia is an acquired impairment of communication, which may include expressive (speaking) ability, receptive (comprehension) ability, or both. *Aphasia* is the term more frequently used in the clinic for this disorder, although that term more accurately refers to the complete loss of these communication abilities.

The brain's cortex contains 2 areas, Broca's and Wernicke's, which are primarily responsible for communication. Communication is a lateralized brain function, meaning that different components of communication are controlled predominantly on each side of the brain. In most people, spoken language is lateralized to the left hemisphere of the brain and nonverbal communication is lateralized to the right hemisphere (although this rule does not apply to about half of the people who are left-handed). The communication impairments observed after a stroke vary depending on the location(s) affected by the stroke.

Following a stroke that involves Broca's area of the left cerebral cortex, a person will have trouble verbally expressing him- or herself. The impairment is with the process of motor programming for the production or the organization of spoken words. This may present as slow or nonfluent speech, poor articulation, or grammatically incorrect speech.

When a stroke affects Wernicke's area of the left cerebral cortex, an individual will be impaired with the receptive components of communication. The impairment is in the comprehension of language; therefore, these individuals may have difficulty following the PTA's spoken instructions. The person with this lesion will retain the ability to speak fluently, but the use of words is impaired, and the patient may demonstrate the use of meaningless words or phrases. In addition to the anticipated frustration that accompanies a disorder of communication, this type of lesion will also contribute to agitation and related emotional reactions.[54]

Nonverbal communication may be impaired following a stroke in the right hemisphere. If Broca's area is involved, the person will be impaired with expression, such as the use of emotional gestures, or with the intonation of speech. If Wernicke's area is involved, the individual will have trouble interpreting nonverbal signals (eg, facial expressions or gestures) from others. A lesion to this area will also cause a deficiency in comprehending spatial relationships (eg, distances).[55]

The following list includes additional communication disorders the PTA will encounter[56]:

- Anomia: Naming and word-finding impairments

- Dysarthria: Impaired articulation during speech (from incoordination or weakness of the oral-facial muscles)

- Dyslexia or alexia: Impaired reading (comprehension of written communication)

- Dysgraphia or agraphia: Impaired ability to communicate through writing
- Paraphasia: The inappropriate substitution of words when speaking

Communication impairments will adversely affect a patient's response to therapeutic interventions and his or her ability to function. Because of the complexity of these disorders, the PTA should consult with the PT, and possibly the speech-language pathologist, to identify the communication strategy that is optimal for each individual.

Affective Disorders

Affect refers to mood or the emotional component of behaviors. It is expected that there will be emotional reactions among patients who have had a stroke, and these may include sadness, denial, passivity, agitation, mood swings, indifference, or the inability to control impulsive or socially inappropriate behaviors.[57] However, the location or type of injury from the stroke may contribute to severe or persistent affective changes that need to be managed within the context of the health care team. Due to the medical management options that may need to be used, the PTA should consult with the PT when the following behaviors are encountered: abulia (extreme apathy), anxiety, emotional lability (rapid swings among emotional states), pathological laughing and crying, and depression (also called *post-stroke depression*).

One challenge for some patients is demonstrating behaviors that are in keeping with the social and cultural expectations for a situation. Stroke may result in a loss of this ability, which is called a *loss of inhibitions* or *disinhibition*. When disinhibition occurs, a patient may act in a manner that would have been unacceptable to him or her before the stroke (eg, telling off-color jokes or physically grabbing at others). The PTA should address the inappropriate behavior when it occurs because the action is not acceptable whether it is the patient's typical behavior or a symptom of stroke, and the PTA should also clarify the behavioral expectations. A patient with disinhibition may require a comprehensive behavioral shaping program, applied by all members of the health care team, to achieve an appropriate response to typical situations or improvements of behavior.

Dysphagia

Dysphagia is a disorder of swallowing that may result from incoordination or weakness of the oral, pharyngeal, laryngeal, or esophageal muscles. A patient with dysphagia may benefit from treatment to improve control or strength in these muscles. Until this is achieved, the patient may be on a restricted diet to prevent pulmonary aspiration. A common restriction related to dysphagia is the person is only allowed to drink fluids that have had a thickener added, which slows the swallowing process and makes it easier for the individual to swallow correctly. The PTA assisting a person at this stage of rehabilitation must comply with the dietary restriction because a variation may result in aspiration, which can lead to complications (eg, pneumonia).

Impaired Somatosensation

The somatosensory system conveys information to the brain from the musculoskeletal system and the skin. When a portion of the brain responsible for processing or interpreting this information is affected by a stroke, the person will have an impairment of somatosensation. This will affect safety because the person will be delayed or unable to sense pain and withdraw from harm. It will also impair movement, coordination, and balance because somatosensation informs us about the position(s) and rate(s) of movement of our limbs and body. Without this information, we cannot move accurately, and this is one of the causes of ataxia (incoordination of movement that is not a result of weakness).

Another symptom that may develop is learned nonuse, in which the absence of sensation from a limb contributes to the adaptive behavior of relying on the limb with intact sensation to assist with all functions while the limb with impaired somatosensation is not used to assist with functions. Interventions directed at improving somatosensation may include tactile stimulation through electrical stimulation or stroking of the skin or training for tactile perception through recognition of objects, discrimination of textures, or recognition of positions.[58]

Impaired Vision

A stroke that interrupts the pathways for transmitting or interpreting visual information will cause an impairment of vision. Homonymous hemianopia is a commonly encountered visual impairment following stroke and results in defective or lost vision in the right or left half of the visual field. This visual field loss occurs in both eyes and should not be confused with unilateral neglect. Homonymous hemianopia is an impairment of visual sensation, and unilateral neglect is an impairment of attention or awareness. These different disorders may present concurrently or alone.

Visual acuity may also be impaired following stroke, with symptoms such as blurred vision or diplopia (double vision). These develop because of disruption in the ability to stabilize gaze (ie, maintain visual fixation on an object), which is a prerequisite for normal vision. One cause for gaze instability is disruption of the brainstem nuclei responsible for stabilization (which is mediated by the vestibulo-ocular and optokinetic reflexes) or from loss of vestibular or visual sensory input to these nuclei. Another cause is disruption of the movement system for the eyes and control of the muscles that move the eye or the brainstem locations that innervate these muscles, which can result in diplopia or blurred vision.[56]

GOALS AS SET BY THE PHYSICAL THERAPIST

Information gathered about the patient's current status should be considered in light of the goals set by the PT. The goals will provide an outline for the PTA regarding the expected timing of and activities related to progression of the patient. For example, a patient whose current status includes ambulating with minimal assistance from the therapist along with the use of a small-based quad cane, and whose goal indicates he or she should be ambulating independently with no assistive device within 3 weeks, helps the PTA recognize the expected rate of progression and to anticipate the progression (small-based quad cane to straight cane to no assistive device).

Goals common to the acute care setting during the initial stages of therapy include maintaining ROM and protecting the shoulder joint of the more involved UE, educating the patient regarding safety and positioning issues, and facilitating a smooth transition to the subacute setting. Goals in the subacute setting include preventing or minimizing secondary complications, improving movement control with functional tasks, improving postural control and balance, increasing independence with functional tasks such as ADL and gait, and increasing cardiovascular endurance.

PATIENT'S DIAGNOSIS

A natural part of the PTA's clinical decision-making process includes considering the implications of the medical diagnosis of CVA. One basic principle that should be considered is the fact that because a stroke is an acute event, it is normal to expect that the patient will have at least some recovery of function. In the *Guide*,[3] CVAs fall under Practice Pattern 5D: Impaired Motor Function and Sensory Integrity Associated With Nonprogressive Disorders of the Central Nervous

Table 12-10
Cerebral Circulation and Common Deficits Associated With Cerebrovascular Accident

Artery	Cerebral Area Supplied	Common Deficits Associated With a Lesion
Middle cerebral artery	Lateral cortex of temporal lobe, anterolateral frontal lobe, and parietal lobe	• Contralateral hemiparesis • Contralateral sensory loss • Global aphasia (if dominant side) • Upper > lower extremity involvement • Perceptual deficits
Anterior cerebral artery	Medial portions of the frontal lobe, superior medial parietal lobe, basal ganglia, and corpus callosum	• Contralateral hemiplegia • Contralateral sensory loss • Lower > upper extremity involvement • Mental impairment • Apraxia • Behavioral changes
Posterior cerebral artery	Occipital lobe, medial and inferior temporal lobe, thalamus, and midbrain	• Abnormal sensation of pain, temperature, and proprioception • Hemiplegia • Contralateral ataxia • Drowsiness • Lack of interest in movement • Disturbance in memory
Vertebral and posterior inferior cerebral arteries	Brainstem, medulla, and cerebellum	• Vertigo • Ipsilateral ataxia • Ipsilateral sensory deficit • Contralateral hemiparesis • Gait ataxia

System—Acquired in Adolescence or Adulthood. As is indicated in this practice pattern, CVA is an acute focal event that leads to acquired deficits (as opposed to those that are congenital in origin). Although the deficits associated with a stroke may be permanent, the pathology itself is limited. Additionally, because of the normal, neuroplastic capabilities of the brain, the PTA should expect a patient who has had a stroke to recover all or some of the body functions and abilities in the absence of confounding factors (discussed later in this chapter).

Although individuals who have had a stroke generally have common deficits (motor control impairments, sensory deficits, etc [see Table 12-1]), specific patterns of deficits depend on the area of vascular compromise. Therefore, it is important for the PTA to have a general understanding of the typical pattern of deficits associated with the major cerebral blood vessels (Table 12-10) as well as which deficits are common with each hemisphere (Table 12-11). This will allow the PTA to contextualize the information found in the PT's evaluation and to anticipate the patient's presentation. While each person with a stroke will present a unique combination of symptoms, recognizing these general patterns of symptoms will improve the PTA's ability to recognize and respond to the complexities involved with the treatment of patients who have had a stroke.

Table 12-11
Impairments Based on Side of Lesion

Right Hemisphere	Left Hemisphere
Left hemiparesis	Right hemiparesis
Left hemisensory loss	Right hemisensory loss
Trouble perceiving emotions and nonverbal communication	Speech-language impairments
Trouble sustaining movements	Trouble planning/sequencing movement
Quick and impulsive	Slow, cautious, anxious
Poor judgment	Difficulty processing
Difficulty with abstract concepts	Trouble expressing positive emotion
Visual-perceptual deficits	

PATIENT'S PROGNOSIS

Recovery after an ischemic stroke follows a fairly predictable pattern. Initial recovery of body functions and abilities occurs within the first few days to weeks after the stroke event. This recovery of neurological function is attributed to reduction of edema and improvement in local blood flow to the cerebral tissues. Recovery after this initial time frame is attributed to unmasking of neuropathways and collateral sprouting among surviving neurons. This recovery tends to follow a pattern of improvement over the course of the first 6 months post-stroke. After the 6-month time frame, improvements in function can occur for patients who are motivated and prepared to work diligently to meet their individual goals.

Because of this typical course of recovery, the PTA's expectation is that the patient will demonstrate improvement in functional abilities in response to physical therapy interventions; this will usually be observed as progress toward, or achievement of, the goals established in the PT's plan of care. The rate of improvement should be communicated to the PT. In some cases, the PTA may note a deterioration of functional abilities, and this also should be communicated to the PT. This is particularly important when there is a notable deterioration in functioning or cognitive ability, or when the patient becomes more lethargic, because the patient may be experiencing complications that require acute medical services. Specific expectations related to rate of improvement are highly individualized. The PTA should refer to the physical therapy goals to determine what the expected rate of recovery is for each patient. Patient prognosis and rate of recovery are affected by and frequently depend on the presence of comorbidities and confounding problems.

Comorbidities/Confounding Problems

When caring for an individual who has had a CVA, the PT's and PTA's major emphasis will be on the impairments of body functions and limitations in abilities that are results of the stroke. Most individuals who are recovering from a stroke, however, have preexisting medical problems that cannot be ignored. These medical problems can directly affect the patient's ability to participate and progress with physical therapy interventions.

Common cardiovascular diseases found in patients recovering from a stroke include hypertension, coronary artery disease with a history of a heart attack or a coronary artery bypass surgery

(CABG), and peripheral vascular disease. The PTA will need to monitor the cardiovascular status of the individual during therapeutic activities. If the individual has a history of a heart attack or CABG, it is important to know when these occurred so that the appropriate precautions related to exercise intensity can be taken. For example, a patient who recently underwent a CABG and subsequently had a CVA will have precautions related to the amount of pressure that can be put through the UEs during functional activities. This will lead to the need for alternative strategies for sit-to-stand transfers because the patient cannot push through the hands on the chair.

Common musculoskeletal conditions that may be encountered include arthritis, joint replacement, amputation, osteoporosis, pathologic fractures (hip, wrist, back), back pain, and rotator cuff injury and repair. Again, impairments and limitations related to these conditions can affect the patient's progress during recovery after a CVA. For example, a patient who has had a transfemoral amputation of the left leg and who now demonstrates hemiparesis of the right side may require a one-arm drive w/c for functional mobility. Precautions related to preexisting conditions must be taken into consideration during provision of interventions (eg, weight-bearing restrictions or total joint precautions).

Other common conditions that are encountered in this patient population are diabetes and chronic obstructive pulmonary disease (COPD). When working with individuals with diabetes, it is important for the PTA to be able to recognize symptoms of hypoglycemia so that appropriate action can be taken. A patient with a diagnosis of COPD may need oxygen supplementation during therapeutic activities. The PTA will need to monitor the patient's response to exercise by noting the respiratory rate and monitoring oxygen saturation. The patient may need verbal cues for appropriate breathing strategies during the physical therapy session. The patient may be limited in his or her endurance for therapy, and the session may need to be divided to allow the patient to rest in between different activities.

Contraindications/Precautions

The PTA must keep in mind any precautions associated with stroke and any accompanying diagnosis that the patient has when interventions are being provided. Although there is no direct contraindication when working with patients who have had a stroke, there are several conditions that are precautions and should be monitored for patient safety. Most of these have been discussed earlier in this chapter but will be mentioned again to highlight their importance.

As noted previously, it is common for the hemiparetic UE to demonstrate joint subluxation due to "inadequate muscular support to compensate for the tractioning effect of gravity."[42] It is essential for the PTA to monitor the limb at all times. Positioning strategies and using slings and electrotherapeutic modalities to address this concern have been described. It is also imperative that the patient, the patient's family, and all caregivers be made aware of the concern and be taught to monitor the positioning of the limb at all times. For example, when assisting the patient into standing, that arm should not be used to pull the patient up from a chair. Similarly, the LE can be at risk for injury because of weakness and sensory deficits. It is important to monitor the limb placement and positioning with all activities. This is of special concern during transfers; if the foot is not positioned appropriately and monitored, the ankle may roll as weight is transferred to the limb, resulting in soft tissue injury.

Also discussed earlier was the importance of monitoring the patient's cardiovascular response to activities. Stroke may be the result of underlying cardiovascular disease that could reduce the patient's capacity for exercise, and hemiplegia will create new methods of moving that increase the physical demands imposed on the patient. It is the PTA's responsibility to protect the patient through vigilant measuring of vital signs for interpreting the patient's response to interventions.

Although dysphagia is a condition that is primarily treated by speech therapy rather than physical therapy, it is imperative that PTAs be aware of the potential for aspiration and seek clarification of any swallowing restrictions. When working with a patient who has had a stroke, it is common for the

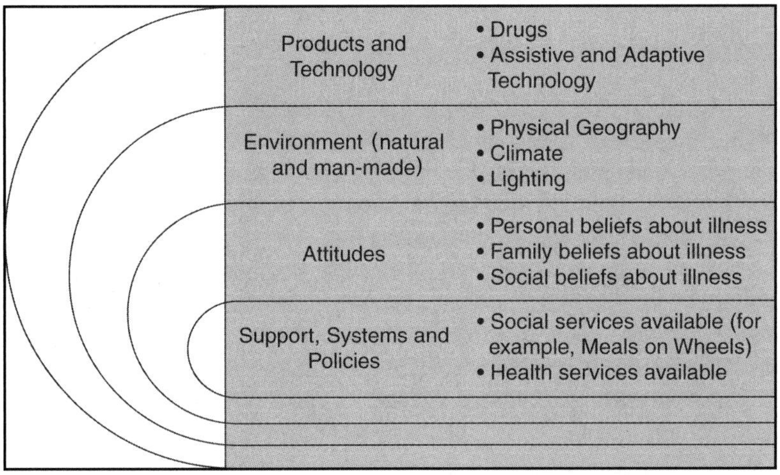

Products and Technology	• Drugs • Assistive and Adaptive Technology	
Environment (natural and man-made)	• Physical Geography • Climate • Lighting	
Attitudes	• Personal beliefs about illness • Family beliefs about illness • Social beliefs about illness	
Support, Systems and Policies	• Social services available (for example, Meals on Wheels) • Health services available	

Figure 12-13. Examples of environmental factors based on the International Classification of Functioning, Disability and Health categories.

patient to ask for a drink of water during the physical therapy session. The PTA must confirm and comply with the patient's dietary restrictions, which may change day to day, to protect the patient.

Finally, patients who have had an ischemic stroke are typically on anticoagulation therapy. Anticoagulation therapy can make patients more susceptible to bruising; therefore, extra care should be taken to ensure patients are handled carefully.

PERSONAL/ENVIRONMENTAL FACTORS

When beginning to work with a patient who is recovering from a CVA, the PTA must not only consider the limitations due to preexisting medical conditions but also should have an idea of the patient's prior level of functioning as reported in the PT's initial evaluation. Each patient is unique regardless of the diagnostic label(s). Many individuals with multiple medical conditions continue to be active and are reportedly healthy, while other patients have a sedentary lifestyle with obesity and generalized weakness due to inactivity but may not have any diagnosed medical conditions. Therefore, an understanding of the patient's prior level of function will help to shape the expectations for therapeutic intervention. In addition, knowledge of the patient's prior functional activity will provide insight into the patient's perception of exercise or activity and can guide the PTA in determining how to best approach the patient to ensure optimal participation in therapy.

Psychosocial issues that can affect the provision of physical therapy must also be recognized. The patient's cultural background and belief system related to disability and medical intervention must be considered. For example, a social and cultural background that views disability as a personal weakness that must be hidden can result in differing responses. One patient may be motivated to overcome the disability to be able to reenter his or her previous social role, whereas another individual may become depressed and lose interest in participation with therapy. Regardless of the belief system or response, it is the responsibility of all health care providers to be sensitive to these issues and to work within the patient's belief system to ensure optimal recovery. Family and social support can often make the difference in a patient being able to return home or needing alternate discharge arrangements. The PTA should review the initial evaluation to gain insight into the social support that is available to the patient and note the prognosis for the discharge environment. Figure 12-13 provides examples of environmental considerations per categories outlined in the International Classification of Functioning, Disability and Health. A patient with mild limitations in functional mobility may not be able to return to independent living, but if a spouse or other family member is available, this could mean the difference between the individual returning home or needing to move into an assisted living facility. Care must be taken to determine the abilities and the willingness of the family to provide the needed assistance. Patients who have a CVA are often elderly, and many times their spouses are not in good health; it may be dangerous to the patient as well as the spouse if the patient were to return home.

IMPLEMENTING THE INTERVENTION

As Skinner and McVey state in their text *Clinical Decision Making for the Physical Therapist Assistant,* "Effective PTAs do not simply perform a set of PT prescribed interventions. Instead, they fashion those prescribed interventions into a coherent and logical treatment sequence that best meet the rehabilitation goals. This requires PTAs to make clinical decisions based on a clear understanding of the conditions and the various factors that influence rehabilitation."[59] Therefore, we have spent the majority of this chapter discussing a model for clinical decision making and describing various factors the PTA must consider to be an effective PTA. It is only after taking the multiple factors into consideration that the PTA will be ready to engage the patient and initiate implementation of selected interventions as directed by the PT. However, during the implementation process, the PTA will continue to encounter decisions that need to be made regarding how to proceed with patient care tasks. These decisions include how to determine whether the patient is safe to participate in the planned interventions, how to ensure patient comfort and safety during the intervention, how and when to progress activities, and when to communicate with the PT regarding the patient's response to care. The remainder of this chapter will consider these clinical decisions and discuss factors for the PTA to consider when making them.

Determine Patient Readiness to Participate

Prior to initiating any intervention, a PTA must always assess the patient to determine if the patient is medically stable and physiologically and psychologically stable enough to engage in the planned activities. In an inpatient environment (acute care, subacute rehab, SNF), this includes reviewing the medical chart to verify that there have not been any changes in the patient's medical status that would affect participation in physical therapy. Direct observation of the patient through measurement of the patient's vital signs (heart rate and BP at a minimum) and monitoring for changes in the patient's cognitive status are essential to determine whether it is appropriate to initiate physical therapy interventions. These assessments should occur prior to each therapy session. To make appropriate decisions related to the patient's vital signs, the PTA will need to become familiar with the patient's typical vital sign readings found in the medical record. In the days following a stroke, the medical management often includes maintaining a moderately elevated BP to promote blood flow to the brain tissue immediately around the damage from the stroke. These patients may be allowed to have BPs as high as 230/120 mm Hg.[1] Other patients with cardiovascular conditions will have specific parameters that must be maintained. In general, however, the PTA can follow basic guidelines for cardiovascular status as listed here to determine whether the patient is responding safely during physical therapy interventions:

- Heart rate less than 130 beats per minute with regular rhythm
- Respiratory rate less than 40 breaths per minute
- Oxygen saturation above 88%
- BP below 140/90 mm Hg, with diastolic pressure remaining above 60

It is not unusual for a patient and his or her family to respond to a stroke with the request to allow the patient time to rest and recover from this devastating medical event. However, physical therapy is the preferred treatment to promote recovery. The PTA should clarify that close monitoring of the patient's vital signs will ensure that the patient is safe and responding appropriately to the challenges of therapy.

During this process, it is important to recognize the potential for cognitive and communication deficits. Excellent strategies for modifying treatment to accommodate a cognitive impairment have been described by Shumway-Cook and Woollacott[31]:

1. Reduce confusion: Make sure the task goal is clear to the patient

2. Improve motivations: Work on tasks that are relevant and important to the patient

3. Encourage consistency of performance: Be consistent with goals, and reinforce only those behaviors that are compatible with those goals

4. Reduce confusion: Use simple, clear, and concise instructions

5. Seek a moderate level of arousal to optimize learning: Moderate the sensory stimulation in the environment; agitated patients require decreased intensity of stimulation (soft voice, low lights, slow touch) to reduce arousal levels; stuporous patients require increased intensity of stimulation (use brisk, loud commands and fast movements, working in a vertical position)

6. Provide increased levels of supervision, especially during the early stages of retraining

7. Recognize that progress may be slower when working with patients who have cognitive impairments

8. Improve attention: Accentuate perceptual cues that are essential to the task, and minimize the number of irrelevant stimuli in the environment

9. Improve problem-solving ability: Begin with relatively simple tasks, and gradually increase the complexity of the task demands

10. Encourage declarative as well as procedural learning: Have a patient verbally and/or mentally rehearse sequences when performing a task

Implement Selected Interventions

In inpatient settings, patients are frequently seen twice a day for physical therapy. In acute care settings, the time frame is typically limited to the patient's endurance. In the inpatient rehab setting, physical therapy sessions are often an hour long. Because there are frequently several different deficits that need to be addressed, the PTA should consider how to prioritize each session based on factors such as (1) which interventions will target body functions foundational to function (ie, trunk control), (2) which goals are most significant to the patient, (3) how close is the patient to discharge, and (4) what activities previous interventions have focused on. Taking these types of factors into consideration will allow the PTA to prioritize and structure each session.

During each session, the PTA should begin by clearly communicating the significance of the activity to the patient. As Dutton states, "Explicit knowledge of the task goals before practice for individuals post-stroke appears to improve implicit learning of motor skills."[5] As part of this process, the PTA may need to demonstrate the motion or activity desired to provide a visual example. These steps, of course, may be inappropriate for patients with cognitive, visual perceptual, or communication deficits. All patients can, however, be guided through the movement to provide the patients with a kinesthetic input regarding the desired movement. As stated previously, guided movement should be limited for appropriate motor learning to occur. At this point, the PTA will use the motor-learning principles discussed above to modify and/or advance the activities appropriately based on the patient's response.

During each individual session, a variety of activities at a variety of levels may be practiced. This variability, when chosen intentionally, can be helpful in the motor learning process. It is important at some point in each session to significantly challenge the patient; however, it is best to end each session with an activity the patient is able to complete, thus ending on a positive note.

Determine Patient's Response to Interventions

Another great challenge when providing physical therapy interventions to the patient who has had a stroke is the dynamic presentation of the symptoms of the stroke. The PTA should expect that changes in symptoms will occur and, therefore, rigorously collect data to inform the process of modifying the intervention(s) to the patient. Changes in response to physical therapy interventions for the symptoms from a stroke may be subtle and observed over several days or may be sufficient to require intervention progressions to occur repeatedly within a single physical therapy session with the patient.

Much of the assessment will occur through observation of the patient's response rather than through any formal test. The PTA will monitor the patient's movements to note muscle substitutions or degradation of movement patterns that indicate fatigue. The PTA should also note changes in the patient's attention and cognitive function, which can also indicate fatigue.

Formally assessing vital signs during a therapy session is important for patients who have cardiovascular conditions or when the patient is engaged in therapeutic exercise for aerobic/capacity and endurance. Other formal assessment processes such as strength measures, standardized tests, etc, will occur based on the plan of care to note progress.

Progress, Modify, or Discontinue

Based on the assessment through observation and data from tests, the PTA will make decisions to progress, modify, or discontinue aspects of procedural interventions. The PTA will progress the intervention based on the expectations outlined in the plan of care when the patient is demonstrating the expected response. Progression may include changing assistive devices (from a hemi cane to a quad cane) or advancing activities (moving from a focus on static sitting balance to dynamic sitting balance). If the patient has met all the established goals, the PTA will consult with the PT to determine whether further goals should be established.

Throughout a therapy session, the PTA will make multiple modifications to the intervention to challenge the patient as well as to ensure the safety and comfort of the patient. Modification can include the various aspects described related to motor learning. Modification can also be made when the patient is not responding as desired during a therapy session. For example, when attempting to teach a patient how to perform a sit-to-stand transfer, if the patient is unable to perform the task without significant assistance, the PTA may choose to raise the surface the patient is sitting on to allow the patient to work through a shortened range and thus experience more autonomy in movement and better tap into the appropriate motor program.

Finally, there will be times when a PTA will need to decide to discontinue with the current intervention tasks at hand. This should occur any time the patient displays a negative physiological response, a decrease in cognitive functioning, or significant psychological distress as evidenced by inappropriate heart rate and BP response. Exercise should be stopped any time the systolic BP drops 20 mm Hg or more or is greater than 260 mm Hg, or if the diastolic BP is greater than 115 mm Hg.[60]

Notify the Physical Therapist

To ensure that the most effective and efficient care is being provided, it is imperative that the PTA communicate regularly with the PT regarding the patient's response to interventions. The type and frequency of communication will vary based on the patient's needs, the PT's preferences, and the setting where care is being provided. In an inpatient environment where the PT and PTA may be working side by side, the PT may be able to observe and monitor the care being provided by the PTA and provide guidance when needed without making specific plans for scheduled communication. The PTA's documentation will act as an additional form of communication between the PTA and the PT. Some state practice acts regulate the frequency of PT/PTA interaction regarding patient care. However, regardless of these issues, the PTA should ensure the PT is kept up to date regarding the patient's status and progress. The PTA should inform the PT any time the patient has met a goal or when the patient's progress is not proceeding as expected (whether it is faster or slower than expected). The PTA should also make sure the PT is aware of any changes that could affect the patient's goals or plan of care. For example, if the plan was based on the patient being discharged to an assisted-living environment but the patient's family has decided to take the patient home instead, the PT needs to determine whether there are needed alterations to the plan of care. Finally, as described earlier, the PTA should immediately inform the PT of any negative responses the patient may display.

CONCLUSION

Providing interventions for a patient with a CVA is based on the plan of care and considers the individual patient's goals, functional capabilities, and discharge plan. Data collection is critical because the symptoms of the stroke may be changing between, and even within, the physical therapy sessions. While providing skilled interventions, the PTA must identify when changes occur and appropriately modify those interventions provided within the treatment plan established by the PT. Particular attention must be paid to the progression of interventions, such as therapeutic exercise or gait-training techniques, so that the patient is challenged appropriately and advanced toward achieving optimal functional abilities.

Finally, value the role of the patient, the patient's family, and the other caregivers in this process. The selected physical therapy interventions provided will involve only a small portion of the patient's day, but when others are encouraged to be involved in the process, a team effort is available to support the rehabilitation of the patient. This will extend and reinforce the activities and exercises necessary for the patient to achieve an optimal outcome from the process.

CASE STUDIES

CASE #1

A 64-year-old man was admitted to an acute rehabilitation facility 6 days after having a CVA, which was diagnosed as a left internal capsule infarction. The patient displayed mild right extremity and trunk weakness. The patient also displayed diminished sensation throughout the right extremities. He demonstrated impaired balance and motor control and required minimal assistance for gait activities due to apraxia. The patient required constant verbal cues when ambulating and became easily distracted in cluttered environments or when other individuals walked past him. He had poor insight into his deficits and demonstrated impulsivity that placed him as a safety risk. The patient previously lived alone in a home with 5 steps to enter, and his goal was to return to that environment. The PT's plan of care called for therapeutic exercise to improve strength and motor control, gait training on level and uneven surfaces, and patient education.

QUESTIONS

1. List the impairments of body functions, limitations in activities, and restrictions in participation this patient demonstrates.

2. Within the plan of care, what activities could be used to address the right LE strength deficits? What parameters would be used (frequency, intensity, etc)?

3. This patient demonstrates safety issues during gait due to motor apraxia and anosognosia. How do you want to progress the environmental context in which this patient is practicing gait activities?

4. Discuss feedback strategies to utilize related to the patient's functional mobility deficits.

5. Utilizing the concepts of movement sequencing, discuss other postures and activities you might choose to use with this patient to address the deficits of motor apraxia noted during gait.

6. What are you (the PTA) going to observe in this patient's movements to determine if the intervention strategies being used are effective?

CASE #2

A 72-year-old woman was on vacation with her sister when she had a left middle cerebral artery CVA. She was transported from her hotel room to the hospital via an ambulance. The patient displayed strength of 0/5 throughout the right UE. The patient had sufficient strength to initiate the movements of hip extension and adduction but demonstrated severe weakness and decreased tone throughout the right LE musculature. The patient required maximal assistance with all mobility, including rolling, supine-to-and-from-sit and sit-to-and-from-stand transitions, as well as transfers from bed to and from the w/c. When standing, she needed maximal assistance and a hemi cane and was unable to support weight through her right leg. The patient's sitting balance was diminished, requiring minimal to moderate assistance to maintain an upright posture. The patient demonstrated mild pusher behavior and required frequent verbal cues to shift her weight to the left. The patient also demonstrated global aphasia. She did not attempt to speak and communicated only with head nods and shakes. The speech therapist's notes indicated the patient had only 50% accuracy with head nods and shakes. The patient was able to follow simple commands with physical and visual cues with 90% accuracy. Discharge plans are for the patient's son to come to assist with transporting the patient back to her hometown, where she will enter an inpatient rehabilitation unit. She will travel by commercial air. The son will need to be taught how to transfer the patient from a w/c into and out of a car and needs to practice a simulated transfer from a w/c into and out of an airplane seat.

QUESTIONS

1. List the impairments of body functions, limitations in activities, and restrictions in participation this patient demonstrates.

2. Describe how this patient will need to be positioned when sitting in a w/c.

3. Discuss how you will approach this patient in relation to her aphasia.

4. Describe activities that can be utilized to help facilitate the patient's use of her right leg.

5. Discuss what parameters would be appropriate when addressing transitional movements (variability, components of movement, etc).

6. Detail the approach you will use when teaching the patient's son how to assist the patient in transfers.

REFERENCES

1. Fuller KS. Stroke. In: Goodman CV, Fuller KS, eds. *Pathology: Implications for the PT.* 3rd ed. St Louis, MO: Saunders-Elsevier; 2009.

2. Gordon NF, Gulanick M, Costa F, et al. Physical activity and exercise recommendations for stroke survivors: an American Heart Association scientific statement from the Council on Clinical Cardiology, Subcommittee on Exercise, Cardiac Rehabilitation, and Prevention; the Council on Cardiovascular Nursing; the Council on Nutrition, Physical Activity, and Metabolism; and the Stroke Council. *Circulation.* 2004;109(16):2031-2041.

3. American Physical Therapy Association. Interactive Guide to Physical Therapist Practice With Catalog of Tests and Measures. Version 1.1. 2003. http://guidetoptpractice.apta.org/. Accessed August 7, 2013.

4. Fell DW. Progressing therapeutic intervention in patients with neuromuscular disorders: a framework to assist clinical decision making. *J Neurol Phys Ther.* 2004;28(1):35-46.

5. Dutton LL. Adult nonprogressive central nervous system disorders. In: Cameron MH, Monroe LG, eds. *Physical Rehabilitation: Evidence-Based Examination, Evaluation and Intervention.* St. Louis, MO: Saunders; 2007:405-435.

6. Gentile AM. Skill acquisition: action, movement and neuromotor processes. In: Carr J, Shepherd R, Gordon J, et al, eds. *Movement Science: Foundations for Physical Therapy in Rehabilitation.* Rockville, MD: Aspen Publishers; 1987:93-154.

7. Carr J, Shepherd R. *Stroke Rehabilitation: Guidelines for Exercise Training to Optimize Motor Skill.* Edinburgh, Scotland: Butterworth-Heinemann; 2003.

8. Katalinic OM, Harvey LA, Herbert RD. Effectiveness of stretch for the treatment and prevention of contractures in people with neurological conditions: a systematic review. *Phys Ther.* 2011;91(1):11-24.

9. Hesse S. Rehabilitation of gait after stroke: evaluation, principles of therapy, novel treatment approaches, and assistive devices. *Top Geriatr Rehabilitation.* 2003;19(2):109-126.

10. Visintin M, Barbeau H, Korner-Bitensky N, Mayo NE. A new approach to retrain gait in stroke patients through body weight support and treadmill stimulation. *Stroke.* 1998;29(6):1122-1128.

11. Kisner C, Colby LA. *Therapeutic Exercise: Foundation and Techniques.* 5th ed. Philadelphia, PA: FA Davis; 2007.

12. Ryerson S, Levit K. *Functional Movement Reeducation.* Philadelphia, PA: Churchill Livingstone; 1997.

13. Ouellette MM, LeBrasseur NK, Bean JF, et al. High-intensity resistance training improves muscle strength, self-reported function on disability in long-term stroke survivors. *Stroke.* 2004;35(6):1404-1409.

14. Farrarello F, Baccini M, Rinaldi LA, et al. Efficacy of physiotherapy interventions late after stroke: a meta-analysis. *J Neurol Neurosurg Psy.* 2011;82(2):136-143.

15. Jørgensen JR, Bech-Pedersen DT, Zeeman P, Sørensen J, Andersen LL, Schönberger M. Effect of intensive out-patient physical training on gait performance and cardiovascular health in people with hemiparesis after stroke. *Phys Ther.* 2012;90(4):527-537.

16. Bean JF, Kiely DK, LaRose S, O'Neill E, Goldstein R, Frontera WR. Increased velocity exercise specific to task training versus the National Institute on Aging's strength training program: changes in limb power and mobility. *J Gerontl A Biol Sci Med Sci.* 2009;64(9):983-991.

17. Ryerson S. Hemiplegia. In: Umphred DA, Lazaro RT, Burton GU, eds. *Umphred's Neurological Rehabilitation.* 5th ed. St Louis, MO: Mosby; 2007.

18. Faghri PD, Rodgers MM, Glaser RM, Bors JG, Ho C, Akuthota P. The effects of functional electrical stimulation on shoulder subluxation, arm function recovery, and shoulder pain in hemiplegic stroke patients. *Arch Phys Med Rehabil.* 1994;75(1):73-79.

19. Price CI, Pandyan AD. Electrical stimulation for preventing and treating post-stroke shoulder pain: a systematic Cochrane review. *Clin Rehabil.* 2001;15(1):5-19.

20. Gritsenko V, Prochazka A. A functional electrical stimulation-assisted exercise therapy system for hemiplegic hand function. *Arch Phys Med Rehabil.* 2004;85(6):881-885.

21. Sullivan JE, Hedman LD. A home program of sensory and neuromuscular electrical stimulation with upper-limb task practice in a patient 5 years after a stroke. *Phys Ther.* 2004;84(11):1045-1054.

22. Newsam CJ, Baker LL. Effect of an electric stimulation facilitation program on quadriceps motor unit recruit-ment after stroke. *Arch Phys Med Rehabil.* 2004;85(12):2040-2045.

23. Burridge JH, Taylor PN, Hagan SA, Wood DE, Swain ID. The effects of common peroneal stimulation on the effort and speed of walking: a randomized controlled trial with chronic hemiplegic patients. *Clin Rehabil.* 1997;11(3):201-210.

24. Taub E, Uswatte G, Pidikiti R. Constraint-induced movement therapy: a new family of techniques with broad application to physical rehabilitation—a clinical review. *J Rehabil Res Dev.* 1999;36(3):237-251.

25. Blanton S, Wolf SL. An application of upper-extremity constraint-induced movement therapy in a patient with subacute stroke. *Phys Ther.* 1999;79(9):847-853.

26. Kunkel A, Kopp B, Müller G, et al. Constraint-induced movement therapy for motor recovery in chronic stroke patients. *Arch Phys Med Rehabil.* 1999;80(6):624-628.

27. Jette DU, Warren RL, Wirtalla C. The relation between therapy intensity and outcomes of rehabilitation in skilled nursing facilities. *Arch Phys Med Rehabil.* 2005;86(3):373-379.

28. Page SJ, Sisto S, Levine P, McGrath RR. Efficacy of modified constraint-induced movement therapy in chronic stroke: a single-blinded randomized controlled trial. *Arch Phys Med Rehabil.* 2004;85(1):14-18.

29. Saposnik G, Levin M. Virtual reality in stroke rehabilitation: a meta-analysis and implications for clinicians. *Stroke.* 2011;42(5):1380-1386

30. Saposnik G, Teasell R, Mamdani M, et al. Effectiveness of virtual reality using Wii gaming technology in stroke rehabilitation: a pilot randomized clinical trial and proof of principle. *Stroke.* 2010;41(7):1477-1484.

31. Shumway-Cook A, Woollacott MH. *Motor Control Theory and Practical Applications.* 2nd ed. Philadelphia, PA: Lippincott Williams & Wilkins; 2001.

32. Adams RD, Victor M, Ropper AH. *Principles of Neurology.* 6th ed. New York, NY: McGraw-Hill; 1997:57.

33. Kertesz A, Nicholsom I, Cancelliere A, Kassa K, Black SE. Motor impersistence: a right-hemisphere syndrome. *Neurology.* 1985;35(5):662-666.

34. Donkervoort M, Dekker J, van den Ende E, Stehmann-Saris JC, Deelman BG. Prevalence of apraxia among patients with a first left hemisphere stroke in rehabilitation centers and nursing homes. *Clin Rehabil.* 2000;14(2):130-136.

35. van Heugten CM, Dekker J, Deelman BG, Stehmann-Saris JC, Kinebanian A. Rehabilitation of stroke patients with apraxia: the role of additional cognitive and motor impairments. *Disabil Rehabil.* 2000;22(12):547-554.

36. Kelly JO, Kilbreath SL, Davis GM, Zeman B, Raymond J. Cardiorespiratory fitness and walking ability in sub-acute stroke patients. *Arch Phys Med Rehabil.* 2003;84(12):1780-1785.

37. Mackay-Lyons MJ, Makrides L. Exercise capacity early after stroke. *Arch Phys Med Rehabil.* 2002;83(12):1697-1702.

38. Bernhardt J, Dewey H, Thrift A, Donnan G. Inactive and alone: physical activity within the first 14 days of acute stroke unit care. *Stroke.* 2004;35(4):1005-1009.

39. Hendricks HT, van Limbeck J, Geurts AC, Zwarts MJ. Motor recovery after stroke: a systematic review of the literature. *Arch Phys Med Rehabil.* 2002;83(11):1629-1637.

40. Andrews AW, Bohannon RW. Distribution of muscle strength impairment following stroke. *Clin Rehabil.* 2000;14(1):79-87.

41. Vuagnat H, Chantraine A. Shoulder pain in hemiplegia revisited: contribution of functional electrical stimulation and other therapies. *J Rehabil Med.* 2003;35(2):49-56.

42. Turner-Stokes L, Jackson D. Shoulder pain after stroke: a review of the evidence base to inform the development of an integrated care pathway. *Clin Rehabil.* 2002;16(3):276-298.

43. Murphy MA, Roberts-Warrior D. A review of motor performance measures and treatment interventions for patients with stroke. *Top Geriatr Rehabilitation.* 2003;19(1):3-42.

44. Roller ML. The "pusher syndrome." *J Neurol Phys Ther.* 2004;28(1):29-34.

45. Pérennou DA, Amblard B, Laassel EM, Benaim C, Hérisson C, Pélissier J. Understanding the pusher behavior of some stroke patients with spatial deficits: a pilot study. *Arch Phys Med Rehabil.* 2002;83(4):570-575.

46. Lewis CB, McNerney T. *The Functional Toolbox: Clinical Measures of Functional Outcomes.* Washington, DC: Learn Publications; 1994.

47. Lewis CB, McNerney T. *The Functional Toolbox II: Clinical Measures of Functional Outcomes.* Washington, DC: Learn Publications; 1997.

48. Bohannon RW. Measurement, nature, and implications of skeletal muscle strength in patients with neurological disorders. *Clin Biomech (Bristol, Avon).* 1995;10(6):283-292.

49. Pierce SR, Buxbaum LJ. Treatments of unilateral neglect. *Arch Phys Med Rehabil.* 2002;83(2):256-268.

50. Swan L. Unilateral spatial neglect. *Phys Ther.* 2001;81(9):1572-1580.

51. Stone SP, Wilson B, Wroot A, et al. The assessment of visuo-spatial neglect after acute stroke. *J Neurol Neurosurg Psychiatry.* 1991;54(4):345-350.

52. Maeshima S, Dohi N, Funahashi K, Nakai K, Itakura T, Komai N. Rehabilitation of patients with anosognosia for hemiplegia due to intracerebral hemorrhage. *Brain Inj.* 1997;11(9):691-697.

53. Pedersen PM, Jørgensen HS, Nakayama H, Raaschou HO, Olsen TS. Frequency, determinants, and consequences of anosognosia in acute stroke. *Neurorehabil Neural Repair.* 1996;10(4):243-250.

54. Ross ED. Acute agitation and other behaviors associated with Wernicke aphasia and their possible neurological basis. *Neuropsychiatry Neuropsychol Behav Neurol.* 1993;6(1):9-18.

55. Lundy-Ekman L. *Neuroscience: Fundamentals for Rehabilitation.* Philadelphia, PA: WB Saunders; 2002.

56. Waxman SA. *Correlative Neuroanatomy.* 23rd ed. Stamford, CT: Appleton and Lange; 1996.

57. Ghika-Schmid F, Bogousslavsky J. Affective disorders following stroke. *Eur Neurol.* 1997;38(2):75-81.

58. Bohannon RW. Evaluation and treatment of sensory and perceptual impairments following stroke. *Top Geriatr Rehabil.* 2003;19(2):87-97.

59. Skinner SB, McVey C. *Clinical Decision Making for the Physical Therapist Assistant*. Sudbury, MA: Jones and Bartlett; 2011.

60. Elokda AS, Helgeson K. Deconditioning. In: Cameron MH, Monroe LG, eds. *Physical Rehabilitation: Evidence-Based Examination, Evaluation and Intervention*. St Louis, MO: Saunders; 2007:635.

Please see accompanying Web site at

www.healio.com/books/neuroptavideos

Clients With Degenerative Diseases

Parkinson's Disease, Multiple Sclerosis, and Amyotrophic Lateral Sclerosis

Rolando T. Lazaro, PT, PhD, DPT, MS, GCS
Amanda A. Forster, PT, DPT, NCS

KEY WORDS

- Amyotrophic lateral sclerosis
- Degenerative disease of the central nervous system
- Multiple sclerosis
- Parkinson's disease
- Physical therapy examination
- Physical therapy intervention
- Therapeutic exercises

CHAPTER OBJECTIVES

- Discuss the signs and symptoms of Parkinson's disease, multiple sclerosis, and amyotrophic lateral sclerosis, and explain their implications to physical therapy examination and intervention.

- Discuss common intervention strategies for patients and clients with degenerative diseases of the central nervous system (CNS).

- Identify some clinical pearls that can assist a physical therapist assistant in treating patients and clients with degenerative conditions of the CNS.

Umphred DA, Lazaro RT, eds.
Neurorehabilitation for the Physical Therapist Assistant,
Second Edition (pp 375-391).
© 2014 SLACK Incorporated.

INTRODUCTION

Many of the patients and clients referred for physical therapy intervention have conditions caused by the degeneration of specific portions of the central nervous system (CNS), specifically those that involve or influence movement. The degeneration may be caused by the normal aging process, mediated by genetic abnormalities, exacerbated or hastened by harmful environmental agents, or a combination of 2 or more of these factors. As movement specialists, physical therapists (PTs) and physical therapist assistants (PTAs) have an important and unique role in helping patients and clients with degenerative neuromuscular diseases achieve and/or maintain their highest functional capacity and optimum health and well-being. A thorough understanding of the specific functions of the structures of the CNS will allow the clinician to make inferences on potential movement disorders based on the structures involved in the disease process. This knowledge will facilitate appropriate clinical decision making and allow the PTA to determine what to expect (assuming a typical presentation of the condition) and will empower the PTA to communicate to the PT possible changes in the patient's condition that do not follow the specific presentation for the disease. For example, if the PTA who is treating a patient with Parkinson's disease (PD) notices that this patient has developed paralysis on one side of the body, the PTA should communicate this finding to the PT because this is not consistent with a medical diagnosis of PD.

Impairment in motor performance is a common problem seen in patients with degenerative conditions. The PTA can use several intervention approaches to improve this problem. It is important for the PTA to monitor the patient's response to these interventions because this will indicate whether the overall plan of care is meeting the anticipated goals and expected outcomes. In people with degenerative conditions, it is important to be aware of undesired responses, especially in relation to fatigue and further loss of strength. This will be discussed in more detail later in the chapter.

This chapter will focus on the 3 most common degenerative diseases in adults: PD, multiple sclerosis (MS), and amyotrophic lateral sclerosis (ALS).

PARKINSON'S DISEASE

PD is a medical condition that results in a variety of movement disorders that impair an individual's ability to perform normal everyday tasks. In the United States, 100 to 150 of every 100,000 people are affected by PD, with 1% of those over 60 years of age afflicted by the condition.[1] Sources indicate that approximately 50,000 people are diagnosed with PD annually in the United States.[2]

A person with PD may exhibit one or more of the following motor impairments: bradykinesia (extreme slowness of movement), rigidity, resting (unintentional) tremors, postural instability, and festinating gait.[3] Bradykinesia in PD is also associated with "on-off phenomenon," characterized by freezing episodes in which the person appears to be fixed or "stuck" in space, usually seen during a gross motor activity.[4] Other physical traits associated with PD include increased thoracic kyphosis and decreased lumbar lordosis, producing a stooped and flexed posture.[3] This posture can also be a compensatory mechanism to account for loss of stability when weight is shifted posteriorly, as is often indicated on the pull test.[5] A person with PD may feel as though he or she is losing balance posteriorly and thus exaggerate the anteriorly shifted posture. Each of these manifestations of PD impairs the gross motor function of all extremities, thus negatively affecting balance. Poor balance leads to falls that, when combined with other comorbidities associated with aging, can create life-threatening results. One study, which used a questionnaire that reported on the frequency of falls in patients with PD, stated that more than one-third of these patients had fallen and more than 10% fall at least once a week. Causes of these falls were attributed to postural instability, movement dysfunction, gait abnormalities, and difficulty with transfers.[6] Falls may occur because of the delayed motor responses when standing, walking, turning, and sitting without back support.[7] As normal individuals age, falls become an increasing problem. With age and a preexisting diagnosis of a disease such as PD, an individual may not only be at risk of falling, but the resulting problems following a fall may have greater consequences.

Because PD is due to a progressive degeneration of the basal ganglia, people with PD present with increasingly altered posture, rigidity, and bradykinesia, which become more significant over time and lead to a decreased ability to balance. Eventually, movement requires so much energy that the individual may become bedridden, with a fixed trunk and flexion contractures. In the advanced stages, inspiration is decreased, coughing is difficult, and bronchopneumonia may be one of the reasons for morbidity.[3]

Traditionally, drug therapy has been the primary intervention to delay the progression of impairments, activity limitations, and participation restrictions related to PD. The general effect of these PD medications is to replenish the brain's supply of dopamine, a neurotransmitter that is important in basal ganglia function. Common medications for PD include Sinemet, a levodopa-carbidopa combination. The "next-generation" medications that have been approved include Permax (pergolide mesylate) and Mirapex (pramipexole), which are dopamine agonists that bind to and stimulate cerebral dopamine receptors to improve motor performance.[8] While on these medications, patients may experience motor fluctuations causing unpredictable on-off episodes, which interfere with performance of activities of daily living (ADL) and ambulation. Recent research indicates that physical exercise can also alter the disease process and allow medications to work more effectively.[9,10] Many new studies[9-11] are being conducted to further evaluate the effect of physical exercise on the underlying health condition of PD, as well as the changes in outward physical presentation of persons with PD. This information is exciting and pertinent to rehabilitation professionals working with persons with PD and an indication for specific physical therapy intervention with these patients and clients.

Several stages classify the progression of PD, called Hoehn and Yahr stages.[12] This scale was modified in 2004 to include intermediate stages in the progression of the disease.[13] These stages are medically diagnosed by a physician or other health care provider licensed to determine medical diagnoses. Physical therapy interventions and goals will vary depending on the stage of PD. Several screening instruments and scales for PD can be found at the National Parkinson Foundation Web site (www.parkinson.org/Professionals/Professional-Resources/Screening-Instruments).

MULTIPLE SCLEROSIS

MS is the most common neurological condition affecting young adults. It is characterized by degeneration and subsequent loss of myelin scattered throughout the CNS, primarily in the white matter. In this condition, plaques of demyelination are accompanied by destruction and inflammation of oligodendroglia, which form part of the supporting structure of the CNS. Because of the degeneration of the myelin, neurotransmission is disrupted and will manifest as delayed or absent transmission of nerve impulses.[14]

Since demyelination can occur anywhere in the CNS, the resulting signs, symptoms, and clinical manifestations can vary based on the areas affected. These symptoms can develop slowly over days and weeks or rapidly within hours. Common symptoms include fatigue, motor weakness, paresthesias, unsteady gait, double vision, tremor, and bladder and/or bowel dysfunction. Fatigue is the most common symptom of MS and is frequently misunderstood by family, friends, and employers because it is not a visible symptom. Some researchers and clinicians have noted that the fatigue experienced by patients with MS increases as the day progresses and can also vary depending on the climate and environmental temperature.[14]

Figure 13-1. Types of multiple sclerosis. (Reprinted with permission from Exercise as it relates to disease/aerobic or resistance training for multiple sclerosis? Wikibooks. http://en.wikibooks.org/wiki/Exercise_as_it_relates_to_Disease/Aerobic_or_Resistance_training_for_Multiple_Sclerosis%3F.)

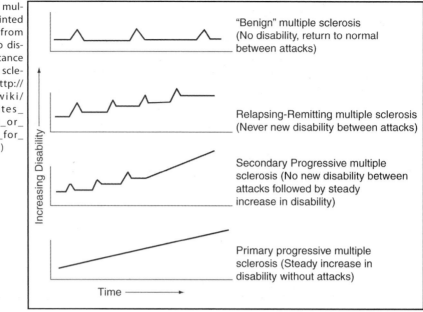

In terms of the pattern of the disease, the classic presentation is characterized by periods of exacerbations (relapses) and remissions (partial or total disappearance of symptoms). As the disease progresses, the periods of exacerbations become more frequent and longer, while the periods of remissions become more limited. Individuals afflicted with this disease then demonstrate progressive deterioration of function. Factors that have been associated with exacerbations include excessive fatigue, hot weather, and rise in body temperature due to fever, trauma, and hot baths or showers.[14] Figure 13-1 illustrates the types of MS.

Fatigue and heat intolerance are 2 important symptoms that are common in people with MS. Fatigue is reported by 65% to 97% of people with MS, with almost half of them stating that this symptom most significantly affects their functional performance.[15] Primary fatigue, otherwise known as *lassitude*, is a direct result of the demyelination process, causing abnormalities in nerve conduction. Secondary fatigue often results from deconditioning and other associated conditions from the disease (infections, disturbances in sleep, inadequate nutrition, etc).[15] A significant proportion of people with MS also report worsening of symptoms following an increase in core body temperature due to physical exercise or a hot climate.[15]

Over the past 2 decades, treatment with disease-modifying agents has been developed. These agents have been found to reduce the frequency and severity of relapses, reduce the numbers of brain lesions as shown on magnetic resonance imaging, and possibly reduce future impairments, activity limitations, and participation restrictions. The medications are divided into 2 categories: (1) immunomodulators, which modify the immune system and include interferon beta 1a-intramuscular (Avonex), interferon beta 1a-subcutaneous (Rebif), interferon beta 1b (Betaseron), and glatiramer acetate (Copaxone); and (2) immunosuppressants, which shut down the immune system temporarily and include mitoxantrone (Novantrone).[16]

AMYOTROPHIC LATERAL SCLEROSIS

ALS, also known as *Lou Gehrig's disease*, is the most common progressive neurodegenerative disease affecting adults. This disease involves the progressive degeneration of the motor neurons in the brain and spinal cord. Progression of the disease is rapid, and death due to compromise of the respiratory system is typically noted within 2 to 5 years.[17]

Clinical symptoms include fasciculations (involuntary twitching of muscle fibers), muscle cramps, fatigue, weakness, and atrophy. There is a highly varied pattern of onset in ALS, with the most common pattern being lower extremity (LE) onset, followed by upper extremity (UE) onset and bulbar onset; the least common pattern demonstrates symptoms in the distal musculature of the UEs and LEs. With each pattern of onset, the eventual progression of ALS is similar for most patients, with a spread of weakness to other muscle groups ultimately leading to complete paralysis. The cause of death is usually related to respiratory failure.[17]

Several phases and stages characterize the progression of ALS.[17] Depending on the stage of the disease, physical therapy interventions and goals will vary.[18]

Phase I

Phase I is termed *independent* phase and is characterized by the patient's ability to perform most everyday activities without any limitation. There are 3 stages under phase I. In stage 1, the patient exhibits mild weakness and complaints of clumsiness. Stage 2 is characterized by more evident weakness affecting certain muscle groups, often in the extremities. It is also in this stage that a noticeable decrease in the ability to perform ADL appears. Stage 3 shows more severe selective weakness in the distal portions of the extremities. Respiration is also starting to be affected in this stage, as shown by increased fatigue and slight increase in breathing effort.[17,18]

Phase II

Phase II is termed *partially independent*. As the name implies, the patient requires assistance in several ADL in this phase. Phase II has 2 stages: stages 4 and 5. In stage 4, the patient is still able to perform most ADL but tires easily. In terms of locomotion, the patient is mostly using a wheelchair (w/c) at this point. Muscular weakness is present, and tone abnormalities (spasticity) may be evident. More affectation in functional performance due to progression of the disease is evident in stage 5, which is characterized by significant weakness of the LEs and moderate to severe weakness of the UEs. Because of decreased mobility, the risk of skin breakdown is also evident in this stage.[17,18]

Phase III

Phase III is termed the *dependent* phase of the disease. There is one stage under this phase: stage 6. In this stage, the patient is bed bound and requires maximal assistance in ADL. Respiratory function is severely compromised in this stage.[17,18] (Refer to Box 13-1 for a summary of these 3 phases and the 6 stages within them.)

EXAMINATION AND EVALUATION: THE ROLE OF THE PHYSICAL THERAPIST ASSISTANT

The physical therapy examination of a patient with degenerative disease must be guided by several factors. First, it is important to identify from the patient's perspective the impact of the presenting signs and symptoms on his or her ability to function. It is important to determine, in terms of activity, what the patient can and cannot do and then hypothesize the impairments that may be causing the identified activity limitations. The *Guide to Physical Therapist Practice*[19] (the *Guide*) is a helpful tool to guide the clinician in identifying the pertinent tests and measures that

---

Box 13-1

Summary of the Stages of Amyotrophic Lateral Sclerosis

Phase I: Independent

Stage 1: Patient exhibits only mild weakness with no limitation in function.

Stage 2: Patient exhibits definite weakness in some muscle groups.

Stage 3: Patient's muscle weakness affects activities of daily living (ADL), especially in the extremities, although independence is still demonstrated and compensation observed.
Respiratory function is beginning to be compromised.

Phase II: Partially Independent

Stage 4: Patient able to perform most ADL with adaptations, but fatigues quickly. Mobility is primarily through the use of a w/c.

Stage 5: Both upper and lower extremities demonstrate severe weakness, limiting the individual's ability to function independently.

Phase III: Dependent: Final Phase

Stage 6: Patient is bed dependent and requires maximal assistance for all activities.

---

will provide the best representation of the patient's functional level. The PTA may be delegated portions of a reexamination (see Chapter 5), and it is of the utmost importance for the PTA to clearly communicate the results of the tests and measures to the PT.

As a PTA, it is important to identify the specific signs and symptoms associated with the condition, to monitor these signs and symptoms, and to communicate to the supervising PT any significant changes in the patient's presentation, which may indicate the progression of symptoms, ineffectiveness of the prescribed physical therapy intervention, medication issues, or the possibility of other comorbidities. The rehabilitation team must be cognizant of other signs and symptoms that may necessitate referral to other medical practitioners. For example, symptoms of chest congestion, difficulty breathing, increased coughing, and mucus may be indicative of aspiration pneumonia and must be resolved expediently. This congestion may have been precipitated by decreased respiratory function (chest expansion, decreased inability to clear secretions, or ineffective cough) and is a fairly common complication in patients with degenerative neuromuscular disorders.

In looking at examination, it is important to identify the patient and family goals in making the determination regarding exercises and activities that will be implemented. Standardized functional tests often provide the clinician useful information regarding the impact of the disease progression on the patient's function. Serial testing of function allows the clinician to generate objective documentation of function; however, it should always follow a thoughtful interpretation of the results afforded by the PT. Examples of general functional tests that could be administered to patients with PD, MS, or ALS include the Performance-Oriented Mobility Assessment (POMA),[20] Berg Balance Scale (BBS),[21] Functional Reach Test (FR),[22] or Timed Up and Go (TUG).[23] These tests give the clinician insight regarding the patient's level of function and risk of falls. Several disease-specific tests have also been developed: for PD, the United Parkinson's Disease Rating Scale (UPDRS),[24] and for MS, the Kurtzke Extended Disability Status Scale (EDSS).[25] It is also important to include measures of participation, self-efficacy, and quality of life. Examples of these measures include the Parkinson's Disease Quality of Life Questionnaire,[26] Multiple Sclerosis Quality of Life Inventory (MSQLI),[27] and ALS-specific quality of life instrument (ALSSQOL).[28]

All the examination areas mentioned in Chapter 4 must be assessed in patients with degenerative diseases to provide the clinician with a clear picture of the patient's impairments, activity limitations, and participation restrictions.

Intervention

Physical therapy intervention for patients with degenerative disorders should be based on the correction of, remediation of, or compensation for the identified activity limitations and impairments. The *Guide*[19] identifies procedural interventions PTs commonly use when treating patients with PD, MS, and ALS. All of the following interventions could be delegated to a PTA as long as the patient is stable and does not need ongoing (formal) assessment during the intervention period.

Aerobic and Endurance Conditioning and Reconditioning

The ability of the patient to have the cardiopulmonary capacity to be able to perform functional activities is central to optimal health and well-being. Graded exercise must allow the patient to perform activities within the safe levels of cardiopulmonary functioning to allow the patient to tolerate increased activities. ADL training, gait, and locomotion activities can be incorporated into therapeutic intervention, as appropriate. Aquatic exercise programs also allow the patient to perform these activities with less impact on the joints; however, increased workload due to increased hydrostatic pressure must be monitored accordingly. Examples of aerobic and endurance conditioning and reconditioning include the use of an upper body ergometer, LE pedal exerciser or exercise bike, treadmill training, or walking using an appropriate assistive device, increasing distance as tolerated while making sure that vital signs are within safe limits. In terms of ADL training, the therapist can start with facilitation of simple ADL tasks (eg, maintaining sitting balance while the patient puts on socks and shoes) and then progress to those activities that require higher demands on the system in terms of postural control, coordination, endurance, and safety. The use of progressive resistance exercise has been shown to improve mobility and muscular strength in people with PD, so this is a consideration when performing physical therapy interventions and prescribing a home exercise program for these patients and clients.[29] Similar types of resistive exercises need to be carefully monitored with individuals diagnosed with ALS, while individuals with MS may benefit as long as prolonged fatigue does not set in.

Balance, Coordination, and Agility Training

There must be an emphasis on decreasing the risk of falls to avoid the deleterious effects of decreased activity and the medical complications following such an incident. Task-specific performance training could be used to improve performance of everyday tasks, increase confidence in mobility activities, and improve quality of life. Vestibular training might be indicated to heighten the role of the vestibular system in balance tasks and compensate for loss in somatosensory and visual systems. Examples include standing weight-shifting activities with eyes open and eyes closed, standing or balancing on foam, tandem walking, braiding, tai chi, and maintaining balance while performing functional tasks such as brushing teeth, getting something from the refrigerator or kitchen cabinets, or putting on socks and shoes. Some of these activities can be performed in groups, which helps to increase the socialization of these individuals and make them feel included as a whole. Thus, when working on balance, multiple individuals can be throwing and catching balls, which causes weight shifting as well as perturbations as the individual catches the ball. Increasing and decreasing the weight of the ball can change the activity. In a group setting, multiple balls can be used and switched to increase the challenge and enjoyment of these interactions.

Balance exercises may be performed by incorporating them with ADL, gait training, or endurance training. The therapist could start by having the patient sit upright, providing adequate support as necessary, instructing the patient to "sense" the upright position, improving stability in this position via compression (approximation through the shoulder will allow co-contraction and, therefore, stability) or proprioceptive neuromuscular facilitation (PNF) rhythmic stabilization, and then strengthening the postural muscles using PNF or progressive resistance using manual and machine-generated resistance. Once the patient achieves relative stability in the static sitting position, the therapist can progress to working on dynamic sitting. To achieve this, the therapist could incorporate ADL training. For example, the therapist could ask the patient to reach for an object that is outside his or her base of support and then guide the patient to make sure that the patient maintains balance. Performing isometric holds when the patient is in varying degrees of leaning will allow the patient to be stable in those increments of motion and achieve improved proprioceptive input in that position. The patient can then use the newly learned balance strategies in more ADL (eg, putting on shoes and socks while sitting) or in recreational activities (eg, tossing a balloon, playing beanbag basketball, or throwing darts). These same principles can be performed while facilitating static and dynamic standing balance. Regardless of the degenerative disease, it is important for the PTA to monitor the patient's response to the activity to determine its value to the patient's therapeutic environment. Oftentimes, maintaining function is the goal of therapeutic intervention, rather than regaining function. Physical therapy cannot prevent the progressive nature of a degenerative disease, but often function can be maintained for a period of time in spite of the progressive nature of the disease process by maintaining the highest level of motor performance possible.

Flexibility Exercises

It is important for patients with degenerative diseases to maintain or improve their range of motion (ROM) and flexibility to allow for normal excursions of the body during functional tasks, thereby decreasing the risk of falls. Flexibility exercises also allow for easier transfers from one surface to another or easier performance of ADL, such as lower-body hygiene and grooming. These exercises can also potentially improve or normalize tone, which is commonly a major issue for patients with PD, MS, or ALS. Because daily ROM is important, the patient must be taught how to perform self-assisted ROM activities, and the family must also be instructed on performing these activities. If the patient has cognitive deficits that prevent him or her from performing a self-ROM program, family members and caregivers should be performing these activities. It is imperative that they understand the importance of adequate joint mobility and muscle length on the patient's functional abilities. Examples include passive to active-assisted to active ROM of shoulder (flexion, abduction, and internal-external rotation), elbow (flexion and extension), forearm (pronation and supination), wrist and hand (flexion, extension, abduction, and adduction), hip (flexion, extension, abduction, and internal-external rotation), knee (flexion and extension), and ankle and foot (dorsiflexion, plantarflexion, inversion, and eversion) movements.

Muscle Performance

The PTA must incorporate interventions that increase muscle performance, including activities that improve muscular strength, power, and endurance. Often, activity limitations result from lack of strength, power, or endurance to perform an activity. Weakness in the LEs has also been associated with increased fall risk, decreased gait velocity, and decreased functional performance.

The PTA must appropriately apply the principles of therapeutic exercise in terms of accurately identifying the patient's threshold, dosing, and response to ensure that the exercise prescription achieves the goal of improving muscular performance while preventing excessive overheating and fatigue (especially for persons with MS) or extreme muscle soreness. All modes of strengthening exercise can be applied to these patients. In patients with MS, the recommended protocol for strengthening includes 2 to 3 training sessions every week, with 1 to 3 sets of 8 to 15 repetitions for major muscle groups, with the patient in the seated position if necessary. The resistance is increased by 2% to 4% when 15 repetitions are easily performed.[30] There are no specific recommendations for people with PD; however, several studies have confirmed the importance of strengthening exercises to facilitate muscle hypertrophy, improve mobility, and decrease fall risk. The exercise modes vary from low- to high-intensity activities, performed with supervision in the clinic or home as part of a home program.[31-33] There are also no suggested protocols regarding exercise in people with ALS, but evidence also supports the benefits of exercise in this population.[34] However, caution must be exercised to not overfatigue the patient; therefore, submaximal exercise dosage has been suggested when working with this population.[35] There is evidence that indicates that submaximal exercise is beneficial in delaying the decline in motor performance in people with ALS.[36]

Relaxation

An often forgotten, but nevertheless important, component of a successful rehabilitation program for patients with degenerative disorders is relaxation training. Relaxation in the form of breathing exercises allows for increased oxygenation of the muscles and vital organs, thereby leading to increased performance and endurance, which may lead to improved swallowing and speech while allowing chest expansion and improved posture in the process. Examples of activities include rhythmic breathing, progressive relaxation by contracting and relaxing muscle groups, and using imagery or music. Since diminished respiratory capacity can be a factor in PD, MS, and ALS, the importance of diaphragmatic breathing should be emphasized with these patient populations. There are many ways to teach patients to breathe using their diaphragm. For example, the patient lies supine on a firm but comfortable bed or mat with a pillow to support the head, and another pillow under the knees. The therapist instructs the patient to put one hand on the diaphragm and another on the sternum. The patient is then asked to breathe in through the nose and breathe out using pursed lips. The patient is instructed to feel the rise of the hand placed on the diaphragm, to indicate correct technique. The therapist further instructs the patient to make sure that the upper chest does not rise with inspiration; if it does, the patient is using accessory muscle, and the technique must be corrected. Once the patient has gained the correct techniques, the therapist then instructs the patient to feel the shoulders and then the back and the neck relax while breathing deeply.

Neuromuscular Education or Reeducation

It is important to maintain the patient's ability to run normal functional motor programs to optimize functional performance. If this is impaired because of PD, MS, or ALS, the PTA could facilitate the performance of these functions using various neurological approaches that aim to allow for a window by which more normal tone is achieved. These approaches facilitate the performance of normal movement while that window is open and consciously and consistently open that window so the patient might eventually run an entire program sequence in the most efficient, effective, and functional manner possible. Examples of these neurological approaches include the use of PNF or Neuro-Developmental Treatment to strengthen muscle and facilitate functional mobility, transfers, or gait. If the PT has specific methods or strategies that employ these approaches, open communication with the PTA will help improve continuity of care and improve intervention outcomes. An example of how to narrow and then open a window to a functional activity might be analyzing the activity of sit to stand to sit. If an individual cannot sit down in a controlled and safe manner (as often seen in people with PD), the PTA can start the activity in standing. If a high/low mat table is available, the PTA could start by having that patient sit on the mat, elevate the mat to a height where the patient is almost standing, then ask the patient to perform several sit-to-stands from this table height. This way, the PTA narrows the available range to allow the patient to perform this activity safely and correctly. Once the patient is able to perform this activity correctly, the PTA may decide to lower the mat so the patient is now performing the activity with a wider range and a greater challenge to improve strength, range, balance, and skill. The mat is lowered further until the patient reaches a mat height that is similar to a regular chair. To facilitate task-specific training, the same principle can then be used, but this time using bar stools of varying heights, from tallest to shortest, and then transitioning to performing sit-to-stands using a regular armless chair. Once the entire fluid movement is within the capability of the patient, then he or she should sit back in the chair, relax, and then come back to stand. Many functional activities can be narrowed into programs that patients can control and then reintroduced with a wider ROM or need for additional power or other variables that aim to improve motor performance.

Gait and Locomotion Training

In addition to the benefits stated above, gait or locomotion training is important to the patient's functional independence. Being able to ambulate functional distances will allow the patient more freedom in movement (eg, the ability to walk from the bedroom to the dining room or bathroom), as well as allowing him or her to be a more social and productive member of the community. A PTA might be asked to perform gait training with any of these individuals with degenerative CNS problems. Certainly maintaining functional gait will empower the patient. How best to regain or maintain ambulation skill varies based on the balance, strength, endurance, speed of ambulation, ability to run feed-forward programs for walking, ROM, desire to ambulate, and dysfunction caused by the disease itself. All of these variables can lead to variance in the specific treatment protocol. Whether the individual needs assistive devices, such as a quad cane, a walker, or a single upright cane,[37] or whether the PT thinks using a body weight–support system while ambulating on a treadmill or over ground[38] is the best selection for intervention, the PTA must be able to sequence the intervention toward the established goals. If gait is not realistic, the ability of the patient to safely and independently use an appropriate mobility device (eg, a w/c) will improve endurance while allowing the patient to be as functional as possible.[39] Examples include w/c mobility training and gait training using the appropriate assistive device on level or uneven surfaces while progressively decreasing assistance, as appropriate. Selection of noncompliant surfaces as the training site (eg, hardwood, tile, or linoleum) versus compliant surfaces (eg, rugs, grass, or dirt) can vary the training environment and demands placed on the patient's CNS.[40]

Activities of Daily Living Training

All of the activities mentioned earlier must have the ultimate goal of facilitating improvements in the performance of ADL to allow the patient the highest level of independence possible. Examples include training for activities, such as dressing, grooming, bathing, transfers, and bed mobility.

Monitoring Response to Exercise Interventions and Level of Fatigue

As mentioned in the beginning of the chapter, it is important for the PTA to always monitor the patient's response to the plan of care. In people with degenerative conditions, it is especially important to look for abnormal responses to interventions that should improve motor performance. Degenerative conditions that result in damage to the lower motor neuron could present with muscle weakness because of the decrease in the amount of functioning motor units. Strenuous strengthening exercise in this case may lead to further deterioration of the remaining intact motor units, thereby causing a further decline in strength. It is suggested that moderate exercise could still be an effective way of maintaining or improving strength. However, with damage to motor units resulting in grades below a fair (3/5) grade, improvement is unlikely; therefore, the PTA is advised to focus on stronger muscles.[41]

Other degenerative conditions show a similar abnormal response to strengthening exercises. It is hard to differentiate whether loss of muscle function is due to a progressive disease process or due to overwork. For that reason, the PTA must be aware that exercises at a level to cause a positive effect in a normal muscle may damage diseased muscle. Thus, keeping exercise at a functional level and not too strenuous is important. Exercise will not prevent the progression of the disease, but it will often maintain the functional skills for a longer period of time as well as keep the individual interacting with the physical world. Mild or gentle exercises often increase ROM and maintain muscle function, which often can decrease pain and muscle stiffness.[42]

In individuals with degenerative diseases, there are additional recommendations with regard to exercise interventions.[41] First, a combination of individual and group exercises may improve adherence to the therapeutic programs. Group exercises are of particular importance in creating opportunities for social interaction and a feeling of accomplishment or success. It has also been suggested that strengthening should focus on concentric more than eccentric contractions, with adequate rest periods to avoid fatigue. Finally, muscle strength should be closely monitored in those individuals who participate in unsupervised movement activities (home treadmill exercises, elliptical machines, or other available gyms) because these individuals may be exercising too strenuously and causing further decline in their muscular strength.

CLINICAL PEARLS

The following are suggestions from the field for approaches that might help patients with degenerative diseases.

Focus 1: Parkinson's Disease

- Rotation is important. Trunk rotation should be part of any physical therapy intervention for PD unless contraindicated because of spinal conditions or surgery or other conditions that contraindicate trunk rotation. Rotation decreases the tone of the axial musculature, thereby decreasing trunk rigidity, and opens a window that will allow the patient to perform movements that are more normal and functional.[43] Rotation can be performed supine in bed in the morning (lower trunk rotations) before the patient gets up, in sitting throughout the day, and in standing (as long as the patient is safe in this position). Rocking also decreases tone.

- Encourage the patient to participate in group exercises. Group exercises allow the patient to engage in social activities, talk to other individuals who may have a similar condition or situation, and improve flexibility, strength, and endurance. Using a ball while throwing and catching with others in the group will encourage rotation, total body activities, and eye-hand coordination while interacting with other people.[40] Tai chi is becoming a more recognized form of group exercise and can also be incorporated into a person's individual home exercise program.[11,44,45]

- Imagery may help. Incorporating visual imagery may assist in motor performance, whether contraction or relaxation. Teaching the patient to visualize being "strong and stable like a tree" may assist in improving standing balance; also, visualization may assist in relaxation ("imagine that you are relaxing in your favorite place…").[46]

- Music and rhythm may help. Music often gives the individual a rhythmical beat that overrides the freezing episodes and can be used very effectively with walking or gait interventions.[47]

- Incorporate large amplitude movements in interventions and recommend safe performance of these movements as part of a home exercise program. Recent research has indicated that amplified movements during specific exercises can have a positive and prolonged effect on tasks, such as walking, arm swing, and the ability to turn around.[10]

Focus 2: Multiple Sclerosis

- Encourage the patient to achieve optimum health and well-being.[48] Together with the goal of maintaining the strength of the unaffected muscles to compensate for loss of strength of other muscle groups, encourage the patient to maintain a high overall level of fitness. In this regard, allow the patient to take the responsibility for his or her health and well-being through daily exercise, appropriate nutrition and hydration, following the medical advice provided by the physician, and maintaining a positive and optimistic mental outlook. Patients need to learn to not only maintain a daily exercise routine but also to recognize when they have exercised too much and weakness overcomes them.

- Watch out for fatigue and overheating.[49] As mentioned earlier, one precaution for patients and clients with MS is fatigue and decreased tolerance to heat. Always consider the environment where the treatment occurs. Regulate the temperature as to minimize overheating, which will cause fatigue of the patient. Timing and sequencing of the treatment are also important. Encourage the patient to perform the more difficult and potentially more fatiguing activities early in the day and to conserve energy where possible. Many patients like to exercise in water, but they need to make sure the water is not too warm and does not cause fatigue.

- Improve balance and coordination. An optimum level of balance and coordination decreases the risk of falls and prevents the development of secondary complications, which may be detrimental to the patient.[50] Examples of exercise were provided previously; it is suggested that these exercises be performed with the incorporation of functional training that will improve the quality of life.

- Normalize or improve tone (decrease spasticity) before training for functional tasks. Performance of functional tasks will have a longer carryover if performed over the foundation of as normal a tone and pattern as possible.[51] In this regard, abnormal tone must be decreased first to open a window by which the foundation of normal movement can occur. Using stretching, relaxation, and tone-inhibiting postures are some examples of interventions that can decrease spasticity.

- Compensate for impaired sensation by teaching the patient frequent skin checks for skin breakdown, using appropriate footwear when walking, and being cognizant of situations where lack of protective sensation may be dangerous (such as cooking, taking a bath, or walking on uneven surfaces).[52] Discourage people with MS from walking and standing without appropriate footwear, even inside the home.

- Adapt the environment and use appropriate orthotic appliances to protect the joint and improve function and safety. The patient's environment can be modified to assist in energy conservation and more efficient movement. Orthotic devices like an ankle-foot orthosis may allow the patient to transfer and ambulate more safely and more efficiently while protecting the joint from injury.[53]

- Discuss with the supervising PT the need to refer the patient to appropriate medical professionals as necessary.[54] The patient may present with other signs and symptoms that can be better managed by other health care professionals. Referral to a neuropsychiatrist, speech therapist, or occupational therapist may assist the patient in improving function.

Focus 3: Amyotrophic Lateral Sclerosis

- Optimize cardiopulmonary function.[55] Maintaining good cardiopulmonary health is very important in patients with ALS to avoid the rapid decline in functional level due to secondary complications arising from decreased oxygenation. (Refer to Chapter 14 for additional recommendations.) Examples of interventions include diaphragmatic breathing exercises, assisted cough (as necessary), and postural exercises to maintain optimal trunk alignment, which is important in efficient breathing. More complex equipment and intervention may be necessary with some patients or with patients in the more advanced stages of the disease, and a referral to a physician and a respiratory therapist may be appropriate.

- Maximize functional performance.[56] While maximizing functional performance may be important when discussing the rehabilitation of all patients, maintaining the highest functional performance is of utmost importance with patients and clients with ALS. Emphasis must be on achieving and maintaining the ability to perform vital activities, such as mobility in bed, transferring, locomotion, sitting and standing balance, and toileting and hygiene activities. Patients will benefit from a ROM and muscle-strengthening program to prevent contractures and to maintain and improve strength. A home program consisting of these exercises, performed independently by the patient initially or assisted by the caregiver, is appropriate. The use of adaptive equipment may allow for performance of activities without assistance and should be considered. This equipment ranges from orthotic appliances to assist in ambulation or improve ROM to reacher sticks and dressing aids. Adaptive equipment also includes personal care aids, which will assist in optimizing function when used.

- Discuss with the PT the options available to improve communication. Because patients with ALS eventually lose the ability to communicate verbally because of paralysis of the muscles of speech, alternative communication strategies may be considered.[57] These communication aids may be in the form of a basic communication board or more complex computer equipment.

- Optimum psychological health is important.[58] Maintaining a positive mental outlook decreases stress, which is detrimental to the body's immune response. Examples of approaches to achieving good psychological health include daily exercise, participating in support groups, psychological consultation, and good nutrition, among others. It is important to remember that a potential reason for an observed decline in functional performance is depression. The PTA should communicate this finding to the PT.

CONCLUSION

Patients and clients with degenerative diseases of the CNS often access and can benefit from physical therapy services. Appropriate intervention is based on the identified activity's limitations and impairments. An individualized treatment program developed by the PT can be effectively carried out by the PTA. A variety of treatment approaches have been presented in this chapter. Communication between the PT and the PTA is important to ensure that the patient receives care that is appropriate and evidence based to optimize the patient's level of health and wellness.

CASE STUDIES

CASE #1

MG is a 72-year-old man who was diagnosed with PD 12 years ago. Current medical diagnosis indicates that MG is at Hoehn and Yahr stage 3 when his medications are at their optimum. The client resides in an independent living facility with his wife. The environment provides the client with a wide spectrum of social interaction and cognitive challenges as well as good access to health care. MG is cognitively aware of his surroundings and the effects of his illness. He cites unsteadiness when walking and dressing, poor night vision, and occasional drooling as symptoms that he experiences.

The client currently takes Sinemet and Mirapex. He reports that he experiences freezing episodes when his medications wear off. As a result, he and his wife carefully plan outings around peak medication times. The client reports increasing difficulty with ambulation and ADL, such as transfers, dressing, and bathing. The client also reports increased falls in the past several weeks. He is afraid that he might sustain severe injuries following a serious fall in the future. He owns a single-point cane and a front-wheeled walker, both of which he intermittently uses.

The client presents with a stooped posture, rounded shoulders, and thoracic kyphosis. He ambulates to the department carrying (not using) a single-point cane in the left hand, with a festinating gait pattern. He also presents with pill-rolling tremor in the right greater than the left UE at rest. He transfers from the bed to the mat with minimal assistance. Functional mobility testing shows that the client is independent with bed mobility but requires minimal assistance to sit from the supine position. He requires minimal assist to perform sit to stand. Sitting balance is Good, while standing balance is Fair. ROM is within functional limits to all 4 extremities. He demonstrates weakness in his bilateral LEs, as well as truncal rigidity. The client scored a 17/28 in the Tinetti balance and gait tests, indicating risk for falls. He scored 6 inches in the Functional Reach test, and this also indicates a risk for falls. The Berg Balance Test was also administered, and the client scored a 38/56, also indicating a risk for falls.

QUESTIONS

1. Identify the impairments and activity limitations presented.
2. What potential interventions can be performed by the PTA to assist in improving the patient's functional performance?

CASE #2

PJ is a 45-year-old woman who was diagnosed with MS 5 years ago. She works part-time as a telemarketer and has a phone and computer setup that allow her to work at home. She reports progressive decline in functional ability in the past few years. She has had several periods of exacerbations and remissions since the diagnosis. She lives with her husband and teenaged daughter, who both help her with her ADL. Her current complaints include weakness of the LEs, fatigue, and bouts of vision disturbances (double vision). She reports lack of sleep at night due to leg cramps. She also mentions falling several times, usually during the night when she gets up to go to the bathroom.

The client is able to ambulate independently at home, holding onto walls and furniture for support as needed. In the community, she is able to ambulate short distances using a front-wheeled walker but fatigues easily. She uses a w/c as her primary mode of locomotion when outside.

ROM testing reveals tightness of bilateral hamstrings and calf muscles. Tone assessment using the Modified Ashworth Scale reveals a grade of 2 in the LEs. The patient demonstrates impaired UE and LE light touch and proprioception sensation, with the LEs more affected than the UEs.

Bed mobility, supine to sit, and transfers to the w/c are independent, but the patient performs these movements slowly. Sitting balance is Good for static and Fair+ to Good for dynamic. Balance in standing is Good for static and Fair for dynamic. She scored a 16/28 on the Tinetti/Performance-Oriented Mobility Assessment and a 41/56 on the Berg Balance Test. Both of these tests indicate the patient's increased risk for falls.

QUESTIONS

1. Identify the impairments and activity limitations presented.

2. What potential interventions can be performed by the PTA to assist in improving the patient's functional performance?

CASE #3

RW is a 58-year-old man with a medical diagnosis of ALS. He reports that he was diagnosed with the condition 2 years ago. He is a retired truck driver and lives in a double-wide trailer with his girlfriend, who is his primary caregiver. He receives home health supportive services: a nurse visits every month and a home health aide visits every other day to assist him with self-care activities.

The client is still capable of speech communication, but his caregiver reports that his speech is getting worse. The client also reports difficulty in breathing at night and gets supplemental oxygen via nasal cannula. During the time of the examination, the client's vital signs are as follows: blood pressure is 120/90, pulse is 88, and respiration is 20. The client is incontinent of bladder and has a Foley catheter in place. Inspection of the skin reveals a slightly reddened sacral area.

He is able to move in bed with minimal assistance and use of the overhead trapeze bar. He requires minimal assistance to get up from supine to sit and to transfer from the bed to the w/c using a slideboard. The client demonstrates poor sitting and standing balance. He is able to stand with minimal assist and a front-wheeled walker and take a few steps with moderate assistance, but he is unable to functionally ambulate. The client uses a manual w/c as his primary mode of locomotion, with his girlfriend or caregiver pushing the w/c. He is unable to afford a power w/c.

The client demonstrates bilateral plantarflexion contractures and some tightness of both hamstrings. He has spasticity of both LEs (grade 2 on the Modified Ashworth Scale). Strength of both LEs and UEs is generally 3 to 3+/5. The client demonstrates absent proprioception for both LEs and impaired light touch sensation bilaterally.

QUESTIONS

1. Identify the impairments and activity limitations presented.

2. What potential interventions can be performed by the PTA to assist in improving the patient's functional performance?

REFERENCES

1. Schenkman M, Cutson TM, Kichibhatla M, Chandler J, Pieper C. Reliability of impairment and physical performance measures with Parkinson's disease. *Phys Ther.* 1997;77(1):19-27.

2. US Department of Health & Human Services. National Institutes of Health. Parkinson's disease. http://report. nih.gov/NIHfactsheets/ViewFactSheet.aspx?csid=109. Accessed June 21, 2012.

3. Melnick ME. Basal ganglia disorders: metabolic, hereditary, and genetic disorders in adults. In: Umphred DA, ed. *Umphred's Neurological Rehabilitation.* 4th ed. St Louis, MO: Mosby; 2001:669-670.

4. Marsden CD. On-off phenomena in Parkinson's disease. In: Rinne UK, Klinger M, Stamm G, eds. *Parkinson's Disease: Current Progress, Problems, and Management.* Amsterdam, The Netherlands: Biomedical Press; 1990.

5. Mille ML, Creath RA, Prettyman MG, et al. Posture and locomotion coupling: a target for rehabilitation interventions in persons with Parkinson's disease. *Parkinsons Dis.* 2012;2012:754186.

6. Koller WC, Glatt S, Vetere-Overfield B, Hassanein R. Falls and Parkinson's disease. *Clin Neuropharm.* 1989;12(2):98-105.

7. Aita JF. Why patients with Parkinson's disease fall. *JAMA.* 1982;247(4):515-516.

8. New Parkinson's drug receives marketing clearance. Mirapex is the first new Parkinson's drug cleared in US this decade. http://www.prnewswire.com/news-releases/new-parkinsons-drug-receives-marketing-clearance-mirapex-is-the-first-new-parkinsons-drug-cleared-in-us-this-decade-74603477.html. Accessed September 6, 2013.

9. Ahlskog JE. Does vigorous exercise have a neuroprotective effect in Parkinson's disease? *Neurology.* 2011;77(3):288-294.

10. Fox C, Ebersbach G, Ramig L, Sapir S. LSVT LOUD and LSVT BIG: behavioral treatment programs for speech and body movement in Parkinson's disease. *Parkinsons Dis.* 2012;2012:391946.

11. Li F, Harmer P, Fitzgerald K, et al. Tai chi and postural stability in patients with Parkinson's disease. *N Engl J Med.* 2012;366(6):511-519.

12. Hoehn MM, Yahr MD. Parkinsonism: onset, progression and mortality. *Neurology.* 1967;17(5):427-442.

13. Goetz CG, Poewe W, Rascol O, et al. Movement Disorder Society Task Force report on the Hoehn and Yahr staging scale: status and recommendations. *Mov Disord.* 2004;19(9):1020-1028.

14. Frankel D. Multiple sclerosis. In: Umphred DA, ed. *Umphred's Neurological Rehabilitation.* 4th ed. St Louis, MO: Mosby; 2001:595-599.

15. Widener G. Multiple sclerosis. In: Umphred D, Lazaro R, Roller M, Burton G, eds. *Umphred's Neurological Rehabilitation.* 6th ed. St Louis, MO: Elsevier; 2012.

16. National Multiple Sclerosis Society. The National MS Society's disease management consensus statement. https://www.google.com/url?sa=t&rct=j&q=&esrc=s&source=web&cd=1&cad=rja&ved=0CC4QFjAA&url=http%3A%2F%2Fwww.nationalmssociety.org%2Fdownload.aspx%3Fid%3D8&ei=brybUdCII5Cu8ATW0IGgDA&usg=AFQjCNG5SH2wRRv1ATcThn99DblF8nJmlQ&sig2=SK1LbTaJkQ7YLoEe7a9RDQ. Accessed September 6, 2013.

17. Hallum A. Neuromuscular diseases. In: Umphred DA, ed. *Umphred's Neurological Rehabilitation.* 4th ed. St Louis, MO: Mosby; 2001:377-378.

18. Dal Bello-Haas V, Kloos A, Mitsumoto H. Physical therapy for a patient through six stages of amyotrophic lateral sclerosis. *Phys Ther.* 1998;78(12):1312-1324.

19. *Guide to Physical Therapist Practice.* 2nd ed. Alexandria, VA: American Physical Therapy Association; 2001.

20. Tinetti ME. Performance-oriented assessment of mobility problems in elderly patients. *J Am Geriatr Soc.* 1986;34(2):119-126.

21. Berg K. Measuring balance in the elderly: validation of an instrument. *Physiother Can.* 1989;41:304.

22. Duncan PW, Weiner DK, Chandler J, Studenski S. Functional reach: a new clinical measure of balance. *J Gerontol.* 1990;45(6):M192-M197.

23. Podsiadlo D, Richardson S. The timed "up and go": a test of basic functional mobility for frail elderly persons. *J Am Geriatr Soc.* 1991;39(2):142-148.

24. Stebbins GT, Goetz CG. Factor structure of the Unified Parkinson's Disease Rating Scale: Motor Examination section. *Mov Disord.* 1998;13(4):633-636.

25. Kurtzke JF. A new scale for evaluating disability in multiple sclerosis. *Neurology.* 1955;5(8):580-583.

26. de Boer AG, Wijker W, Speelman JD, de Haes JC. Quality of life in patients with Parkinson's disease: development of a questionnaire. *J Neurol Neurosurg Psychiatry.* 1996;61(1):70-74.

27. National Multiple Sclerosis Society. The Multiple Sclerosis Quality of Life Inventory. http://www.nationalmssociety.org/ms-clinical-care-network/researchers/clinical-study-measures/msqli/index.aspx. Accessed November 15, 2012.

28. Simmons Z, Felgoise SH, Breme BA. The ALSSQOL balancing physical and nonphysical factors in assessing quality of life in ALS. *Neurology.* 2006;67(9):1659-1664.

29. David FJ, Rafferty MR, Robichaud JA, et al. Progressive resistance exercise and Parkinson's disease: a review of potential mechanisms. *Parkinsons Dis.* 2012;2012:124527.

30. White LJ, Dressendorfer RH. Exercise and multiple sclerosis. *Sports Med.* 2004;34(15):1077-1100.

31. Hirsch MA, Toole T, Maitland CG, Rider RA. The effects of balance training and high-intensity resistance training on persons with idiopathic Parkinson's disease. *Arch Phys Med Rehabil.* 2003;84(8):1109-1117.

32. Dibble LE, Hale TF, Marcus RL, Droge J, Gerber JP, LaStayo PC. High-intensity resistance training amplifies muscle hypertrophy and functional gains in persons with Parkinson's disease. *Mov Disor.* 2006;21(9):1444-1452.

33. Ashburn A, Fazakarley L, Ballinger C, Pickering R, McLellan LD, Fitton C. A randomised controlled trial of a home based exercise programme to reduce the risk of falling among people with Parkinson's disease. *J Neurol Neurosurg Psychiatry.* 2007;78(7):678-684.

34. de Almeida JP, Silvestre R, Pinto AC, de Carvalho M. Exercise and amyotrophic lateral sclerosis. *Neurol Sci.* 2012;33(1):9-15.

35. Kent-Braun JA, Miller RG. Central fatigue during isometric exercise in amyotrophic lateral sclerosis. *Muscle Nerve.* 2000;23(6):909-914.

36. Carreras I, Yuruker S, Aytan N, et al. Moderate exercise delays the motor performance decline in a transgenic model of ALS. *Brain Res.* 2010;1313:192-201.

37. Constantinescu R, Leonard C, Deeley C, Kurlan R. Assistive devices for gait in Parkinson's disease. *Parkinsonism Relat Disord.* 2007;13(3):133-138.

38. Frenkel-Toledo S, Giladi N, Peretz C, Herman T, Gruendlinger L, Hausdorff JM. Treadmill walking as an external pacemaker to improve gait rhythm and stability in Parkinson's disease. *Mov Disord.* 2005;20(9):1109-1114.

39. Karmarkar AM, Dicianno BE, Graham JE, Cooper R, Kelleher A, Cooper RA. Factors associated with provision of wheelchairs in older adults. *Assist Technol.* 2012;24(3):155-167.

40. Kluding P, McGinnis PQ. Multidimensional exercise for people with Parkinson's disease: a case report. *Physiother Theory Pract.* 2006;22(3):153-162.

41. Kilmer DD, Aitken S. Neuromuscular disease. In: Frontera WR, Dawson DM, Slovik DM, eds. *Exercises in Rehabilitation Medicine.* Champaign, IL: Human Kinetics; 1999:253-266.

42. Aksu S, Citak-Karakaya I. Effects of exercise therapy on pain complaints in patients with amyotrophic lateral sclerosis. *Pain Clin.* 2002;14(4):353-359.

43. Schenkman M, Donovan J, Tsubota J, et al. Management of individuals with Parkinson's disease: rationale and case studies. *Phys Ther.* 1989;69(11):944-955.

44. Corcos DM, Comella CL, Goetz CG. Tai chi for patients with Parkinson's disease. *N Engl J Med.* 2012;366(18):1737-1738, author reply 1738.

45. Liu T, Lao L. Tai chi for patients with Parkinson's disease. *N Engl J Med.* 2012;366(18):1737-1738, author reply 1738.

46. Tamir R, Dickstein R, Huberman M. Integration of motor imagery and physical practice in group treatment applied to subjects with Parkinson's disease. *Neurorehabil Neural Repair.* 2007;21(1):68-75.

47. McIntosh GC, Brown SH, Rice RR, Thaut MH. Rhythmic auditory-motor facilitation of gait patterns in patients with Parkinson's disease. *J Neurol Neurosurg Psychiatry.* 1997;62(1):22-26.

48. Wilhite B, Keller MJ, Hodges JS, Caldwell L. Enhancing human development and optimizing health and well-being in persons with multiple sclerosis. *Ther Recreation J.* 2004;38(2):167-187.

49. Bakshi R. Fatigue associated with multiple sclerosis: diagnosis, impact and management. *Mult Scler.* 2003;9(3):219-227.

50. Petajan JH, White AT. Recommendations for physical activity in patients with multiple sclerosis. *Sports Med.* 1999;27(3):179-191.

51. Brar SP, Smith MB, Nelson LM, Franklin GM, Cobble ND. Evaluation of treatment protocols on minimal to moderate spasticity in multiple sclerosis. *Arch Phys Med Rehabil.* 1991;72(3):186-189.

52. Di Fabio RP, Soderberg J, Choi T, Hansen CR, Schapiro RT. Extended outpatient rehabilitation: its influence on symptom frequency, fatigue, and functional status for persons with progressive multiple sclerosis. *Arch Phys Med Rehabil.* 1998;79(2):141-146.

53. Finlayson M, Guglielmello L, Liefer K. Describing and predicting the possession of assistive devices among persons with multiple sclerosis. *Am J Occup Ther.* 2001;55(5):545-551.

54. Storr LK, Sørensen PS, Ravnborg M. The efficacy of multidisciplinary rehabilitation in stable multiple sclerosis patients. *Mult Scler.* 2006;12(2):235-242.

55. Mutluay FK, Demir R, Ozyilmaz S, Caglar AT, Altintas A, Gurses HN. Breathing-enhanced upper extremity exercises for patients with multiple sclerosis. *Clin Rehabil.* 2007;21(7):595-602.

56. Dal Bello-Haas V, Kloos AD, Mitsumoto H. Physical therapy for a patient through six stages of amyotrophic lateral sclerosis. *Phys Ther.* 1998;78(12):1312-1324.

57. Adams MR. Communication aids for patients with amyotrophic lateral sclerosis. *J Speech Hear Disord.* 1966;31(3):274-275.

58. Rowland LP, Shneider NA. Amyotrophic lateral sclerosis. *N Engl J Med.* 2001;344(22):1688-1700.

Please see accompanying Web site at

www.healio.com/books/neuroptavideos

Cardiopulmonary Issues Associated With Patients Undergoing Neurorehabilitation

Ronald De Vera Barredo, PT, DPT, EdD, GCS

KEY WORDS

- Aerobic exercise
- Breathing retraining
- Cardiovascular system
- Chronic obstructive pulmonary disease
- Congestive heart failure
- Dyspnea
- Exercise intolerance
- Progressive deconditioning
- Pulmonary system
- Restrictive lung disease

CHAPTER OBJECTIVES

- Describe the basic anatomy and physiology of the cardiovascular and pulmonary systems.

- Explain how neuromuscular pathologies can affect cardiovascular and pulmonary function.

- Discuss common cardiovascular and pulmonary comorbidities that may affect patients undergoing neurorehabilitation.

- Describe physical therapy examination procedures and common diagnostic tests used with individuals with primary or secondary cardiovascular and pulmonary problems.

- Describe procedural interventions that are used to manage patients with cardiovascular and pulmonary conditions.

Umphred DA, Lazaro RT, eds.
Neurorehabilitation for the Physical Therapist Assistant,
Second Edition (pp 393-410).
© 2014 SLACK Incorporated.

INTRODUCTION

Oxygen delivery and carbon dioxide elimination are important to sustaining life. Normal body functioning requires the presence of oxygen for cell metabolism and energy production. Without enough oxygen, the cells will not work properly, eventually impairing neuromuscular and musculoskeletal function. A byproduct of cell metabolism and energy production is carbon dioxide. Carbon dioxide is transported to the lungs so that it may be eliminated from the body through the process of exhalation.

The entire process of oxygen delivery and carbon dioxide elimination are mediated through the cardiovascular and pulmonary systems. The cardiovascular and pulmonary systems are complementary systems that participate in gas exchange, oxygen transport, and carbon dioxide elimination. Problems with either or both systems may interfere with the rehabilitation process by limiting muscle performance, exercise tolerance, and functional capacity. Likewise, conditions of the neuromuscular and musculoskeletal systems that affect the cardiovascular and pulmonary systems can impair the latter's ability to deliver oxygen and eliminate carbon dioxide.

The purpose of this chapter is 3-fold: first, to describe how impairments resulting from neuromuscular pathologies can alter cardiovascular and pulmonary function; second, to discuss how cardiovascular and pulmonary comorbidities affect neurorehabilitation; and third, to outline examination and intervention strategies appropriate for the physical therapist assistant (PTA) to perform commensurate to his or her scope of practice. A sufficient understanding of the dynamics between the neuromuscular system and the cardiovascular and pulmonary systems will allow the PTA to employ appropriate strategies within the established plan of care.

REVIEW OF ANATOMY AND PHYSIOLOGY OF CARDIOVASCULAR AND PULMONARY SYSTEMS

The cardiovascular and pulmonary systems are complementary systems that participate in gas exchange, oxygen transport, and carbon dioxide elimination. The pulmonary system is integral to gas exchange and carbon dioxide elimination. The cardiovascular system transports oxygenated blood from the lungs to the various cells, tissues, and organs in the body. Waste products, including carbon dioxide from the cells, tissues, and organs, are transported back to the lungs for waste elimination. In supplying oxygen to and eliminating carbon dioxide from the body, the pulmonary system is able to regulate the pH balance of the body.

The pulmonary system is composed of a network of airways that begins in the nose and mouth; proceeds inferiorly to the pharynx, larynx, trachea, and airways; and terminates into the alveoli, which are surrounded by capillaries. Inhaled air passes through these airways until it reaches the alveoli, where gas exchange occurs. Oxygen from the inhaled air diffuses through the alveoli into the arterial system, while carbon dioxide from the venous system diffuses into the alveoli and exits the body through the same network of airways during exhalation.

Essential in the mechanics of breathing is the integrity of the chest wall mechanics and respiratory muscle function. The chest wall should be able to expand and return to its resting position without compromise. The primary and accessory muscles of respiration should function appropriately to the needs of the person and the demands of the body. Consequently, neuromuscular and musculoskeletal pathologies and impairments that interfere with the normal functioning of the chest wall and the respiratory muscles may affect the mechanics of breathing, which would manifest itself in difficulty inhaling, exhaling, or both.

The cardiovascular system is composed of the heart and the blood vessels that not only supply oxygenated blood to the various parts of the body (systemic circulation), but also transport

Table 14-1
Cardiovascular and Pulmonary Responses to Sympathetic and Parasympathetic Stimulation

System Component	Sympathetic Response	Parasympathetic Response
Heart	↑ Heart rate and contractility	↓ Heart rate and contractility
Peripheral vessels	Vasoconstriction	Vasodilation
Lungs	Bronchodilation	Bronchoconstriction

deoxygenated blood from the various parts of the body to the lungs for oxygenation and waste elimination (pulmonary circulation). The heart is central to both systemic and pulmonary circulation. It is a 4-chambered organ consisting of 2 atria and 2 ventricles. The atria act as a temporary storage chamber as the blood is transmitted to the ventricles. The ventricles function to eject the blood to either the lungs or the rest of the body. Between the atria and ventricles are valves that prevent the backflow of blood from one chamber to another.

The right side of the heart participates in pulmonary circulation. Deoxygenated blood coming from systemic circulation passes through the right atrium, the tricuspid valve, and the right ventricle and is ejected to the lungs via the pulmonary arteries. The left side of the heart participates in systemic circulation. Oxygenated blood coming from the lungs is transported back to the heart via the pulmonary veins. The blood then passes through the left atrium, the mitral valve, and the left ventricle and is ejected to the body via the aorta, systemic arteries, arterioles, and capillaries.

Both the parasympathetic and sympathetic nervous systems innervate the heart, lungs, and blood vessels. Parasympathetic innervation is effected primarily through the vagus nerve, while sympathetic innervation is effected through the pre- and post-ganglionic neurons that extend through the thoracolumbar regions of the spinal cord. The effects of these systems on the cardiovascular and pulmonary systems are outlined in Table 14-1. Consequently, neuromuscular pathologies and impairments that interfere with the normal functioning of the parasympathetic and sympathetic systems would affect the response of the cardiovascular and pulmonary systems.[1]

NEUROMUSCULAR PATHOLOGIES AFFECTING CARDIOVASCULAR AND PULMONARY FUNCTION

Neuromuscular pathologies and impairments have the potential of affecting cardiovascular and pulmonary function. The PTA needs to be aware of this potential to address issues of a cardiovascular or pulmonary nature when working with patients undergoing neurorehabilitation. For example, changes in muscle tone may affect muscle performance. Upper motor neuron lesions generally result in increased muscle tone, while lower motor neuron lesions generally result in decreased muscle tone. Such changes in muscle tone may not only affect motor performance but also contribute to impairments in posture. Consequently, impairments in muscle performance and postural control can affect the mechanics of breathing. The impact of changes in muscle tone on the mechanics of breathing is outlined in Table 14-2.

Neuromuscular pathologies such as stroke and amyotrophic lateral sclerosis may also result in impairments of bulbar functions or cranial nerve involvement, which include chewing, swallowing, and speech. Paralysis of the muscles involved with bulbar function may result in the patient aspirating fluid and food particles to the lungs, resulting in aspiration pneumonia. The PTA

Table 14-2 *Effects of Changes in Tone on the Mechanics of Breathing*			
Location of the Lesion	**Change in Muscle Tone**	**Musculoskeletal Effect**	**Cardiopulmonary Consequence**
Upper motor neuron lesion (eg, stroke, spinal cord injury, Parkinson's disease)	Increased	Decreased motor control	• Postural impairment due to weakness or increased tone • Altered chest movement
Lower motor neuron lesion (eg, poliomyelitis, neuropathy, muscle dystrophy)	Decreased	Muscular weakness	• Difficulty recruiting accessory muscles • Inability to produce an effective cough

should recognize signs that point to problems with chewing, swallowing, or aspiration. These include excessive drooling, especially at mealtime; pocketing of food in the cheeks; choking or trouble swallowing certain foods or liquids; having a gurgling voice during or after a meal; coughing before or after swallowing; and frequent throat clearing during or after a meal.

In addition to their impact on respiratory muscle function, breathing mechanics, and bulbar function, neuromuscular pathologies may also result in impairments of autonomic nervous system function. Patients with spinal cord injuries (SCIs), for example, may have problems regulating blood pressure (BP), but these tend to change with time following the injury. During the spinal shock stage (hours to days), there is massive dilation of the blood vessels, resulting in profound hypotension. As time progresses (days to weeks), spinal shock diminishes; however, patients experience frequent bouts with hypotensive episodes during changes in position or prolonged sitting, including lightheadedness, dizziness, and syncope. Conversely, instead of hypotensive episodes, patients with SCIs above T5 or T6 may experience bouts of hypertensive episodes brought about by noxious stimuli below the level of the lesion (autonomic dysreflexia), such as a distended bladder, a blocked catheter, or tight clothing. During these instances, the presence of noxious stimuli activates the sympathetic nervous system, resulting in increased BP, flushing of the face and upper body, and complaints of pounding headache. Current studies show that autonomic dysreflexia occurs more frequently during the early phases of SCI, while hypotensive episodes can persist for years after the injury.[2] The PTA should recognize signs and symptoms of hypertension as well as hypotension with this population, especially during neurorehabilitation, to avert any untoward consequences to the patient, such as falls during hypotensive episodes and stroke during hypertensive episodes. Table 14-3 outlines signs and symptoms associated with hypotensive and hypertensive episodes that the PTA needs to be familiar with.

PRIMARY CARDIOVASCULAR AND PULMONARY PATHOLOGIES AFFECTING NEUROREHABILITATION

Cardiovascular Pathologies

Patients undergoing neurorehabilitation may have cardiovascular comorbidities that require attention during the development and implementation of the plan of care. Some of these

Table 14-3	
Common Signs and Symptoms Representative of Hypotensive and Hypertensive Episodes	
Hypotensive Episode	*Hypertensive Episode*
Lightheadedness	Pounding headache
Dizziness	Flushing of face
Syncope	Sweating
Shortness of breath	Goose pimples
Irregular heartbeat	Nausea

Table 14-4	
Ranges of Blood Pressure	
Condition	*Blood Pressure Reading*
Optimal	Systolic less than 120 mm Hg; diastolic less than 80 mm Hg
Prehypertensive	Systolic 120 to 139 mm Hg; diastolic 90 to 89 mm Hg
Hypertensive	Systolic 140 mm Hg and above; diastolic 90 mm Hg and above

comorbidities may have been preexisting conditions that contributed to the development of the neurological condition. A classic example of this is the role of hypertension (BP greater than 140/90 mm Hg) in the development of stroke. Consistently high BP weakens the blood vessels and damages the flow to organs such as the brain, thereby resulting in a stroke. Table 14-4 outlines the BP readings considered optimal, prehypertensive, and hypertensive.

PTAs working with patients who are hypertensive need to be familiar with the signs and symptoms of hypertension. Additionally, they should consider taking BP readings in the unaffected arm, since BP readings are unreliable if taken in the affected arm. Studies have shown that muscle tone in the affected arm can influence the BP reading in that extremity. Spastic extremities yield higher BP readings, while flaccid extremities yield lower BP readings.[3,4]

Atherosclerosis refers to the hardening of arteries usually caused by deposition of fat, cholesterol, and other substances that harden and form structures called *plaques*. The narrowing of the arteries results in decreased blood flow, starving cells and tissues of oxygen-rich blood. Decreased blood flow to the cardiac muscles results in chest pain, also known as *angina*. Angina may feel like pressure or squeezing in the chest and can radiate to the shoulders, chest, jaw, or back. Sometimes, in the absence of chest pain, other symptoms are present, such as dyspnea, profuse sweating, extreme fatigue, and belching; these are known as *anginal equivalents* that also indicate decreased blood flow to the cardiac muscles. Stable angina occurs with activity or stress. This type of angina is predictable because symptoms are absent at rest or with mild activity. However, in the presence of increasing activity, decreased blood flow is unable to meet the oxygen demands of the heart, thereby eliciting angina. A decrease in activity or the administration of nitroglycerin may minimize the symptoms. On the other hand, unstable angina does not follow a predictable pattern. Angina may occur at rest and may not respond to medication. Therefore, unstable angina is a medical emergency. The PTA should be able to recognize the signs and symptoms of angina. Should anginal onset occur during neurorehabilitation, the PTA needs to cease the activity and

Table 14-5
Clinical Model for Predicting Pretest Probability for Deep Vein Thrombosis

Clinical Feature	Score
Active cancer (treatment ongoing or within previous 6 months or palliative)	1
Paralysis, paresis, or recent plaster immobilization of the lower extremities	1
Recently bedridden for more than 3 days or major surgery, within 4 weeks	1
Localized tenderness along the distribution of the deep venous system	1
Entire leg swollen	1
Calf swelling by more than 3 cm when compared with the asymptomatic leg (measured 10 cm below tibial tuberosity)	1
Pitting edema (greater in the symptomatic leg)	1
Collateral superficial veins (nonvaricose)	1
Alternative diagnosis as likely or greater than that of DVT	−2

Low probability 0 or less, moderate probability 1 to 2, high probability 3 or more.
(Reprinted from *The Lancet*, 350 (9094), Philip S. Wells,David R. Anderson, Janis Bormanis, Fred Guy, Michael Mitchell, Lisa Gray, Cathy Clement, K. Sue Robinson, Bernard Lewandowski, Value of assessment of pretest probability of deep-vein thrombosis in clinical management, 1795-1798, Copyright 1997, with permission from Elsevier.)

notify the physical therapist (PT) immediately. Additionally, if nitroglycerin has been prescribed, the patient needs to be instructed to take the medication as prescribed by the physician.

Arrhythmias refer to problems with the rate and/or rhythm of the heart. Patients undergoing neurorehabilitation may report having palpitations, fluttering, or pounding in the chest. This may be accompanied by other symptoms, such as lightheadedness, dizziness, dyspnea, chest discomfort, or fatigue. In addition to recognizing the signs and symptoms of arrhythmias, the PTA who works with a patient who has arrhythmia should continually monitor the patient's pulse and BP. Additionally, the PTA should be trained not only in cardiopulmonary resuscitation but also in the use of an automated external defibrillator should the need arise for this device to be used.

Deep vein thrombosis (DVT) refers to a blood clot in the legs. The blockage causes pain, swelling, and warmth in the legs. DVT may be caused by prolonged bed rest or immobility, such as those caused by stroke or during the acute phase of SCI. DVT is an important consideration, especially during the early phases of rehabilitation, because a medically unmanaged DVT may result in the release of an embolus from the site of the DVT, which eventually lodges itself in the lungs, causing a pulmonary embolism. Because Homan's sign is of no clinical use,[5] using the Wells Prediction Rule is a better alternative to determining the probability of a DVT. By determining the clinical presentation of the patient and assigning scores to the clinical features, the rule classifies patients as having either low, moderate, or high probability of having a DVT.[6] Table 14-5 outlines the specifics of the Wells Prediction Rule.

The PTA needs to be familiar with the risk factors for and the signs and symptoms of DVT. Additionally, the assistant should be familiar with the signs and symptoms of pulmonary embolism, should this occur during neurorehabilitation. Signs and symptoms include sudden and unexplained shortness of breath, difficulty with breathing, chest pain, tachypnea, palpitations, coughing, or coughing up blood. Individuals with DVT should not participate in physical therapy until otherwise cleared by the physician.

Table 14-6

Representative Signs and Symptoms Associated With Right- and Left-Sided Heart Failure

Left-Sided Heart Failure		Right-Sided Heart Failure	
Forward Failure	*Backward Failure*	*Forward Failure*	*Backward Failure*
Hypotension Lightheadedness Dizziness Cool extremities	Pulmonary edema Dyspnea Orthopnea	Hypoxemia	Dependent edema Hepatomegaly Visible neck veins Ankle swelling

Like hypertension, congestive heart failure (CHF) has been recognized as a risk factor for stroke. CHF occurs when the heart is unable to pump adequately to meet the needs of the body. The heart's inability to pump adequately can result from coronary artery disease, valvular diseases of the heart, and hypertension. Right-sided heart failure occurs when the right ventricle is unable to eject blood to the pulmonary circuit, which is involved with gas exchange. Left-sided heart failure occurs when the left ventricle is unable to eject blood to the systemic circuit, which is involved with supplying oxygenated blood to various parts of the body.

Regardless of which side of the heart is involved, the signs and symptoms of heart failure may be classified as the result of either forward failure (consequences resulting from blood not moving forward) or backward failure (consequences resulting from blood backing up from whence it came). In right-sided heart failure, for example, the right ventricle is unable to eject a sufficient amount of blood for gas exchange, thereby resulting in hypoxemia (forward failure). Concurrently, since the right ventricle is unable to fully eject blood from the right ventricle, blood is dammed back to the right atrium, then to the superior and inferior vena cava, and back to the venous system, thereby resulting in distended neck veins, dependent edema, and hepatomegaly (backward failure). On the other hand, in left-sided heart failure, the left ventricle is unable to eject a sufficient amount of blood for systemic circulation, which may result in lightheadedness and hypotension (forward failure). Additionally, since the left ventricle is unable to eject a sufficient amount of blood forward, blood is dammed back to the left atrium, then back to the lungs, thereby resulting in pulmonary edema, shortness of breath, and wheezing (backward failure). Table 14-6 outlines the representative signs and symptoms associated with right- and left-sided heart failure.

The PTA needs to be familiar with the signs and symptoms of heart failure alluded to earlier. Additionally, the PTA should remember that patients undergoing neurorehabilitation who have CHF as a comorbidity may also report having dyspnea, fatigue, exercise intolerance, and weight gain. The assistant should report these findings to the PT or to other appropriate personnel.

Pulmonary Pathologies

Patients with pulmonary comorbidities may exhibit exercise and activity limitations while undergoing neurorehabilitation. The PTA needs to be familiar with the impairments resulting from these pathologies to implement strategies that will allow the patient to maximize the rehabilitation process while operating within his or her pulmonary limitations. Chronic obstructive pulmonary disease (COPD) and restrictive lung diseases represent 2 types of pulmonary pathologies. Obstructive lung conditions make it difficult for patients to expel air (expiration), while restrictive lung conditions make it difficult for patients to expand the lungs (inspiration). Despite these differences, obstructive and restrictive lung conditions result in patients having dyspnea or shortness of breath. During the early stages of obstruction or restriction, dyspnea would limit the performance of exercises and other activities and may limit the person's ability to participate in social interactions. As the condition progresses, dyspnea worsens to the point that it interferes with normal functioning and activities of daily living (ADL).

Patients with obstructive conditions experience dyspnea because they are unable to expire the air that is trapped in the lungs. Air trapping can result from the destruction of the alveolar walls, such as seen in emphysema. When the lining of the alveolar walls are destroyed, the alveoli permanently expand, causing air to be trapped within it. The more chronic the condition, the more alveolar destruction is present and the more air trapping takes place, causing the patient to exhale slowly and longer in an effort to expel the air. Another cause of air trapping is the narrowing of the airways. The presence of mucus, such as seen in chronic bronchitis, or a state of bronchoconstriction, such as seen in asthma, makes the diameter of the airways narrower. Because resistance to air movement is greater on expiration than inspiration, air can get in the lungs but has difficulty getting out. Like in emphysema, air trapping takes place, causing the patient to exhale slowly and longer in an effort to expel air.

Patients with restrictive conditions experience dyspnea because they are unable to fully inspire air because of some type of pulmonary or extrapulmonary restriction. This restriction may be related to the inability of the lung tissue to fully expand, such as seen in pneumothorax (air in the intrapleural space) or pleural effusion (fluid in the intrapleural space); stiffness of the lung parenchyma, such as seen in interstitial lung disease; structural defects of the thoracic cage, such as seen in kyphoscoliosis; weakening of the respiratory muscles, such as seen in muscular dystrophy; increased tone of the muscles of the thorax, such as seen in hemiplegia; or damage to nerves that assist with breathing, such as in phrenic nerve compression.

Because of the increased respiratory effort and work associated with dyspnea, patients with obstructive and restrictive conditions may limit their food intake. Their use of accessory muscles contributes to higher energy expenditure. These 2 factors result in unintended weight loss. In addition to dyspnea and unintended weight loss, cough may also present among patients with pulmonary pathologies. For patients with obstructive conditions, cough is usually productive; for patients with restrictive conditions, cough is usually dry. Finally, for more chronic conditions, patients manifest with hypoxemia and may require supplemental oxygenation to meet the demands of the body. Hypoxemia may, in turn, cause restlessness, altered mental status, tachycardia, and diaphoresis.

Despite body system impairments caused by pulmonary comorbidities, patients undergoing neurorehabilitation need not stop exercising. Exercise can increase physical capacity, decrease anxiety, reduce fatigue, and improve independence. The PTA needs to communicate closely with the PT on the exercise parameters appropriate for the patient. Pacing and rest breaks are also important considerations during therapy. Finally, the PTA should be able to recognize the signs and symptoms of respiratory distress and respond appropriately to the needs of the patient within the established plan of care.

COMMON PARTICIPATION RESTRICTIONS, FUNCTIONAL ACTIVITY LIMITATIONS, AND BODY SYSTEM IMPAIRMENTS OF THE CARDIOPULMONARY SYSTEM

Participation limitations for patients with cardiopulmonary pathologies are largely a result of progressive deconditioning. Because dyspnea is central to most cardiopulmonary conditions, patients who experience this and other symptoms, such as leg fatigue and discomfort, minimize or avoid physical activity.[7] Patients become sedentary, and the resulting decrease in physical activity contributes to continued physical deconditioning, resulting in dyspnea on minimal exertion and

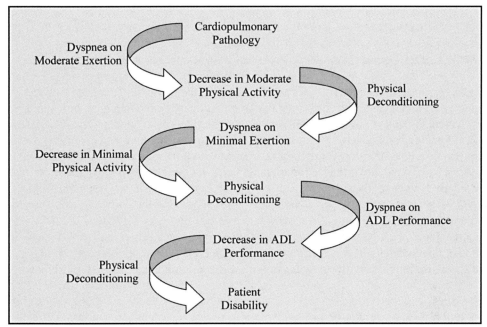

Figure 14-1. Dyspnea—Deconditioning spiral.

eventual inability to participate in normal life activities and loss of function performing ADL. The loss of function in social participation and ADL also results in depression.[8] Figure 14-1 illustrates the role of dyspnea in deconditioning.

In addition to dyspnea, exercise intolerance is evident in patients with cardiopulmonary conditions, particularly those with CHF.[9] Exercise intolerance is defined as the reduced ability to perform activities that involve dynamic movement of large skeletal muscles because of symptoms of dyspnea, muscle weakness, or fatigue.[10] For a patient undergoing neurorehabilitation, exercise intolerance is a primary consideration. The PTA should accommodate for dyspnea and muscle weakness or fatigue while implementing the established plan of care.

The PTA should always be aware and cognizant of cardiac decompensation, which is indicative of the sudden worsening of symptoms related to heart failure. Symptoms may be manifested as increasing shortness of breath; onset of coughing and wheezing; worsening fatigue; and the development of hypotension, lightheadedness, cyanosis, angina, or arrhythmias.

EXAMINATION TOOLS, TESTS, AND MEASURES USED TO EVALUATE CARDIOVASCULAR AND PULMONARY FUNCTION

Physical Examination

For patients undergoing neurorehabilitation, neurological assessment should include an examination of the cardiopulmonary system, especially since impairments in cardiovascular and pulmonary function may interfere with the rehabilitation process. While the PT of record should perform the initial examination/evaluation, parts of the reexamination are often delegated to the PTA. Similarly, a problem might develop during any intervention, and the PTA needs to be aware of the signs and symptoms of a cardiopulmonary problem. For that reason, the PTA needs to understand and be skilled at examining the cardiopulmonary system. If a problem develops and the PTA does not feel comfortable with the reexamination, the PT of record should be contacted immediately to prevent a delay in recognizing potential life-threatening dangers in the patient's cardiopulmonary system.

Physical therapy examination of the cardiovascular and pulmonary systems encompasses 4 areas: observation, palpation, percussion, and auscultation.[1,11,12] *Observation* refers to the visual inspection of the patient, which includes an assessment of the patient's general appearance, integumentary status, and breathing pattern. When observing the patient's general appearance, the PTA should recognize signs of respiratory distress. The assumption of a tripod posture is characteristic of a patient having respiratory distress. In the tripod posture, a patient leans forward in sitting or standing and supports the upper body with the hands on the knees or on another surface. In this position, with the head and upper extremities (UEs) fixed, the accessory muscles in the neck and chest are able to contract in reverse origin insertion to expand the chest when breathing. Another observable sign of respiratory distress is the increased work of breathing, manifested not only in the use of accessory muscles but also in the increased rate of breathing (tachypnea). Nasal flaring or the widening of the openings of the nose during breathing may also be observed.

When observing the patient's integumentary status, the PTA should be aware of changes in the skin that may result from cardiovascular and pulmonary pathologies. Cyanosis or bluish discoloration of the skin occurs when the patient is not receiving adequate amounts of oxygen. This may occur centrally (ie, around the mouth and lips) or peripherally (ie, in the fingers). On the other hand, pallor or paleness of the skin occurs when there is decreased blood flow to the area, such as seen in arterial occlusion. Another observable skin condition is digital clubbing. Digital clubbing is characterized by changes in the base of the nails that result in the formation of convex distal phalanges. The condition may be seen among patients with lung neoplasms, chronic pulmonary infections, cor pulmonale (right-sided heart failure), or chronic CHF.[13] For patients with CHF, edema may be observed in the lower extremities (LEs) due to the damming of blood from the right ventricle to the peripheral venous circulation. Edema is usually manifested by swelling caused by fluid accumulating in the tissues. In prolonged upright postures, swelling accumulates in the LEs, causing dependent edema.

When observing the patient's breathing pattern, the PTA should be aware of changes in the type, symmetry, rate, and depth of breathing. As stated earlier, patients in respiratory distress may manifest with tachypnea and accessory muscle use. Depending on the pulmonary condition, both the rate and depth of breathing may increase. An important consideration in observing the patient's breathing pattern may also include the neurological impairments that the patient has. In hemiplegia, for example, symmetry of breathing may be compromised because of changes in muscle tone and posture. Hemiparesis of the diaphragm causing involvement of one side of the diaphragm is almost always present following a middle cerebral artery stroke. Paradoxical breathing may be observed in patients whose SCI occurs at a high level. Paradoxical breathing occurs because of the loss of thoracic muscle tone and the paralysis of the thoracic muscles whose innervations come from the thoracic segments. The work of quiet breathing is borne solely by the diaphragm whose innervation comes from C3 to C5. When the patient inhales, the abdomen rises while the upper chest retracts. This type of paradoxical breathing is opposite that of patients in the latter stages of COPD. For these patients, the diaphragm has descended inferiorly because of air trapping, so the work of breathing is performed largely by the accessory muscles. When the patient inhales, the upper chest rises while the abdomen retracts. Figure 14-2 illustrates the difference between both types of paradoxical breathing.

Palpation represents the second area of physical examination. Palpation involves touching the patient to feel for and examine structures underneath. Palpation may be performed to determine the presence of tenderness. When patients report being short of breath but it is not noticeable to anyone else, palpation may be used to feel for accessory muscle use. Edema may also be palpated to determine whether it is pitting or nonpitting. When pressure applied over an edematous area causes an indentation in the skin that persists after the pressure is released, then the edema is

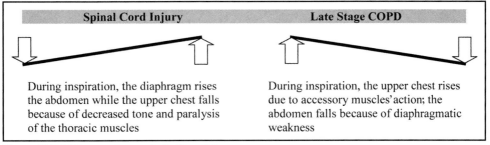

Figure 14-2. Differences in paradoxical breathing.

considered pitting. Conditions involving the heart and kidneys result in salt and fluid retention, usually leading to pitting edema. Additionally, skin turgor may also be assessed to determine the level of hydration. Skin that remains elevated after being pulled up and released indicates decreased turgor, which is indicative of decreased hydration.

Palpation is essential when taking the pulse. By palpating the pulse, the PTA can determine not only the heart rate but also the rhythm and amplitude of the pulses. By determining the pattern of pulsations (rhythm), the PTA can confirm the presence of arrhythmias and describe the pulses as regular, regularly irregular, or irregularly irregular. The amplitude or strength of the pulsations may be described as either absent, faint, weak, strong, and bounding. Unfortunately, because a description of amplitude comes with subjectivity, determining amplitude should take into consideration the patient's condition, presentation, and comorbidities.[14] Outside of determining the heart rate, palpation can also be used to determine the presence of peripheral pulses. In the presence of peripheral vascular disease, the absence of peripheral pulses may indicate compromised blood flow.

Percussion represents the third area of physical examination. It involves the tapping of the thorax and abdomen to determine the condition of structures underneath it. Since thoracic and abdominal structures have different densities, the vibrations they generate during percussion vary. For example, air-filled structures, such as the lungs, normally produce resonance during percussion. However, when the lung tissue is consolidated (pneumonia), resonance changes to dullness on percussion. In the presence of increased air (air trapping), resonance changes to hyperresonance on percussion.

Auscultation represents the fourth area of physical examination. During auscultation, a stethoscope is used to listen to heart and lung sounds. Lung sounds are produced with the movement of air in and out of the lungs during each breath (breath sounds). Conditions that result in air trapping, such as emphysema, make it difficult for air to move in and out of the lungs; this results in decreased breath sounds. At other times, additional lung sounds are heard in addition to the breath sounds (adventitious sounds). These adventitious sounds indicate lung pathologies. Wheezing, for example, is an adventitious lung sound generated by air moving through narrowed airways, such as in asthma. Crackles (rales) is another example of an adventitious lung sound generated when air moves through pus, fluid, or mucus, such as in chronic bronchitis.

Heart sounds are produced by blood flow and valve closure. During cardiac auscultation, the closure of the atrioventricular valves produce the "lub" in the lub-dub sound of the heart, while the closure of the semilunar valves produce the "dub" in the lub-dub sound of the heart. The former represents the S1 sound, while the latter represents the S2 sound. The presence of an S3 sound (heard immediately after S2) may be normal in children but may also indicate cardiac failure in adults. The presence of an S4 sound (prior to S1) may indicate a pathological condition such as myocardial infarct. In addition to the closure of the valves, a heart sound may be produced by turbulent blood flow. These are called *murmurs*. Murmurs may be classified as innocent or abnormal murmurs. Innocent murmurs are not caused by heart conditions but are nonetheless common in children. On the other hand, abnormal murmurs are caused by heart problems. They are generated when blood flows through either narrowed valves (stenosis) or incompetent valves (regurgitation).

Tests and Measures to Evaluate Cardiopulmonary Function

A number of diagnostic tests and outcomes measures are used to measure cardiovascular and pulmonary function. Although details on the administration of some of these tests and measures may be beyond the scope this text, the PTA needs to be familiar with what these tests do and what type of information they provide to understand the test result found in the chart and the effect those results may have on exercise or performance of ADL. The following tests will be covered in this section: pulmonary function tests, oximetry, arterial blood gases, activity and endurance evaluation, and stress testing.

Pulmonary function tests are used to determine how well the lungs function. More specifically, they measure the lungs' ability to: (1) hold air, (2) move air in and out, and (3) exchange oxygen and carbon dioxide from the blood. During testing, a patient breathes in and out of a mouthpiece into a recorder that measures the actual lung volumes and capacities and compares these values with predicted values that are based on the patient's age, sex, and height. Patients who undergo pulmonary function testing may be asked to breathe in and out normally and quietly. At other times, they may be asked to breathe in or out forcefully after taking a deep breath. An example of the latter is performed when measuring forced vital capacity (FVC). Since FVC involves maximum air exhalation after maximum air inhalation, the test reveals how fast and how much air patients can expire. Normally, a healthy individual can exhale between 75% and 80% of air during the first second of the FVC maneuver (FEV1). For patients with obstructive conditions, the value of FEV1/FVC is lower (ie, it takes longer for them to exhale). On the other hand, for patients with restrictive conditions, the value of FEV1/FVC is higher (ie, the patients are able to expire most of the air quickly). Another use of pulmonary function tests is to determine the efficacy of pulmonary medications in improving lung function. Baseline measures of lung function are taken and compared with values taken after administering pulmonary medications, such as bronchodilators. Should there be sufficient improvement in lung function, the medications become part of the patient's regimen, especially during functional activities that increase the demand on the pulmonary system.

Oximetry measures the concentration of oxygen in the blood by determining how saturated the hemoglobin is with oxygen molecules. The more saturated the hemoglobin with oxygen molecules, the higher the oxygen saturation. Oxygen saturation can be measured using a pulse oximeter or through arterial blood gas analysis. When a pulse oximeter is used, oxygen saturation is labeled SpO_2; when arterial blood gas analysis is used, oxygen saturation is labeled SaO_2. Normal oxygen saturation is 97% to 99%, with 95% representing a clinically acceptable level of saturation for patients with a normal hemoglobin level. Generally speaking, activity should be stopped when oxygen saturation falls below 90%.[15,16] While working with a patient undergoing neurorehabilitation, the PTA should ensure that the patient is above the clinical threshold determined by the PT. When oxygen saturation falls below this threshold, the PTA needs to cease the activity and consult with the PT.

Arterial blood gas measurements determine not only the amount of oxygen and carbon dioxide in the blood but also maintain the acid-base balance of the body through buffer mechanisms between the respiratory and renal systems. During instances of hypoventilation (such as in COPD), levels of carbon dioxide increase in the body and result in a condition known as *respiratory acidosis*. During instances of hyperventilation (such as in anxiety hyperventilation), carbon dioxide levels decrease in the body and result in a condition known as *respiratory alkalosis*.[8] When the underlying cause of either respiratory acidosis or alkalosis is untreated, the patient may manifest multisystemic signs and symptoms, such as those outlined in Table 14-7.

For patients who have been bedridden or are just starting to get out of bed, an activity evaluation may be in order. An activity evaluation is used to determine whether the patient is able to

Table 14-7
Signs and Symptoms of Respiratory Acidosis and Respiratory Alkalosis

Respiratory Acidosis	Respiratory Alkalosis
Confusion	Blurred vision
Disorientation	Dizziness
Dyspnea	Hypocapnea
Headache	Inability to concentrate
Hypercapnea	Muscle cramps
Respiratory distress	Muscle twitching and weakness
Restlessness	Numbness and tingling
Shallow respirations	Palpitations

tolerate a variety of self-care activities performed first in supine, then progressed to sitting and then to standing. During the performance of these self-care activities, the patients are monitored for symptoms including shortness of breath, lightheadedness, fatigue, fainting, and chest pain. Additionally, their heart rate and BP are monitored with each change in position. A drop of >20 mm Hg systolic BP and a drop of >10 mm Hg diastolic BP accompanied by a 10% to 20% increase in heart rate indicates postural hypotension.[13] Should postural hypotension be present, care should be taken for the patient to accommodate changes in position through gradual adaptation to changes in position. Once the patient is able to assume the standing position without any symptoms of or objective measures indicating hypotension, then the patient is cleared for an endurance evaluation.

An endurance evaluation is used to determine whether the patient is able to perform an activity for a prolonged period of time. During an endurance evaluation, the patient walks a predetermined circuit for 2 to 3 minutes, after which his or her vital signs are taken while the patient is marching in place. During this time, the patient is also monitored for symptoms such as shortness of breath, lightheadedness, fatigue, fainting, and chest pain. In the absence of physiological changes or subjective complaints that warrant termination of the test, the patient continues for a series of 2- to 3-minute intervals of walking and monitoring. The evaluation ends when the patient's perceived exertion is rated as "somewhat hard" (13/20) using the Borg Rating of Perceived Exertion (RPE) Scale. At the conclusion of the test, the distance walked by the patient is recorded as a baseline measure.[1]

Whereas an endurance evaluation is a symptom-limited measure of exercise capacity, the use of the 6-minute walk test is a time-limited, submaximal exercise test that provides an objective measure of functional exercise capacity. The test measures the distance that a patient can quickly walk in 6 minutes. During the administration of the test, the patient is monitored for symptoms similar to those identified in the endurance test. At the conclusion of the test, the distance covered is recorded as a baseline measure.

Stress testing provides information on how the heart functions during conditions of physical stress. Patients who are able to perform exercise stress tests (graded exercise tests) usually walk on a treadmill or pedal a bicycle. As the heart contracts harder and beats faster, its demand for oxygenated blood increases. However, in the presence of coronary artery disease, the narrowed arteries are unable to supply the needs of the heart, thereby resulting in symptoms such as angina, shortness of breath, and changes in the heart's rate, contraction, and rhythm. Because of myriad physiological responses taking place in response to physical stress, the patient is monitored using a number of equipment and devices, including an electrocardiogram to record and monitor changes in cardiac activity; a spirometer to record and monitor changes in breathing and gas exchange; a pulse oximeter to record and monitor oxygen saturation; and a sphygmomanometer to record and monitor changes in BP.[17] Additionally, the patient may be asked to respond to the level of effort or exertion being expended during the stress test using a perceived exertion scale, such as the Borg RPE Scale.[18]

The Borg RPE Scale goes from 6 ("minimal exertion") to 20 ("maximal exertion") and has been shown to correlate linearly with oxygen uptake and heart rate.[16] Perceived exertion ratings of 12 to 14 (13 is "somewhat hard") usually indicate a moderate level of intensity. This table can be found on the Web site of the Centers for Disease Control and Prevention (www.cdc.gov/physicalactivity/everyone/measuring/exertion.html).

INTERVENTIONS

PTAs provide physical therapy services under the direction and supervision of a PT. The PTA implements selected interventions, obtains data related to the interventions provided, and makes modifications within the plan of care to progress the patient or to ensure that patient safety and comfort is maintained. When working with patients who are undergoing neurorehabilitation, the PTA may be directed to implement interventions specific to body system impairments and functional limitations resulting from cardiovascular and pulmonary comorbidities that may interfere with or have an impact on the neurorehabilitation process. These may include breathing exercises, coughing exercises, chest mobilization exercises, respiratory resistance training, bronchial hygiene techniques, and aerobic exercise training.[1,11,12]

Breathing exercises have numerous purposes. Deep breathing exercises help promote chest expansion and ventilate underventilated areas of the lung. This is especially important with patients who are bedridden. Patients who have recently had chest surgery are also encouraged to perform deep breathing exercises; oftentimes, an incentive spirometer is used to promote sustained inspiration. Diaphragmatic breathing exercises help promote the use of the diaphragm instead of accessory muscles to minimize energy expenditure. Patients who use accessory muscles when breathing are taught to use the diaphragm to minimize the work of breathing. Pursed-lip breathing exercises help create backpressure in the airways to prevent them from closing prematurely. By expiring through pursed lips (such as when blowing a candle or whistling), expiration is prolonged. Because patients with COPD use accessory muscles and have air trapping in the lung, they are often instructed to perform diaphragmatic breathing with pursed lip expiration. Segmental breathing exercises help promote ventilation to underventilated areas; facilitation strategies, such as the use of tactile stimuli over the area to be ventilated, usually precede instructions to breathe into or toward the area of the tactile stimulus.

Research indicates that breathing exercises and ventilatory training alter both the rate and depth of breathing. However, despite using these breathing techniques as interventions, they do not have an impact on alveolar oxygenation or gas exchange.

Coughing exercises help promote expectoration of mucus from the lower airways. Patients who are bedridden benefit from coughing exercises as a prophylactic intervention against pneumonia. Patients with pulmonary conditions that result in excessive secretions, such as chronic bronchitis or cystic fibrosis, also benefit from coughing exercises because coughing helps remove the secretions that are accumulating in the lungs. Finally, patients who have a weak cough, such as those with neuromuscular weakness or those who recently had chest surgery, benefit from coughing exercises for their prophylactic and therapeutic effects.

To perform an effective cough, a person should be able to inhale deeply, hold his or her breath momentarily, and expel the air forcefully. Sometimes, however, patients are unable to perform any or all of this sequence of events. Therefore, patients need to learn techniques that compensate for or facilitate coughing. Huffing is performed by forcefully exhaling air through an open airway.

For patients who are unable to perform an effective cough, huffing may be the first step in training the patient to do so. Self-assisted coughing is performed when the UEs are thrust inward and upward on the upper abdomen in Heimlich-like fashion. Another method of self-assisted coughing is by having the patient flex the trunk forward during the expulsive phase of the cough. With hands behind the neck, the patient doubles down on him- or herself in either the short sitting or long sitting positions. Patients who have weak abdominals, for example, can benefit from these examples of self-assisted coughing. During instances when a patient is unable to perform self-assisted coughing, therapist-assisted coughing is used. The hand of the therapist is placed over the upper abdomen and pushed upward and inward during the expulsive phase of the cough. Splinting is a coughing technique used by patients who have had chest surgery. By placing a towel or pillow over the surgery site, the patient is able to support and relieve the pressure on the suture during the cough.

Chest mobilization exercises help improve chest mobility by incorporating chest wall, trunk, and/or arm movements with breathing. For example, a patient whose trunk muscles are tight on one side, such as those with hemiplegia, may not expand that side of the trunk during inspiration. Another patient who manifests with a kyphotic posture and pectoral muscle tightness, such as seen among patients with Parkinson's disease, may not be able to retract the shoulders and extend the trunk during inspiration. In the former example, the patient may be instructed to perform side-bending and rotation exercises away from the side of tightness during inspiration. In the latter example, the patient may be instructed to perform bilateral UE flexion or horizontal abduction with trunk extension during inspiration.

Care should be exercised when performing chest or trunk mobilization exercises. Sometimes the patient's spine is purposely being exposed to conditions that would cause the spine to tighten to maintain an upright posture. The PTA should continually confer with the PT regarding questions or concerns about the plan of care.

Respiratory resistance training is used to strengthen and improve the endurance of respiratory muscles of patients who have weak abdominal and chest wall musculature. Patients with SCI, for example, may have reduced respiratory function because of the weakness of the respiratory muscles around the chest and abdomen. By using respiratory resistance training flow devices, patients are able to strengthen the respiratory muscles. Respiratory resistance training flow devices provide a training stimulus by decreasing the diameter through which air flows, thereby increasing the resistance to it. Inspiratory resistance loading provides resistance on inspiration, while concurrent flow devices provide resistance on inspiration and expiration. Over time, the muscles become stronger and more efficient when breathing.[19,20]

Bronchial hygiene techniques consist of noninvasive airway-clearance techniques that are designed to facilitate gas exchange by mobilizing and clearing secretions from the airways. Bronchial hygiene techniques include postural drainage and a variety of manual techniques, such as chest percussion, vibration, and shaking. Postural drainage involves placing the patient in positions that would allow the affected lung segments to be placed in the most vertical position, thereby allowing gravity to mobilize the secretions. Patients are required to assume the position for several minutes, after which they are instructed to cough voluntarily to expel any secretions that have been drained. To facilitate the mobilization of secretions, manual techniques may also be applied to the chest while the patient is in a postural drainage position. Percussion is performed by tapping on the chest over the lung segment being drained. After 2 to 3 minutes of chest percussion, vibration is applied while the patient exhales. In so doing, secretions that have been drained by positioning and/or percussion are moved centrally and superiorly for expectoration.

Aerobic exercise training is a hallmark of any cardiac or pulmonary rehabilitation program. Aerobic exercise training involves the exercising of large muscle groups for an extended period of time. Initially, the program may start at a low level and progress to a longer duration as the patient's cardiopulmonary fitness improves. An aerobic exercise program begins with a warm-up phase, followed by the aerobic phase, and finally a cool-down phase. The aerobic phase may involve

	Table 14-8 **Principles of Exercise Training**
Principle	**Description**
Specificity	The type of exercise chosen should be appropriate for the type of improvement expected.
Progression	Because the body adapts to exercise intensity, the amount and intensity of exercise should be increased gradually.
Overload	Fitness improves when workloads are greater than those normally encountered in daily life.
Reversibility	Any gains in physical fitness due to exercise can be reversed when physical activity ceases.
Tedium	A variety of exercises need to be incorporated in a training program to prevent the onset of tedium.

continuous training, interval training, circuit training, or circuit-interval training. Continuous training requires sustained effort until the exercise has been completed. Interval training involves alternating sessions of exercise and recovery. Circuit training allows for the training of specific muscle groups as the patient moves through the various stations in the circuit. Circuit-interval training involves the use of stations to train specific muscle groups and to provide recovery. In developing the exercise program, the PT should consider the following principles of exercise training—specificity, progression, overload, rest/recovery, and tedium—and apply them to the specific needs of the patient.[11,21] Table 14-8 provides a brief description of these principles.

When a patient is participating in an aerobic exercise training program, the PT should determine baseline measures and tailor an appropriate program for the patient, including the duration, intensity, and frequency of the program. The PT needs to determine acceptable parameters of physiological response, including heart rate, BP, and oxygen saturation, and communicate these to the PTA. Concurrently, the PTA needs to continually communicate with the PT regarding the status of the patient, including progress toward established goals. During the treatment session, the PTA should be able to recognize signs and symptoms of respiratory failure and cardiac decompensation, including dyspnea, angina, exercise intolerance, and others, and terminate the session as needed.

CONCLUSION

PTAs provide physical therapy services under the direction and supervision of a PT. When working with patients who are undergoing neurorehabilitation, the PTA may be directed to implement interventions specific to body system problems and functional limitations resulting from cardiovascular and pulmonary comorbidities that may interfere with or have an impact on the neurorehabilitation process. Toward this end, the PTA should be familiar with the anatomy and physiology of the cardiovascular and pulmonary systems and the impact of neuromuscular pathologies on the cardiovascular and pulmonary systems, and vice versa. Additionally, the PTA should be familiar with examination procedures and diagnostic tests that measure cardiovascular and pulmonary function. Finally, the PTA should be able to implement selected interventions, obtain data related to the interventions provided, and make modifications within the plan of care to progress the patient or to ensure that patient safety and comfort are maintained.

CASE STUDIES

CASE #1

A 74-year-old patient sustained a stroke 3 days ago and is currently in acute care. The patient has type 2 diabetes and has a history of coronary artery disease. The medical record indicates that the patient has dysarthria (slurred speech) and requires thickened liquids as part of the meal. For the past 3 days, the patient has been bedridden and is just now getting out of bed. Before doing so, however, the PT directs the PTA to take the vital signs of the patient in supine, then in sitting on the side of the bed, and finally in standing.

QUESTIONS

1. What cardiovascular and pulmonary complications should the PTA expect?

2. What is the rationale for monitoring vital signs in supine, sitting, and standing?

3. Is the information gathered from taking vital signs sufficient to progress the patient from one position to another? Why or why not?

4. When taking the vital signs, what parameters would be indicative of orthostatic hypotension?

5. How would the PTA determine the patient's tolerance for the activity?

CASE #2

A patient sustained an SCI at the level of T4 6 weeks ago. The patient is currently in inpatient rehab undergoing intensive physical therapy and occupational therapy. While performing wheelchair/mat transfers in the gym, the patient reports having a pounding headache. This is accompanied by redness of the face and upper body along with hypertensive readings on the sphygmomanometer.

QUESTIONS

1. Is the patient's current condition a medical emergency? Why or why not?

2. What steps should the PTA take initially to address the patient's current condition?

3. What relationship, if any, does the patient's SCI have to do with his current condition?

4. Is there anything that the PTA can do in the future to minimize the likelihood of events such as this?

5. What other cardiovascular and pulmonary complications should the PTA expect?

REFERENCES

1. Watchie J. *Cardiovascular and Pulmonary Physical Therapy: A Clinical Manual.* 2nd ed. St Louis, MO: Saunders; 2009.
2. Claydon VE, Steeves JD, Krassioukov A. Orthostatic hypotension following spinal cord injury: understanding clinical pathophysiology. *Spinal Cord.* 2006;44(6):341-351.
3. Dewar R, Sykes D, Mulkerrin E, Nicklason F, Thomas D, Seymour R. The effect of hemiplegia on blood pressure measurement in the elderly. *Postgrad Med J.* 1992;68(805):888-891.
4. Uijen AA, Hassink-Franke LJA. Blood pressure measurements in hemiparetic patients: Which arm? *Fam Med.* 2008;40(8):540.

5. Tovey C, Wyatt S. Diagnosis, investigation, and management of deep vein thrombosis. *BMJ.* 2003;326(7400): 1180-1184.

6. Wells PS, Anderson DR, Bormanis J, et al. Value of assessment of pretest probability of deep-vein thrombosis in clinical management. *Lancet.* 1997;350(9094):1795-1798.

7. Rochester CL. Exercise training in chronic obstructive pulmonary disease. *J Rehabil Res Dev.* 2003;40(5):59-80.

8. Dressendofer RH, Haykowsky MJ, Eves N. Exercise for people with chronic obstructive pulmonary disease. *ACSM Commentary.* http://www.acsm.org/docs/current-comments/exerciseforpersonswithcopd.pdf. Accessed September 29, 2012.

9. Fleg JL. Improving exercise tolerance in chronic heart failure? A tale of inspiration. *J Am Coll Cardiol.* 2008; 51(17):1672-1674.

10. Piña IL, Apstein CS, Balady GJ, et al. Exercise and heart failure a statement from the American Heart Association Committee on Exercise, Rehabilitation, and Prevention. *Circulation.* 2003;107(8):1210-1225.

11. Kisner C, Colby LA. *Therapeutic Exercise Foundations and Techniques.* 5th ed. Philadelphia, PA: FA Davis; 2007.

12. Hillegass E. *Essentials of Cardiopulmonary Physical Therapy.* 3rd ed. St Louis, MO: Saunders; 2011.

13. Karnath B. Digital clubbing: a sign of underlying disease. *Hospital Physician.* 2003;39:25-27.

14. Higgens D. Patient assessment part 5—measuring pulse. *Nurs Times.* 2008;104(11):24-25.

15. American Association of Critical Care Nurses. *Oxygen Saturation Monitoring by Pulse Oximetry.* 4th ed. Philadelphia, PA: Saunders; 2001.

16. Goodman CC, Fuller KS. *Pathology Implications for the Physical Therapist.* 3rd ed. St Louis, MO: Saunders; 2009.

17. US Department of Health & Human Services. National Heart, Lung and Blood Institute. 2011. What to expect during stress testing. http://www.nhlbi.nih.gov/health/health-topics/topics/stress/during.html. Accessed September 26, 2012.

18. Utter AC, Kang J, Robertson RJ. Perceived exertion. *ACSM Commentary.* http://www.acsm.org/docs/current-comments/perceivedexertion.pdf. Accessed September 29, 2012.

19. Piepoli MF, Conraads V, Corra U, et al. Exercise training in heart failure: from theory to practice. A consensus document of the Heart Failure Association and the European Association for Cardiovascular Prevention and Rehabilitation. *Eur J Heart Fail.* 2011;13(4):347-357.

20. Litchke LG, Russian CJ, Lloyd LK, et al. Effects of respiratory resistance training with a concurrent flow device on wheelchair athletes. *J Spinal Cord Med.* 2008;31(1):65-71.

21. Powers SK, Dodd SL. *Total Fitness & Wellness.* 3rd ed. San Francisco, CA: Pearson/Benjamin Cummings; 2009:32-42.

Please see accompanying Web site at
www.healio.com/books/neuroptavideos

15

Complementary Therapies or Integrative Health Care

Carol Davis, PT, DPT, EdD, MS, FAPTA
Megan E. Petrosky, PT, DPT

KEY WORDS

- Body talk
- Body work
- Ch'i
- Complementary therapies
- Energy work
- Holistic
- Integrative medicine
- Mind work

CHAPTER OBJECTIVES

- Identify the various types of complementary or integrative therapies.

- Differentiate traditional allopathic from holistic medicine.

- Identify various complementary therapies integrated within a traditional physical therapy intervention program.

- Discuss appropriate roles of the physical therapist assistant when taught or asked to use complementary therapies as part of intervention within both traditional and alternative environments.

INTRODUCTION

The 21st century has brought many changes to health care. Many individuals have advanced from knowing they have control over their health care (whether it is through their political choices or through their daily health habits) to actively owning the responsibility to change. The mentality of Americans has undergone a paradigm shift due to rising health care costs and has resulted in

Umphred DA, Lazaro RT, eds.
Neurorehabilitation for the Physical Therapist Assistant,
Second Edition (pp 411-424).
© 2014 SLACK Incorporated.

many people taking active steps to change not only how they take care of themselves but how they view their health. Health care in the coming years will focus more on the personal responsibility of the individual to manage health. Whether it is through monitoring our bodies, eating right, avoiding stress as much as possible, or partaking in exercises such as yoga that call for body awareness, individuals will no longer be passive participants in their health but will hold the control to make changes.

The face of rehabilitation in health care has changed as well. The increasing prevalence of patients seeking complementary and alternative therapies for acute and chronic illness[1,2] and the increasing number of health care professionals practicing complementary and alternative therapies have influenced the practice of rehabilitation in a major way. Complementary and alternative therapies embrace the concept of self-responsibility and allow individuals control over their health. Sixty-eight percent of people who responded to a survey reported trying at least one form of complementary therapy in their life, and 4 out of 10 individuals are currently using some form of complementary or alternative therapy.[3,4] Even if physical therapist assistants (PTAs) are not practitioners of alternative and complementary therapies themselves, having a rudimentary understanding of the various therapies that exist will enrich their practice and ability to connect with patients. PTAs, along with other therapists, are able to use holistic therapies to augment their practice with patients. When integrating a complementary therapy with traditional intervention, the physical therapist (PT) and PTA need to ask: "What factors make the administration of that therapy a part of rehabilitation?" rather than saying "yoga or tai chi." This chapter will answer that important question regarding justification of complementary therapies as part of physical therapy intervention.

HOLISTIC HEALTH

Complementary therapies are often termed *holistic*. What we mean by holistic therapies and holistic health is that the totality of a person can be seen to incorporate 4 areas of need and function: the physical (traditionally the body and movement), the intellectual (the brain and mind functions), the emotional (feelings and needs), and the spiritual (the eternal questions that help us organize meaning: Who am I? Why have I lived? Why am I ill? What am I to do?).[5] How these 4 areas function while interrelating in the world refers to the social aspect of need and function. This social aspect becomes the fifth area to consider.

In rehabilitation, the focus is on helping patients correct disorders of function that are primarily physical, but PTs and PTAs are strongly influenced by patients' intellectual, emotional, and spiritual needs as well. The PT and PTA who practice holistically question the patient in such a way—most pointedly while taking the history—that illuminates problems and unmet needs in all 5 areas and then advocate to see that all those needs are addressed.[5] Indeed, this is the ethical responsibility of all health care professionals.

Traditionally, fragmented care, in contrast to holistic care, is concerned only with the "part" of the person that falls under each professional's province. One result of this fragmentation is recognized when patients become labeled with their illness or disability, and therapists may respond to the question "Who are you seeing next?" with "The low back at 1:30." In Eisenberg et al's[1] classic study from the early 1990s on the patterns of use of holistic therapies in the United States, the increasing frequency of use of holistic therapies was, in part, reportedly due to patients' objections to the fragmentation and impersonal aspects of traditional health care. Astin's[2] later study found that people were turning to holistic and complementary therapies primarily because these approaches seemed more consistent with their ideas of health and healing.

COMPLEMENTARY AND ALTERNATIVE THERAPIES— INTEGRATIVE HEALTH CARE

In general, complementary and alternative therapies can be termed holistic and focus on using to advantage the inextricable link between mind and body. These therapies are administered in an effort to help a person regain health and stay healthy by facilitating the flow of that person's human energy or ch'i. Holistic theory posits that when human energy is balanced and flowing freely, it contributes to overall homeostasis, but when blocked, it interferes with health and renders the body and mind together vulnerable to pathogens and/or biochemical imbalance. The natural state of the human is to be in balance, to be healthy. Blocks to ch'i can occur from disruptions not just physically but in each of the 4 quadrants of function: physical, intellectual, emotional, and spiritual. Ideally, once a block to homeostasis of the ch'i occurs, a holistic practitioner would be able to detect that blockage and reverse it without the need for medications or major interventions. Evidence that people often heal themselves has made necessary the traditional double-blind, placebo-based clinical trial.[6]

Complementary and alternative therapies are nontraditional interventions that can be administered either as a substitute to (alternative to) traditional allopathic therapies or in conjunction with (complementary with) traditional therapies. As they become more prominently used, they are commonly integrated seamlessly into rehab programs. They can be classified as systems, approaches, or techniques within approaches.[7] Examples of health care systems include chiropractic, Ayurveda, traditional Chinese medicine, homeopathy, and naturopathy. Within systems are approaches such as acupuncture, acupressure, and herbal therapies in traditional Chinese medicine. Even more basic is a technique within an approach, such as auricular acupuncture, found within the system of traditional Chinese medicine, and transcendental meditation and sesame seed oil massage, both found within the system of Ayurveda.[7] One of the first categorizations of holistic approaches was found in the Chantilly report of the National Institutes of Health,[8] which listed the following categories of alternative therapies.

Alternative Systems of Medical Practice

Ironically, 70% to 90% of all health care worldwide is considered an alternative system to Western medical allopathic practice. Popular health care, community-based care, professionalized health care, traditional oriental medicine (including acupuncture and Ayurveda), homeopathy, anthroposophically extended medicine (elements of homeopathy and naturopathy), and naturopathic medicine[6] fall under the category of alternative medical practice.

Mind-Body Interventions

Psychotherapy, support groups, meditation, imagery, hypnosis, biofeedback, dance and music therapies, art therapy, prayer, mental healing, yoga, tai chi, Qigong, Alexander Technique, Feldenkrais Method, and Pilates are examples of mind-body interventions. Many interventions used by PTs and PTAs incorporate techniques drawn from the philosophies and techniques of these approaches.[8,9] Although the body of literature with regard to complementary and alternative therapies with neurological populations is small, patients with neurological dysfunctions are seeking complementary and alternative therapies more than individuals without neurological disorders.[10] Some of the most beneficial aspects of mind-body interventions are reductions in stress, anxiety, depression, and pain.[11]

Bioelectromagnetics Application to Medicine

Thermal applications of nonionizing radiation, radiofrequency hyperthermia, laser and radiofrequency surgery, low-energy laser, radiofrequency diathermy, nonthermal applications of pulsed electromagnetic field stimulation for bone repair, magnets, and nerve stimulation fall within this classification.[8,9,12]

Manual Healing Methods

Among this group are touch, manipulation, osteopathy, chiropractic, massage therapy, Rolfing, soma therapy, neuromuscular therapy, and biofield or bioenergy therapeutics, which include healing touch, noncontact therapeutic touch, myofascial release, both osteopathic and sustained release or Barnes Method, craniosacral therapy, Reiki, Jin Shin Do, and manual lymph drainage. Specific Human Energy Nexus therapy, a biofield method of treating psychosomatic disorders by releasing repressed and suppressed debilitation emotions, would also be classified here.[8]

Pharmacological and Biological Treatments

Certain pharmacological and biological treatments can be classified as alternative medications and are not accepted by allopathic medicine. These therapies are not regulated by the Food and Drug Administration. As a PTA, it is important to make sure that the patient knows the possible interactions of alternative therapies while taking medication prescribed by their physician, and they should be informed to notify the physician of any additional medication or treatments. The following list includes some of those alternative medications:

- Chondroitin sulfate derived from shark cartilage has been shown to have a protective effect within joints[13]
- Marijuana is legally prescribed in certain states for pain control and is being studied to evaluating its effectiveness on spasticity in patients with neurological dysfunctions[14]
- Evening primrose oil: Linoleic acid found in sunflower seeds and safflower oil is used to relieve some symptoms of multiple sclerosis[15]
- Biologically guided chemotherapy[8]
- St John's Wart has been shown to assist with depression and anxiety[16]
- Ginkgo biloba is said to improve circulation and prevent ischemia in the central nervous system, leading to a neuroprotective effect. It is also known for improving memory[17]

Diet and Nutrition

For the prevention of chronic disease, Dean Ornish's program, the Pritikin program, Junger's detox plan,[18] and the Atkins plan are based on the philosophy that nutritional intake and, thus, diet are critical for not only maintaining health but also preventing common diseases such as diabetes, cardiovascular disease, cancer, and Alzheimer's.[8,9,19]

COMPLEMENTARY THERAPIES COMMONLY INTEGRATED IN REHABILITATION

Energy medicine is another term given to holistic therapies integrated within traditional rehabilitation therapies such as neuromuscular facilitation, exercise, and work hardening. All medicine and all health care, traditional and holistic, can be seen as energetically based because we are influencing the flows of energy in each of our interventions, whether that flow of energy is found in blood flow, nerve flow, lymph flow, neurotransmitter flow, neuropeptide flow, steroid flow, hormone flow, or the flow of thoughts.[8] The goal of clinicians as facilitators of healing integrating complementary or holistic therapies is to help restore normal function, balance, and rhythm to the body systems so that the body can once again be in homeostasis and a state of healing or self-regulation. As practitioners, therapists become transmitters of a healing energy that surrounds the patient as well as the clinician. By way of intention, the energy is focused through the clinician into patients so that resonance is achieved.[20]

The Third Edition of *Complementary Therapies in Rehabilitation: Evidence for Efficacy in Therapy, Prevention, and Wellness*[7] lists the following as approaches commonly used by therapists in rehabilitation settings. PTAs are able to study and practice these techniques to add to their repertoire of treatment options.

Body Work

Therapeutic Massage

Therapeutic massage is an array of ancient healing practices of manual therapies that include stroking, tapping, stretching, shaking, vibrating, rolling, rubbing, friction, clapping, gliding, kneading, percussion, and manipulation of tissue. This is practiced with the intent of altering the structure of the tissue and the consciousness of the recipient. It engages the musculoskeletal, neurological, lymphatic, and circulatory systems.[21] Many traditional physical therapy techniques, although described according to neuromusculoskeletal research and science, could also be considered body work.

Craniosacral Therapy

This holistic manual therapy that energetically manipulates the flow of the cerebrospinal fluid (CSF) within the craniosacral system promotes self-correction and healing throughout the entire body. The practitioner restricts and then allows movement of CSF according to the rhythm of breath and pulse of the flow of the CSF. This technique has been found to improve pain, sleeping habits, and overall well-being.[22,23]

Myofascial Release (Barnes Method)

Myofascial release is a holistic manual therapy that focuses on releasing inappropriate fascial restrictions that distort tissue and the shape of the body. These restrictions can be found within the macrolevel of muscles and fascial layers down to the cellular level in such a way that flow or normal fascial and muscle gliding is restricted. Fascial tightness causes the body to lose its physiological adaptive capacity, and homeostasis is disrupted because fascia encapsulates muscle, bone, and organs. It is believed that sustained myofascial release facilitates the release of electrons through a piezoelectric effect to restore the length of the fascia by "releasing" primarily the ground substance of the fascia so that soft tissue is restored to its original shape.[24] This release is not only able to be felt by the clinician and patient as a tightness that "melts" or gives way, but it is able to be seen using dynamic ultrasound and is correlated with pain reduction.[25] Individuals with spinal cord injury could benefit from myofascial release due to restrictions secondary to cervical and lumbar fusions.

Complete Decongestive Therapy (Manual Lymphatic Drainage)

Manual lymphatic drainage (MLD) is one component of a comprehensive lymphedema management program termed *complete decongestive therapy*. In many European countries, this approach is considered traditional physical therapy intervention. In the United States, lymph drainage is generally used with postsurgical cancer patients. Molecular and energetic flows are affected. Complete decongestive therapy consists of skin care, lymphatic massage, and bandaging of the swollen limb, followed by active exercises.[26] Individuals who undergo MLD can experience decreases in limb girth and volume that significantly affect the gait and lead to increased quality of life and the ability to perform activities of daily living (ADL).[27]

Rolfing or Structural Integration

Developed by Ida Rolf, this is a manual body-based therapy that mechanically and energetically changes the tissues of the body. The myofascial system is aligned so that gravity flows through the body tissues and supports upright posture and movement. In this way, structure and function are realigned to promote health and homeostasis. Structural integration can increase the ability to process sensory information and make a patient more receptive, reduce anxiety, and improve neuromotor organization and overall well-being.[28] Deviations in posture and tissue restrictions serve to locate dysfunction. The therapy consists of 10 systematic and prescribed sessions of both structural integration and intense deep connective tissue manipulation to restore appropriate tissue length and upright posture.[29] The patient takes an active part in the session by moving his or her body part while pressure is applied as tissue gives way.

Mind and Body Work

Tai Chi

Tai chi is described as choreography of body and mind. Originally a martial art, tai chi movements are a response to an attacker. That attacker's own movement and, thus, his or her energy, is used against that person by moving in such a way as to sidestep the attacker and throw him or her off balance. There are numerous forms of tai chi containing as many as 108 postures and movements. Family names are associated with different forms, such as Wu, Ch'en, Ch'uan, and Chih. Each is distinctive but follows classic tai chi principles that are based on integrating the mind and body to facilitate the flow of energy in the movements.[14] Tai chi is a low-impact form of movement exercise that has been shown by well-documented research studies to improve respiratory status, functional balance, and aerobic control.[30] Tai chi has grown in use with the neurological populations, such as individuals with Parkinson's disease, chronic migraines, and multiple sclerosis. The psychological aspects of tai chi are also important, such as stress and anxiety reduction.[31–33]

Biofeedback

Biofeedback is a process of electronically using information from the patient's body to teach that person to recognize processes taking place inside his or her body, brain, nervous system, and muscles. Instruments reveal conscious and unconscious actions that are occurring, and patients or clients are then instructed to use this sensory feedback information to change unwanted activity. In this way, people are able to learn how to control unwanted activity, such as muscle tension, blood pressure, and congestion of blood in the vessels of the brain that cause migraine headaches.[34] Biofeedback is also important with individuals who might have a decreased sense of self and awareness of surroundings, such as people who have had a stroke or have Parkinson's disease. Therapists use verbal, visual, and kinesthetic biofeedback through voice, demonstration, and manual contacts every day and often do not recognize when one system is contradicting the other. With the advent of interactive video gaming, such as the Nintendo Wii, the therapist can integrate this software into the therapy session to give real-time feedback to patients.[35] This type of biofeedback is effective, inexpensive, and easy to access for PTs and PTAs. The use of game-oriented training sessions as biofeedback can easily be used to augment home programs in outpatient rehabilitation. The key to success of this type of intervention is that the patient enjoys the activity and practices often between therapy sessions, and that the feedback can change with improvement in skill and is appropriate to the ability of the person.[36]

Yoga

There are many forms or approaches to yoga. The most commonly used in rehabilitation is hatha yoga. Yoga is derived from a Sanskrit verb meaning to unite, as in uniting the body, mind, and spirit. Classic yoga practice includes more than body movements and positions, or asanas, performed with mindfulness and attention, especially to breathing. It is a broad philosophical model of health based on human experience. Hatha yoga is especially useful in rehabilitation to facilitate patients' attention to the importance of breathing and moving mindfully through a full range of motion (ROM). Bringing attention to the breath unites body and mind, and the meditative movement facilitates the spirit to be "in the now."[37] Integrating movement with body awareness, as practiced in yoga, reduces stress, depression, and anxiety.[38]

Alexander Technique

Based on the study of his own habits of movement that interfered with function, F. M. Alexander developed a technique whereby the teacher helps the student organize the position of the head to the neck and back, redistributing muscle tone and opening up consciousness. Poor habits of movement are identified to the patient by way of touch and direction, and the patient is directed to change in ways that facilitate conscious control of movement, overriding poor habits of motion. Choice is thus given to the patient to move in ways that reinforce an "extended field of consciousness."[39] The Alexander Technique can influence control of voluntary movement and balance and was shown to improve the ability of individuals with Parkinson's disease to conduct ADL.[40]

Feldenkrais Method

Each person develops patterns of movement to maximize his or her basic needs when growing to maturity. Many of these highly individual patterns of movement are limited in skill, flexibility, and practice. Mental and physical aspects are incorporated into these habitual patterns. Some movements optimize physical performance while others are inefficient ways of moving. Moshe Feldenkrais developed a method of movement that would assist people in functioning at a higher level. Efficient postural patterns and movements away from and back toward those postures are taught. Those patterns are performed with a minimal amount of effort accompanied by a well-developed kinesthetic sense of awareness. In this way, a person should easily recover from any movement or postural challenge or trauma. Functional integration is a one-on-one, hands-on approach, and awareness through movement is a verbally directed movement process that can be performed in groups.[41] The Feldenkrais Method can translate to improvements in level of perceived pain, in the ability to perform ADL, and, most importantly, in patients' quality of life.[42] Applying movement principles coupled with self-awareness takes patients beyond their limitations and opens up new possibilities of fluid, pain-free movement.

Pilates

Joseph Pilates overcame his physical frailties by developing this exercise method that is performed on mats and on several types of apparatus that use springs to assist an injured individual in successfully completing movements that would be otherwise restricted. By altering spring tension or increasing the challenge of gravity, an individual can be assisted in strengthening toward functional movement. The Pilates environment consists of various appliances such as the reformer, trapeze table, chair, ladder barrel, and mat. The focus of exercise is on strengthening the core or trunk so that the extremities can be supported in movement. Attention is given to the breath, alignment, and smoothness of movement.[43] Symmetry can be emphasized using the reformer, on which both lower extremities can go through a motion at the same time with graduated springs to assist or resist the movement.

Body Talk

Body talk is the active experience of observing and analyzing the posture, appearance, and movements of an individual to evaluate various factors involved in the patient's health state. Body talk combines concepts and research from Western medicine with techniques of traditional Chinese medicine, yoga, and acupuncture.[44] Body talk works on the premise that the body can be thrown out of homeostasis where internal energy is disrupted, which leads to disease and dysfunction in the body. Along with other complementary therapies, body talk views the patient as an active participant who is capable of directing and channeling energy to encourage healing. The body talk philosophy uses techniques such as breathing, rearranging energy, hands-on analysis of energy blockages, and visualization techniques.[45]

Energy Work

Reiki

Reiki is a Japanese word meaning universal life force that animates all living things. The meaning of Reiki is similar to that of *ch'i*, *prana*, *pneuma*, or *ruah*. Reiki is a healing system that channels the universal life force surrounding all of us through the practitioner's hands into the mind and body of the recipient, promoting energy balance, healing, and a state of well-being within the physical, mental, emotional, social, and spiritual domains. Anyone can learn Reiki, but it must be transferred from a Reiki master to the student during the induction process called *attunement*. The learner opens up to channel the energy to another. Intentionality is critical to this process. Reiki practitioners focus attention of thought or concentration in a specific way to bring about a healing or balance by way of energy flow.[46] Evidence for the use of Reiki for improving function in neurological illnesses is weak, but in one study, Reiki therapy led to improved pain and anxiety associated with chronic illness.[47]

Qigong

Qigong is the foundational energy that underlies all energy techniques, including tai chi. This ancient Chinese medicine philosophy states that health and healing depend on a balance of vital energy, a still mind, and controlled emotions. Physical dysfunction results from disordered patterns of long-standing energy. To balance and restore energy flow, Qigong uses exercises that include slow, controlled, nonimpact-type movements and postures that gain control over the center of gravity. Qigong integrates deep breathing, movement, and postures while stressing expansion of the base of support, trunk control, and improving rotation of the trunk and coordination of isolated extremity motions. The meditative component serves to make an individual more aware of his or her body, enhancing the ability to control muscle tension, posture, and movement and facilitating a peace of mind that leads to an overall sense of well-being.[48] A bounty of literature exists showing improvements in quality of life and balance and a decrease in falls. Studies promote Qigong and tai chi as effective additions to traditional physical therapy practice.[49]

Magnets

Often grouped with crystals, magnets are thought to be worthless in health and healing by most allopathic health practitioners. The research, as limited as it is, indicates that there may indeed be a healing effect of magnetic energy on the body and mind. Magnets exert their influence by way of a magnetic field emanating from them. *Unipolar* and *bipolar* refer to the presence of which poles (north, south, or both) face the surface. Manufacturers claim one or the other is more therapeutically beneficial. In the literature, many claims are made that are not substantiated with good research. However, some studies with patients who are medically diagnosed with pain, wounds, and fibromyalgia indicate that magnets seem to offer a therapeutic effect.[50] The literature must be studied with a careful eye to ascertain the true benefits of which strength of magnet and which polarity seemed to be most beneficial.[50] The therapeutic community needs to be aware of this research to advise patients who are seeking relief. Although there is benefit to magnetic therapy, the quality of magnets that are shown to have benefit are not widely available to the general population.

Acupuncture

Having been in existence as a therapeutic modality for more than 2000 years, acupuncture is one part of the system of traditional Chinese medicine. Its theory is based on the concept that the flow of ch'i can be influenced by mechanically and energetically stimulating acupuncture points that lie along pathways (or meridians) to restore balance and flow. Disease results in and from a deficiency of flow of ch'i. Acupuncture physicians study the signs that indicate an imbalance in one or both forms of ch'i, the yin and yang energy. These clinicians learn how to facilitate flow through needling the acupuncture points, direct stairways to the pathways of flow (or meridians).[51] A study by Hsing et al using electroacupuncture, not traditional acupuncture, on stroke patients found significant improvements in functional ability as measured by the National Institutes of Health Stroke Scale.[52] Like any intervention, the location and application of treatment was extremely important, because the sham electroacupuncture group showed no improvement as compared with the treatment group.[52]

Therapeutic Touch

A manual therapy developed by Delores Kreiger, RN, PhD, and Dora Kunz, therapeutic touch is considered a nursing intervention in which the patient or client is not touched by the practitioner, but the electromagnetic energy field of that person is manually manipulated in such a way as to remove blocks and disturbances in it.[53] In this way, noncontact therapeutic touch facilitates an improvement in energy flow in the environment around the patient so the natural healing powers of the patient can be maximized. This holistic therapy is one of the few that have been taught in college curricula for credit because of Kreiger's position as an academic.[53]

THE ROLE OF THE PHYSICAL THERAPIST ASSISTANT IN THE INTEGRATION OF COMPLEMENTARY AND ALTERNATIVE THERAPIES IN REHABILITATION

Each of these (and other) complementary therapies carries with it a learning process requiring that the person performing the therapy be schooled in the theory and practice of the technique. Some require extensive coursework followed by examination and certification. Others require learning of the technique but do not require official certification. When offered in a rehabilitation setting, the PTA, acting within the scope of practice of an assistant to the PT, must work with the PT in instituting complementary therapies. For a PTA to be delegated the total responsibility of interventions using the following therapies, that PTA must be licensed or certified by agencies providing education in this modality: acupuncture, biofeedback, yoga, Pilates, Reiki, MLD, Alexander Technique, Feldenkrais Method, or Rolfing.

When offering modalities that require certification without the supervision of a PT, the PTA should step outside the boundaries of practice as a PTA and practice according to the stipulations of the license or certification that the complementary therapy offers. In other words, the PTA should perform as a certified or licensed complementary therapy practitioner but not as a PTA. And, for risk management purposes, a PTA should provide these therapies outside of traditional allopathic health care environments. Within an acute care, rehabilitation, or long-term care environment, the PTA will provide interventions delegated by the PT. For that reason, autonomy of practice by the PTA using any of these approaches would not be appropriate and would place the PTA's certification or license at risk. If the PT is licensed or certified to offer the above therapies, then the PTA can assist the PT according to the instructions of the PT in the rehabilitation setting. This is true of all of the complementary therapies described.

There is risk associated with the use of complementary therapies in traditional Western medical management settings. For example, if a PT decides that a patient would benefit from yoga exercises and the PTA has been educated in the application of yoga as exercise, then the PTA is still required to work under the overall supervision of the PT even if the PTA knows more about yoga than the PT. Once a complementary therapy becomes part of the physical therapy program administered within the practice environment of the PT, the PT is still responsible for the process of patient care.

THE IMPORTANCE OF A GOOD COMMUNICATING RELATIONSHIP BETWEEN PHYSICAL THERAPIST AND PHYSICAL THERAPIST ASSISTANT

The optimal relationship between the PT and the PTA requires ongoing communication and decision making for the benefit of the patient or client. This does not change with the integration of complementary and alternative therapies. The application of these energy-based techniques requires special education and development of the intention of the PT and PTA to be successful in using them with patients and clients. Ideally, the PT and PTA will learn, for example, myofascial release or Pilates or craniosacral therapy together and, thus, both will be able to benefit patients with these holistic methods as complementary to their rehabilitation process. Communication is critical to the effective partnership of the PT and PTA. However, in the rehabilitation setting when complementary therapies are offered to patients, whether it is magnets, myofascial release, therapeutic touch, or MLD, the PTA must work under the specific supervision of the PT no matter how skilled he or she is in the application of these complementary therapies.

CONCLUSION

Holistic therapies have a great deal to offer in helping patients regain a higher quality of life and empowerment toward better health. At the least, these approaches offer energy-based methods that are often helpful when all traditional therapies have failed. At the most, holistic therapies require an interaction with patients that restores therapeutic presence to the application of physical therapy; they move both the PT and the PTA out of the business mode of the managed care administration of therapy and back into an emphasis on the whole person and empowerment. Sacrosanct in this process of administering complementary therapies is the mandated supervisory relationship of the PT and PTA. No matter how knowledgeable the PTA is in the administration of holistic therapies, the PT maintains supervisory control of the patient care process when practiced within Western medical environments. As the PTA is delegated additional responsibilities for the intervention of patients receiving physical therapy, having training in complementary approaches should provide an environment that leads to a feeling of wellness and empowerment within the patient. Hopefully, empathic communication among the PT, the PTA, and the patient will round out the treatment so that the experience is fulfilling for each person.

CASE STUDIES

CASE #1

Mrs. J was referred to Dr. Hagen (DPT) for examination and evaluation of balance problems. Dr. Hagen was a staff PT in an outpatient neurorehabilitation center of a large teaching hospital. Upon examination, Dr. Hagen determined that Mrs. J, who was in good health overall, had developed her unsteady gait after moving from her 2-story home to an apartment where she no longer had any stairs to climb. As a result of using the elevator and only walking on flat surfaces, her balance problems began from increasing weakness in her hips and knees. Examination using the Berg Balance Scale, including the forward reach and manual muscle testing, revealed that her problem was muscle weakness. She scored 3(-) in hip extensors, knee extensors, and ankle dorsiflexors bilaterally. No inner ear problems were noted, but she was experiencing some difficulty with her vision and her hearing.

Dr. Hagen consulted with PD, a PTA who worked with her in the neurorehabilitation setting. Together, they devised an exercise program that included systematic strengthening of her pelvis and lower extremities and suggested participation in a group tai chi class taught by PD, the PTA, on Mondays, Wednesdays, and Fridays from 10:30 am to 12:00 pm.

PD had studied tai chi with a tai chi master and had gained skill to the extent that she was able to teach tai chi at the rehabilitation center, as a PTA under the supervision of the director of physical therapy. The state in which they practiced allowed her to practice out of line of sight of the supervising PT, and her group met in a quiet common area near the main rehab gym. PD employed the assistance of several aids and family members as "spotters" for her patients during the group session.

Mrs. J recovered her strength very rapidly with exercises and tai chi. PD did a follow-up assessment of her balance and reported that Mrs. J was functioning safely, and she felt she was ready for the supervising PT to do a final discharge evaluation. Mrs. J liked the tai chi group exercises so much that she enrolled in a wellness center group and continued with tai chi for several months.

Questions

1. Was an appropriate protocol used by both the PT and PTA with the delegation to the PTA of a group class that included the complementary approach referred to as tai chi?

2. Once Mrs. J met the objectives of the traditional interventions as well as the functional balance activities of the tai chi, was it appropriate for the PTA to recommend that Mrs. J go back to the supervising PT for final examination and discharge, or could the PTA, as a tai chi instructor, do this independently?

Case #2

Mr. K, a 65-year-old executive at a local bank, was evaluated by PT Connie W for beginning Parkinson's symptoms that were limiting his participation. Upon examination, Mr. K showed no involvement in his handwriting and moderate rigidity in his back and shoulders. He held his left arm in slightly more flexion at the elbow, and the fingers of his left hand were straight with slight metacarpophalangeal flexion. His head flexed forward 6 inches; his left arm showed diminished swing with gait, and his steps were shortened to a 12-inch stride. His turn-around time to the left was slower than the right, taking several more steps to complete. No shuffling gait was noted. No detectable tremor was found, but Mr. K reported that a slight tremor of his left hand was present upon awakening some mornings. He had full animation of his face, no seborrhea; his speech was clear and easily understood, but quiet. He reported no difficulty in self-care. He was quite concerned about how this diagnosis would affect his career at the bank, which included interaction with many powerful people who trusted him with their money. He was most anxious that he not show any sign of weakness or pathology.

Muscle strength was normal throughout. ROM in left shoulder flexion was slightly diminished to 150 degrees. Trunk rotation and cervical rotation were limited to two-thirds normal. With regard to balance, one-legged stance time was less than 10 seconds on either foot. He was able to stand from a chair 10 times in 30 seconds without using his arms to assist. He was able to pick up a pencil off the floor, but was unable to tandem stand. Connie W, the PT, devised a therapeutic program composed of myofascial release, which she performed focusing on releasing deep fascial restrictions on the psoas area bilaterally, opening up the occipital ridge, the thoracic inlet, and pectoral areas and working to improve fascial length for trunk rotation and shoulder flexion. Exercises were designed to emphasize deep breathing and increasing fluidity of spine rotation and gait. In addition, she had Mr. K practicing one-legged stance and tandem stance at the sink at home and wanted him to start practicing yoga on a regular basis.

Estelle F, a PTA working with Connie W in the rehabilitation center, was also a certified yoga instructor and had a part–time evening and weekend yoga practice in a small storefront location quite near the rehabilitation center. Mr. K's PT knew that Estelle F, PTA, was also an excellent yoga instructor, who specialized in assisting people with disabilities in assuming postures with supporting towels and who emphasized therapeutic breathing. She suggested to Mr. K that he enroll in her yoga classes on Tuesday and Thursday evenings. Thus, Connie W, PT, would see Mr. K as an outpatient in the rehabilitation center on Mondays and Fridays, and Mr. K would take yoga on Tuesday and Thursday evenings. This plan appealed to Mr. K, who sensed that he really must not be "all that disabled" if he could take yoga as part of his physical therapy.

Estelle F (PTA) spoke with Connie W (PT) about Mr. K when he enrolled in her evening yoga class. Connie W was able to share her examination and evaluation information on Mr. K with Estelle F and suggest an emphasis on trunk rotation and upper extremity range in addition to yoga breathing exercises. Estelle F was able to supplement Mr. K's rehabilitation by implementing these suggestions in Mr. K's yoga practice with much success.

QUESTIONS

1. Would the myofascial release techniques and the traditional exercises be considered physical therapy?

2. Would recommending yoga as a life activity be considered physical therapy, and should the PTA consider her class as part of the PT interventions designed by the PT? If so, how would the PT and PTA deal with the concept of supervision? If not, why would the PT recommend the individual enroll in the yoga class?

3. Once the individual completed the intervention aspect of the traditional PT program and continued with the yoga, would it still be considered physical therapy?

REFERENCES

1. Eisenberg DM, Kessler RC, Foster C, Norlock FE, Calkins DR, Delbanco TL. Unconventional medicine in the United States. Prevalence, costs, and patterns of use. *N Engl J Med.* 1993;328(4):246-252.
2. Astin JA. Why patients use alternative medicine: results of a national study. *JAMA.* 1998;279(19):1548-1553.
3. Kessler RC, Davis RB, Foster DF, et al. Long-term trends in the use of complementary and alternative medical therapies in the United States. *Ann Intern Med.* 2001;135(4):262-268.
4. Barnes PM, Powell-Griner E, McFann K, Nahin RL. Complementary and alternative medicine use among adults: United States, 2002. *Adv Data.* 2004;(343):1-19.
5. Davis CM. *Patient Practitioner Interaction: An Experiential Manual for Developing the Art of Health Care.* 5th ed. Thorofare, NJ: SLACK Incorporated; 2011.
6. Davis CM. Complementary therapies in rehabilitation. In: Gonzalez EG, Myers SM, Edelstein JE, Lieberman J, Downey, JA, eds. *Downey and Darling's Physiological Basis of Rehabilitation Medicine.* 3rd ed. Boston, MA: Butterworth-Heinemann; 2001:777-793.
7. Davis CM. *Complementary Therapies in Rehabilitation: Evidence for Efficacy in Therapy, Prevention, and Wellness.* 3rd ed. Thorofare, NJ: SLACK Incorporated; 2009.
8. *Alternative Medicine: Expanding Medical Horizons.* The Chantilly, Virginia, workshop report on alternative medical systems and practices in the United States to the National Institutes of Health. Pittsburgh, PA: Superintendent of Documents; 1992.
9. Spencer JW, Jacobs JJ. *Complementary/Alternative Medicine: An Evidence-Based Approach.* 2nd ed. St Louis, MO: Mosby; 2002.

10. Wells ER, Phillips RS, McCarthy EP. Patterns of mind-body therapies in adults with common neurological conditions. *Neuroepidemiology.* 2011;36(1):46-51.

11. Wahbeh H, Elsas SM, Oken BS. Mind-body interventions: applications in neurology. *Neurology.* 2008;70(24): 2321-2328.

12. Shen WW, Zhao JH. Pulsed electromagnetic fields stimulation affects BMD and local factor production of rats with disuse osteoporosis. *Bioelectromagnetics.* 2010;31(2):113-119.

13. Imada K, Oka H, Kawasaki D, Miura N, Sato T, Ito A. Anti-arthritic action mechanisms of natural chondroitin sulfate in human articular chondrocytes and synovial fibroblasts. *Biol Pharm Bull.* 2010;33(3):410-414.

14. Husseini L, Leussink VI, Warnke C, Hartung HP, Kieseier BC. Cannabinoids for symptomatic therapy of multiple sclerosis [in German]. *Nervenarzt.* 2012;83(6):695-704.

15. Namazi MR. The beneficial and detrimental effects of linoleic acid on autoimmune disorders. *Autoimmunity.* 2004;37(1):73-75.

16. Benzie IFF, Wachtel-Galor S. *Herbal Medicine: Biomolecular and Clinical Aspects.* 2nd ed. Boca Raton, FL: CRC Press; 2011

17. Mdzinarishvili A, Sumbria R, Lang D, Klein J. Ginkgo extract EGb761 confers neuroprotection by reduction of glutamate release in ischemic brain. *J Pharm Pharm Sci.* 2012;15(1):94-102.

18. Junger A. *Clean: The Revolutionary Program to Restore the Body's Natural Ability to Heal Itself.* New York, NY: Harper Collins; 2009.

19. Accardi G, Caruso C, Colonna-Romano G, Camarda C, Monastero R, Candore G. Can Alzheimer disease be a form of type 3 diabetes? *Rejuvenation Res.* 2012;15(2):217-221.

20. Oschman JL. *Energy Medicine: The Scientific Basis.* New York, NY: Churchill-Livingstone; 2000.

21. Kahn J. Therapeutic massage and rehabilitation. In: Davis CM, ed. *Complementary Therapies in Rehabilitation: Evidence for Efficacy in Therapy, Prevention, and Wellness.* 3rd ed. Thorofare, NJ: SLACK Incorporated; 2009: 53-72.

22. Jäkel A, von Hauenschild P. Therapeutic effects of cranial osteopathic manipulative medicine: a systematic review. *J Am Osteopath Assoc.* 2011;111(12):685-693.

23. Wahl DG. Craniosacral therapy. In: Davis CM, ed. *Complementary Therapies in Rehabilitation: Evidence for Efficacy in Therapy, Prevention, and Wellness.* 3rd ed. Thorofare, NJ: SLACK Incorporated; 2009:75-87.

24. Barnes JF. Myofascial release: the missing link in traditional treatment. In: Davis CM, ed. *Complementary Therapies in Rehabilitation: Evidence for Efficacy in Therapy, Prevention, and Wellness.* 3rd ed. Thorofare, NJ: SLACK Incorporated; 2009:89-109.

25. Tozzi P, Bongiorno D, Vitturini C. Fascial release effects on patients with non-specific cervical or lumbar pain. *J Bodyw Mov Ther.* 2011;15(4):405-416.

26. Funk B. Complete decongestive therapy. In: Davis CM, ed. *Complementary Therapies in Rehabilitation: Evidence for Efficacy in Therapy, Prevention, and Wellness.* 3rd ed. Thorofare, NJ: SLACK Incorporated; 2009:113-125.

27. Cohen MD. Complete decongestive physical therapy in a patient with secondary lymphedema due to orthopedic trauma and surgery of the lower extremity. *Phys Ther.* 2011;91(11):1618-1626.

28. Jacobson E. Structural integration, an alternative method of manual therapy and sensorimotor education. *J Altern Complement Med.* 2011;17(10):891-899.

29. Deutsch J. The Ida Rolf method of structural integration. In: Davis CM, ed. *Complementary Therapies in Rehabilitation: Evidence for Efficacy in Therapy, Prevention, and Wellness.* 3rd ed. Thorofare, NJ: SLACK Incorporated; 2009:127-133.

30. Bottomley JM. T'ai chi: choreography of body and mind. In: Davis CM, ed. *Complementary Therapies in Rehabilitation: Evidence for Efficacy in Therapy, Prevention, and Wellness.* 3rd ed. Thorofare, NJ: SLACK Incorporated; 2009:137-157.

31. Li F, Harmer P, Fitzgerald K, et al. Tai chi and postural stability in patients with Parkinson's disease. *N Engl J Med.* 2012;366(6):511-519.

32. Field T. Tai chi research review. *Complement Ther Clin Pract.* 2011;17(3):141-146.

33. Wahbeh H, Elsas SM, Oken BS. Mind-body interventions: applications in neurology. *Neurology.* 2008;70(24): 2321-2328.

34. Bottomley JM. Biofeedback: connecting the body and mind. In: Davis CM, ed. *Complementary Therapies in Rehabilitation: Evidence for Efficacy in Therapy, Prevention, and Wellness.* 3rd ed. Thorofare, NJ: SLACK Incorporated; 2009:159-179.

35. Esculier JF, Vaudrin J, Bériault P, Gagnon K, Tremblay LE. Home-based balance training programme using Wii Fit with balance board for Parkinson's disease: a pilot study. *J Rehabil Med.* 2012;44(2):144-150.

36. Byl K, Byl N, Byl M. Integrating technology into clinical practice in neurological rehabilitation. In: Umphred DA, Lazaro R, Roller M, Burton G, eds. *Umphred's Neurological Rehabilitation.* 6th ed. St Louis, MO: Elsevier; 2013.

37. Taylor MJ. Yoga therapeutics: an ancient practice in a 21st century setting. In: Davis CM, ed. *Complementary Therapies in Rehabilitation: Evidence for Efficacy in Therapy, Prevention, and Wellness.* 3rd ed. Thorofare, NJ: SLACK Incorporated; 2009:183-204.

38. Smith JA, Greer T, Sheets T, Watson S. Is there more to yoga than exercise? *Altern Ther Health Med.* 2011;17(3):22-29.
39. Zuck D. The Alexander technique. In: Davis CM, ed. *Complementary Therapies in Rehabilitation: Evidence for Efficacy in Therapy, Prevention, and Wellness.* 3rd ed. Thorofare, NJ: SLACK Incorporated; 2009:207-224.
40. Woodman JP, Moore NR. Evidence for the effectiveness of Alexander Technique lessons in medical and health-related conditions: a systematic review. *Int J Clin Pract.* 2012;66(1):98-112.
41. Stephens J, Miller TM. Feldenkrais method in rehabilitation: using functional integration and awareness through movement to explore new possibilities. In: Davis CM, ed. *Complementary Therapies in Rehabilitation: Evidence for Efficacy in Therapy, Prevention, and Wellness.* 3rd ed. Thorofare, NJ: SLACK Incorporated; 2009:227-243.
42. Connors KA, Pile C, Nichols ME. Does the Feldenkrais Method make a difference? An investigation into the use of outcome measurement tools for evaluating changes in clients. *J Bodyw Mov Ther.* 2011;15(4):446-452.
43. Anderson B. Pilates rehabilitation. In: Davis CM, ed. *Complementary Therapies in Rehabilitation: Evidence for Efficacy in Therapy, Prevention, and Wellness.* 3rd ed. Thorofare, NJ: SLACK Incorporated; 2009:245-256.
44. Gale NK. From body-talk to body-stories: body work in complementary and alternative medicine. *Sociol Health Ill.* 2011;33(2):237-251.
45. International BodyTalk Association. BodyTalk principles. http://www.bodytalksystem.com/learn/bodytalk/principles.cfm. 2012. Accessed May 19, 2012.
46. Singg S. Reiki: an alternative and complementary healing therapy. In: Davis CM, ed. *Complementary Therapies in Rehabilitation: Evidence for Efficacy in Therapy, Prevention, and Wellness.* 3rd ed. Thorofare, NJ: SLACK Incorporated; 2009:261-277.
47. Lee MS, Pittler MH, Ernst E. Effects of reiki in clinical practice: a systematic review of randomised clinical trials. *Int J Clin Pract.* 2008;62(6):947-954.
48. Bottomley JM. Qi gong for health and healing. In: Davis CM, ed. *Complementary Therapies in Rehabilitation: Evidence for Efficacy in Therapy, Prevention, and Wellness.* 3rd ed. Thorofare, NJ: SLACK Incorporated; 2009:279-302.
49. Jahnke R, Larkey L, Rogers C, Etnier J, Lin F. A comprehensive review of health benefits of qigong and tai chi. *Am J Health Promot.* 2010;24(6):e1-e25.
50. Spielholz NI. Magnets: what is the evidence of efficacy? In: Davis CM, ed. *Complementary Therapies in Rehabilitation: Evidence for Efficacy in Therapy, Prevention, and Wellness.* 3rd ed. Thorofare, NJ: SLACK Incorporated; 2009:305-328.
51. LaRiccia PJ, Galantino ML. Acupuncture theory and acupuncture-like therapeutics in physical therapy. In: Davis CM, ed. *Complementary Therapies in Rehabilitation: Evidence for Efficacy in Therapy, Prevention, and Wellness.* 3rd ed. Thorofare, NJ: SLACK Incorporated; 2009:331-344.
52. Hsing WT, Imamura M, Weaver K, Fregni F, Azevedo Neto RS. Clinical effects of scalp electrical acupuncture in stroke: a sham-controlled randomized clinical trial. *J Altern Complement Med.* 2012;18(4):341-346.
53. Anderson EZ. Therapeutic touch. In: Davis CM, ed. *Complementary Therapies in Rehabilitation: Evidence for Efficacy in Therapy, Prevention, and Wellness.* 3rd ed. Thorofare, NJ: SLACK Incorporated; 2009:347-357.

Please see accompanying Web site at
www.healio.com/books/neuroptavideos

Financial Disclosures

Dr. Fritzie Arce has no financial or proprietary interest in the materials presented herein.

Dr. Ronald De Vera Barredo has no financial or proprietary interest in the materials presented herein.

Claire E. Beekman has no financial or proprietary interest in the materials presented herein.

Dr. Gordon U. Burton has no financial or proprietary interest in the materials presented herein.

Dr. Barbara H. Connolly has no financial or proprietary interest in the materials presented herein.

Dr. Kristine N. Corn has no financial or proprietary interest in the materials presented herein.

Dr. Carol Davis has no financial or proprietary interest in the materials presented herein.

Lisa Ferrin has no financial or proprietary interest in the materials presented herein.

Dr. Amanda A. Forster has no financial or proprietary interest in the materials presented herein.

Dr. Sharon L. Gorman has no financial or proprietary interest in the materials presented herein.

Patricia Harris has no financial or proprietary interest in the materials presented herein.

Cynthia J. Hogan has no financial or proprietary interest in the materials presented herein.

Dr. Bret Kennedy has no financial or proprietary interest in the materials presented herein.

Dr. Dennis Klima has no financial or proprietary interest in the materials presented herein.

Dr. Rolando T. Lazaro has no financial or proprietary interest in the materials presented herein.

Dr. Nelson Marquez has no financial or proprietary interest in the materials presented herein.

Becky S. McKnight has no financial or proprietary interest in the materials presented herein.

Dr. Megan E. Petrosky has no financial or proprietary interest in the materials presented herein.

Esmerita Roceles Rotor has no financial or proprietary interest in the materials presented herein.

Shannon Ryals has no financial or proprietary interest in the materials presented herein.

Dr. Kelly Ryujin has no financial or proprietary interest in the materials presented herein.

Dr. Dale Scalise-Smith has no financial or proprietary interest in the materials presented herein.

Dr. Eunice Shen has no financial or proprietary interest in the materials presented herein.

Dr. James M. Smith has no financial or proprietary interest in the materials presented herein.

Dr. Darcy A. Umphred has no financial or proprietary interest in the materials presented herein.

Index

acquisition of motor skill, 57–58

activities of daily living (ADL) skills, 7, 22, 28, 37, 138, 261, 384

acupuncture, 418–419

adaptive equipment, 97–98, 278–280

adolescence, 35–36

adult head injury, practice patterns, 306

adulthood physiological changes, 37

aerobic capacity, 338–339, 351

affective disorders, 30

aging physiological changes, 16–18
    adolescence, 35–36
    adulthood, 37
    cardiovascular system, 21–22
    childhood, 34–35
    cognitive system, 23–24
    early childhood, 31–34
    innate motor behaviors, 24
    intrinsic, extrinsic factors, interaction between, 17
    middle adulthood, 37
    motor development, 25–27
    motor skill development, 39–40
    musculoskeletal system, 19–21
    neurological system, 22–23
    older adulthood, 37–39
    physiological changes, 19–23
    prenatal, 24–31
    pulmonary system, 21–22

agitated patient, 314

Alexander Technique, 417

altered consciousness, 122

alternative therapy, 411–424

ambiguity of basic indicators, 11

American Heart Association, 339

American Spinal Cord Association Impairment Scale, 254

American Spinal Injury Association, 292–293

amyotrophic lateral sclerosis, 378–379, 387
    stages, 380

anoxia, 179

anoxic injury, 182

anterior cord syndrome, 256–257

apraxia, 349–351

asphyxia, 179

assistive devices, 95

ataxia, 79

ataxic muscle tone, 179

athetoid muscle tone, 179

athetosis, ataxia, 79

attention, 122–123

attitude, 72–73

audiologists, 242

augmented treatment, 96–95

autonomous stage of motor learning, 58

balance, 79, 234–235, 340, 353
    examinations, 138–142
    impairments, 310–311
    measures, 356
    tools, 229

Barnes method, 415

Barthel Index, 146

bed mobility, 273

bedside equipment, 346

Berg Balance Scale, 145

bioelectromagnetics, 414

biofeedback, 416

biological treatment, 414

bladder injury, 259

blast injuries, 317–318

blood pressure ranges, 397

body functions, 118–121

body image, 155

body system impairments, 400–401

body talk, 417–418

body work, 415–418
brain injury, 313–315
    agitated patient, 314
    cognitive intervention, 314–315
    coma emergence, 313–314
    precautions, 315
breathing mechanics, 396
Bruininks-Oseretsky test, 228

canes, 346–347
cardiopulmonary system, 237–238, 393–410
    blood pressure ranges, 397
    body system impairments, 400–401
    breathing mechanics, 396
    cardiovascular pathology, 396–399
    cardiovascular system, 394–395
    deep vein thrombosis, 398
    with Down syndrome, 237–238
    examination tools, 401–406
        physical examination, 401–404
        tests of cardiopulmonary function, 404–406
    exercise training, 408
    functional activity limitations, 400–401
    hypertensive episode, 397
    hypotensive episode, 397
    left-sided heart failure, 399
    neuromuscular pathologies, 395–396
    parasympathetic stimulation, 395
    participation restrictions, 400–401
    primary cardiovascular pathology, 396–400
    pulmonary pathologies, 399–400
    pulmonary system, 394–395
    respiratory acidosis, 405
    respiratory alkalosis, 405
    right-sided heart failure, 399
    sympathetic stimulation, 395
cardiovascular system, 394–395
    changes in, 21–22
    endurance, 356
    pathology, 396–399
career development, 12–13
categories of intervention, 73–97
    dual tasking, 84–85
    functional training, 74–75, 344–345
    impairment training, 75–85
        balance, 79
        hypertonicity, 77

hypotonicity, 77
joint mobility, 76–77
motor tonicity fluctuation, 79
neuromuscular system, 77
nonintentional tremor, 78–79
postural control, 79
range of motion, 76–77
reflexive patient, 78
rigidity, 77
spinal motor generators, 77
stereotypic patient, 78
vestibular rehabilitation, 81–84
    progressing functional training activities, 75
    reaction time, 85
cauda equina syndrome, 257
central bleed, 179
central cord syndrome, 256
central nervous system insult, 177–210
    anoxia, 179
    anoxic injury, 182
    asphyxia, 179
    ataxic tone, 179
    athetoid tone, 179
    central bleed, 179
    cerebellar insult, 179
    cerebral palsy, 178–182
        diplegia, 193
            lower extremities, 193
            quadriplegia, 193
            thorax, 193
            upper extremities, 193
    diencephalon insult, 179
    diplegia, 179
        lower extremities, 193
        lower thorax, 193
        upper extremities, 193
        upper thorax, 193
    distal cortical insult, 179
    extensor tone, 191–192
    facilitation techniques, 193–201
    fluctuating programming, 179
    frontal motor insult, 179
    global ischemia, 179
    hemiplegia, 179
    hemispheric bleed, 179
    high tone, 179
    hypertonic muscle tone, 179

hypotonic muscle tone, 179
hypoxic injury, 182
inhibition techniques, 193–201
low to high tone, 179
low tone, 179
medical prognosis, 182
mixed programming, 179
motor involvement, 179
multisystem involvement, 179
muscle tone classification, 179
neurological impairment, 183–185
parietal lobe insult, 179
periventricular insult, 179
postural tone, 190–191
posture correction, 193–194
quadriplegia, 179
    lower extremities, 193
    lower thorax, 193
    upper extremities, 193
    upper thorax, 193
quadriplegic athetoid involvement, 179
regulatory inconsistencies, 179
spastic/multisystem involvement, 179
technology, 195–197
therapeutic horseback riding, 197–201
total asphyxia, 179
toys, therapeutic use of, 194–195
traumatic injury, 182
treatment, 185–189
triplegia, 179
trunk flexor tone, 192
cerebellar insult, 179
cerebral circulation, 362
cerebral palsy, 178–182
  central nervous system insult, 178–182
  diplegia, 193
  lower extremities, 193
  quadriplegia, 193
  thorax, 193
  upper extremities, 193
cerebrovascular accident, 328
children, 31–35, 177–210
  anoxia, 179
  anoxic injury, 182
  asphyxia, 179
  ataxic tone, 179
  athetoid tone, 179
  central bleed, 179

cerebellar insult, 179
cerebral palsy, 178–182
  diplegia, 193
    lower extremities, 193
    quadriplegia, 193
    thorax, 193
    upper extremities, 193
diencephalon insult, 179
diplegia, 179
  lower extremities, 193
  lower thorax, 193
  upper extremities, 193
  upper thorax, 193
distal cortical insult, 179
extensor tone, 191–192
facilitation techniques, 193–201
fluctuating programming, 179
frontal motor insult, 179
global ischemia, 179
hemiplegia, 179
hemispheric bleed, 179
high muscle tone, 179
hypertonic muscle tone, 179
hypotonic muscle tone, 179
hypoxic injury, 182
inhibition techniques, 193–201
low muscle tone, 179
low to high muscle tone, 179
medical prognosis, 182
mixed programming, 179
motor involvement, 179
multisystem involvement, 179
muscle tone, 179
  hypertonic, 179
  hypotonic, 179
muscle tone classification, 179
neurological impairment, 183–185
parietal lobe insult, 179
periventricular insult, 179
physiological changes, 31–35
postural tone, 190–191
posture correction, 193–194
quadriplegia, 179
  lower extremities, 193
  lower thorax, 193
  upper extremities, 193
  upper thorax, 193
quadriplegic athetoid involvement, 179

regulatory inconsistencies, 179
spastic/multisystem involvement, 179
technology, 195–197
therapeutic horseback riding, 197–201
total asphyxia, 179
toys, therapeutic use of, 194–195
traumatic injury, 182
treatment, 185–189
triplegia, 179
trunk flexor tone, 192
Christopher and Dana Reeve Foundation, 293
client adjustment, 156–157
clinical interaction, 12–13
clinical medical geneticist, 241
cognitive impairments, 357–360
anosognosia, 359
communication disorders, 359–360
unilateral neglect, 357–358
cognitive issues, 151–163
body image, 155
client adjustment, 156–157
crisis, 157–158
cultural influences, 159–160
family issues, 156–157
grief, 157–158
hope, 158–159
loss, 157–158
spiritual outlook, 158–159
stress, 157–158
cognitive system changes, 23–24
cognitive understanding, 72
collaboration, 61, 241–243
coma emergence, 313–314
community integration, 317
community reentry, 278, 315–317
complementary therapies, 411–424
bioelectromagnetics, 414
biological treatment, 414
body work, 415–418
Alexander Technique, 417
biofeedback, 416
body talk, 417–418
complete decongestive therapy, 415
craniosacral therapy, 415
Feldenkrais Method, 417
myofascial release, 415
Pilates, 417

Rolfing, 416
structural integration, 416
tai chi, 416
therapeutic massage, 415
yoga, 416–417
diet, 414
energy work, 418–419
acupuncture, 418–419
magnets, 418
Qigong, 418
Reiki, 418
therapeutic touch, 419
manual healing methods, 414
mind-body interventions, 413
nutrition, 414
pharmacological treatment, 414
complete decongestive therapy, 415
concussion, 317
conscious proprioception, 127
consciousness, 122
consequences, predictability of, 11
constraint-induced movement, 99
control, motor, 49–52
conus medullaris syndrome, 257
cranial nerve examination, 136–138
craniosacral therapy, 415
cri du chat syndrome, 218
criticality of results, 12
cultural influences, 159–160

deciding, doing, continuum between, 10–12
deep vein thrombosis, 398
degenerative diseases, 375–391
activities of daily living, training, 384
amyotrophic lateral sclerosis, 378–379, 387
stages, 380
fatigue, 383–385
multiple sclerosis, 377–378, 386
Parkinson's disease, 376–377, 385–386
delegation strategies, 9–12
roles of PT/PTA, 9–12
development of career, 12–13
developmental-behavioral pediatrician, 241
developmental milestones, 220–221
developmental problems, 219–226
balance, 234–235
balance tools, 229

Bruininks-Oseretsky test, 228
coordination, 234–235
coordination tools, 229
developmental milestones, 220–221
gross motor development test, 228
gross motor function measure, 228
handling techniques, 233
hypertonia, 228–229
hypotonia, 228–229
motor skill development, 222–228
muscular dystrophy, fatigue with, 236
muscular strength, 233–234
Peabody Developmental Motor Scales, 228
soft tissue mobility, 235–236
tone abnormalities, 228–229
tone problems, 230–233
developmental reflexes, 133–136
developmental theories, 16–18
diagnosis of patient, 7
diencephalon insult, 179
diplegia, 179, 193
lower extremities, 193
lower thorax, 193
upper extremities, 193
upper thorax, 193
discharge planning, 285–286, 315–317
blast injuries, 317–318
community integration, 317
concussion, 317
equipment procurement, 315–316
family training, 315–316
home assessment, 316
home programs, 316–317
discriminative touch, 124–127
distal cortical insult, 179
distributed practice, 56
documentation, 165–176, 287
formats, 175–176
guidelines, 166–167
intervention element, 171–174
measuring data, 167–168
organizing tests, 167–168
reimbursement, 174–175
doing, deciding, continuum between, 10–12
Down syndrome, 213–217
cardiopulmonary impairments, 237–238

dual tasking, 84–85
dysphagia, 360

Edwards' syndrome, 219
electrotherapeutic modalities, 348
energy work, 418–419
acupuncture, 418–419
magnets, 418
Qigong, 418
Reiki, 418
therapeutic touch, 419
environmental parameters, 97–98
equipment procurement, 315–316
evaluation of patient, 7
evidence-based treatment, 99–102
body weight–supported treadmill training, 100–102
constraint-induced movement, 99
exoskeletons, 100–102
robotics, 100–102
virtual reality environments, 100–102
examination, 6, 117–150
balance examinations, 138–142
bodily system screening, 120
bodily systems review, 119
body functions, 118–121
cranial nerve examination, 136–138
functional activities, 142–144
functional balance grades, 143
impairment/functional tests, 145–146
Barthel Index, 146
Berg Balance Scale, 145
Functional Independence Measure, 146
Functional Reach, 145
Motor Assessment Scale, 145–146
Performance Oriented Mobility Assessment, 145
Timed Up and Go, 145
measures, 119–146
motor examination, 128–136
components, 128
coordination, 134–136
developmental reflexes, 133–136
Modified Ashworth Scale, 130
muscle strength, 130–131
muscular tone, 129–130

phasic stretch reflexes, 131–132
range of motion, 128
reaction assessment, 135–136
synergy, 132–133
synergy patterns of extremities, 132
observation, 121–123
arousal, 122
attention, 122–123
attention types, 123
consciousness, 122
mental status, 121–122
orientation, 122
states of altered consciousness, 122
pain assessments, 120–121
participation, 146
patient history, 118–119
categories, 119
sensation, 123–128
conscious proprioception, 127
discriminative temperature, 128
discriminative touch, 124–127
fast pain, 127–128
sensory testing, 124
tests, 119–146
vital signs, 120
exoskeletons, 100–102
extensor tone, 191–192
extrinsic, intrinsic factors, interaction between,
17

facilitation techniques, 193–201
family education, 284–285
family issues, 156–157
family training, 315–316
fast pain, 127–128
fatigue, with muscular dystrophy, 236
feedback, 59–60
Feldenkrais Method, 417
flexibility, 340
fluctuating programming, 179
formats, documentation, 175–176
frontal motor insult, 179
functional activities, 142–144
functional balance grades, 143
Functional Independence Measure, 146
functional mobility training, 309
Functional Reach, 145

functional tests, 145–146
Barthel Index, 146
Berg Balance Scale, 145
Functional Independence Measure, 146
Functional Reach, 145
Motor Assessment Scale, 145–146
Performance Oriented Mobility Assessment,
145
Timed Up and Go, 145
functional training, 74–75, 344–345

gait, 311, 340–342, 384
gaming, virtual-reality, 238–239
genetic conditions, 212–219
cri du chat syndrome, 218
Down syndrome, 213–217
Edwards' syndrome, 219
muscular dystrophy, 219
Prader-Willi syndrome, 217
Rett syndrome, 218–219
trisomy 21, 213–217
genetic counselor, 241
Gentile's taxonomy of tasks, 337
Glasgow Coma Scale, 302
global ischemia, 179
grief, 157–158
gross motor development test, 228
gross motor function measure, 228
group balance activities, 85
guidelines for documentation, 166–167

hand splints, 347–348
handling techniques, 88–94, 233
hands-on intervention, 96–95
assistive devices, 95
handling techniques, 88–94
relaxation techniques, 86–88
hemiparesis, 341
hemiplegia, 179
hemispheric bleed, 179
hemorrhagic stroke, 328
high muscle tone, 179
hippotherapy, 197–201
history of patient, 118–119
holistic health, 411–424
home assessment, 316
home evaluation, 285

home programs, 316–317
hope, 158–159
hypertensive episode, 397
hypertonia, 228–229
hypertonic muscle tone, 179
hypertonicity, 77
hypotensive episode, 397
hypotonia, 228–229
hypotonic muscle tone, 179
hypotonicity, 77
hypoxic injury, 182

impairment training, 75–85
    balance, 79
    hypertonicity, 77
    hypotonicity, 77
    joint mobility, 76–77
    motor tonicity fluctuation, 79
    neuromuscular system, 77
    nonintentional tremor, 78–79
    postural control, 79
    range of motion, 76–77
    reflexive patient, 78
    rigidity, 77
    spinal motor generators, 77
    stereotypic patient, 78
    vestibular rehabilitation, 81–84
indicators
    ambiguity of, 11
    observability of, 11
inhibition techniques, 193–201
innate motor behaviors, 24
inpatient rehabilitation, 286–287
integrative health care, 411–424
    bioelectromagnetics, 414
    biological treatment, 414
    body work, 415–418
        Alexander Technique, 417
        biofeedback, 416
        body talk, 417–418
        complete decongestive therapy, 415
        craniosacral therapy, 415
        Feldenkrais Method, 417
        myofascial release, 415
        Pilates, 417
        Rolfing, 416
        structural integration, 416

        tai chi, 416
        therapeutic massage, 415
        yoga, 416–417
    diet, 414
    energy work, 418–419
        acupuncture, 418–419
        magnets, 418
        Qigong, 418
        Reiki, 418
        therapeutic touch, 419
    manual healing methods, 414
    mind-body interventions, 413
    nutrition, 414
    pharmacological treatment, 414
intensive care unit, 301–302
International Classification of Functioning, Disability and Health, 3–5
International Classification of Impairments, Disabilities and Handicaps, 3–4
intervention procedures, 69–115
    adaptive equipment, 97–98
    attitude, 72–73
    augmented treatment, 96–95
    categories of intervention, 73–97
        dual tasking, 84–85
        functional training, 74–75, 344–345
        impairment training, 75–85
        progressing functional training activities, 75
        reaction time, 85
    cognitive understanding, 72
    designing, 72–73
    environmental parameters, 97–98
    evidence-based treatment, 99–102
        body weight–supported treadmill training, 100–102
        constraint-induced movement, 99
        exoskeletons, 100–102
        robotics, 100–102
        virtual reality environments, 100–102
    group balance activities, 85
    hands-on intervention, 96–95
        assistive devices, 95
        handling techniques, 88–94
        relaxation techniques, 86–88
    impairment training
        balance, 79

hypertonicity, 77
hypotonicity, 77
joint mobility, 76–77
motor tonicity fluctuation, 79
neuromuscular system, 77
nonintentional tremor, 78–79
postural control, 79
range of motion, 76–77
reflexive patient, 78
rigidity, 77
spinal motor generators, 77
stereotypic patient, 78
vestibular rehabilitation, 81–84
Neuro-Developmental Treatment, 102–107
participation training, 96–97
proprioceptive neuromuscular facilitation,
102–106
sensory system, 95–96
intrinsic, extrinsic factors, interaction between,
17
intrinsic feedback, 59–60
ischemic stroke, 326–328

joint mobility, 76–77

lacunar infarction, 327
lateral pain system, 127–128
left-sided heart failure, 399
levels of cognitive function, Rancho Los Amigos,
303
levels of recovery, 302–304
locomotion training, 311, 340–342, 384
low muscle tone, 179
low to high muscle tone, 179
lower motor neuron lesions, 255
lymphatic drainage, 415

magnets, 418
manual healing methods, 414
manual lymphatic drainage, 415
mass practice, 55–56
massage, 415
medical team collaboration, 241
mental status, 121–122
middle adulthood, 37
mind-body interventions, 413
mixed programming, 179
models of neurorehabilitation, 3–5

Modified Ashworth Scale, 130
Motor Assessment Scale, 145–146
motor control, 49–52, 352
motor development, 24–39
adolescence, 35–36
adulthood, 37
aging, 18
childhood, 34–35
early childhood, 31–34
innate motor behaviors, 24
intrinsic, extrinsic factors, interaction between,
17
middle adulthood, 37
motor development, 25–27
motor skill development, 39–40
older adulthood, 37–39
physiological changes, 19–23, 28–23
cardiovascular system, 21–22
cognitive system, 23–24
musculoskeletal system, 19–21
neurological system, 22–23
pulmonary system, 21–22
play, as therapy, 40
prenatal, 24–31
theories of development, 16–18
motor examination, 128–136
components, 128
coordination, 134–136
developmental reflexes, 133–136
Modified Ashworth Scale, 130
muscle strength, 130–131
muscular tone, 129–130
phasic stretch reflexes, 131–132
range of motion, 128
reaction assessment, 135–136
synergy, 132–133
synergy patterns of extremities, 132
motor involvement, 179
motor learning, practice contexts, 52–61
associative stage/refinement, 58
autonomous stage/retention, 58
cognitive stage/acquisition of motor skill,
57–58
progressive/sequential-part learning, 54
pure-part learning, 53–54
whole learning, 53
whole to part to whole learning, 54–55

motor skill development, 39–40, 226–228
    developmental delay, 222–227
motor tonicity fluctuation, 79
movement development, 15–43
    adolescence, 35–36
    adulthood, 37
    aging, 18
    cardiovascular system, 21–22
    childhood, 34–35
    cognitive system, 23–24
    early childhood, 31–34
    innate motor behaviors, 24
    intrinsic, extrinsic factors, interaction between, 17
    middle adulthood, 37
    motor development, 25–27
    motor skill development, 39–40
    musculoskeletal system, 19–21
    neurological system, 22–23
    older adulthood, 37–39
    physiological changes, 19–23
        infancy, 28–23
    play as therapy, 40
    prenatal, 24–31
    pulmonary system, 21–22
    theories, 16–18
multiple sclerosis, 377–378, 386
multisystem involvement, 179
muscle strength, 130–131
muscle tone, 129–130, 179
    ataxic, 179
    athetoid, 179
    classification, 179
    high tone, 179
    hypertonic, 179
    hypotonic, 179
    low to high tone, 179
    low tone, 179
muscular dystrophy, 219
    fatigue with, 236
muscular strength, 233–234
musculoskeletal system, changes in, 19–21
myofascial release, 415

Nagi models, 3–4
National Spinal Cord Injury Association, 293
neurodevelopmental conditions, 239–240
    early intervention, 239–240
    medical team collaboration, 241

Neuro-Developmental Treatment, 106–107
neurological impairment, 183–185
neurological injury, 253–257
neurological level, 253–254
neurological system, changes in, 22–23
neuromuscular pathologies, 395–396
neuromuscular system, 77
neuroplasticity, 46, 61–63
nonintentional tremor, 78–79
nutrition, 414

observation, 121–123
    arousal, 122
    attention, 122–123
    consciousness, 122
    mental status, 121–122
    orientation, 122
older adulthood, physiological changes, 37–39
orientation, 122
orthotics, 347

pain assessments, 120–121
paraplegia, 255
parasympathetic stimulation, 395
parietal lobe insult, 179
Parkinson's disease, 376–377, 385–386
participation training, 96–97
Patient/Client Management Model, 6
patient history, 118–119
    categories, 119
Peabody Developmental Motor Scales, 228
Performance Oriented Mobility Assessment, 145
periventricular insult, 179
pharmacological treatment, 414
phasic stretch reflexes, 131–132
physiological changes, 19–23
    cardiovascular system, 21–22
    cognitive system, 23–24
    musculoskeletal system, 19–21
    neurological system, 22–23
    pulmonary system, 21–22
Pilates, 417
play as therapy, 40
postural control, 79
postural tone, 190–191
posture correction, 193–194
practice areas, 8–9
practice schedule, 55–57
    distributed practice, 56

mass practice, 55–56
random practice, 57
Prader-Willi syndrome, 217
predictability of consequences, 11
pressure sores, 280–285
primary cardiovascular pathology, 396–400
procurement of equipment, 315–316
progressing functional training activities, 75
proprioceptive neuromuscular facilitation, 102–106
psychosocial issues, 151–163
body image, 155
client adjustment, 156–157
crisis, 157–158
cultural influences, 159–160
family issues, 156–157
grief, 157–158
hope, 158–159
loss, 157–158
spiritual outlook, 158–159
stress, 157–158
pulmonary pathologies, 399–400
pulmonary system, 21–22, 394–395
pure-part learning, 53–54

Qigong, 418
quadriplegia, 179, 193
lower extremities, 193
lower thorax, 193
upper extremities, 193
upper thorax, 193
quadriplegic athetoid involvement, 179

Rancho Los Amigos levels of cognitive function, 303
random practice, 57
range of motion, 76–77, 128
reaction time, 85
reentry into community, 315–317
refinement of motor learning, 58
reflexive patient, 78
regulatory inconsistencies, 179
Reiki, 418
reimbursement documentation, 174–175
relaxation techniques, 86–88
respiratory acidosis, 405
respiratory alkalosis, 405

retention of motor learning, 58
Rett syndrome, 218–219
right-sided heart failure, 399
rigidity, 77
robotics, 100–102
Rolfing, 416

schedule for practice, 55–57
distributed practice, 56
mass practice, 55–56
random practice, 57
screening bodily system, 120
seating, 307
sensation, 123–128
conscious proprioception, 127
discriminative temperature, 128
discriminative touch, 124–127
fast pain, 127–128
sensory testing, 124
sensory system, 95–96
sensory testing, 124
sequential-part learning, 54
sexual dysfunction, 259
shoulder pain after stroke, 352–353
slings, 347–348
soft tissue mobility, 235–236
somatosensation, 360–361
spasticity, 179
speech-language pathologist, 242
spinal cord injury, 251–296
American Spinal Cord Association Impairment Scale, 254
anterior cord syndrome, 256–257
autonomic dysreflexia, symptomology, 260
autonomic dysreflexia or autonomic hyper-reflexia, 259–261
bowel dysfunction, 259
cauda equina syndrome, 257
central cord syndrome, 256
complete, vs. incomplete injury, 254
complications, 261–262, 300–301
conus medullaris syndrome, 257
epidemiology, 252–253
etiology, 252
extent of lesion, 253–254
incidence, 252
level of injury, 255

life expectancy, 252
lower motor neuron lesions, 255
motor loss, 257
neurological injury, 253–257
neurological level, 253–254
pain, 261
paraplegia, 255
pathophysiology, 252–253
psychological reaction to loss, 261
respiratory muscles, 257–258
sensory loss, 258
spasticity, 259
tetraplegia, 255
upper motor neuron lesions, 255
Spinal Cord Injury Model System Information
    Network, 293
spinal motor generators, 77
spiritual outlook, 158–159
stabilization of spine, 263–264
    develop endurance, 268–269
    head-hips relationship, 270–278
    learn functional skills, 270
    range of motion, 265–266
    respiratory program, 269–270
    strengthen weak muscles, 267–268
stages of motor learning, 57–58
    associative stage/refinement, 58
    autonomous stage/retention, 58
    cognitive stage/acquisition of motor skill,
        57–58
stereotypic patient, 78
strategies of delegation, 11
stress, 157–158
stroke, 325–373
    aerobic capacity endurance, 338–339
    attention, 335
    balance, 340
    cerebrovascular accident, 328
    cognitive impairments
        anosognosia, 359
        communication disorders, 359–360
        unilateral neglect, 357–358
    coordination, 340
    current status, 354
    electrotherapeutic modalities, 348
    endurance, 343–344
    environmental factors, 365–366

environmental progression, 336–337
equipment, 346–348
    bedside equipment, 346
    canes, 346–347
    hand splints, 347–348
    orthotics, 347
    slings, 347–348
    wheelchairs, 346
examination tools, 354–356
    affective disorders, 30
    balance measures, 356
    cardiovascular endurance, 356
    cerebral circulation, 362
    cognitive impairments, 357–360
    dysphagia, 360
    flexibility, 355
    functional limitations, 355
    motor control, 354–355
    somatosensation, impaired, 360–361
    vestibular sensation, 357
    vision, impaired, 361
exercise interventions, 333–339
exercise programming, 339
feedback, 335
flexibility, 340
functional limitations, 349–353
    aerobic capacity, 351
    apraxia, 349–351
    balance deficits, 353
    functional limitations, 353
    motor control, 352
    shoulder pain after stroke, 352–353
    strength, 352
gait, 340–342
gait deviations, 341
Gentile's taxonomy of tasks, 337
hemiparesis, 341
hemorrhagic stroke, 328
ischemic stroke, 326–328
lacunar infarction, 327
locomotion training, 340–342
prognosis, 363–365
    comorbidities, 363–364
    contraindications, 364–365
strength, 343–344
stroke rehabilitation, 348–349
transient ischemic attack, 327

structural integration, 416
sympathetic stimulation, 395
synergy, 132–133

tai chi, 416
tetraplegia, 255
therapeutic exercise, 307–309
therapeutic horseback riding, 197–201
therapeutic massage, 415
therapeutic touch, 419
Timed Up and Go, 145
tone, 179, 228–229
    hypertonic, 179
    hypotonic, 179
    problems, 230–233
total asphyxia, 179
toys, therapeutic use of, 194–195
training family, 315–316
transfers, 274–275
transient ischemic attack, 327
traumatic brain injury, 297–324
    adult head injury, practice patterns, 306
    brain injury, 313–315
        agitated patient, 314
        cognitive neuromuscular intervention, 314–315
        coma emergence, 313–314
        precautions, 315
    community reentry, 315–317
    diagnosis, 306
    discharge planning, 315–317
        blast injuries, 317–318
        community integration, 317
        concussion, 317
        equipment procurement, 315–316
        family training, 315–316
        home assessment, 316
        home programs, 316–317
    evaluation, 306
    examination, 304–305
    functional limitations, 307–313

Glasgow Coma Scale, 302
impairments, 307–313
    balance impairments, 310–311
    functional mobility training, 309
    gait, 311, 384
    locomotion training, 311, 384
    seating, 307
    therapeutic exercise, 307–309
intensive care unit, 301–302
interventions, 306
levels of recovery, 302–304
mechanisms of injury, 299–300
prognosis, 306
Rancho Los Amigos levels of cognitive function, 303
treadmill training, 100–102, 238–239
tremor, nonintentional, 78–79
triplegia, 179
trunk flexor tone, 192

upper motor neuron lesions, 255

vestibular rehabilitation, 81–84
vestibular sensation, 357
virtual reality environments, 100–102, 238–239
vision, impaired, 361
vital signs, 120

water therapy, 189
Wernicke's area, stroke affecting, 359–360
Western Neuro Sensory Stimulation Profile, 314
wheelchair mobility, 276–278
wheelchairs, 279–280, 346
whole learning, 53
whole to part to whole learning, 54–55
Williams syndrome, 214
World Health Organization (WHO), disablement model of, 4

yoga, 412–413, 416–417, 419